CIRCUMPOLAR HEALTH 84

SIXTH INTERNATIONAL SYMPOSIUM ON CIRCUMPOLAR HEALTH

SPONSORED BY

The American Society for Circumpolar Health
The University of Alaska
The Alaska Public Health Association
The North Slope Borough, Alaska
The Alaska Department of Health and Social Services

SUPPORTED BY

The Alaska Council on Science and Technology
The Office of Naval Research, Washington, D.C.
Exxon Corporation
RCA Alascom
Sohio Alaska Petroleum Company
The Arctic Institute of North America
Wien Air Alaska

THE NATIONAL ORGANIZING COMMITTEE

Frederick A. Milan, President
Helen D. Beirne, Secretary General
Wayne W. Myers, Secretary General
C. Earl Albrecht, Founder of the Symposium
Robert Fortuine, Editor of the Proceedings
Edward M. Scott, Chairman of the Scientific Programs
Carl Hild, Member
Theodore A. Mala, Member
John Middaugh, Member
Frank Pauls, Member
Chester Pierce, Member

CONFERENCE COORDINATION

Conferences and Institutes, University of Alaska-Fairbanks

CIRCUMPOLAR HEALTH 84

VOLUME PREPARATION

PRODUCTION EDITING, GRAPHICS

David W. Norton and Sue Keller
University of Alaska Press, Fairbanks

DISTRIBUTION

University of Washington Press
Seattle & London

CIRCUMPOLAR HEALTH 84

Proceedings
of the
Sixth International Symposium on
Circumpolar Health

Edited By
Robert Fortuine

University of Washington Press
Seattle and London

Six contributions to this volume were written and prepared primarily
by U.S. government employees on official time and are therefore
in the public domain. These contributions (with inclusive page numbers) are:

Study of a cohort of Yukon-Kuskokwim Delta Eskimo children:
An overview of accomplishments and plans for the future (115-119);

Communicable disease control in the early history of Alaska I. Smallpox (187-190);

Communicable disease control in the early history of Alaska II. Syphilis (191-194);

Increased prevalence of hepatitis B surface antigen in pregnant Alaska Eskimos (206-208);

Pertussis: A study of incidence and mortality in a Yukon-Kuskokwim Delta epidemic
(229-234); and

Alcohol-related health problems in Alaska--preventive strategies (322-326).

Library of Congress Cataloging-in-Publication Data

International Symposium on Circumpolar Health
(6th : 1984 : Anchorage, Alaska)
Circumpolar health 84.

Based on a symposium held in Anchorage, Alaska,
13-18 May 1984, sponsored by the American Society for
Circumpolar Health and others.
Includes index.
1. Circumpolar medicine--Congresses. I. Fortuine,
Robert. II. American Society for Circumpolar Health.
III. Title. [DNLM: 1. Cold Climate--congresses.
2. Communicable Diseases--congresses. 3. Environmental
Exposure--congresses. 4. Epidemiology--congresses.
5. Health Services--congresses. 6. Mental Disorders--
congresses. 7. Public Health--congresses.

W3 IN916VE 6th 1984c / WA 100 I618 1984c]
RC955.2.I57 1984   616.9'88'1   85-50874
ISBN 0-295-96202-X

Proceedings of the Sixth International Symposium on Circumpolar Health,
held in Anchorage, Alaska, 13-18 May 1984

CONTENTS

SECTION 3. Demography, Morbidity and Mortality

SECTION 4. Infectious Disease

SECTION 5. Non-Infectious and Chronic Disease

SECTION 6. Acculturation, Mental Health, and Substance Abuse

SECTION 7. Health Programs and Manpower

CONTRIBUTORS

(Please see Index for pages on which the authors' contributions begin.)

C. EARL ALBRECHT, M.D., Affiliate Professor of Medical Science, University of Alaska, Palmer, Alaska, U.S.A.

W. ALBRITTON, University of Manitoba, Winnipeg, Manitoba, Canada

NILS O. ALM, M.D., Institute of Work Physiology, Kysthospitalet, Oslo, Norway

MARY G. ALTON MACKEY, Extension Service, Memorial University of Newfoundland, St. John's, Newfoundland, Canada

WALLACE ALWARD, M.D., Arctic Investigations Laboratory, Center for Infectious Diseases, Centers for Disease Control, U.S. Department of Health and Human Services, Public Health Service, Anchorage, Alaska, U.S.A.

J.H. ANDERSON, Ph.D., Institute of Arctic Biology, University of Alaska, Fairbanks, Alaska, U.S.A.

BEN ANDREW, Naskapi Montagnais Innu Association, Sheshashit, Labrador, Newfoundland, Canada

J. AXELSSON, Department of Physiology, University of Iceland, Reykjavik, Iceland

C. BACKMAN, M.D., Department of Clinical Physiology, University of Umeå, Umeå, Sweden

JAMES D. BAXTER, M.D., Professor and Chairman, Department of Otolaryngology, McGill University, Montreal, Quebec, Canada

ROGER BELLEAU, Centre de Pneumologie, Université Laval, Quebec City, Quebec, Canada

THOMAS R. BENDER, M.D., M.P.H., Arctic Investigations Laboratory, Center for Infectious Diseases, Centers for Disease Control, U.S. Department of Health and Human Services, Public Health Service, Anchorage, Alaska, U.S.A.

J.W. BERRY, Psychology Department, Queen's University, Kingston, Ontario, Canada

A. BIRT, M.D., F.R.C.P.(C), Department of Dermatology, University of Manitoba, Winnipeg, Manitoba, Canada

PETER BJERREGAARD, M.D., Department of Epidemiology, State Serum Institute, Copenhagen, Denmark

JANICE DANI BOWMAN, Ph.D., Center for Alcohol and Addiction Studies, University of Alaska, Anchorage, Alaska, U.S.A.

S.A. BRIDGMAN, M.B., Ch.B., British Antarctic Survey and Centre for Offshore Health, Robert Gordon's Institute of Technology, Aberdeen, Scotland, U.K.

J. CARSON, M.D., Northern Medical Unit, University of Manitoba, Winnipeg, Manitoba, Canada

JOSEPH CONNOR, Faculty of Medicine, Communication Systems, University of Manitoba, Winnipeg, Manitoba, Canada

PENELOPE M. CORDES, Department of Anthropology, Stanford Univeristy, Palo Alto, California, U.S.A

WILLIAM M. DANN, M.P.A., Dann and Associates, Inc., Anchorage, Alaska, U.S.A.

R.D.O. DEVINE, University of Alberta, Edmonton, Alberta, Canada

RAY A. DIETER, JR., M.D., Glen Ellyn Clinic, Glen Ellyn, Illinois, U.S.A.

MARTI DILLEY, Ph.D.,   Alaska Department of Health and Social Services, Juneau, Alaska, U.S.A.

J. DOOLEY, M.B., B.Ch., B.A.O.,   Northern Medical Unit, University of Manitoba, Winnipeg, Manitoba, Canada

CHARLES DUMONT,   Department of Community Health, Montreal General Hospital, Montreal, Quebec, Canada

BERNARD DUVAL,   Projet Nord, D.S.C., C.H.U.L., Quebec City, Quebec, Canada

ALISON C. EDWARDS, B.Sc.,   Program of Northern Medicine and Health, Memorial University of Newfoundland, St. John's, Newfoundland, Canada

JOEL R.L. EHRENKRANZ, M.D.,   Department of Medicine, Columbia University, Morristown, New Jersey, U.S.A.

DAVID T. ESTROFF, M.D.,   Alaska Native Hospital, Alaska Area Native Health Service, U.S. Department of Health and Human Services, Public Health Service, Mt. Edgecumbe, Alaska, U.S.A.

G. WILLIAM N. FITZGERALD, M.D., F.R.C.S.(C),   Grenfell Regional Health Services, Charles S. Curtis Memorial Hospital, St. Anthony, Newfoundland, Canada

PETER M. FOGGIN,   Département de Géographie, Université de Montréal, Montréal, Québec, Canada

HARRIET FORSIUS, Associate Professor,   Department of Pediatrics, University of Oulu, Oulu, Finland

HENRIK FORSIUS, Professor, Head, Department of Ophthalmology, University of Oulu, Oulu, Finland

ROBERT FORTUINE, M.D., M.P.H.,   Family Medicine Service, Alaska Native Medical Center, U.S. Department of Health and Human Services, Public Health Service, Anchorage, Alaska, U.S.A.

B. FRIESEN, M.D.,   Northern Medical Unit, University of Manitoba, Winnipeg, Manitoba, Canada

G.J. FROESE,   University of Alberta, Edmonton, Alberta, Canada

WINNIE GIESBRECHT,   Community Consultant, Winnipeg, Manitoba, Canada

ANNE GILLAN, B.Sc., D.I.C., Ph.D.,   Coordinator, Laboratory Services, Stanton Yellowknife Hospital, Yellowknife, Northwest Territories, Canada

JANE GREEN, M.Sc.,   Program of Northern Medicine and Health, Memorial University of Newfoundland, St. John's, Newfoundland, Canada

JACQUELINE A. GREENMAN, R.N., M.P.H.,   Office of Maternal and Child Health, Alaska Area Native Health Service, U.S. Department of Health and Human Services, Public Health Service, Anchorage, Alaska, U.S.A.

C. GREENSMITH, M.D., F.R.C.P.(C),   Northern Medical Unit, University of Manitoba, Winnipeg, Manitoba, Canada

LORNA GUSE,   Evaluation of Maternal and Child Health Outreach Seminar, Winnipeg, Manitoba, Canada

JAMES A. HAHN,   Dann and Associates, Inc., Anchorage, Alaska, U.S.A.

DAVID B. HALL, Ph.D.,   Arctic Investigations Laboratory, Center for Infectious Diseases, Centers for Disease Control, U.S. Department of Health and Human Services, Public Health Service, Anchorage, Alaska, U.S.A.

J.P. HART HANSEN,   Department of Pathology, Gentofte Hospital, Copenhagen, Denmark

JENS C. HANSEN, Institute of Hygiene, University of Aarhus, Århus, Denmark

PEDER KERN HANSEN, M.D., Department of Obstetrics and Gynecology, Hvidovre Hospital, Hvidovre, Denmark

SIXTEN S.R. HARALDSON, Dr. Med., M.P.H., D.H.E., C.F.P., Professor of International Development, Clark University, U.S.A. (affil.)

G.K.M. HARDING, University of Manitoba, Winnipeg, Manitoba, Canada

H. HUNTLEY HARDISON, M.D., Arctic Investigation Laboratory, Center for Infectious Diseases, Centers for Disease Control, U.S. Department of Health and Human Services, Public Health Service, Anchorage, Alaska, U.S.A.

BENT HARVALD, Department of Internal Medicine C, Odense University Hospital, Denmark

J. HASSI, Oulu Regional Institute of Occupational Health, Oulu, Finland

MARGARIDA HERMANN, Danish Cancer Society, Copenhagen, Denmark

E.S. HERSHFIELD, M.D., F.R.C.P.(C), Department of Medicine, University of Manitoba, Winnipeg, Manitoba, Canada

WILLIAM L. HEYWARD, M.D., Arctic Investigations Laboratory, Center for Infectious Diseases, Centers for Disease Control, U.S. Department of Health and Human Services, Public Health Service, Anchorage, Alaska, U.S.A.

PAIVI HIRVONEN, M.A., Department of Pediatrics, University of Oulu, Oulu, Finland

H. HODES, M.B., B.Ch., B.A.D., South Zone, Manitoba Region, Medical Services Branch, Health and Welfare Canada, Winnipeg, Manitoba, Canada

J.H. HOOFNAGLE, National Institute of Arthritis, Diabetes and Digestive and Kidney Disease, National Institutes of Health, Bethesda, Maryland, U.S.A.

A. PAUL HORNBY, Environmental Carcinogenesis Unit, British Columbia Cancer Research Centre, Vancouver, British Columbia, Canada

J.M. HORNE, Department of Social and Preventive Medicine, University of Manitoba, Winnipeg, Manitoba, Canada

ANNIE HUBERT, GIS Epidémiologie et Immunovirologie des Tumeurs, Lyon, France

HOLGER HULTIN, M.D., M.P.H., Department of Public Health Science, University of Helsinki, Espoo, Finland

G.L. HURST, M.B., Ch.B., British Antarctic Survey and Centre for Offshore Health, Robert Gordon's Institute of Technology, Aberdeen, Scotland, U.K.

H.J. ILECKI, Institute of Otolaryngology, Royal Victoria Hospital, McGill University, Montreal, Quebec, Canada

BELINDA IRELAND, M.D., M.S., Arctic Investigations Laboratory, Center for Infectious Diseases, Centers for Disease Control, U.S. Department of Health and Human Services, Public Health Service, Anchorage, Alaska, U.S.A.

P.A. JARVINEN, Department of Obstetrics and Gynecology, University of Oulu, Oulu, Finland

BJARNE BO JEPPESEN, M.D., Department of Clinical Chemistry, Slagelse County Hospital, Denmark

GORDON J. JOHNSON, M.D., Ph.D., Program of Northern Medicine and Health, Memorial University of Newfoundland, St. John's, Newfoundland, Canada

I.L. JOHNSON, M.D., University of Manitoba, Winnipeg, Manitoba, Canada

MARK S. JOHNSON, Emergency Medical Services Section, Alaska Department of Health and Social Services, Juneau, Alaska, U.S.A.

BRUNO M. KAPPES, Psychology Department, University of Alaska, Anchorage, Alaska, U.S.A.

M. KARLSSON, Preventive Heart Clinic, Reykjavik, Iceland

C. KATO, Department of Community and Pediatrics, McGill University, Montreal, Quebec, Canada

JOSEPH M. KAUFERT, Department of Social and Preventive Medicine, University of Manitoba, Winnipeg, Manitoba, Canada

A. KAUPPILA, Department of Obstetrics and Gynecology, University of Oulu, Oulu, Finland

LISA KNUTSON, M.S., Arctic Investigations Laboratory, Center for Infectious Disease, Centers for Disease Control, U.S Department of Health and Human Services, Public Health Service, Anchorage, Alaska, U.S.A.

EEVA-RIITA KOKKONEN, M.D., Department of Pediatrics, University of Oulu, Oulu, Finland

WILLIAM W. KOOLAGE, Department of Anthropology, University of Manitoba, Winnipeg, Manitoba, Canada

ANDREW KOSTER, Independent Media Producer, Winnipeg, Manitoba, Canada

B. LAGERKVIST, Department of Clinical Physiology, University of Umeå, Umeå, Sweden

K. LAPINLEIMU, M.D., National Public Health Institute, Helsinki, Finland

G.J. LARKE, M.D., Provincial Laboratory of Public Health, University of Alberta, Edmonton, Alberta, Canada

JOHN F. LEE, M.D., M.P.H., Anchorage, Alaska, U.S.A.

V.P. LEE, University of Alberta, Edmonton, Alberta, Canada

J. LEPPÄLUOTO, Nordic Council for Arctic Medical Research, Department of Physiology, University of Oulu, Oulu, Finland

HÅKAN LINDERHOLM, M.D., Professor, Department of Clinical Physiology, University Hospital, Umeå, Sweden

N. LING, B.N., Northern Medical Unit, University of Manitoba, Winnipeg, Manitoba, Canada

E. LL. LLOYD, M.B., F.R.C.P.E., F.F.A.R.C.S., Princess Margaret Rose Orthopaedic Hospital, Edinburgh, Scotland, U.K.

THOMAS D. LONNER, Ph.D., Center for Alcohol and Addiction Studies, University of Alaska, Anchorage, Alaska, U.S.A.

W. LOSNO, Instituto de Biología Andina, Universidad Nacional Mayor de San Marcos, Lima, Peru

D.J. LUGG, M.D., Antarctic Division, Department of Science and Technology, Kingston, Tasmania, Australia

D.W. MCCULLOUGH, M.D., F.R.C.S.(C), Department of Otolaryngology, University of Manitoba, Winnipeg, Manitoba, Canada

FREDERICK MCGINNIS, Department of Human Resources, State of Georgia, Atlanta, Georgia, U.S.A.

L. LYNN MCINTYRE, M.D., Division of Community Health, Faculty of Medicine, University of Toronto, Toronto, Ontario, Canada

JILL G. MCKELVY, Ph.D., University of Alaska, Anchorage, Alaska, U.S.A.

DONALD M. MCLEAN, M.D., F.R.C.P.(C), Department of Medical Microbiology, University of British Columbia, Vancouver, British Columbia, Canada

BRIAN J. MCMAHON, M.D., Medicine Service, Alaska Native Medical Center, Alaska Area Native Health Service, U.S. Department of Health and Human Services, Public Health Service, Anchorage, Alaska, U.S.A.

THEODORE A. MALA, M.D., M.P.H., Department of Biological Sciences, University of Alaska, Anchorage, Alaska, U.S.A.

J. MANFREDA, M.D., University of Manitoba, Winnipeg, Manitoba, Canada

G. MARCHESSAULT, R.D., B.H.Ec., Medical Services Branch, Health and Welfare Canada, Winnipeg, Manitoba, Canada

JOHN R. MARTIN, M.D., F.R.C.P.(C), Program of Northern Medicine and Health, Faculty of Medicine, Memorial University of Newfoundland, St. John's, Newfoundland, Canada

JOHN T. MAYHALL, D.D.S., Ph.D., Professor, Faculty of Dentistry, University of Toronto, Toronto, Ontario, Canada

JAMES G. MESSER, B.D.S., F.D.S., R.C.P.S., D.D.S., Grenfell Regional Health Services, St. Anthony, Newfoundland, Canada

WILLIAM J. MILLS, High Latitude Study, University of Alaska, Anchorage, Alaska, U.S.A.

G.Y. MINUK, M.D., Department of Medicine, University of Calgary Health Sciences Centre, Calgary, Alberta, Canada

M.E.K. MOFFATT, Northern Medical Unit and Department of Pediatrics, University of Manitoba, Winnipeg, Manitoba, Canada

ESTHER MOORE, Native Services, St. Boniface Hospital, Winnipeg, Manitoba, Canada

SIMO NÄYHÄ, M.D., Department of Public Health Science, University of Oulu, Oulu, Finland

L.E. NICOLLE, Department of Medical Microbiology and Infectious Diseases, University of Calgary, Calgary, Alberta, Canada

N. HØJGAARD NIELSEN, M.D., Department of Pathology, Rigshospitalet, Copenhagen, Denmark

YURI P. NIKITIN, Deputy Chairman, Siberian Branch of the Academy of Medical Sciences, U.S.S.R.

LYDIA NOVAK, President, Medical Workers' Union, Moscow, U.S.S.R.

F. O'DONOGHUE, Regional Education Office, Government of the Northwest Territories, Frobisher Bay, Northwest Territories, Canada

JOHN D. O'NEIL, Ph.D., Department of Social and Preventive Medicine, University of Manitoba, Winnipeg, Manitoba, Canada

P.H. ORR, M.D., Northern Medical Unit, University of Manitoba, Winnipeg, Manitoba, Canada

ROBIN D. ORR, Faculty of Medicine, Memorial University of Newfoundland, St. John's, Newfoundland, Canada

J.G. ÓSKARSSON, University of Iceland, Reykjavik, Iceland

R. PÄÄKKÖNEN, Oulu Regional Institute of Occupational Health, Oulu, Finland

GUDRUN PÉTURSDÓTTIR, Institute of Physiology, University of Oslo, Oslo, Norway

JACKIE PFLAUM, R.N., School of Nursing, University of Alaska, Anchorage, Alaska, U.S.A.

C. POKRANT, Northern Medical Unit, University of Manitoba, Winnipeg, Manitoba, Canada

B. POSTL, M.D., F.R.C.P.(C), Northern Medical Unit, University of Manitoba, Winnipeg, Manitoba, Canada

JUKKA PUOLAKKA, M.D., Department of Obstetrics and Gynecology, University of Oulu, Oulu, Finland

ROBERT L. RAUSCH, Division of Animal Medicine, University of Washington, Seattle, Washington, U.S.A.

LISE RENAUD, M.Sc., Department of Community Health, Montreal General Hospital, Montreal, Quebec, Canada

LOUIS REY, Ph.D., President, Comité Arctique International, Monaco

BILL RICHARDS, M.D., Chief, Area Mental Health, U.S. Public Health Service, Alaska Area Native Health Service, Anchorage, Alaska, U.S.A.

JOËLLE ROBERT-LAMBLIN, Ph.D., Laboratoire d'Anthropologie du Musée de l'Homme, Paris, France

ELIZABETH ROBINSON, M.D., M.Sc., C.C.F.P., Department of Community Health, Montreal General Hospital, Montreal, Quebec, Canada

K. RODAHL, M.D., Institute of Work Physiology, Oslo, Norway

ANDRIS RODE, M.Sc., Ph.D., Eastern Arctic Scientific Resource Centre, Igloolik, Northwest Territories, Canada

J. RODRIGUES, M.D., Northern Medical Unit, University of Manitoba, Winnipeg, Manitoba, Canada

A.R. RONALD, University of Manitoba, Winnipeg, Manitoba, Canada

DALEE SAMBO, Alaska Director, Inuit Circumpolar Conference, Anchorage, Alaska, U.S.A.

NANCY SANDERS, R.N., M.N., School of Nursing, University of Alaska, Anchorage, Alaska, U.S.A.

PETER SARSFIELD, M.D., Cambridge Bay, Northwest Territories, Canada

OTTO SCHAEFER, M.D., F.R.C.P.(C), Northern Medical Research Unit, Medical Services Branch, Health and Welfare Canada

BERNARD SEGAL, Ph.D., Center for Alcohol and Addiction Studies, University of Alaska, Anchorage, Alaska, U.S.A.

LEILA SEITAMO, Chief Psychologist, Department of Pediatrics, University of Oulu, Oulu, Finland

ROY J. SHEPHARD, M.D., Ph.D., School of Physical and Health Education, University of Toronto, Toronto, Ontario, Canada

N. SIGFUSSON, Preventive Heart Clinic, Reykjavik, Iceland

J.D. SILVER, B.A., Northern Medical Unit, University of Manitoba, Winnipeg, Manitoba, Canada

PETER SKINHØJ, M.D., Medical Department A, Rigshospitalet, Copenhagen, Denmark

MARGARET SMITH, Services to Native People Program, Health Sciences Centre, Winnipeg, Manitoba, Canada

SØREN FRIIS SMITH, Psychologist, Social Pediatric Clinic, Department of Pediatrics, Rigshospitalet, University of Copenhagen, Copenhagen, Denmark

L. SOININEN, Health Center, Inari, Finland

D. SPADY, M.D., F.R.C.P.(C), Department of Pediatrics, University of Alberta, Alberta, Canada

JOHN W. STAMM, D.D.S., D.D.P.H., M.Sc.D., Faculty of Dentistry, University of Toronto, Toronto, Ontario, Canada

FREJ STENBÄCK, Secretary General, Nordic Council for Arctic Medical Research, Oulu, Finland

M. STENVIK, National Public Health Institute, Helsinki, Finland

M.C. STEPHENS, M.D., Ph.D., Northern Medical Unit, University of Manitoba, Winnipeg, Manitoba, Canada

HANS F. STICH, Environmental Carcinogenesis Unit, British Columbia Cancer Research Centre, Vancouver, British Columbia, Canada

VERNER STILLNER, M.D., M.P.H., Department of Psychiatry, University of Kentucky Medical School, Lexington, Kentucky, U.S.A.

M. THOMSON, R.N., University of Manitoba, Winnipeg, Manitoba, Canada

JENS JØRGEN THORN, D.D.S. Lic. Odont., Department of Oral Medicine and Oral Surgery, Rigshospitalet, Copenhagen, Denmark

JEAN-PIERRE THOUEZ, Département de Géographie, Université de Montréal, Montréal, Québec, Canada

J.G. WAGGONER, National Institute of Arthritis, Diabetes and Digestive and Kidney Diseases, National Institutes of Health, Bethesda, Maryland, U.S.A.

G.V. WATTERS, Departments of Community Medicine and Pediatrics, McGill University, Montreal, Quebec, Canada

ANTHONY B. WAY, University Health Sciences Center, Texas Tech University, Lubbock, Texas, U.S.A.

GLORIA HOUSTON WAY, M.P.H., Emergency Medical Services Section, Alaska Department of Health and Social Services, Juneau, Alaska, U.S.A.

ISABEL WHITFORD, Services to Native People, Health Sciences Centre, Winnipeg, Manitoba, Canada

RUSSELL WILKINS, Department of Community Health, Montreal General Hospital, Montreal, Quebec, Canada

CHRISTOPHER J. WILLIAMS, M.S., Arctic Investigations Laboratory, Center for Infectious Diseases, Centers for Disease Control, U.S. Department of Health and Human Services, Public Health Service, Anchorage, Alaska, U.S.A.

J.H. WILLIAMS, M.B., F.R.C.Path., F.R.C.P.(C), Programme of Northern Medicine and Health, St. Anthony, Newfoundland, Canada [Deceased]

JOSEPH F. WILSON, M.D., Surgery Service, Alaska Native Medical Center, Alaska Area Native Health Service, U.S. Department of Health and Human Services, Public Health Service, Anchorage, Alaska, U.S.A.

TERESA WOLBER, M.A., F.N.P., Alaska Native Medical Center, U.S. Department of Health and Human Services, Public Health Service, Anchorage, Alaska, U.S.A.

K.A. WOTTON, M.D., M.P.H., F.R.C.P.(C), Nairobi, Kenya

T. KUE YOUNG, M.D., M.Sc., Northern Medical Unit and Department of Social and Preventive Medicine, University of Manitoba, Winnipeg, Manitoba, Canada

Conrad Earl Albrecht, M.D., undeniably did us a great service 18 years ago by establishing the series of International Symposia concerned with the health of the human populations in the circumpolar parts of the world. These populations include many of us enthusiastically relocated southerners, and the people who have been here in the circumpolar regions for countless generations before us. The symposium and this Proceedings volume document the common focus of the two groups, newcomers and the original peoples, in seeking good health for all.

Although there was a World Health Organization Conference on Medicine and Public Health in the Arctic and Antarctic in Geneva in 1962, it had no successors. Dr. Albrecht's First International Symposium in Fairbanks, Alaska, in 1967, attended by Soviets, Scandinavians, Canadians and Alaskans, among others, was such a good idea, that other symposia followed regularly every three or four years. The second symposium took place in Oulu, Finland, in 1971. The third symposium was held in Yellowknife, Northwest Territories, Canada, in 1974, and the fourth in Novosibirsk, USSR, in 1978. The fifth symposium was held in Copenhagen, Denmark, in 1981, and the Sixth International Symposium on Circumpolar Health, the Proceedings of which follow, was held in Anchorage, Alaska, during the week of 13 May 1984. Planning for the seventh symposium, to be held in Umeå, Sweden, in 1987, is presently progressing.

I had participated in all of the previous symposia, but to my surprise, I was elected President of this symposium at the business meeting in Copenhagen at the fifth symposium. Fortunately, Wayne W. Myers, M.D., then Director of the WAMI Medical Education Program in Fairbanks, and Helen D. Beirne, Ph.D., then Commissioner of the Department of Health and Social Services of the State of Alaska, were present at that business meeting and they immediately volunteered to serve as "Secretaries General." Dr. Myers had also brought with him an invitation from Dr. Jay Barton, then President of the University of Alaska, to hold the next symposium in Alaska. Upon returning to Alaska from Copenhagen, we put together a hard-working National Organizing Committee, any member of which could have served as the president. Their names are listed in the front of this volume. Previous symposia served as models and inspiration for the Organizing Committee.

In organizing this symposium, the committee found that raising money through solicitation was the most difficult task. Given the climate of fiscal austerity in the United States and in Alaska these days, no single large component of the federal or state governments could entirely subsidize the hosting of such a major symposium as this one. Instead, the National Organizing Committee had to seek numerous small- and medium-sized appropriations from federal, state, and local agencies, as well as from private enterprise, to defray the symposium's considerable expenses. Our solicitations succeeded because of the appeal of the subject matter for which we requested support. The University of Alaska, for example, contributed financially through the President's Office, through the University of Alaska Press, through the Chancellor's Office of the Fairbanks Campus, and through the Director of the Division of Life Science. The total of these various forms of financial support from the University of Alaska, plus the non-financial support of faculty time, advice, and encouragement, amounted to a large commitment of resources from one small university to help the symposium succeed. Another significant source of financial support was the North Slope Borough. Eugene Brower, Mayor in 1984 of that municipality in arctic Alaska, populated by Iñupiaq-speaking Eskimos, wrote to the National Organizing Committee:

I have consulted with my Health Department Director and we both agree that this kind of information exchange is critical to any effort to provide quality health care for all Arctic peoples. The North Slope Borough, therefore, would like to commit $50,000 to this effort and is proud to be listed as one of the sponsoring organizations. (Letter, 2 May 1983)

Contributions from organizations that could not provide direct funds have also helped the symposium and *Circumpolar Health 84* along the way. The Arctic Institute of North America, for example, is acknowledged by a number of authors in this volume for its help as a source of grant-in-aid support for field research. The Arctic Institute has also agreed to review critically this Proceedings volume in the pages of the society's quarterly journal, *Arctic*.

Much of the funding and other forms of support the committee raised have been directed to the completion of this book, because it constitutes the publication of record for this series and will reflect the success of the Organizing Committee and the 1984 symposium. Out of about 280 paper and poster presentations at the symposium, half were submitted as manuscripts, and the scientific editor, Robert Fortuine, M.D., made the difficult selections that resulted in the 108 papers published here. Once the selections were made, Dr. Fortuine was assisted by David W. Norton, Ph.D. and Sue Keller, serving as production editors from the University of Alaska, Fairbanks. Before they could deliver the camera-ready copy to the University of Washington Press, a great deal of work had to be done to prepare a book of quality worthy of the attendees at the symposium. Virtually all illustrations and figures were re-drafted and photographed to provide a standard quality and size of characters. The three editors also rose to the challenge posed by the multilingual backgrounds of authors. They persisted at bringing forth clear technical English text from authors whose first languages were as varied as Russian, Swedish, French, Finnish, and even North American variants of English. The editors were meticulous at preserving original orthography of western European languages (see, for example, pp. 22-31).

With the Index, and the Appendix containing the essentials of the symposium's original program, the Organizing Committee has fashioned what we hope will be a solid, scholarly, and useful reference text. The Sixth International Symposium passes this legacy to our successors in Umeå with every hope that they will add their own improvements to the publishing tradition of the series.

The contents of *Circumpolar Health 84* document our contention that much progress in health fields continues to be made, even since the Copenhagen Symposium three years earlier. Major strides in health care delivery, immunization, self-determination in health programs, and historical analyses of past experiences in circumpolar health are evident. Changes in demographic patterns, occupational pursuits, and cultural identities are better understood now as determinants of the health and illness picture in different communities in high latitude settings. Such changes are occurring rapidly, and we are likely to see continued transitions in the foreseeable future. The future of the series of International Symposia on Circumpolar Health presently appears favorable. Policy for circumpolar health and science seems to be taking shape. It is gratifying that the host nation for the 1984 symposium enacted the National Arctic Research and Policy Act, and the American Public Health Association adopted the National Arctic Health Science Policy both within months of the Symposium itself (see footnote, p. 39).

Finally, I must observe that the essence of this series of symposia is its focus on interdisciplinary science and international collaboration. The fraternal multidisciplinary challenge is as exciting today as when Dr. Albrecht opened the first Symposium in 1967. After all, this is more than a medical congress. Throughout this volume, authors cite evidence of real advances in circumpolar health care, health status, health delivery, and preventive strategies for health maintenance. In virtually every case, underlying such progress is a coordinated interdisciplinary study or approach. Without the inclusion of ethnography, anthropology, demography, local political tacticians, and many other types of expertise in various combinations, the medical professions alone might still be limited to struggling with "illness care" in circumpolar regions, and this series might be designated with some negative title. I much prefer the positive, and with due respect to Lydia Novak, I paraphrase her words of greeting to the Symposium: "Good health to you all."

Frederick A. Milan, Ph.D.
President of the Symposium

PREFACE

This volume brings together a selection of the papers and addresses presented at the Sixth International Symposium on Circumpolar Health held in Anchorage, Alaska, May 13-18, 1984. Scientists, administrators, and health workers assembled from 21 countries for the conference, at which some 199 papers were read in the scientific sessions and another 84 presented as posters. In addition, several invited scientists and guests, including Nobel Laureate Baruch Blumberg, addressed the two major plenary sessions and other special Symposium events.

Because of limitations of space, not every worthy paper submitted for publication could be used. As editor, I have tried to make reasonable selections of manuscripts based on such attributes as significance, originality, their clarity of expression, and length. I have also endeavored to keep the overall theme of the Proceedings volume in perspective while making some of the more difficult decisions respecting individual manuscripts. For example, a few otherwise excellent papers are not included because they are only peripherally related to the polar regions. Some other contributions were outstanding, but of such a specialized nature that they were better suited to publication in technical journals. In making these uncomfortable choices, I have been ably assisted by the Scientific Section Chairpersons and others, but the ultimate responsibility for decisions and for the minor editorial amendments cannot be laid at their door.

The papers were diverse in their length, style, and content. Not all followed the traditional organizational pattern of a scientific paper, nor was it appropriate that they should. They have been arranged in the book by subject matter, although their sequence here differs somewhat from that used at the Symposium itself.

An abbreviated program is printed as an appendix to this volume so that the reader may recall the original context of each paper and note the titles of papers presented at the Symposium but not included in the Proceedings.

This program also allows the reader to appreciate the breadth of subject matter presented at the Sixth Symposium. As with most such conferences, not every abstract was followed up by a presented paper; moreover, several papers in their final form had a new title or a different sequence of authors from those listed in the original program. These last-minute changes have been reflected as accurately as possible in the program printed here.

To follow in the tracks of one's eminent editorial predecessors is never easy, and my respect for their accomplishment is even greater now that I have limped along their path. I especially appreciate the assistance of not one, but two, university presses in preparing this book. The University of Alaska Press, represented by Dr. David W. Norton and Ms. Sue Keller, provided copy-editing, correspondence with authors, design, graphics, and layout of the camera-ready copy. The staff of the University of Washington Press, particularly Mr. Richard Barden, Assistant Director and Controller, encouraged and advised throughout the early production process, then supervised the printing and binding of the book and now serve as the agents for its distribution.

Finally, my personal gratitude to the staff of the Alaska Area Native Health Service for their indulgence of my preoccupations with this task, and to my wife Sheila for her continuing forbearance and support.

Robert Fortuine, M.D.
Editor, *Circumpolar Health 84*

SECTION 1. INTRODUCTORY STATEMENTS AND GENERAL SURVEYS

WORDS OF WELCOME FROM THE INUIT CIRCUMPOLAR CONFERENCE

DALEE SAMBO

Ladies and Gentlemen, fellow speakers, and the National Organizing Committee, I am very happy and very honored to have the opportunity to speak before the 6th International Symposium on Circumpolar Health.

I work for the Inuit Circumpolar Conference here in Anchorage, Alaska, as Director of the Alaskan Office and a Special Assistant to the ICC president, Hans-Pavia Rosing. We also have a Canadian Regional Office in Ottawa, Ontario, and our headquarters office is in Nuuk, Greenland.

The ICC is an international organization with United Nations non-governmental organization status. We represent the Inuit of Alaska, Canada and Greenland, who are approximately 100,000 strong. Our purpose is to promote unity amongst the Inuit of the arctic rim countries and furthermore, with that unity speak out in protection of our culture and environment.

The ICC was first organized in 1977 at Barrow, Alaska. This conference was hosted by the North Slope Borough and the people of Barrow. Our founder was the late mayor of the North Slope Borough, Eben Hopson, Sr. Eben Hopson felt a need to establish a comprehensive international arctic policy to address concerns of the arctic people which range from health and welfare to environmental protection. He felt the only way to do this effectively was to organize the Inuit on an international level because of our common culture and common environment.

The Inuit of Greenland hosted the second General Assembly in 1980 and most recently the Canadian Inuit hosted our third General Assembly held in the summer of 1983 at Frobisher Bay, NWT, Canada. Throughout these 3 Assemblies the appointed delegates have addressed, by resolution, the concerns of Inuit health and welfare. Past ICC resolutions have discussed the health and welfare of the elders in Inuit communities, alcohol and drug abuse among Inuit, and the high rate of teenage pregnancy. An issue cited at our 1983 conference was the need for more Inuit professionals and paraprofessionals in health and welfare services in the circumpolar regions. Other resolutions range from a call for an arctic nuclear-free zone to improvement of communications and transportation and education and environmental protection. The 1983 conference delegates primarily focused on the development of an arctic policy. We will continue to work on the declaration of our policies and priorities with regard to an arctic policy and hope to have the final and formal declaration adopted at the 1986 General Assembly. The 1986 General Assembly will be our fourth and is scheduled for the summer of 1986 in Kotzebue, Alaska.

It is from the ICC and its membership that I warmly welcome you, and especially those of you from countries afar, to Alaska for this most important and useful symposium.

The first international gathering of health and medical experts and scientists took place in Fairbanks, Alaska, in 1967. Thus, the International Symposium on Circumpolar Health precedes the ICC by 10 years. It is an organization that has brought many diverse countries and cultures together, and its work is of the utmost importance and significance to the circumpolar peoples, Native and non-Native. This is a most opportune time to express our appreciation to the Founder, Dr. C. Earl Albrecht, for organizing a symposium to focus on health conditions of the arctic peoples.

The environment and climate of the arctic and sub-arctic countries are unique, thus making the health problems unique. The exchange of health related information, problems, and solutions is very important and valuable not only to those who live in the Arctic but also to people all over the world. The research, work, and accomplishments of those who have gathered at each preceding symposium have made significant contributions to the field of health in the Arctic. We are very grateful to this organization and its membership for their contribution to the northern peoples.

It is my hope that the ICC and the International Symposium on Circumpolar Health can align their concerns and begin to work cooperatively on arctic health matters in the coming years. I would encourage the blending of traditional tribal medicine and healing practices of all indigenous peoples with those of modern medicine and further hope that this type of work can be done soon, as we need to explore this idea before we no longer can. I would support and endorse this type of work. This international sharing of information may provide mutual answers to our common problems much sooner than working independently.

I want to thank the National Organizing Committee, the sponsors, and also the supporters of this symposium for making it possible, and wish them and each of you the best for a successful and educational week. I trust that this week of activities will produce an even greater contribution to not only the Inuit but to mankind in general. Again, on behalf of the Inuit of Alaska, Canada, and Greenland, welcome to Alaska! Quyaanah.

Dalee Sambo
Alaska Director
Inuit Circumpolar Conference
429 D Street
Suite 211
Anchorage, Alaska 99501
U.S.A.

GREETINGS FROM THE MEDICAL WORKERS' UNION OF THE USSR

LYDIA NOVAK

First of all, I would like to express our sincere gratitude to the National Organizing Committee and the leadership of the Alaska Public Health Association for their decision to invite representatives of our union to this important international gathering and for the opportunity to address its participants.

I am greatly honored and pleased to bring you all warm greetings and best wishes from the seven million members of the Medical Workers' Union of the USSR. While honored by the invitation to participate in this major scientific assembly, I feel I am bound to explain briefly why and how we have come.

One, we see our coming to Anchorage, once again, both as a direct result and a fresh step forward in the development of the recently established but already firm and fruitful relations between our union and the following organizations--the Alaska Public Health Association, University of Alaska, Anchorage, and the Alaska Department of Health and Social Services.

Two, our delegation's participation in this international scientific conference is explained by the nature of our union, which brings together all categories of physicians, nurses, and other medical, administrative and technical personnel in the public health field, as well as all medical researchers. As a result, our organization is directly involved in the planning and implementation of public health and medical science development programs covering, in particular, the regions of Siberia and the Far North which are so vast and rich in natural resources.

Three, we were grateful to have received your kind invitation to attend this symposium in view of our own rich experience of international contacts which we believe to be of great practical value and relevance in many respects. Not the least of these is our having a further opportunity to exchange professional views and experiences in this field, to promote bilateral ties and multilateral cooperation, to establish friendly relations on a personal level and to promote better mutual understanding between peoples.

Whatever the problems we may have come to discuss at a meeting like this, be they the problems of circumpolar or general health care, maternal and child health, the social and health problems of the aged, environmental pollution or industrial health, we must not neglect the single most important problem facing public health today, namely, the threat of a world nuclear war capable of destroying all living things on earth.

More than anyone, we representatives of public health professionals--workers in the most humane occupation of all--should stand for the preservation of peace, in the full realization that the current arms drive, especially the nuclear arms race, is a heavy burden on the nations of the world as they pursue the path of social and economic progress, and is pushing the world ever closer to the dangerous brink of nuclear disaster.

We know that in the front ranks of the unprecedented campaign against this nuclear madness are physicians and other public health workers, many of whom will meet in the Fourth World Congress of Physicians of the World Against Nuclear War in Helsinki in early June 1984.

I am firmly convinced that, by uniting and by forging closer ties of friendship and cooperation, we should be able, for the greater benefit of our respective nations, to develop and improve medicine and public health and, still more important, make a greater contribution to the effort to preserve peace and life on earth.

Finally, I wish this conference every success and fruitfulness in the spirit of friendship and cooperation; I also wish all delegates happiness and the best of health.

Lydia Novak
President
Medical Workers' Union
Lenin Avenue 42
Moscow 117-119
U.S.S.R.

Circumpolar Health 84:4-7

THE ARCTIC CHALLENGE

LOUIS RFY

NEW INDUSTRIAL VENTURES

An interesting feature of global policy, within the last 2 or 3 decades, has been the progressive opening of the arctic regions to advanced industrial development. As a consequence, their economic significance has increased substantially, thus reinforcing the strategic importance of an area which is still considered as a highly critical zone in the delicate military balance between the major Eastern and Western alliances.

The discovery of huge natural resources and, more precisely, of large fossil fuel deposits within the arctic lands and the adjacent continental shelf offshore easily explains the sudden interest demonstrated by governments and private enterprise for the desolate northern wastes and it is at the origin of a fantastic revolution in traditional mining, drilling, and industrial practices.

Indeed, the vast, remote, cold, boreal lands present a continuous and multifocal challenge to the massive deployment of advanced technology. Adverse climatic conditions make any operation extremely difficult, and sometimes hazardous, both on unstable permafrost and in ice-infested waters. In the harsh and often unpredictable arctic environment, men are exposed to constant stress and strain and they can easily lose their bearings and wreck their reactional patterns in a raging blizzard, or in the depths of the demanding continuous polar night. Moreover, the immensity of the arctic regions and, therefore, the huge distances which lie between the tiny, scattered camps or settlements, generate enormous logistic difficulties for routine transportation and supply, as well as for emergency situations. As for that particular issue, curiously enough it has not been possible to resort to the clever techniques developed over millennia by the first arctic native settlers since the nature and size of the operations make it compulsory to follow entirely new approaches geared to their specific requirements.

Temporary winter camps and airfields built on reinforced sea ice, supporting lines of barges sailing in the narrow channels opened in the summer pack by powerful icebreakers, full-size modular buildings shipped by air cargo or sea lanes and erected on elevated piles driven deep into the hard but sensitive permafrost, air cushion vehicles gliding on uneven barren grounds or on the chaotic sea ice of the shear zone, heavy massive structures trucked along thousands of miles of rugged haul roads--these are some of the developments which had to be achieved to implement numerous arctic resource-oriented exploration ventures.

In those conditions, the construction of large permanent exploitation complexes in remote sites has proven to be even more difficult and involved many new pioneering technologies. Directional drilling, for instance, allowed packing wellheads on selected pads while highly elaborate thermoactive support frames helped insulate the pipeline from underlying permafrost while still giving to the line the appropriate flexibility through its zigzag design to withstand wide summer/winter temperature variations and earthquakes.

Needless to say, prices rocketed to yet unknown levels and the financial load was further aggravated by the long delays in clearance and construction procedures, requiring large amounts of up-front unproductive investment.

THE LAST FRONTIER

The development of an appropriate technology is not the only issue in arctic industrial development and many other steps are required in order to achieve a harmonious integration of the new structures within the pristine, still fragile, wilderness.

Indeed, under polar and circumpolar conditions, the biophysical environment as well as the different ecosystems are extremely sensitive and demonstrate very little adaptation or reclaiming capacities. As such, any operation carried out in the Arctic is bound to interact strongly and in a durable way with the existing natural patterns and, if improperly managed, can leave open scars which might never heal: collapsed trails in the Ogoturuk Valley and deep gullies on the arctic slopes are sad reminders of the utmost sensitivity of permafrost to overload and repeated abuses.

In the polar sea itself, marine mammals show a great reactivity to outside disturbance of their usual acoustic environment and should not be challenged during sensitive periods as is the case for the bowhead whale during its spring migration through the Bering Strait along the Alaskan North Slope coastline. Moreover, the massive release of foreign chemicals by accidental spills or improper waste management can seriously alter the feeding layers of sea mammals and even, at sub-threshold levels, impair the behavior of anadromous fish and prevent mating in crustacea. On land, the erection of bulky structures and especially the development of extensive piping may interfere with the migration of wandering caribou and, accordingly, these networks will have to be built in such a way that they do not present impassable obstacles for the herds heading north in spring or back south toward the interior tundra in October.

THE PEOPLE OF THE NORTH

Last but not least, man himself is obviously involved in this process either because, as an arctic operator, he is subjected to strenuous work and exposed to severe environmental pressure, or because, as a permanent settler, the development schemes encroach in part on his own hunting or fishing grounds or interact with his traditional sociocultural and economic patterns.

The Modern Sourdoughs: The Arctic Operators

Whether they constitute a transient or stable labor force, the selected teams who operate in the arctic regions have to face altogether hard duty, adverse working conditions, and continuous environmental stress. Moreover, being isolated from major centers, they have to rely on their own judgment and skills to challenge any arising hazards and make the best use of their limited resources to protect their people, their installations, and the surrounding environment. As such, they diverge widely from the early western pioneers, hunters, trappers, or gold miners since today they have to endure the far-reaching consequences of wrong or accidental maneuvers and are thus endowed with an extended personal responsibility.

Further, if appropriate logistics can provide comfortable housing, varied foods and substantial recreational facilities, health and emergency services still remain limited and depend entirely upon prevailing meteorological and operational conditions, both on-site and at the main support centers.

Along the same lines, special garments, vehicles, and miscellaneous arctic gear definitely help the workers to alleviate, as much as possible, the harsh outdoor conditions, but nevertheless the major environmental factors specific to the polar regions still exert considerable pressures on both men and equipment.

Low temperatures, strong winds (sometimes violent gales and blizzards), and extreme dryness of the air are particularly hard on skin, upper airways and lungs, and thus impair respiration and contribute to a constant overload upon the cardiovascular system. They also impose the need for elaborate thermal protection, and boost substantially the physical strain through increased numbness and added unproductive

weight. Under those conditions sustained efforts are difficult to maintain.

Violent winds can also demonstrate some more subtle effects on man by the pumping (Venturi) action they exert on closed vehicles and habitats which become the sites of cyclic depressions and low-frequency air vibrations, accompanied by irritating, battering noises. This often induces psychotic disorders in wintering parties and can be correlated to the more acute form of "arctic hysteria."

It is even felt that on a larger scale, steady prevailing air streams, impinging on regular occasional geographic structures like mountain ranges or sequenced isolated hills, are likely to generate leeward side atmospheric pressure-waves with associated infrasounds which might influence human reactions and thus add a new load onto the already stressed organism.

Among the different environmental factors, however, special emphasis should be placed on the effects of light. It is, indeed, a practical experience that most arctic operators are seriously challenged by the changing photoperiods in the upper latitudes and by the progressive outphasing of circadian rhythms and biological clocks. The resulting de-synchronization might induce, in sensitive individuals, serious impairment of sleep cycles and of sleep structure, peaking at the time of the several months' continuous daylight or in the middle of the equally long polar night. An interesting side effect of this continuously changing day length is that it also provokes differential responses to occasional therapy, as demonstrated in recent chronopharmacological studies.

Finally, it is more than likely that the strong magnetic disturbances which occur around the geo-magnetic poles and within the wider auroral zone (as a result of the irregular flux into the magnetosphere of the charged particles released from solar spots) interact with brain activities and impair sleep.

The obvious conclusion is that the arctic environment is very demanding and that it exerts a profound and diversified action on man which might affect not only his physical health but also his mental health through increased anxiety, abnormal sleep patterns, and disturbed metabolic and glandular functions due essentially to the cyclic de-synchronization of the biological and circadian rhythms. These changes can explain many odd reactions which are known to occur in circumpolar regions, mainly in transition periods, like the "ruska reaction" in the autumn in Finland or the "spring crazy period" in Alaska and Canada. It is equally self-evident that they might have serious effects, not only on behavior, mood, and emotion, but also, for sensitive individuals, on their performance rate as well as on their memory, vigilance, and aptitude for making rapid decisions in emergency situations with all their obvious consequences.

To this should also be added the still unknown physiological effects of regular commuting to arctic sites from southern latitudes, with the associated abrupt changes in living conditions and time budget.

The Irreversible Involvement of Permanent Arctic Dwellers

Contrary to the Antarctic situation, the boreal polar regions have been inhabited by ancient man for more than 15,000 years, since the end of the last ice age (Wurm-Wisconsin period). There, over thousands of years, arctic cultures have demonstrated a remarkable adaptation to one of the harshest climates on earth and have developed fairly advanced technologies to secure survival, family life, and even permanent settlements.

For centuries, these people remained at the rim of the western world and were not involved in its evolution. They were equally in close balance with their environment and shared in common resources and lands. Despite the fact that they vastly outnumbered any other ethnic group, however, they were not alone and many "Western" southerners also settled in circumpolar regions, sometimes as early as the 6th century A.D. (Finland, northern Norway). In some instances it is not even unlikely that the first inhabitants of the virgin arctic lands were not the Natives but the wandering Vikings as in southern and southwestern Greenland.

The situation remained almost unchanged until very recent times and most arctic people maintained intact their original cultures, languages, and economies.

Today, the abrupt intrusion of Western man and of his all-purpose technologies directly challenges the equilibrium painfully established between man and nature over thousands of years, and thus isolated arctic communities are irreversibly being driven into the powerful maelstrom of an advanced industrial civilization. This is a difficult and often frustrating experience since it endangers seriously the pre-existing cultures and equally impedes the implementation of a comprehensive global policy in the area.

In this rapidly evolving situation, domestic and professional activities are drastically remodelled and this results in major sociocultural and political tensions. In the search for an appropriate balance between traditional values and the newly introduced "occidental lifestyle," education and public health issues appear quite critical. Indeed, in the latter case, marked changes in nutritional patterns and in time budgets have been known to impair individual performance and lead to character instability.

At the same time, the basic roots of a former purely oral culture are undermined by the incipient fading out of the use of native languages, further aggravated by the progressive spin-off of the younger arctic dwellers toward the main focal urban areas in southern latitudes.

Quite certainly, responsible statesmen are trying to fight this evolution to achieve, on-site, the transformation of a stone-age culture into a modern community, and the role played in this regard by such organizations as the Inuit Circumpolar Conference should be acknowledged. It is, however, an extremely complex process with highly emotional issues and major political undercurrents and it seldom obeys rational rules.

Cultural clash and socioeconomic adjustment are not the only political effects of industrial development on arctic dwellers; there are also some important environmental constraints which might affect public health in the upper latitudes.

Atmospheric pollution, for instance, is becoming a source of growing concern in the high Arctic and more particularly in Spitsbergen, northern Greenland and Canada with a regular occurrence, during the late winter months, of a pervasive, extended "arctic haze." This problem has not been well documented and it has been found that the thick, stable aerosol has a continental basis and is derived from the atmospheric pollution generated by mid-latitude industrial activities over Europe and the western USSR. Coal and fuel-fired power stations bear the primary responsibility in this process despite the fact that some major smelting industries, like the Siberian operations in Norilsk also contribute.

The resulting air-borne chemicals released in the cold, dry, air masses are driven east and northeast by the general circulation over an extensive continental pathway and enter the polar highs and the Arctic Ocean near Novaya Zemlya. They then follow the main air-streams and eventually get trapped on the northern flank of the cold North American lands where they finally settle. Their radioactive properties, nucleation behavior, and depositional effects are still unknown but it looks highly probable that they interfere with the overall land-atmosphere-space energy balance and that they, equally, build up in the trophic chain.

Another highly regrettable similar case deals with the progressive uptake of radionuclides by the scarce northern vegetation. Indeed, during the 1950s and 1960s atmospheric testing of nuclear weapons, large amounts of long-life radioactive material were released in the upper atmosphere and from there were driven into the "arctic sink" and picked up by the lichens, acting as "bio-accumulators." In Alaska, they moved to the caribou foraging in winter in the Brooks Range area and, through the flesh of the animals killed during the spring migration and eaten during the following month, stockpiled into the bodies of the Natives (mainly into bones as Strontium-90) during the following summer period.

This was most unfortunate because it had long-lasting effects and, even today, despite the long-standing ban on atmospheric nuclear testing, lichens still provide, indirectly, a substantial amount of radionuclides in the diet of the Inuit. That particular issue, however, is somewhat less spectacular now because, as a consequence of the construction of the trans-Alaska pipeline and the development of the Prudhoe Bay oil-field, the previously isolated inhabitants of Anaktuvuk Pass have considerably altered their traditional lifestyle. Caribou meat is no longer the major element in the diet and this results in a sharp decrease in the total body count of radionuclides and in the associated radiation load on the organism. Unfortunately, many good things have their negative counterpart and it is equally true that, as a result of the same outside contacts, tuberculosis spread quickly over the population and this, in turn, implied numerous regular health controls, including frequent chest X-ray examinations, which, finally, deliver annually a much larger cumulative dose of radiation than the consumption of meat loaded with radionuclides did previously!

An almost identical situation exists with agrochemicals and, especially, with organo-chlorinated compounds, which, by successive distillation and redeposition mechanisms, migrate from the tropical belt and temperate regions toward the upper latitudes and are captured by the vegetative cover and subsequently stored in the fat of reindeer, foxes, and birds. So also for mercury and many other chemicals which meet their ultimate fate in the Arctic, transforming the area into a vast pollution sink despite the absence of any significant local industrial or urban activities!

This long distance transfrontier atmospheric transport is a difficult problem which has not yet been addressed properly by international law and requires an in-depth international assessment and regulation.

Whatever unfortunate consequences the industrial development of mid-latitudes may have on the remote, sensitive arctic environment, it is not, however, the only source of concern in the area and rising attention is now given to the impact of indoor microclimates and pollution on the health of permanent settlers.

The absolute necessity of maintaining decent temperatures within the living quarters as well as having appropriate cooking facilities impose, in arctic homes, more or less continuous use of local heat sources which are, generally, wood or peat stoves. These rather primitive combustion systems release large amounts of carbon dioxide, carbon monoxide, and particulate carbon and this, coupled with the fact that windows and doors are hermetically sealed because of the harsh climate, create a most unfavorable polluted indoor microclimate. Unfortunately, for the same climatic reasons, people spend the greater part of their time at home, especially newborns, young children, and housewives, and thus soak in this pollution bath which has, quite clearly, the worst effect on their health.

It is interesting to note, at this point, that this is by no means a new problem and that in the beautifully preserved Eskimo mummies found near Umanak in Greenland, a fair amount of soot has been found in the lungs of the young children and of adult females.

In this particular issue, industrial development can undoubtedly improve the situation drastically by providing, through natural gas, a steady, safe source of energy even in the most remote isolated homes. This, in fact, has already been achieved in Barrow.

This last example, as well as those which have been discussed previously, show, according to the evidence, that extreme care has to be taken before making any definitive statement on the goods and evils of industrial development. There is, certainly, no easy answer to the problem and in any industrial impact assessment we should put in proper perspective all the different relevant physical, chemical, biological, sociocultural, economic, and political issues and exercise our best judgment to reach sound conclusions and avoid emotional reactions.

Thus, maybe, we shall be able to achieve Job's prophecy--Aurum ab aquilone venit--and find in a balanced, harmonious development of the North a source of mutual prosperity, reward, and satisfaction for both its permanent settlers and southern entrepreneurs.

Louis Rey
President
Comité Arctique International
Monaco

Circumpolar Health 84:8-10

SOME HEALTH PROBLEMS OF MAN IN THE SOVIET FAR NORTH

YURI P. NIKITIN

Areas lying north of 66°33'N, as you know, have been designated as "high latitudes" by a recommendation of the Geneva Conference. Other no less well known terms are "arctic," trans-polar" and "sub-polar" regions. The name Far North is used with a very similar meaning in the Soviet Union. The Far North lies mostly in the permafrost areas, which account for close to 50% of the entire Soviet land mass. At the same time, this vast territory is peopled by just over 5% of the population of the Soviet Union, with population density averaging 1 person per 1.5 square kilometers.

Siberia and the Far North are very rich in many mineral resources such as oil, natural gas, coal, iron ore, gold, diamonds, and many more. This has been one of the main reasons for the fast growth of the Siberian economy in both its southern regions and the Far North. New towns and settlements have grown up beyond the Arctic Circle. All this has brought about a number of serious ecological and health problems, including the problems of environmental protection, settlement and adaptation of large numbers of migrant workers, problems of optimal development of the indigenous populations against the backdrop of accelerating industrial and urban development of the arctic areas, and more. Evidently, to solve all these problems will take far more than what medical science and practice can offer. But they cannot be expected to find adequate solution without a contribution by the medical profession.

Four years ago, the Government decided to establish the Siberian Branch of the National Academy of Medical Sciences which today is made up of the following medical research institutes in Siberia and the Far East: Epidemiological Institute of Vladivostok, Maternal and Child Care Institute in Khabarovsk, Respiratory Physiology and Pathology Institute in Blagoveschensk, Institute of Arctic Medical Problems in Krasnoyarsk, Laboratory of Polar Medicine in Norilsk, Complex Hygiene Problems Institute in Kuzbass, and Institutes of Physiology, Experimental Medicine, Immunology, and Internal Medicine Research in Novosibirsk. Research Institutes of Oncology, Cardiology, and Mental Health are located in Tomsk. Apart from that, Siberia is the home of 15 medical schools and training institutes, all engaged in training physicians, plus 2 special institutes and a further 7 departments of medical schools, all offering advanced refresher training courses to the medical profession. The National Ministry of Health maintains a further 13 research institutes specializing in public sanitation, hygiene, surgery, traumatology, etc.

Basically, what all these research institutes are involved in is, first, research into the differences in disease in the settler and indigenous populations, and identification of the role played by environmental, climatic, geochemical, industrial, social, and other factors, and, second, research in the field of disease prevention, new types of treatment, and management of the health service for the populations of Siberia and the Far North.

First of all, I would like to discuss some matters relating to the health of the settler populations. Often, these people are described as migrants, that is, people migrating to the Far North from other climatic and geographic regions.

Given the rapid pace of economic growth of Siberia and the Far North, these areas are currently experiencing considerable labor shortages. Over the past few years, these regions have seen a substantial influx of migrant workers from the European Soviet Union, the Caucasus, and Central Asian Republics. Some of the migrants settle for good in both established and newly-founded towns and settlements while others, due to some reason or other, fail to adapt and leave before too long. Some work under the rotating shift plan whereby they alternate 3 or 4 week periods of work in the Far North with rest periods in their established homes in other parts of the country.

The medical profession is faced with a whole range of problems of a medical, biological, social, and hygiene nature. These include the problems of medical statistics, acclimatization and adaptation to the subarctic conditions, occupational health, housing, clothing, and transport, problems of the most rational nutrition and recreation, and a host of others. Even such a seemingly simple matter as vacations presents a number of questions such as who should get them, and how often, where and when annual paid leave should occur, whether to go to the warm Southern seas or spend the holidays in one's own climatic zone--all these questions need to be answered in the best possible way. Then there is the very urgent problem of the environment and ecology of the Far North being affected by man's activities and increasing industrialization of the region.

Health statistics show the settler populations in the arctic region to be better off than the populations in the European Soviet Union and southern Siberia. The reason is simple enough: it is mostly healthy young people that come to settle in the Arctic. Still, a more careful study of the health pattern of people spending varying lengths of times in the Far North reveals that, in the first months and generally during the first 2 years of life in the Far North, the human body is affected by a complex set of temporary changes in the nervous and mental spheres, hormonal balance, bioenergetics and thermoregulation, body metabolism, and functioning of the respiratory and cardiovascular systems. By now, fairly detailed studies have been made of numerous aspects of man's adaptation to subarctic conditions and of various temporary changes in the state of health.

In the first 3 months following their arrival in the Far North, about a half, and according to some estimates more than half, of the new arrivals come with complaints about a deteriorating general condition--increased tiredness, sleepiness, insomnia, headaches, chest pains and the like. Later, these conditions taper off gradually as the body adapts to the new environment. However, in many cases longer periods of life in the Far North tend to drain the body's reserves and various pathological conditions begin to manifest themselves after about 10 to 15 years in the Far North.

Studies of the populations settled in the subarctic areas for over 10 years have shown them to display a higher incidence of hypertension, ischemic heart disease, chronic bronchitis, pneumonia, and neurocirculatory dystonia than population groups of the same age in the European part of the Soviet Union. I could go on discussing sickness patterns of the arctic settler populations. Some of these matters might require a separate discussion, including such matters as differences in the clinical picture, symptomatology, and the course of cardiovascular, respiratory, and gastrointestinal conditions in the settler populations, peculiarities of disease in non-indigenous people born in the Arctic and many more interesting questions. But I would like to reserve my remaining time for the second part of my report, which deals with the health of the indigenous population of the Far North.

In the arctic regions of the European and Asian parts of the Soviet Union, there are over 30 different nations and nationalities totalling just over 1 million people. The Yakut number some 350,000, while the combined total of the so-called "smaller" nationalities of the Far North stands at about 150,000.

Census figures and annual statistical reports show all nationalities of the North to be growing appreciably. In the period between the national census of 1970 and that of 1979, the combined total of all "smaller" nationalities of the North increased by 8,000 to reach a total of 158,000.

However, in respect to the indigenous population there remain a number of specific problems which we are doing our best to

study and help solve. One of these problems is the peculiarities of their medical status, that is, possible ethnic differences and the role of genetic and environmental factors in different pathological conditions. Of great importance is the study of trends in morbidity and mortality from different disease categories. Our research institutes do not study all types of disease but those we do study I will now attempt to describe briefly.

My own immediate field is cardiovascular disease which, in earlier days, was relatively rare in the indigenous people of the Far North. They still show a substantially lower rate of hypertension as compared with the settler populations. This may be a result of the indigenous people's better adaptation to the harsh climatic conditions of the Far North. The Chukcha show themselves to be considerably different in terms of hormone levels in the blood. Thus, their cortisol (hydrocortisone) level is much lower than that of the settler populations. It may be possible that the low incidence of hypertension in the indigenous population is a result of low salt intake.

The incidence of ischemic heart disease in some groups of the indigenous population has increased substantially in recent years as compared with the situation of some 10 to 20 years ago. The coastal Chukcha and especially Eskimos show a much lower rate of hypertension and ischemic heart disease compared with the Chukcha tundra dwellers. Their respective diets show substantial differences, with the coastal Chukcha and Eskimo eating a more traditional diet while the tundra Chukcha's diet is distinctly more European, so to speak, containing much saturated fat and sugar.

The incidence of diabetes mellitus in the indigenous Evenk, Yakut, and Chukcha is lower than in the people living in the European part of the Soviet Union.

The indigenous people of the Far North also show some distinct differences in the physiology and pathology of the respiratory system. Morphologically and functionally, the difference is that respiratory tissue has developed a peculiar thermal protection from the cold by increasing the residual volume and substantially diluting the inhaled cold air with the warm alveolar air. Alveolar ventilation efficiency decreases as a result of increased residual volume and "dead space" in the respiratory sections.

The above peculiarities of the respiratory system, especially when compounded by harsh climate, smoking, and specific living conditions, tend to affect the pathology of the respiratory system. Over the last few decades, the indigenous population has shown a dramatic decrease in tuberculosis incidence and fewer complicated pneumonias and suppurative respiratory processes. However, chronic bronchitis and pneumonia are more prevalent than in the southern parts of Siberia. At the same time, the indigenous arctic peoples have much less bronchial asthma than the new settlers in the area. Evidently, the local people have some peculiarities in their immune homeostasis.

Gastrointestinal disease incidence in the indigenous arctic populations is difficult to assess due to the lack of standard research methods, making it impossible to obtain compatible statistics.

Clinical observation makes it possible to conclude that the local people have a somewhat reduced gastric secretion. Many children and adults adapt poorly to the change from the traditional to the "European" diet. Dyspeptic disorders are numerous and, not infrequently, chronic digestive disorders in the indigenous people tend to have a discrete character. In Yakutia, a study involving more than 6,000 people was conducted by A.A. Bezrodnykh to assess the spread of gastric ulcer. The indigenous Yakut have shown a much lower incidence of that disorder than the local Russian population, with 4.2 and 35.2%, respectively, being affected.

Prospectively, oncological disease epidemiology is being studied at its fullest in Yakutia by P.A. Petrov. Over the past 10 years there has been no increase in neoplastic disease in the area, with some downward trend in the rates. The 1972 figures for Yakutia showed 136 malignant tumors per 100,000 coming down to 133 cases in 1982. The indigenous Yakut show a higher mortality from malignant tumors than the settler population. This can be explained by the younger age and higher migration rate of the non-indigenous population, with some leaving the Arctic upon developing the disease.

Over the past few years, adult males have shown a prevalence of lung cancer, even though lung cancer statistics for Yakutia show it falling behind those of the northern provinces of Canada and Scandinavia. Rectal cancer has increased, while cancer of the esophagus and stomach has declined.

In many areas of the Far North, the local population have high rates of dental caries, which may be attributed to the low mineral content of drinking water, especially the low fluoride content. Dental caries is a very serious problem in the Far North.

Otolaryngologists note a number of peculiarities in the disease patterns of the local population who show fewer chronic tonsillitis cases but far more chronic otitis cases. The latter may have some connection to certain peculiarities in the anatomy of the hearing organs.

For their part, ophthalmologists too find some peculiarities in the indigenous people, who show fewer cases of progressive myopia, certain types of glaucoma, retinal vascular pathology, and strabismus. But this pattern lies beyond my scope of competence and I find it somewhat difficult to interpret.

I have had no opportunity, at this point, to discuss various other disease categories. I can only repeat that research done by the medical profession in Siberia shows the indigenous population of the Far North to have certain peculiarities in their patterns of disease which vary in incidence and natural history as compared with both settler populations and those in the European part of the Soviet Union. Obviously, the public health service must take these differences and peculiarities into consideration.

The Soviet Government has done a great deal to bring adequate health care to the people of the Far North, which has the country's highest doctor-to-patient ratio, at 47 and 42 per 10,000 of population in Chukotka and Evenk Autonomous National Regions respectively. In terms of hospital beds available, the Northern Autonomous National Regions are far ahead of the rest of the country, with Evenk and Taimyr Regions having 215, and Koryak Region on the Kamchatka Peninsula 304 beds per 10,000 population respectively. The large specialized hospitals are supplemented by a vast network of medical and health facilities in the smaller communities. Helicopter and amphibious vehicle-borne mobile health teams reach the smallest isolated communities to conduct full periodic physical examination of all people living in the Far North. Local public health bodies have a special fleet of medical aircraft and helicopters.

Much is being done to maintain the health of the indigenous people of the North who, having lived for centuries in the harshest conditions on the globe, have never stopped making their special contribution to the economic and cultural development of our country. They are fully entitled to a special care on the part of the medical profession.

Yuri P. Nikitin
Therapeutic Research Institute
Siberian Branch of the U.S.S.R. Academy
 of Medical Sciences
Sovetskaja Str 18
Novosibirsk
U.S.S.R. 630099

MEDICAL RESEARCH IN REMOTE NORTHERN AREAS AND ISOLATED POPULATIONS: NEEDS, BENEFITS AND LIMITATIONS

OTTO SCHAEFER

INTRODUCTION

Medical research in small population groups dispersed over large areas with tenuous and often uncertain communications is faced with great difficulties and limitations and is very expensive in terms of man-hours, equipment, and travel costs. It may also remain inconclusive due to difficulties in finding statistically valid sample numbers.

We must ask ourselves, therefore, if results and benefits derived either for the local population or for medical science generally warrant such difficult and costly research efforts. This requires a weighing of difficulties, costs, and limitations against the real needs of formerly isolated populations faced first with new infections and then with rapid changes in nutrition, occupation, culture, social structure, and lifestyle.

We should, on the other hand, appreciate opportunities to clarify factors related to epidemiological changes observed in isolated populations during acculturation. Such observations may help us to understand factors contributing to the pathogenesis of diseases of "civilization" such as obesity, hypertension, diabetes, cardiovascular diseases, peptic ulcer, gallbladder ailments and certain types of cancer.

Local conditions must, however, govern our assessment of the needs, benefits, and limitations of medical research in northern areas, as environmental factors not only may create specific health problems and hinder health care delivery, but also may place limitations on medical research by virtue of exorbitant costs, technical difficulties and available sample size. In the Northwest Territories, for example, less than 50,000 people live in an area of 1,253,000 square miles (3,245,000 km) which is comparable to the land mass of India. About half of the population is concentrated in the more accessible southwestern rim, but many still remain scattered with difficult, expensive, time-consuming and often uncertain communications with secondary and tertiary diagnostic and treatment facilities, due to hostile terrain and weather conditions. Further barriers may be posed by language and cultural diversity.

Changes in infection exposure, nutrition, lifestyle plus sociocultural upheaval have all influenced the health of northern Native populations. Recording epidemiological baselines and monitoring changes in their health picture will not only help health care planning for Natives but may also benefit newcomers to these areas and provide clues to the pathogenesis of a number of the diseases of "civilization" listed above. Primitive local facilities, the hostile climate, and uncertain and often delayed transportation may impair collection, processing, transfer or culture of laboratory specimens.

SPECIFIC EXAMPLES

I want to discuss, by means of a few examples, perceived needs and benefits derived from northern medical research for northern residents or from pathogenetic understanding in general, and then address some new areas of concern and in need of more medical and paramedical research in the future.

Frost damage and cold physiology were vigorously studied by numerous physiologists in the Arctic and Antarctic during the 1940s and 1950s and reviewed by Burton and Edholm, 1955 [1]. Physical adaptation to cold was found in humans for peripheral circulation in the hands by Hildes, et al. [2], for cardiovascular responses to facial cold, wind exposure, and hand immersion by Jacques LeBlanc and others [3], and for regional sweating by us [4]. Sweating was found increased in the face, the only non-clothed body part, but diminished elsewhere, most markedly in the frost-endangered feet of the Eskimos.

When primitive man ventured from his tropical areas of origin into cold circumpolar regions, he achieved, however, a remarkable degree of protection against the immediate and life-threatening dangers of freezing his limbs and cooling of the body core. This he accomplished mainly in typical human fashion--by technological innovations, for example, covering himself with fur clothing and constructing shelters such as moss-insulated double tents, semi-subterranean houses, and the superbly simple but ingenious igloo. Physical adaptation to cold remained, perhaps for this reason and due to the, in evolutionary terms, very short period of northern habitation in man, much more limited than in any other circumpolar mammal.

We could not find any examples of effective adaptation of the respiratory system to inhalation of extremely cold and dry arctic air in northern Natives. Clinical and epidemiological observations as well as systematic examinations of respiratory function, chest films, and electrocardiograms, demonstrated impairment of respiratory function, most marked in middle-aged men with a history of extensive midwinter hunting (5). Such exertion often forces open-mouthed panting, thus circumventing protective warming and moistening of inhaled air in the nasopharynx. The insidious progression of the resulting obstructive lung disease in most cases did not seriously incapacitate hunters until middle-age, when a son or son-in-law could take over as main food provider for the extended family, nor did death after age 55 impede group survival chances. Thus no selection stimulus existed for adaptation of the respiratory tract to extremely cold and dry air.

While cold exposure due to hunting activities and traditional lifestyle has diminished for northern Natives, it has become increasingly important to new permanent or transient migrants coming to northern regions for resource development, trade, administration, defense, or other purposes. A growing segment of persons pursuing strenuous physical exercise during severe winter cold e.g., on drilling rigs, road construction, or outdoor sports, may therefore benefit from research originally derived from our observations on northern Natives.

For the latter, however, present research needs are less concerned with adaptation and limits of adaptation to their hostile climatic environment, and instead more with factors influencing their coping with greater infection pressure, different metabolic demands, and other consequences of a profoundly changed physical, occupational, nutritional and social environment. Socioeconomic problems following the loss of traditional nutrition, self-sufficiency and social order, and newly imported infectious diseases have predominated in recent decades in the complex causality of morbidity and mortality in our northern native societies.

In the early post-contact period most native populations, which had been relatively isolated in the circumpolar regions, were reduced by acute (usually viral) or chronic epidemics (in particular tuberculosis). We attribute the devastating extent, rapid progression, and extremely high mortality of these epidemics to the people's lack of past exposure, disturbed nutrition and crowding, all likely to lower resistance and/or increase new infection pressure. Preliminary investigations at the Montreal Children's Hospital (6), and the Camsell Hospital, Edmonton (7), suggest that in these formerly nomadic northern hunters, the T-cell based immune response to viral and chronic infections may be less brisk than in urban populations, and this may explain the frequent complications seen after viral respiratory infections in northern Indian (8), and Inuit (9), infants. I am also wondering if the prevalence of lymphoepithelial tumors in the head-neck area

(nasopharyngeal and parotid gland "cancers") in Inuit and northern Indians is a parallel to the prevalence of lymphoepitheliomata of the gut in recently settled former nomads in Iran (10). In these formerly nomadic Iranians, now urbanized and living under crowded conditions, the gut is under frequent infectious and parasitic assault. In our northern nomads, B-cell aggregations in the head and neck region are more prone to physical and infectious trauma. The persisting infection problems and apparent low immunological resistance of northern Natives emphasize the need for more investigations into their immune responses and possible means to enhance these.

Almost 20 years ago Edward Scott and his colleagues from the Arctic Health Research Laboratory and the Alaska Native Medical Center found a high incidence of pseudo-cholinesterase deficiency in southwestern Alaskan Eskimos (11). Nancy Simpson found subsequently a number of cases in Canadian Inuit and northern Indians, and drew attention to the fact that approximately half of all cases reported in Canada were found in the small population fraction of northern Natives (12). (I remember off-hand 2 cases of post-anesthetic deaths occurring in northern Natives in the early 1960s in small territorial hospitals, compatible with the diagnosis of respiratory arrest after use of succinylcholine.) Although routine screening attempted by us in collaboration with Dr. Simpson over several years has uncovered only relatively few cases at risk, this may serve as an example that the advent of new conditions, in our case muscle-relaxant drugs, necessitates specific screening procedures to identify and protect persons and population groups at particular risk. Widespread prevalence of myopia in young Indians or Inuit in the face of perfect emmetropia in almost all Canadian Natives of the foregoing generation necessitates a modification of our concept of familial inheritance of myopia.

Isoniazid (INH) has an extremely short half-life in Eskimos (13,14). This became important when intermittent home medication for tuberculosis came into vogue in the 1960s, and led us to increase the frequency of oral medication or make use of an INH matrix preparation (15).

Other inherited deviations from our norms concern the metabolism of carbohydrates, in particular mono- and disaccharides, and these no doubt will increase in importance with the changes in their nutrition. We found a delayed release of insulin after oral glucose loads which improved by giving a protein meal before the glucose load. This pattern and associated intermittent glycosuria was found in half of the tested Eskimos and 25% of tested northern Indians, and it runs in families (16).

Practical applications clearly exist for dietary consultation in northern Natives and likely to a lesser degree also in other peoples. More research in this field appears warranted as diabetes morbidity is increasing to a frightening degree in modern man, most notably in many acculturated American Indian tribes.

Most American Indians become lactase deficient after the age of four and sucrose intolerance was found in approximately 3% of northern Alaskans but almost 10% of Greenland Eskimos (17,18).

Bang and Dyerberg demonstrated a direct relationship between fatty acid patterns found in local food consumed by Greenlanders and fatty acid patterns prevailing in their platelet walls and the resulting hemostatic function (19,20). They explained the low rates of coronary thrombosis in elderly males and increased bleeding tendencies in traditionally living Greenlanders by this nutritionally conditioned shift in clotting factors. The frequency of severe postpartum hemorrhage observed by us until 10 to 20 years ago in sea mammal-eating Inuit may also be related to this (21).

We demonstrated a remarkable change of neoplastic disease patterns in Canadian Inuit (22,23), and T.K. Young found similar patterns in northwestern Ontario Indians (24), reflecting in local and time gradients quite closely the acculturation history of various groups, and we have discussed the possible etiological contribution of a number of environmental as well as hereditary factors for lung, cervical, kidney,* and breast cancer as well as the above mentioned lymphoepitheliomas of the nasopharynx and salivary glands**.

Alcohol abuse has been proven to be involved in a majority of deaths listed as due to violence, accidents, homicide, suicide or poisoning, accounting for almost 40% of all deaths of Indians and Inuit in the territories and provinces for the last 10 to 20 years. Such deaths were 5 times higher for adolescent and young adult Indians and Inuit compared with other Canadians. Suicide rates in young Indian males have reached truly epidemic proportions. When adding the medical consequences of alcohol abuse and excess morbidity and mortality, particularly of children in families of alcoholic parents, the total direct and indirect cost of alcohol is even much larger in modern Native societies.

We reported in 1971 significantly lower metabolic rates of alcohol after intravenous administration for northern Indians and Inuit compared with Caucasian controls (25), confirming anecdotal reports from northern medical, social and law enforcement workers that "sobering-up" took longer for Indians and Inuit than for Whites following arrest for drunken behavior. Sociocultural and psychological identity problems contribute, in my opinion, more than biochemical metabolic factors, however, to the immensity of the alcohol problem in transition Native societies (26). There is no easy solution to this very complex problem. Frequent public statements that the financial hardship of the recent recession contributed to, and exacerbated, alcohol and drug addiction problems are contradicted by the worldwide historical experience in earlier periods and specifically in the North. The oil boom and financial bonanza of land claim settlements in the 1960s and 1970s in Alaska were associated with a five-fold increase of suicidal death, most related to alcohol abuse, and a ten-fold increase of deaths directly attributed to alcohol in Alaska Natives between 1960 and 1974 as reported by Robert Kraus, et al. in Yellowknife, 1974, and subsequently (27,28).

Medical research cannot deal with the sociocultural root causes of alcohol abuse in northern Native populations, but it can define medical consequences and point to special risk groups on whom we should concentrate our surveillance and efforts for medical and educational intervention. We found, for examples, that Indian females of childbearing age run an extraordinarily high risk of suffering and dying early from alcoholic cirrhosis of the liver, much higher than Indian men from the same area who had a much higher hospitalization rate for alcohol-related accidents and violence (29). This may be explained by relatively early beginning of heavy drinking in Indians, poor eating habits (particularly during drinking binges) and the high rates of pregnancies in drinking Indian teenagers and young women, as well as the particular vulnerability of the liver to toxic and infectious insults during pregnancy and periods of high or fluctuating sex hormone levels.

---

* T.K. Young found an even higher proportion of renal cancers in northwestern Ontario Indians, living mainly on fish and game, i.e., also a high protein diet with highly acidic urine.

** A.P. Lanier in Alaska and N.H. Nielsen and J.P.Hart Hansen in Greenland pursue NPC and salivary cancers for epidemiological and histological clues. H. Stich of British Columbia Environmental Cancer Research is searching for dietary factors in the Canadian Arctic suspected to be related to esophageal salivary and other typical Eskimo tumors.

The need to concentrate our preventive efforts on the young Native females has been confirmed and given particular urgency by the large proportion of alcohol-damaged Indian infants reported in recent years. The rate of hospitalization for congenital conditions rose for Indian infants born in the N.W.T. during the last decade to more than twice the rate for other ethnic groups (30), many of these likely related to the fetal alcohol syndrome.

Degenerative cardiovascular diseases have been for many decades at the center of intensive research by clinicians, pathologists, and epidemiologists. They are the leading cause of death in Western societies and are becoming increasingly important also for northern Natives. Despite tremendous research efforts, medical opinion as to the relative importance of various nutritional and lifestyle factors is today still almost as divided as it was a century ago, when Virchow, Rokitansky, and others launched their theories. I believe here again clear geographical and time gradients demonstrated in western and central Arctic population groups, reflecting their stepwise acquaintance with certain civilization factors (31,32,33), allow us better differentiation of the impact of suspected pathogenic factors than is possible in longer-urbanized populations. To some degree this also applies to the worldwide phenomenon of secular growth acceleration, generally ascribed to better, and in particular more protein, nutrition, but observed over the last generation most markedly in those Inuit groups changing their diet from a high protein to high sugar and carbohydrate content but still sufficient in protein (31,34).

Observations in Canadian Inuit provided the first clear evidence linking bottle feeding to otitis media, a common problem of transitional societies in the entire world (35). We also were able to demonstrate that shortening of traditionally prolonged lactation clearly was associated with shortening of birth intervals in Inuit. I believe that the decline of lactation was primarily responsible for the population explosions first in Europe during the Industrial Revolution and then during the last half century in the Third World.

DISCUSSION

Most of the examples shown are quite parochial, influenced mainly by my own interests, and I must apologize for omitting much important work by other Canadian, American, Russian, and Scandinavian researchers. Discussion of benefits and critical remarks concerning those difficulties and limitations are, however, easier when based on personal experiences.

I should, however, stress 2 areas of increasing importance and potentially great medical concern which may need top priority in future environmental and medical research planning for circumpolar regions, namely:

(a) Pollution of air, water, and land from industrial, traffic and military sources;

(b) Fallout of radionuclear substances accumulating in traditional Native food chains.

Local sources of pollution may come from mining and milling but a greater general load in particular of airborne pollution is based on aerial drift from heavy industries and power plants in Europe and North America, as demonstrated in a map of aerosol sulfate concentrations published by Rahn and McCaffey and quoted by Arne Semb (36). While reported concentrations of various air pollution indices appear to be still fairly insignificant for human health in most arctic regions, we should be aware that low precipitation, temperature inversions and ice fog in cold periods tend to delay natural "scrubbing" of air pollutants and their dissipation from local industrial and urban centers during winter.

Lichens and mosses in the arctic tundra avidly absorb, accumulate and store for years toxic or radioactive fallout products, which may find their way in mounting concentrations toward the top of the food chain: man via reindeer and caribou. A good example, and warning for the future, was the finding of quite significant levels of strontium-90 and cesium-137 in reindeer herders in Scandinavia and caribou hunters in the American Arctic in the mid-1960s following multiple atmospheric atomic test series of the late 1950s and early 1960s.

I should add here also a note of concern. We have experienced in several Inuit settlements an increasing research fatigue and we had to establish some precautionary rules to avoid duplications of research, and in particular too frequent blood sample collections and to guarantee observation of not only strict but sensible ethics preceding and following research projects, which include proper explanations· in locally understandable terms of purpose, benefits and dangers or inconvenience of procedures and thereafter practical conclusions for (a) individuals, and (b) the community. Only thus can we hope to maintain or regain the collaboration of these originally very friendly and extremely cooperative people for the sake of their own benefit as well as that of medical knowledge in general.

SUMMARY

Overwhelming acute and chronic infectious epidemics, reducing northern Native populations during the post-contact periods, have been effectively controlled in the course of the last generation. Further research is, however, required of factors influencing resistance to infection and oncogenesis, in particular with regard to cellular-based immunity.

Benefits from research in formerly isolated populations derive for all of us from investigation of specific epidemiological peculiarities found in Northern populations and changes in such patterns consequent to nutritional and lifestyle changes. They may provide important clues to pathogenic factors, for example, with regard to certain cancer forms and degenerative cardiovascular diseases. Small population samples impose, on the other hand, serious statistical limitations on research. These and the logistical difficulties and financial costs of travel to, and collection of samples from remote places with poor communications have to be carefully weighed against above described benefits.

Some precautionary rules became necessary to avoid duplications of research and, in particular, to lessen the frequency of blood sample collections, and to provide individuals and settlement councils with fully understood explanations before and after the examinations. Medical research not hinging on specific local arctic factors is discouraged for certain arctic settlements showing signs of research fatigue.

Pollution of the particularly sensitive arctic air, water and soil from local and global (by aerosol drift) sources is increasing and the need for monitoring of environmental indices and effects on human health must be stressed.

REFERENCES

1. Burton AC, Edholm OG. Man in a cold environment. London: Edward Arnold Publishers Ltd., 1955.
2. Hildes JA, Irving L, Hart JS. Estimation of heat flow from hands of Eskimos by calorimetry. J Appl Physiol 1961; 16:617-623.
3. LeBlanc J. Personal communication and LeBlanc J, Côté J, Jobin M, Labrie A. Plasma catecholamines and cardiovascular responses to cold and mental activity. J Appl Physiol 1979; 47(6): 1207-1211.
4. Schaefer O, Hildes JA, Greidanus P, Leung D: Regional sweating in Eskimos compared to Caucasians. Can J Physiol & Pharmacol 1974; 52:960-965.
5. Schaefer O, Eaton RDP, Timmermans FJW, Hildes JA. Respiratory function impairment and cardiopulmonary consequences in long time residents of the Canadian Arctic. Can Med Assoc J 1980; 123:997-1004.
6. Reece ER, Brotton TS. In vitro studies of cell-mediated immunity in Inuit children. In: Harvald B, Hart Hansen JP, eds. Circumpolar Health 81. Nordic Council for Arct Med Res Rep 1982; 33.
7. Godel JC, Pabst HF. Personal communication.
8. Houston CS, Weiler RL, Harrick BF. Severity of lung disease in Indian children. Can Med Assoc J 1979; 120:1116-1118.
9. Herbert FA, Mahon WA, Wilkinson D, et al. Pneumonia in Indian and Eskimo infants and children I: A clinical study. Can Med Assoc J 1967; 96:257.
10. Dutz W. Personal communication and Dutz W. In: Stacher A, Hocker P, eds. Gastrointestinale Lymphome-- Typen, Verbreitung und mögliche Pathogenese in Lymphknotentumoren. München-Wien: Urban & Schwarzenberg, 1979.
11. Gutsche BB, Scott EM, Wright RC. Hereditary deficiency of pseudocholinesterase in Eskimos. Nature 1976; 215:322-323.
12. Simpson NE. The load of genetic disease and genetic predisposition to disease in the Canadian North. In: Harvald B, Hart Hansen JP, eds. Circumpolar Health 81. Nordic Council for Arct Med Res, 1982; 33.
13. Scott EM, Wright RC, Weaver DD. The discrimination of phenotypes for rate of disappearance of isomicotinoyl hydrazide from serum. J Clin Invest 1969; 48:1173.
14. Jeanes CWL, Schaefer O, Eidus L. Inactivation of isoniazid by Canadian Eskimos and Indians. Can Med Assoc J 1972; 106:331-335.
15. Jeanes CWL, Schaefer O, Eidus L. Comparative blood levels and metabolism of INH and an INH-matrix preparation in fast and slow inactivators. Can Med Assoc J 1973; 109:483-487.
16. Schaefer O, Crockford PM, Romanowski B. Normalization effect of preceding protein meals on "diabetic" oral glucose tolerance in Eskimos. Can Med Assoc J 1972; 107:733-738.
17. Bell RR, Draper HH, Bergan JG. Sucrose, lactose and glucose tolerance in northern Alaskan Eskimos. Am J Clin Nutr 1973; 26:1185-1190.
18. McNair A, Gudmand-Hoyer, Jarnum S, Orrild L. Sucrose malabsorption in Greenland. Brit Med J 1972; 2:19-21.
19. Bang HO, Dyerberg J, Hjørne N. The composition of food consumed by Greenland Eskimos. Acta Med Scand 1976; 200:69-73.
20. Dyerberg J, Bang HO. Hemostatic function and platelet polyunsaturated fatty acids in Eskimos. Lancet 1979; 2:433-435.

21. Schaefer O. Knud Rasmussen Memorial Lecture: Ethnology, demography and medicine in the Arctic. In: Harvald B, Hart Hansen JP, eds. Circumpolar Health 81. Nordic Council for Arct Med Res Rep 1982; 33.
22. Schaefer O, Hildes JA, Medd LM, Cameron DG. The changing pattern of neoplastic disease in Canadian Eskimos. Can Med Assoc J 1975; 112:1399-1404.
23. Hildes JA, Schaefer O. The changing picture of neoplastic disease in the western and central Arctic 1950-80. Can Med Assoc J 1984; 130:25-32.
24. Young TK, Frank JW. Cancer surveillance in a remote Indian population in northwestern Ontario. Am J Publ Health 1983; 73:515-520.
25. Fenna D, Mix L, Schaefer O, Gilbert JAL. Ethanol metabolism in various racial groups. Can Med Assoc J 1971; 105:472-475.
26. Schaefer O. Socio-cultural change and health in Canadian Inuit. In: Tremblay M-A, ed. The Patterns of Amerindian identity. Québec: Presses de l'Université Laval, 1976: 229-293.
27. Kraus RF, Buffler P. Suicide in Alaskan Natives; a preliminary report (abstract). Paper presented at the Third International Symposium on Circumpolar Health, Yellowknife NWT, July 1974.
28. Kraus RF, Buffler P. Intercultural variation in mortality due to violence. Paper read at Annual Meeting of Am Psychiatr Assoc, Miami, May 1976.
29. Romanowski E, Schaefer O. Alcoholic liver cirrhosis in Indian and non-Indian patients of Charles Camsell Hospital, 1950-80. Chron Dis in Canada 1981; 2:17-18.
30. Schaefer O, Spady DW. Changing trends in infant feeding patterns in the Northwest Territories 1973-1979. Can J Publ Health 1982; 73:304-309.
31. Schaefer O, Timmermans JFW, Eaton RDP, Matthews AR. General and nutritional health in two Eskimo populations at different stages of acculturation. Can J Publ Health 1980; 71:397-405.
32. Schaefer O. The relative roles of diet and physical activity on blood lipids and obesity. Am Heart J 1974; 88:673.
33. Schaefer O. Diet, physical activity, blood lipids and incidence of cardiovascular abnormalities in elderly male Eskimos of the Canadian eastern Arctic. Paper presented at the VIIIth International Congress on Nutrition, Prague, 1969.
34. Schaefer O. Pre- and post-natal growth acceleration and increased sugar consumption in Canadian Eskimos. Can Med Assoc J 1970; 103:1059-1068.
35. Schaefer O. Otitis media and bottle-feeding: An epidemiological study of infant feeding habits and incidence of recurrent and chronic middle ear disease in Canadian Eskimos. Can J Publ Health. 1971; 62:478-489.
36. Semb A. Air pollutants in the Arctic. Nordic Council Arct Med Res Rep 1983; 35:7-14.

Otto Schaefer
Northern Medical Research Unit
Health and Welfare Canada
c/o Charles Camsell Hospital
12815-115 Ave.
Edmonton, Alberta T5M 3A4
Canada

WHAT DO WE EXPECT FROM FRONT-LINE HEALTH SERVICES FOR ADVERSELY SITUATED POPULATIONS?

SIXTEN S.R. HARALDSON

INTRODUCTION

In the WHO program "Health for All by the Year 2000," rural health services are given highest priority. This emphasis applies to poor as well as to rich nations, to tropical as well as to arctic regions, and in particular to thinly populated areas--many of them inhabited by nomadic peoples--and presently rather neglected regarding health services. There is, however, an obvious difference in one important respect between tropical and arctic regions of low population density, in that the latter are in a position to be supported by relatively wealthy nations which are capable of providing services to all their provinces. Otherwise there are evident similarities between scattered population groups all over the world, and a fruitful exchange of ideas and experiences should therefore not be limited by geography or climate, but may be discussed in a global context.

WHO ACTIVITIES

In its ambitious program "Health for All by the Year 2000," WHO at an early stage identified certain population groups which would be likely to provide health planners with particular difficulties. Apart from rural areas in general and everywhere, these population groups are two.

The first group is in the uncontrollable and rapidly mushrooming slums around the great cities of the world, such as Calcutta, Mexico City, Hong Kong, and Lagos to mention just a few.

The second group is the 50 to 100 million nomads of the world, who tend to inhabit inhospitable areas with great distances separating small tribal groups. Nomadism by itself is not necessarily the main problem. The health planner must bear in mind not only the factor of distances, but also the nature of traditional cultures in each case. Thus it seems more appropriate to speak of "adversely situated population groups", as constituting both the challenge and the denominator. Such groups everywhere demand both exceptional and unorthodox solutions for health care, solutions which will involve unusually high per capita costs both in capital and recurrent expenditures. These factors explain why scattered population groups are frequently neglected, especially in poor developing countries in the tropics, and most of all in the 25 to 30 Least Developed Nations of the world where resources are minimal and conditions often hard to understand for development expert advisers. Naturally one must take into account national and local health priorities, and also the extent to which nationals can be involved in the creation and operation of health services.

The Least Developed Nations constitute economically the lower strata of the poor world, those which are caught in the vicious circle of slow economic and technical development, where poor health and deficient health services are both a cause and a consequence of the situation. Even if their limited resources are used to the best effect, one can only expect urban dwellers to be provided with tolerable health services. Exceptions to this general rule indicate, however, that other factors are involved, for in spite of a handicapped economy, certain countries such as China, Tunisia, Sri Lanka and Jordan have developed health care systems with reasonable coverage even for marginal rural and pastoral populations. In its definition of health, WHO has stressed that there are 3 aspects to well-being: the physical, the mental, and the social. It is an unfortunate fact that Western health services have been preoccupied with physical health and well-being, each system and organ of the body being examined and treated in turn. But when one comes to consider social, mental, and particularly spiritual or psychological well-being, one has to admit that the industrialized world is in this respect under-developed and has little to contribute in this sphere to those parts of the world in need of advice in the development of their health services.

Such areas, perhaps even more than the Western world, require a philosophy of medicine which is concerned with "the total man in his total environment," that is to say, with the whole man in his physical, social, mental, and psychological or spiritual dimensions. In such situations there is a natural place for multidisciplinary measures, that is situations where medical problems may require non-medical solutions.

Health Services

There exists a somewhat sophisticated definition of health services as follows: "a permanent country-wide system of established institutions, the purpose of which is to cope with the various health needs and demands of the population, and thereby provide health care to individuals and the community, including a broad spectrum of preventive and curative activities, such as environmental sanitation, immunization procedures, and mother and child welfare; and in addition, as its foremost objectives, health education in nutrition and family planning." In such a situation curative activities are limited to the treatment of common and well-known diseases, with the selection of others for transportation to a central health service unit.

A former WHO declaration proclaimed that health is a fundamental right of all human beings, irrespective of race, religion, and socio-economic conditions; this proposition gave birth to the ideal of "Health for All by the Year 2000." But a careful look at the rural areas in most developing countries reveals the need for a radical re-evaluation of health service priorities. Poor countries have not only a marked shortage of trained personnel, but also an appalling imbalance in the distribution of services between town and country. In addition, there is often a disproportionately large number of highly qualified doctors who carry out advanced and expensive techniques, when the demand for elementary and large scale curative procedures is far from supplied.

Accessibility Rate

It goes without saying that the most important aspect of a service unit is that it should actually exist, and that it be reachable by the people it is intended to serve. The accessibility rate depends on the careful siting of the dispensary in relation to the area to be covered. It depends also on the presence or absence of all-weather roads for bicycles and motor vehicles. In Africa, in the absence of motor cars, it has been estimated that 15 kilometers is the maximum distance for ambulatory patients, or for carrying the sick. In impoverished areas, mules, camels, or bicycles provide the chief means of transport. In more developed areas, 4-wheel drive vehicles and buses are available, while in arctic regions increasing use is made of air transport where the additional convenience and comfort justifies the expense.

Acceptability Rate

This term is perhaps a better and more realistic indication of the degree to which a dispensary for example is actually used. Although accessible, a service unit may for various reasons not be accepted and trusted by the local people. Perhaps the staff may not provide the expected standard of services, or patients may bypass the local unit and seek treatment at a better equipped health center or hospital.

Difficulties may arise if the local unit is staffed by members of other tribes or natives of distant provinces. They may well be regarded as foreigners, if they are not fluent in local language or fail to understand and appreciate the local culture and traditional life. Frequently such staff do not stay long enough to become integrated into the local society. Their behavior and way of life may be considered alien to the local people, and their influence may even prove to be detrimental to their culture. Moreover, villagers may prefer their own traditional healers and their time-honored native medicine. Traditional medicine may in fact compete favorably with the mediocre services offered at rural dispensaries in some areas. In other areas, however, Western medicine is appreciated by the local people as a valuable complement to their own folk medicine, while in certain countries, the 2 systems may be practiced harmoniously side by side, and even by the same staff in the one institution. Examples are China, India, and Sri Lanka.

The Utilization Rate

The utilization of a given service facility naturally depends on its accessibility and its acceptability to the local people, who may well prefer traditional medicine, which in fact is estimated to cover as much as two-thirds of all health services in the developing countries of the world. Studies in Tunisia have also proved the effect of primary education, increasing the use of services provided by authorities, particularly in the case of immunization procedures. The educational level of mothers is of special importance in this respect. In other words, people need some basic education in order to stimulate their interest in the creation, operation and utilization of health services. This means that primary education ought to be given a high priority when the development of national, and especially rural health services, is being considered. This is a good example of the principle of "non-medical methods for the solution of medical problems." Education is also profoundly important in providing for the staffing of local health service units as school leavers become available for training as auxiliary health workers. In addition, secondary education opens up the way for the ultimate training of nurses and doctors.

Design of Front-Line Health Services

In developing countries, and particularly in the case of scattered populations with nomadic peoples, services must be adapted to these totally different and extreme local conditions. Health planners must adopt an unorthodox approach. Communication and transportation mostly dominate planning in such outlying regions, and the actual cost of the unusually high per capita figures must be assessed and accepted. Non-medical solutions may also be more urgent and also be a more profitable use of scarce financial resources than curative services, as for instance the provision of hygienic latrines or piped water supply, though the local people may prefer additional curative facilities.

A rigid copying of Western-style medicine will in all probability waste scarce financial resources and provide little lasting improvement. Curative, preventive, and environmental facilities are needed everywhere, of course. Consequently, the relative financial priority given to each is an important and responsible task for the planners. There is also often considerable pressure by senior officials as well as from the general public for better curative services, influenced as they are by impressions gained from the Western world. But a realistic pattern of peripheral rural health services must consist of a large number of small village dispensaries staffed by locally recruited auxiliaries. These will form the basis of the national health service network, constituting a peripheral chain of front-line service units. Naturally, nomadic people cannot receive full and permanent coverage, but from time to time during their migrations, they will be able to utilize the dispensaries of remote settled rural populations. Mobile immunization units, for example, play only a minor role in health services for scattered populations.

Evaluation

The effectiveness of health service units can be estimated from attendance rates, if figures are available. But more difficult to discover are long-term health benefits, such as increased life expectancy, and reduced infant and child mortality. Physical health is also easier to estimate than social, mental, and spiritual well-being, the latter factors being at least equally important in contributing to the quality of life, which itself is probably more important than increased life expectancy. Many attempts have been made to define quality of life. One suggestion is the "physical quality of life index" (PQLI) which is expressed by the sum of indices: one for infant mortality, one for life expectancy, and one for the rate of adult literacy. Each component can vary from zero, for example, for the country with the highest rate of infant mortality, to 100 for the lowest known rate. Thus, the PQLI can be compared between different countries. It needs to be stressed that per capita income as calculated from GNP statistics often provides misleading information on actual living standards, particularly in communities depending largely on a self-sufficient household economy, as is the case in most of the sparsely populated areas of the world.

Prolonged life expectancy and a reduction in the mortality rate are lasting consequences of genuine development everywhere, and infant mortality rates in particular have proved to be an accurate and sensitive indicator of socioeconomic progress, in which health service improvements are one result. Other indications of progress are, for example, an increase in the rate of institutional deliveries and realization of systematic immunization programs. Yet, the assessment of the actual quality of life and happiness of the community is a good deal more elusive, if not quite impossible although in fact these are real goals in all development. Generally, it needs to be stressed constantly that the existence of hospitals and the promotion of treatment for the sick really contribute very little to the standard of health in the community, that is, to the national health. Far more important is a rise in general socioeconomic condition which is associated with improved education, housing and nutrition, as well as personal and environmental hygiene. Health is a welcome side effect in a gradual general development. Consequently, there is an inevitable time factor which is measured in decades or even centuries rather than in years. What many rich countries of today have achieved in 150 years cannot be reached in a few years time in today's poor countries of the world.

The Profitability Rate

The profitability or cost-efficiency of any particular service may refer to the average cost of individual treatments, or may indicate the annual average cost per capita of the population aimed at being covered. It is axiomatic that everywhere resources for any kind of social service are in fact limited. For example, in Ethiopia the health budget calculated on a per capita basis is about 2,000 times lower than in industrialized countries. In densely populated or urban areas, the per capita cost for primary health care is low, but in thinly populated areas the comparable cost is bound to be high, for the daily turnover of patients is often 40 to 50 times less than in urban areas. The immunization of nomads (1) costs 11 times more than the immunization of a comparable number of sedentary or urbanized people.

The time-honored slogan "help for self-help" is certainly worth revival and could be practicable even in impoverished areas. Local people should be involved in the early planning stages and later, in the running of their own dispensary. That is the significance of a more recent slogan, "health by the people." A spirit of self-reliance and self-determination stimulates local interest in the standard and utilization of services. At the same time, economic problems may be shared and easily solved, and mistakes avoided.

A recent and welcome initiative by WHO to clear the appalling jungle of innumerable drugs available or in use has been the preparation of a list of some 200 to 300 essential drugs. For most rural dispensaries, a reduced list with 20 to 30 drugs is adequate for most local needs. Substantial public and private money may be saved this way, and probably also in the health field. For comparison, India and the USA have each marketed approximately 20,000 drugs, while Sweden has only 2,400.

Another comparable and worldwide "disease of health services" is the widespread tendency to seek treatment at an unnecessarily high level in the health service pyramid by avoiding the local dispensary and perhaps the nearest health center, and instead attending a well-equipped hospital for the treatment of minor illness, which could have been treated satisfactorily and cheaply at the village dispensary. This is an uneconomic procedure, as has been demonstrated in New Guinea where the cost of treatment for a case of ordinary pneumonia at a health center is 10 times greater than it is at the village dispensary, and 50 times higher at the regional hospital. This widespread abuse of financial resources, though less noticeable in rich countries, is everywhere a subject for discussion. For example in Sweden, about 30% of patients attending at hospital outpatient departments could be adequately treated at peripheral units by less qualified personnel and at considerably lower cost. This situation can be epitomized by the suggestion, "treatment at the lowest effective care-taking level."

Problems and Bottlenecks

The lack of reliable statistics in many developing countries is a profound handicap in health planning. This deficiency is partly due to inadequate and imperfectly trained staff, but also to insufficient and irregular reporting; hence the lack of factual knowledge on which to base planning. A recent trend in primary health care recommends concentrating efforts on controlling a few of the most important local diseases. This seems to be a very profitable method, but naturally reduces the resources available for the rest of the health service particularly on the curative side, and this situation may easily be misunderstood by the local people.

An atmosphere of mutual cooperation seems to be a fundamental requirement particularly in rural areas. This involves staffing peripheral units with locally recruited young men and women, who have completed primary school and been trained as health workers. Five to 6 years of primary schooling, followed by 6 to 12 months of medical training, can produce health auxiliaries for dispensaries and health centers. This category of native staff constitutes an important link between villagers and professional medicine. They can interpret to the local people totally new ideas and concepts such as family planning, nutrition, environmental hygiene, and other health education topics.

Medical training of 2 to 3 years after primary schooling produces the medical assistant category qualified for more responsible work. In the case of both these categories, the selected students need to be acceptable to their own people, and better still, selected by them. They must also be motivated for their work. If these prerequisites are fulfilled, such staff are likely to continue working among their own people indefinitely.

From the foregoing discussion, primary schooling is obviously a *sine qua non* in the development of health services, particularly in remote rural regions. Furthermore, to ensure a sound and economic utilization of services, a high average literacy rate among mothers and girls is essential. In the almost absent rural development in sub-Saharan Africa, lack of primary education, no doubt, is a dominating factor.

The "barefoot doctor" idea, put into practice in New Guinea as "aid post orderlies" before it was "invented" in China, is sound and adequate. The idea has been tried in many poor countries, though not always with success in regions where primary education is undeveloped, illiteracy rate high, and consequently the local people have been unable to provide suitable students for training.

Close supervision of rural auxiliary health workers by visiting nurses and doctors is an essential factor in the success of the whole scheme. The auxiliary staff have the opportunity for discussing cases regularly, while such visits enhance the villagers' confidence in their local staff and at the same time add to the prestige of the staff. In the eyes of their patients, they are identified with "their master's voice." Reliable radio or telecommunication has the same effect and seems to be an inexpensive way to raise the standard of services, as do efficient transport facilities (2). Daily radio or telecommunication with supervising staff at central health units, although the simplest and cheapest method for improving services in distant places, is unfortunately seldom utilized. Finally, frequent refresher courses for village health aides are necessary for maintaining high standards.

The above-mentioned requirements are largely neglected in many poor countries,and consequently available front-line health services often gradually degenerate to such a low standard that they can hardly compete with local traditional healers. This state of affairs is due not only to limited financial resources, but rather to lack of primary education facilities, and to a general neglect and lack of interest among responsible authorities and among supervising staff.

It is worthwhile to compare the primary health care of scattered tropical populations with those in the Arctic. Successful methods may be adopted and adapted from one to the other. In the case of the Eskimos, the fact that relatively wealthy nations support their health services, ensures that experimentation with new ideas is practicable, and this may result in an adequate coverage of high standard, such as in Alaska (3). Certain aspects of successful arctic health services do not depend so much on abundant financial resources, and may therefore very well be adopted by rural regions in poor countries. The most expensive item in the arctic services is usually air transport. But even in poor countries much could be achieved cheaply with mules as the main means of transport. Concepts developed in the Alaskan village health system, such as using some 200 Eskimo girls as health aides, should be considered for adoption in thinly populated regions in the Tropics in order to establish a reasonable standard of front-line primary health care services.

In contrast to many tropical countries, the development of village health services, such as in Alaska, has not contributed greatly to disturbances of traditional patterns or to acculturation. The retention of traditional culture surely contributes to a natural self-confidence and with it an unusual willingness to cooperate with "foreigners."

To summarize: The rather spectacular success of well-organized health service in thinly populated regions, such as in Eskimo settlements of rural Alaska, is mainly due to the following factors:
-- a generous cooperation of the village people
-- well-utilized primary schools, resulting in almost total literacy
-- a rather generous budget, permitting, for example, frequent air transport
-- and finally, the employment of non-Native professionals from the "lower 48," who are interested in planning, organization and development of a village health aide system with high quality and full coverage.

These "foreigners" are well motivated, have a sympathetic understanding of, and approach to the local Native culture and tend to give long service, resulting in low turnover rates of qualified personnel.

REFERENCES

1. Imperato PJ et al. Mass campaigns and their comparative costs for nomadic and sedentary populations in Mali. Trop Geog Med 1973; 25:416-422.

2. Kreimer O. Health care and satellite radio communication. Alaska Institute for Communication Research, Stanford University and The Lister Hill National Center for Biomedical Communication, USA. 1974

3. Haraldson SSR. Evaluation of Alaska Native Health Service (WHO assignment). Alaska Med 1974; 16:51-60.

Sixten S.R. Haraldson
P.O. Box 5
432 03 Träslövsläge
Sweden

Circumpolar Health 84:22-31

WHEN BEING SMALL IS YOUR STRENGTH: A SURVEY OF ICELAND AS A FORUM FOR POPULATION STUDIES

GUDRUN PÉTURSDÓTTIR

INTRODUCTION

Small communities generally have difficulties in supporting research activities of any dimension, and the chances of making significant contributions as a scientist often seem proportional to the size of one's community. Sometimes, however, smallness can in itself be an advantage, and examples of that are found in the fields of genetics, anthropology, and demography.

I shall outline the possibilities that exist for population research in Iceland-- possibilities which in my opinion are unique, due to the fact that the nation is small and unusually homogeneous genetically and enjoys a high standard of health care. Moreover, a great deal of information is available on the people of Iceland from the time the country was settled 1,100 years ago to the present. I shall mention the main sources of demographic information on the Icelanders, and the main projects that are currently in progress in genetics, anthropology and epidemiology.

Iceland is a volcanic island in the North Atlantic Ocean, bordering on the Arctic Circle, some 300 km south of the east coast of Greenland and 800 km north of Scotland. It is a sparsely populated country with close to 240,000 inhabitants, two-thirds of whom live in the capital city, Reykjavik, and the surrounding area on the southwestern corner of the island. This leaves the rest of the country with less than one inhabitant per square kilometer.

DISCOVERY AND SETTLEMENT OF ICELAND

The permanent settlement of Iceland took place around the year A.D. 900, but the time of its actual discovery is not known. In old Greek and Roman literature the northernmost island in the world was called Ultima Thule. The meaning of the word Thule is unknown and it is debated which country is being referred to, but many believe that it is Iceland.

There is some evidence indicating that Iceland was known to British seafarers in the 4th century B.C. (1), but the oldest remains found in Iceland are some 700 years more recent than that. These are a few Roman coins, stamped during the years A.D. 270-305. Britain was then under Roman rule, and it has been argued that the coins were in the possession of seafarers who drifted to the island at that time, rather than that they were brought there by a later visitor (2). Fantastic accounts exist of the travels of the Irish monk Saint Brendan in

the 6th century. Tim Severin and his crew showed in 1976, when, inspired by the accounts of Saint Brendan, they sailed in a leather curragh from Ireland to Newfoundland, that the monk may well have come close to Iceland and seen what to the modern eye are volcanic eruptions both on sea and land, while to Saint Brendan and his crew these phenomena were of a distinct satanic and soul-destroying nature (3).

Several sources mention sailings between Ireland and Iceland in the 8th century. Around 825 the Irish monk Dicuil wrote about monks and hermits he had met who 30 years earlier had stayed on an island so far north that around summer solstice the sun disappeared only briefly in the night and a man could do whatever he wished, even pick lice from his shirt, as if the sun were there. Iceland certainly seems a strong candidate in this case. Irish hermits are also described in later Icelandic accounts of the colonization, such as Landnamabok (The Book of Settlements) (4) and Islendingabok (The Book of the Icelanders) (5), which state that the hermits soon left the country, choosing not to associate with the pagan settlers.

According to these books, the first colonists arrived in the late 9th century, and the settlement was completed by 930. Recent archaeological findings in the Westman Islands, off the south coast, indicate that people of Nordic origin were living there at least in the 9th century and perhaps even earlier (6).

Landnamabok names and partly traces the genealogy of 444 settlers, most of whom came from Norway. Many of the settlers were Vikings who plundered neighboring countries, not least the British Isles, and brought captives as slaves with them to Iceland. Meanwhile they were influenced culturally by the local people, with whom they interbred. They were therefore genetically mixed when they came to Iceland.

Several methods have been applied to estimate the Irish and British genetic contribution to the Icelandic population, with varying results (7-16). On the basis of serological studies (7), Thompson concluded that Icelanders are almost entirely of "celtic" origin (15). Palsson has pointed out that a considerable selective genetic differentiation may have occurred in Iceland since the settlement, and that it is preferable to study many, including polyfactorial, traits when estimating ethnogenetic relations. His anthropometric and pigmentation studies of over 10,500 living Icelanders and several thousand Norwegians,

Danes, Irishmen, and Scotsmen reveal that, on the whole, Icelanders bear a closer resemblance to Scandinavian peoples than to the Irish or British (9-13). These findings are in accordance with historical, archaeological, and linguistic evidence. Dr. Arnason, Head of the Department of Genetic Research at the Icelandic Blood Bank, has compared various genetic markers, including HLA, among Icelanders, Norwegians, Irishmen, and Hebrideans. His results show that Icelanders do not consistently resemble any of the other groups. He concludes that inbreeding and other "founder effects" have influenced the present genetic composition of Icelanders, and that therefore no quantitative conclusions about the original distribution of these markers can yet be drawn from the present distribution (17).

GENETIC HOMOGENEITY OF THE NATION

The question of the exact origin of the Icelanders is therefore left unresolved. On the other hand, there is no doubt about the fact that the nation is unusually homogeneous genetically, due to external isolation for 1,100 years and to a continuous and ever-increasing interbreeding between people from different parts of the country.

Soon after the settlement, the Icelanders realized the necessity of ruling the country by common legislation. In the year 930 Iceland was declared an independent state and a parliament founded, which was to be held yearly at Thingvellir, a place considered to be equally accessible from all parts of the country. These gatherings were not only important politically, but also for commerce and personal negotiations of various kinds, including marriages.

Later, men from inland farms moved to the south coast for work in the fishing season. Priests and other functionaries often moved with their families from place to place during their years of service. Finally, natural disasters occasionally caused mass migrations within the country. Thus, people from different parts of the country interbred. In later times, improved means of transportation and a steady migration to the more densely populated areas have greatly increased the genetic homogeneity of the nation.

Migration into and out of the country has been minimal, with the exception of a substantial emigration at the turn of the century, when some 18,000 people (about a fifth of the population) moved to North America. Present immigration and emigration rates are less than 0.2% per year.

Thus, the nation is unusually homogeneous, being small, having interbred and remained in virtual external isolation for 1,100 years. This fact, together with the wealth of information, old and new, available on the Icelanders, supports my opening statement about the opportunities for population research in Iceland.

EARLY DEMOGRAPHIC INFORMATION

Icelanders have from the start been great collectors of personal data. The Book of Settlements and the Book of the Icelanders contain much information on the people who settled in Iceland in the late 9th century. The stage is set in Icelandic sagas by tracing the genealogy of the characters who enter the story. Knowing their origin helps us to understand their reactions as much as knowing their interests and obligations. With the Icelanders, the recounting and recording of genealogies is an abiding national sport that makes available a wealth of information in the form of printed and unprinted family trees reaching many centuries back, some comprising tens of thousands of people.

Demographic information on the past is also available in parish records kept by pastors from the 17th century onwards, and from various censuses. In 1106 the Bishop of Skalholt, Gizur Isleifsson, recorded all farmers liable to taxation. On the basis of this census the population is estimated to have been close to 70,000. No census was taken during the Middle Ages. The first general census dates from 1703 (18). There, individuals are listed by name and address, with information on age, occupation, and often marital status and health. The population was then just over 50,000. Shortly afterwards a terrible volcanic eruption took place, followed by plague and famine, which killed off a third of the population. The next general census was taken in 1801, and from 1835 to 1860 censuses were taken every fifth year, followed by ten-yearly intervals until 1960. The latest general census was taken in 1981 and contains information on education, work and sources of income, marital status and number of children, residence, and a description of the present accommodation and the familial relations of those living there.

Thus, census records exist on most Icelanders from 1703 to the present day. These comprise about 700,000 people over 10 generations. Parish records are still kept by ministers of the church. The oldest continuous records (from the parish of Reykholt in Borgarfjordur) date back to 1664. After 1735 records of births and deaths were, by decree, kept in every parish. Later, the information included marriages and often social position and cause of death. Most of these records have been preserved to the present day and are kept in the National Archives.

RECENT DEMOGRAPHIC AND MEDICAL RECORDS

The collection and publication of demographic information became centralized with the establishment of the Statistical Bureau in 1916. It has collected detailed demographic records dating back to 1911 (19). In 1952 a National Registry was formed and identification numbers for the citizens were introduced. This was a major improvement, because it prevents the confusion of individuals who bear the same name. Every person in the country is recorded by name and number, date of birth, sex, marital status, religion, address, and local residence. The registry also obtains all birth certificates, including still-births, with names and birthdates of both parents; marriage certificates which also name place of birth and consanguinity (the incidence of first-cousin marriages is 0.3%) and death certificates stating cause of death. The registry has been linked with various other records.

In 1965 a special committee was established whose main aims are to carry out studies in population genetics by using the unusual facilities available in Iceland for linking people into families as well as linking together various records on individual persons. So far, the Genetic Committee has computerized the general census from 1910 and traced back to 1840 the ancestors of those alive in 1910. Furthermore, all birth records from 1911 to 1952 (when the National Registry was formed) have been computerized. All these data have been linked to the National Registry or to death records, thus providing a basis for continuous computerized records on the nation from 1840 to the present.

To facilitate the generation of computerized genealogies, which will eventually be developed, all marriage records have been computerized. These have in turn been linked to birth records in some pilot studies (e.g., a study on first-cousin marriages). Records on the family triangle, consisting of a child and its parents, are being constructed for all Icelanders born after 1840 (20-23). The computerized information of the Genetic Committee can be linked to various other records, such as those of the Cancer Registry, as will be mentioned below (24,25).

The Genetic Research Department of the Icelandic Blood Bank has gathered extensive information on genetic markers in Iceland. The blood groups of some 150,000 persons have been determined, frequencies of Gc alleles studied and nearly 4,000 individuals have been HLA typed, for up to 21 markers, most giving haplotype information. About 500 persons have been genotyped (17,26-33). Needless to say, the records of the Genetic Committee and the Genetic Research Depart-

ment are highly confidential and great care is taken to maintain discretion regarding information on individual persons and families (21,22).

The director of the Anthropological Institute of the University, Dr. Palsson, has studied anthropometric characteristics and collected demographic, genealogical, social, and historical information on more than 40,000 Icelanders. The aim of the Institute is to investigate all Icelanders 6 years and older. Variations in several anthropometrical markers have been studied with respect to age, sex, region of residence and degree of urbanization, occupation, and social group. Among other projects are studies on the origin of the Icelanders and their kinship with other European nations; and a comparative study of Icelanders living in Iceland and in North America, of which more later (34-38).

APPLICATIONS TO HEALTH RESEARCH

Some special records have been developed for research purposes. Among them is a file on all psychiatric patients from 1908, which was compiled by collecting information on all those who have been seen by a psychiatrist, either on an outpatient basis or as hospitalized patients (39-44).

Data on achievement in elementary school from 1932 to 1964 have also been computerized. These have been linked with social anthropometric parameters and with mental health records (45-49).

A central register of criminality is available. Research workers have gained access to this with the permission of the State Prosecutor and the Ministry of Justice. Again, great care is taken to maintain confidentiality of the information and the registers are only available to specially authorized individuals for research purposes.

Before turning to the medical records, I should briefly characterize Iceland's health service. We have socialized health care, and most medical treatment is virtually free of charge. In 1980 the number of physicians who worked full-time equalled one per 500 inhabitants, and there were 15 hospital and nursing home beds per thousand inhabitants. Mean life expectancies at birth in Iceland are among the highest in the world: 73 years for men and nearly 80 years for women. They have increased by about 15 years in the last 5 decades.

The main medical records include the Cancer Registry, which has been in operation for 30 years under the auspices of the Icelandic Cancer Society. Its computerized records contain information on all tumors diagnosed in the country since 1954. The records are based on information from 3 sources. Firstly, information on all histologically diagnosed cases, including those found at autopsy, is obtained from the University Department of Pathology. This institute covers the whole country with respect to histopathological diagnoses of human material, since practically all autopsies on humans in Iceland are performed at this laboratory or under its auspices. The centralization of histopathologic diagnoses to one institute ensures consistency in classification and is advantageous for the nationwide registration of cancer. In addition all hospitals report to the Registry on every diagnosed case of cancer and subsequent treatment. Finally, all death certificates are scrutinized by the staff of the Registry. This provides objective records of cancer in the entire population since 1954 (50,51). In addition, a survey has been made of all cases of breast cancer diagnosed in Iceland from 1911 till the founding of the Registry (52).

IMPLICATIONS FOR PREVENTIVE MEDICINE

A large scale follow-up health survey was initiated in 1967 by the Icelandic Heart Association. Its primary aims are to detect cardiovascular and various other diseases in their early stages, to determine their prevalence and incidence, and to study their etiology in search of preventive measures. Originally, only people between 34 and 61 years of age were included, but the survey has now been extended to other age groups. About 45,000 people have been investigated, half of them in Reykjavik.

In addition to data supplied by the National Registry, all individuals surveyed answer some 300 questions concerning their health and social situation. Anthropological measurements, along with a blood film, X-ray, spirometry, tonometry, EKG, clinical chemistry, and various other data are collected. All these data have been computerized from the beginning and are continuously analyzed and published (53).

In the general health service the so-called problem-oriented medical records and computerized information, noting all contacts between the health center and its clients, have been adopted in several places, both in outlying districts and in Reykjavik. Besides improving health care, this will alter the nature of the information available for epidemiological research (54,55).

Although the genetic, anthropological, and demographic information on the Icelanders is obviously of great importance for various purposes, I am personally most concerned with its possible utilization in medical research, where it can help discern the patterns of health and disease and thus improve preventive medicine. I will now briefly mention how such information has been used in this context in Iceland. Space does not allow any detailed descriptions of the studies, but they can be found in the references listed.

The extensive screening of about 45,000 Icelanders by the Icelandic Heart Association mentioned above resulted in the detection of risk factors or symptoms of disease in thousands of apparently healthy individuals, and is of major preventive importance.

The Blood Bank and the Genetic Committee have cooperated with clinicians on studies on the heredity of rheumatic (56-64), hematological (65-73), immunological (74-76), and mental disorders (77-79), as well as of cardiac and cerebrovascular diseases (80-84), endocrine (85-92) and neurological disorders (93-99), enzyme deficiencies (100), and osteopathies (101-103).

In ophthalmology, Sveinsson followed up a unique case of familial helicoidal chorioretinal degeneration (104) and Forsius and Eriksson have, in cooperation with Icelandic ophthalmologists, anthropologists, and genealogists, conducted investigations on ophthalmology and population genetics in Iceland (105). An interdisciplinary study on the families of all recorded first-cousin marriages from 1916 to 1964, 378 in number, has been in progress for some years (78,79).

The completeness of the Icelandic Cancer Registry removes many of the biases that are commonly found in studies on the incidence of cancer, such as undefined or selected populations or unreliable recall. The Icelandic cancer study is based on objective records and covers the entire population. From the register, groups that seem at particular risk of developing cancer can be identified, resulting in guidelines for further research into risk factors, and for intensive screening of the high-risk sector of the population.

The incidence of and mortality from breast cancer has been increasing in Iceland as in other countries (106,107). Icelandic studies confirm what has been found elsewhere, that young age at first delivery decreases the risk of developing breast cancer. They have also found that multiparity, independently, has the same effect. The increase in incidence of breast cancer cannot be explained entirely by these reproductive factors, because although parity is decreasing, the number of childless women and the age at first birth are falling (108).

The familial risk of developing breast cancer is currently being studied by Tulinius and his colleagues in cooperation with the Genetic Committee. Their study, based on 499 families, shows that after adjusting for reproductive factors, women who have a first degree relative with breast cancer run an almost threefold higher risk of developing the disease than women with no cases of breast cancer in the family (110-112). These studies are now being extended to 700 families. To obtain information on hereditary patterns, the incidence of breast cancer is being investigated among the descendants of 30 women born in the 19th century and who are known to have had breast cancer (113).

The Cancer Registry cooperates with a cancer detection clinic that has been in operation for 20 years. Its first project was a mass screening for breast and cervical cancer. Since 1964, 83% of Icelandic women between ages 25 and 69 have been examined at least once. The effect is impressive. In the years 1967 to 1978 mortality from cervical cancer remained between 20 and 30 per 100,000 in the group of women who had never been screened, whereas the rates in the screened group were between 2 and 5 per 100,000. Early detection and improved treatment presumably explain the fact that since this clinic began operation, the number of patients who survive for at least 5 years after the diagnosis of cervical cancer has more than doubled (from 33% to 69%) (114-120).

Finally, I would like to mention a study that I have taken part in myself. This is a comparative study of Icelanders and the descendents of Icelanders who emigrated to Canada at the turn of this century. Between 1870 and 1914 approximately 18,000 Icelanders emigrated to Canada and the USA. Many of these people, chiefly those from northern and eastern Iceland, settled in the area north of Winnipeg that is often referred to as the Interlake District, including "New Iceland." A record has been compiled of all the people who emigrated, stating their age and occupation, where they came from, when and where they left Iceland, and their destination (121). Most of the Icelandic inhabitants of the Interlake District today are descendents of the original settlers, and consequently, the possibility exists of linking them genealogically with relatives in Iceland. There has been marriage between the Icelandic and non-Icelandic residents of the district, of course, but our investigation will only comprise those that are solely of Icelandic descent.

Obviously, the situation described provides a unique opportunity for anthropological and epidemiological research, and for assessing the relative importance of genetic and environmental factors in chronic disease. In order to utilize these possibilities, the University's Department of Physiology in Iceland has joined forces with the Anthropological Institute and the Icelandic Heart Association, as well as with scientists in Manitoba and Dr. Anthony B.

Way of Texas Tech University. At present, the main emphasis is put on cardiovascular risk factors. The first phase of the study began in 1975, when Dr. Palsson conducted demographic, genealogical, and anthropological research on people of pure Icelandic descent living in Canada. He has investigated about 700 adults and 300 school children (37). The second phase was an interdisciplinary study on the inhabitants of a region in eastern Iceland, whence a great many of the emigrants stemmed. The results already obtained have been reported in numerous publications, some at this and previous symposia on circumpolar health (37,38,122-137).

Great opportunities for further research lie in the possible linkage of the various computerized registers that I have described; and I think that they warrant the conclusion that the Icelandic population provides unique opportunities for population research and that we have the possibility of contributing significantly to preventive medicine. But it is not enough to collect information and connect information; the point is to put it to use. We must make efforts to bridge the gap between the epidemiologists and the clinicians, so that our knowledge may be applied to the benefit of the people from whom we have gathered the information. Anything else is exploitation and alienation from what must be the main aim of those who work in preventive medicine.

*REFERENCES**

1. Bárdarson HR. Iceland, a portrait of its land and people. Reykjavik 1968.
2. Eldjarn K. Gengid á reka, tólf fornliefathaettir. Reykjavik 1948.
3. Severin T. The Brendan voyage. London 1978.
4. Benediktsson J, ed. Landnámabók. Reykjavik 1968.
5. Ari fródi Thorgilsson. In: Benediktsson J, ed. Íslendingabók. Íslensk fornrit I. Reykjavik 1968.
6. Hermannsdóttir M. Fornleifarannsóknir í Herjólfsdal-Vestmannaeyjum 1971-1981

*(Editors' Note: To assist those who may use this literature survey in bibliographic research, we have made an extra effort to be faithful to the orthography of original languages for authors' names, and titles of articles and journals. Unavoidably, however, the following transliterations from Icelandic were neccessary:

þ   þ   become Th and th;
ð   becomes d;
Æ   æ   become Ae and ae.)

(Excavations in Herjolfsdal-Vestman-naeyjum 1971-1981). Eyjaskinna 1982; 1:83-127.

7. Bjarnason O, Bjarnason V, Edwards JH, Fridriksson S, Magnússon M, Mourand AE, Tills D. The blood groups of Icelanders. Ann Hum Genet 1973; 36:425-458.

8. Brekkan A. Blódflokkar 3962 íslenzkra kvenna (The blood-groups of 3962 Icelandic women). Laeknabladid 1954; 38:134-144.

9. Pálsson JOP. Anthropologische Unter-suchungen in Island unter besonderer Berücksichtigung des Vergleichs mit den Herkunftsländern der islandischen Siedler. Inaug Diss Mainz 1967.

10. Pálsson JOP. Die Herkunft der island-ischen Bevölkerung in anthropo-logischer Sicht. In: Bernhard W, Kandler A, eds. Bevölkerungsbiologie, Beiträge zur Struktur und Dynamik menschlicher Populationen in anthropo-logischer Sicht. Stuttgart 1974; 213-240.

11. Pálsson JOP. Island. In: Schwidetzky I, ed. Rassengeschichte der Menschheit 4, Europa II, Ost-und Nordeuropa. München-Wien 1976; 147-155.

12. Pálsson JOP. Some anthropological characteristics of Icelanders analyzed with the problem of ethnogenesis. J Hum Evol 1978; 7:695-702.

13. Pálsson JOP. A report on an anthro-pometric survey of the Icelanders. VIIme Congrès international des Sciences anthropologiques et ethno-logiques (Moscow 1964) 1968; 3:298; 301.

14. Steffensen J. The physical anthropol-ogy of the Vikings. J Royal Anthropol Inst Great Brit and Ir 1953; 83:86-97.

15. Thompson EA. The Icelandic admixture problem. Ann Hum Gen 1973; 87:69-80.

16. Torgersen J. Rassengeschichte von Skandinavien. In: Schwidetsky I, ed. Rassengeschichte der Menschheit 4, Europa II: Ost-und Nordeuropa. München-Wien 1976; 103-145.

17. Árnason A. Personal communication.

18. Magnússon A, Vídalín P. Manntal á Íslandi árid 1703 (General census in Iceland 1703). Hagstofa Islands. Gutenberg 1924-1947.

19. Hagskýrslur. (The Statistical Bulle-tin) published monthly by the Statis-tical Bureau of Iceland.

20. Fridriksson S. The Icelandic demo-graphic records and their linking. Conference on Methods of Automatic Family Reconstitution, Florence 1977.

21. Fridriksson S. The origin of the Icelanders and trends in the Icelandic population. Reykjavik 1971.

22. Helgason T. Studies in epidemiology of mental disorder, population genetics,

and record linkage in Iceland: a brief outline. In: Medwick SA, Baert AE, Bachmann BP, eds. Prospective longi-tudinal research. Oxford: Oxford University Press, 1981.

23. Thorsteinsson Th. Íslenzk hagskýr-slugerd fyrir stofnun hagstofunnar (Statistical records in Iceland before the establishment of the Statistical Bureau). Hagtídindi 1964; 49:33-36.

24. Bjarnason O, Fridriksson S, Magnússon M. Record linkage in a self-contained community. Record linkage in medicine. Oxford 1967.

25. Bjarnason O, Magnússon M. Linkage of the Icelandic Cancer Registry to an Icelandic population file. In: Grunde-man E and Pettersen E, eds. Recent results in cancer research. 1975; 50.

26. Árnason A. Association of HLA and disease in Iceland. Nordic Council Arct Med Res Rep 1980; 26:83-91.

27. Árnason A, Larsen B, Marshall WH, et al. Very close linkage between HLA-B and Bf inferred from allelic associa-tion. Nature 1978; 268:527-528.

28. Thorsteinsson J, Teitsson I, Árnason A, Sigurbergsson K. LED á Íslandi og HLA flokkun og anti-DNA-antibody maelingar (LED in Iceland, HLA typing and measurements of anti-DNA-anti-body). Laeknabladid 1977; 7-8:181.

29. Ásmundsson P, Árnason A. Vefjaflokkun á Íslandi fyrir nýra-ígraedslu (Tissue typing for kidney-transplants in Iceland). Laeknabladid 1977; 11-12:249-252.

30. Karlsson S, Árnason A, Jensson O. GLO polymorphism in Iceland. Hum Hered 1980; 30:383-385.

31. Karlsson S, Árnason A, Thórdarson G, Olaisen B. Frequency of Gc alleles and a variant Gc allele in Iceland. Hum Hered 1980; 30:119-121.

32. Karlsson S, Skaftadóttir I, Árnason A, Thórdarson G, Jensson O. Gc subtypes in Icelanders. Hum Hered 1983; 35:5-8.

33. Tulinius H, Hauksdóttir H, Bjarnarson O. Litningarannsóknir á vegum Erfda-fraedinefndar Háskólans og Rannsóknar-stofu Háskólans (Chromosomal studies by the Genetic Committee and the University Laboratory of Pathology). Laeknabladid 1969; 4:169-177.

34. Pálsson JOP. Mannfraedistofnun Háskóla Íslands (The Anthropological Institute of the University of Iceland). Árbók Háskóla Íslands 1973-1976. Reykjavik 1978.

35. Pálsson JOP. Mannfraedistofnun Háskóla Íslands. Árbók Háskóla Íslands 1976-1979. Reykjavik 1981.

36. Pálsson JOP. Mannfraedistofnun Háskóla Íslands. Ársskýrsla Rannsóknaráds Ríkisins 1980-1981. Reykjavik 1982.

37. Pálsson JOP. Comparative anthropo-

logical studies on Icelanders in two hemispheres. Homo 1982; 32.

38. Pálsson JOP. Anthropometrical studies of Icelandic women. In: Harvald B, Hart Hansen JP, eds. Circumpolar Health 81. Nordic Council Arct Med Res Rep 1983; 33:194-200.

39. Helgason L. Psychiatric services and mental illness in Iceland. Acta Psychiatr Scand 1977; Suppl 268.

40. Helgason T. Prevalence and incidence of mental disorders estimated by a health questionnaire and a psychiatric case register. Acta Psychiatr Scand 1978; 58:256-266.

41. Helgason T. Epidemiology of mental disorders in Iceland. Acta Psychiatr Scand 1964; Suppl 173.

42. Helgason T. Epidemiological investigations concerning affective disorders. In: Schou M, Strømgren E, eds. Origin, prevention and treatment of affective disorders. London 1979.

43. Helgason T. Epidemiological follow-up research with a geographically stable population. In: Schimmelpenning GW, ed. Psychiatrische Verlaufsforschung. Bern 1980.

44. Helgason T. Psychiatric problems in a fishing population. Nordic Council Arct Med Res Rep 1977; 18:17-21.

45. Björnsson S. Börn í Reykjavik. Rannsókarnidurstödur (Children in Reykjavik; results of the research project). Idunn, Reykjavik 1980.

46. Björnsson S. Longitudinal research project on Icelandic children. Transnat Mental Health Res News Letter 1979; 21:3-4.

47. Thorlindsson Th, Björnsson S. Some determinants of scholastic performance in urban Iceland. Scand J Educ Res 1979; 23.

48. Björnsson S, Edelstein W. Exploration in social inequality: Stratification dynamics in social and individual development in Iceland. Max Planck 1977.

49. Björnsson S. Mental disorders in Icelandic children. Int Mental Health Res News Letter 1975; 17.

50. Bjarnason O, Tulinius H. Cancer registration in Iceland 1955-1974. Acta Pathol Immunol Scand 1983; 91: Suppl 281.

51. Sigvaldson H, Tulinius H. Human health data from Iceland. Banbury Report 4: Cancer incidence in defined populations. 1980; 257-265.

52. Snaedal G. Cancer of the breast. A clinical study of the treated and untreated patients in Iceland 1911-55. Acta Chir Scand Suppl 338, 1964.

53. Sigfússon N. Publications on the Reykjavik Study (Health Survey in the Reykjavik Area) of the Icelandic Heart Association. Reykjavik 1983. (This list covers one hundred publications and is available on request from the Icelandic Heart Association, Lagmula 9, Reykjavik, Iceland.)

54. Sigurdsson G, Magnusson G, Sigvaldsson H, Tulinius H, Einarsson I, Olafsson O. Egilsstadaprosjektet: problem orienterad journal och individbaserat informationssystem för primärvärd. Nord Med Stat Kom. Stockholm 1980.

55. Sigurdsson G. Egilstadir-projektat, Problemorienterade journaler för bättre patientbehandling vid en primärvårdstation. Nord Med 1981; 96:57-58.

56. Thorsteinsson J. Epidemiology of rheumatic disorders in Iceland. Nordic Council Arct Med Res Rep 1980; 26:77-82.

57. Árnason A, Thorsteinsson J. Studies of HLA and Bf in an Icelandic family where SLE (system lupus erythematosus) AR (rheumatoid arthritis), Reiter's syndrome and AS (ankylosing spondylitis) occur. Clin Genet 1978; 13:102.

58. Árnason A, Thorsteinsson J, Sigurbergsson K. Erfdafraedi og gigtsjúkdómar (The genetics of rheumatic diseases). Laeknabladid 1977; 7-8:182.

59. Árnason A. Erfdir og gigtarsjúkdómar (Genetics and rheumatic diseases). Laeknabladid 1977; Suppl 4:9-15.

60. Árnason A, Thorsteinsson J, Sigurbergsson K. Ankylosing spondylitis HLA B-27 and Bf. Lancet 1978; 1:339-340.

61. Teitsson I, Árnason A, Valdimarsson H, Thorsteinsson J. Studies of an inbred Icelandic family with high incidence of connective tissue diseases. 15th International congress of rheumatology, Paris, 21-27 June, 1981.

62. Árnason A, Jónsson H, Thorsteinsson J, et al. Nokkur erfdamörk í hryggikt (AS) og Reiters sjúkdómi (Some genetic markers in patients with ankylosing spondylitis and Reiters disease). Laeknabladid 1981; 8.

63. Teitsson I, Árnason A, Valdimarsson H, Thorsteinsson J. Íslensk gigtaraett: Kliniskar erfdaedilegar og onaemisfraedilegar athuganir (An inbred family with high incidence of rheumatic disease: Clinical genetic and immunological investigations). Laeknabladid 1982; 9.

64. Árnason A, Fossdal R, Thorsteinsson J, et al. HLA-haplotypes and complotypes in a large inbred Icelandic family with a variety of rheumatological disorders demonstrating duplication of C4A locus, acquired deficiency of C4 proteins, high frequency of C4BQO and HLA B27. Immunobiology 1983; 164 No 3/4.

65. Jensson O. Studies on four hereditary

disorders in Iceland (Doctoral dissertation). Acta Med Scand Suppl 618, Reykjavik 1978.

66. Árnason A, Björnsson OG, Gudmundsson S, Jensson O, Thórdarson G, Valdimarsson H. Macroglobulinaemia in an Icelandic family. Clin Genet 1978; 13:102.

67. Björnsson OG, Árnason A, Gudmundsson S, Jensson O, Ólafsson S, Valdimarsson H. Macroglobulinaemia in an Icelandic family. Acta Med Scand 1978; 203:283-288.

68. Jensson O, Björnsson OG, Árnason A, Birgisdóttir B, Pepys B. Serum amyloid P-component and C-reactive protein in serum of healthy Icelanders with macroglobulinaemia. XVIII Nordisk Kongres i Klinisk Kemi, Reykjavik, June 23-26, 1981.

69. Jensson O, Jónasson JL, Magnússon S. Studies on hereditary sphaerocytosis in Iceland. Acta Med Scand 1977; 201:187-195.

70. Jensson O, Jónasson Th, Ólafsson O. Hereditary elliptocytosis in Iceland. Brit J Haematol 1967; 13,6:844-854.

71. Jensson O, Björnsson OG, Árnason A, Birgisdóttir B, Pepys MB. Serum amyloid p-component of healthy Icelanders and members of an Icelandic family with macroglobulinaemia. Acta Med Scand 1970; 187:229-234.

72. Jensson O, Wallett LH. Von Willebrandt's disease in an Icelandic family. Acta Med Scand 1970; 187: 229-234.

73. Jensson O, Árnason K, Jóhannesson GM, Ulfarsson J. Studies on Pelger anomaly in Iceland. Acta Med Scan 1977; 201: 183-185.

74. Árnason A, Jensson O, Fossdal R, Skaftadóttir I, Birgisdóttir B, Thorsteinsson L. HLA-A, B, C, Bf, C2, C4, GLO-I and C3 in IgA deficient Icelandic individuals and their first degree relatives. Conference on Clinical Aspects of Complement Mediated Diseases 1983.

75. Úlfarsson J, Gudmundsson S, Birgisdóttir B, Kjeld JM, Jensson O. Selective serum IgA deficiency in Icelanders. Acta Med Scand 1982; 211: 481-487.

76. Gudmundsson S, Jensson O. Frequency of IgA deficiency in blood donors and Rh negative women in Iceland. Acta Microbiol Scand Sect C 1977; 85:87-89.

77. Tómasson H. Investigations on heredity of manic-depressive psychosis in Iceland. Proc. 7th International Genetics Congress, Cambridge 1941.

78. Helgason T. Mental disorders and consanguinity. Comparison of first-cousin marriages and matched unrelated marriages. Nordic Council Arct Med Res Rep 1980; 26:107-112.

79. Helgason T. Mental disorders in first cousin marriage families. VIth World Congress of Psychiatry 1977.

80. Thórdarson O, Fridriksson S. Aggregation of deaths from ischaemic heart disease among first and second degree relatives of 108 males and 42 females with myocardial infarction. Nordic Council Arct Med Res Rep 1980; 26:28-29.

81. Thórdarson O, Fridriksson S. Death from ischaemic heart disease among 1st and 2nd degree relatives. Acta Med Scand 1977; 205:6.

82. Árnason A, Bjarnason I, Kristinsson A, Jensson O, Skaftadóttir I, Birgisdóttir B. Rannsóknir á nokkrum erfdamörkum í fjölskyldum med arfgengan ofvöxt á hjartavödva (Investigations of some genetic markers in families with hereditary hypertrophic cardiomyopathy). Laeknabladid 1981; 8.

83. Gudmundsson G, Jensson O, Árnason A. Hereditary factors in intracranial haemorrhage in Iceland. Acta Neurol Scand 1980; 62:suppl 78.

84. Gudmundsson G, Jensson O. Genetics and epidemology of cerebrovascular diseases in Iceland. Nordic Council Arct Med Res Rep 1980; 26:22-27.

85. Árnason A, Gudmundsson STh. Tveir sjúkdómar í nýrnahettum og samband theirra vid vefjaflokka (HLA) a) Addisonsveiki á Íslandi (Two adrenal disorders and their connections with HLA. a) Addison's Disease in Iceland). Laeknabladid 1979; 4:190.

86. Árnason A, Gudmundsson STh, Karlsson S, Skaftadóttir I. Tveir sjúkdómar í nyrnahettum og samband theirra vid vefjaflokka (HLA) b) Congenital adrenal hyperplasia (CAH) á Íslandi (Two adrenal disorders and their connections with HLA. b) congenital adrenal hyperplasia in Iceland). Laeknabladid 1979; 4:190.

87. Danielsen R, Árnason A, Helgason T, Jónasson F. HLA and retinopathy in genotyped type I (insulin-dependent) diabetics in Iceland. Laeknabladid 1982; suppl 15.

88. Árnason A, Helgason T, Jensson O. High risk HLA-Bf haplo- and genotypes in type 1 diabetes in Iceland. Laeknabladid 1982; suppl 15.

89. Árnason A, Helgason Th, Jensson O. Vefjaflokkar (HLA) og insulinhad sykursýki (HLA and insulin dependent diabetes). Laeknabladid 1979; 189-190.

90. Sigurdsson GA, Árnason G, Gudmundsson TV, Kjeld M, Sigurdsson G. An Icelandic family with elevated thyroxin binding globulin with X chromosome linked inheritance. Laeknabladid 1982; suppl 15.

91. Eyjólfsson G, Sigurdsson H, Árnason A, Jensson O. Thyrotoxicosis, arthritis, autoimmune phenomena and malignancies of the reticuloendothelial system in an Icelandic family. Laeknabladid 1982; suppl 15.

92. Árnason A, Jensson O, Eyjólfsson G, Sigurdsson H, Birgisdóttir B, Fossdal R. HLA-Bf and other genetic markers in a family with thyrotoxicosis, arthritis, autoimmune phenomena and malignancies of the reticulo-endothelial system. Laeknabladid 1982; suppl 15.

93. Árnason A, Jensson O, Skaftadóttir F, Birgisdóttir B, Gudmundsson G, Jóhannesson G. HLA types, Gc protein and other genetic markers in multiple sclerosis and two other neurological diseases in Iceland. Acta Neurol Scand Suppl 78 1980; 62.

94. Gudmundsson G. Genetics and epidemiology of multiple sclerosis in Iceland. Nordic Council Arct Med Res Rep 1980; 26:12-15.

95. Árnason A, Jensson O, Skaftadóttir F, Birgisdóttir B, Gudmundsson G, Jóhannesson G. HLA types, Gc protein and other genetic markers in multiple sclerosis and two other neurological diseases in Iceland. Acta Neurol Scand Suppl 78 1980; 62:78.

96. Thorsteinsson A, Árnason A, Jensson O, et al. Optic neuritis, HLA-Bf and three other genetic marker systems in MS and non-MS patients. Laeknabladid 1982; Suppl 15.

97. Árnason A, Thorsteinsson A, Gudmundsson G, Jensson O, Skaftadóttir I, Birgisdóttir B. Genetic markers and Parkinsonism in Iceland. Laeknabladid 1982; suppl 15.

98. Gudmundsson G, Jensson O, Árnason A. Huntingtonsveiki (Chorea) í íslenskri aett (Huntington's chorea in an Icelandic family). Laeknabladid 1982; 9.

99. Gudmundsson K. Epidemiological studies of neurological disease in Iceland (Doctoral dissertation). Reykjavik 1973.

100. Árnason A, Jensson O, Gudmundsson S. Serum esterase of Icelanders. 1. A "silent" pseudocholinesterase gene in an Icelandic family. Clin Gen 1975; 7:405-412.

101. Jensson O, Árnason A, Skaftadóttir I, Linnet H, Jónmundsson GK, Snorradóttir M. Osteopetrosis recessiva: Arfgeng marmarabeinveiki. Laeknabladid 1982; 9.

102. Jensson O, Árnason A, Skaftdóttir I, Linnet H, Jónmundsson GK, Snorradóttir M. Arfgeng marmarabeinveiki (osteopetrosis) í ungbörnum (Hereditary osteopetrosis in infants). Laeknabladid 1983; 69:35-41.

103. Jensson O, Árnason A, Fridriksson S. Osteogenesis imperfecta í Íslendingum (Osteogenesis imperfecta in Icelanders). Laeknabladid 1982; 9.

104. Sveinsson K. Helicoidal chorioretinal degeneration. Nordic Council Arct Med Res Rep 1980; 26:58-59.

105. Forsius H, Eriksson A. Investigation in ophthalmology and population genetics in Iceland. Nordic Council Arct Med Res Rep 1980; 26:40-47.

106. Bjarnason O, Day NE, Snaedal G, Tulinius H. The effect of year of birth on the breast cancer age-incidence curve in Iceland. Int J Cancer 1974; 13:689-696.

107. Tulinius H, Sigvaldason H. Trends and incidence of female breast cancer in the Nordic countries. In: Magnus K, ed. Trends in cancer incidence--causes and practical implications. Oslo 1982; 235-247.

108. Tulinius H, Day NE, Jóhannesson G, Bjarnason O, Gonzales M. Reproductive factors and risk for breast cancer in Iceland. Int J Cancer 1978; 21:724-730.

109. Magnússon SS. Research on the epidemiology of breast cancer in Iceland. Paper given at symposium: Kvinnosjukdomar i nordliga glesbygden. Umeå 1982.

110. Tulinius H, Day NE, Bjarnason O, et al. Familial breast cancer in Iceland. Int J Cancer 1982; 29:365-371.

111. Tulinius H, Day NE, Sigvaldsson H, et al. A population-based study on familial aggregation of breast cancer in Iceland, taking some other risk factors into account. In: Gelboin Hv et al., eds. Genetics and environmental factors in experimental and human cancer. Tokyo: Japan Sci Soc Press 1980; 303-312.

112. Tulinius H. Genetics and epidemiology of cancer of the breast. Nordic Council Arct Med Res Rep 1980; 26:113-116.

113. Tulinius H. Personal communication.

114. Thórarinsson A, Jensson O, Bjarnason O. Screening for uterine cancer in Iceland. Acta Cytologica 1969; 13:305-308.

115. Jóhannesson G, Geirsson G, Day NE. The effect of mass screening in Iceland 1965-1974, on the incidence and mortality of cervical carcinoma. Int J Cancer 1978; 21:418-425.

116. Magnússon SS. Research on the detection of cervical cancer in Iceland. Paper given at symposium: Kvinnosjukdomar i nordliga glesbygder. Umeå 1982.

117. Tulinius H, Geirsson G, Sigurdsson K, Day NE. Screening for cervix cancer in Iceland. (In press.)

118. Sigurdsson K. Time trends in cervical cancer rates in Iceland. Talk given at IARC-WHO meeting on screening of cervix cancer. Copenhagen 1983.

119. Jóhannesson G. Resultat av bröstcancer-screening i Island. Symposium: Tidlig upptakt av brystkreft. Stockholm 1979.

120. Tulinius H, Bjarnason O. Morphology specific incidence of breast cancer. In: Correa P, ed. UICC Tech Rep Ser 35, Geneva 1978.

121. Kristjánsson JH. Vesturfaraskrá 1870-1914 (A record of emigrants from Iceland to America 1870-1914). Reykjavik 1983.

122. Axelsson J. Samanburdur a Vestur-Íslendingum og Héradsbúum (Comparative studies of Icelandic people living in Canada and Iceland) Rannsóknir vid Laeknadeild Háskóla Íslands 1981.

123. Pétursdóttir G, Sigfússon N, Way AB, Axelsson J. Blódfita barna á Héradi (Serum lipids in children in Herad). Rannsóknir vid Laeknadeild Háskóla Íslands, March 1981.

124. Axelsson J, Sigfússon N, Way AB, Pétursdóttir G. Blódfita Héradsbúa á aldrinum 21 til 60 ára (Serum lipids in 21 to 60 year old inhabitants of Herad). Rannsóknir vid Laeknadeild Háskóla Íslands 1981.

125. Axelsson J, Pétursdóttir G. Líkamsbygging Héradsbúa a aldrinum 7 til 60 ara (Body build of 7 to 60 year old inhabitants of Hérad). Rannsóknir vid Laeknadeild Háskóla Íslands 1981.

126. Axelsson J, Jónsson S, Oskarsson JG, Pétursdóttir G. Lungastaerdir og loftskiptageta Héradsbúa á aldrinum 7 til 60 ara (Lung size and ventilatory capacity of 7 to 60 year old inhabitants of Hérad). Rannsóknir vid Laeknadeild Háskóla Íslands 1981.

127. Axelsson J, Jónsson B, Skarphedinsson JO. Blódthrystingur Héradsbúa á aldrinum 21 til 60 ára (Blood pressure of 21 to 60 year old inhabitants of Hérad). Rannsóknir Laeknadeild Háskóla Íslands 1981.

128. Axelsson J, Pálsson JOP, Sigfússon N, Pétursdóttir G, Way AB. Comparative studies of Icelandic people living in Canada and in Iceland. In: Harvald B, Hart Hansen JP, eds. Circumpolar Health 81. Nordic Council for Arct Med Res Rep 33:201-205.

129. Pétursdóttir G, Way AB, Sigfússon N, Axelsson J. Serum lipids in children and adolescents from eastern Iceland. In: Harvald B, Hart Hansen JP, eds. Circumpolar Health 81. Nordic Council for Arct Med Res Rep 33:295-299.

130. Axelsson J, Sigfússon N, Way AB, Pétursdóttir G. Serum lipids in 21 to 60 year old people from eastern Iceland. In: Harvald B, Hart Hansen JP, eds. Circumpolar Health 81. Nordic Council for Arct Med Res Rep 33:304-307.

131. Axelsson J, Jónsson B, Skarphedinsson JO, Way AB. Blood pressure in adult females in eastern Iceland. 5th Int Symp on Circumpolar Health, Copenhagen 1981. abstract.

132. Axelsson J, Pétursdóttir G, Óskarsson JG, Sigfússon N. Samanburdur á lungnastaerdum og utþndunargetu íslenskra karla i dreifbýli og théttbýli (Comparison of lung size and forced expiratory volume of Icelandic males in rural and urban areas). Rannsóknir vid Laeknadeild Háskóla Íslands 1982.

133. Steingrímsdóttir L, Pétursdóttir G, Axelsson J. Fituneysla og serum kolesterol barna og unglinga (Lipid consumption and serum cholesterol in children). Rannsóknir vid Laeknadeild Háskóla Íslands 1982.

134. Axelsson J, Pétursdóttir G, Óskarsson JG, Jónsson S. Líkamsthjálfun og threk (Exercise and physical fitness). Rannsóknir Laeknadeild Háskóla Íslands 1982.

135. Axelsson J, Jónsson B, Pétursdóttir G, Skarphedinsson JO. Áhrif áreynslu á blódthrysting (The effect of exercise on blood pressure). Rannsóknir vid Laeknadeild Háskóla Íslands 1982.

136. Axelsson J, Óskarsson JGO, Pétursdóttir G, Way AB, Nikulasson S. Rural-urban differences in lung size and function in Iceland. In: Fortuine R, ed. Circumpolar Health 84. Seattle: University of Washington Press, 1985.

137. Way AB, Axelsson J, Pétursdóttir G, Sigfússon N. Comparison of total serum cholestoral and triglycerides in comparable town-dwelling and farm-dwelling youngsters in Iceland. In: Fortuine R, ed. Circumpolar Health 84. Seattle: University of Washington Press, 1985.

Gudrun Pétursdóttir
Institute of Physiology
University of Oslo
Karl Johans Gate 47
Oslo 1, Norway

Circumpolar Health 84:32-35

U.S. NATIONAL ARCTIC HEALTH SCIENCE POLICY: FINDINGS DEVELOPED BY AMERICAN PUBLIC HEALTH ASSOCIATION TASK FORCE

FREDERICK MCGINNIS

INTRODUCTION

The National Arctic Health Science Policy, developed by the American Public Health Association Task Force, presents a set of guidelines and principles to stimulate:
--   identification of research needs;
--   development, coordination, sustenance and evaluation of research programs;
--   dissemination of research results in order to enhance health and advance biomedical knowledge in regions where arctic environmental living conditions prevail.

The establishment of the Task Force, composed of 28 members, was endorsed by 9 major Alaskan and national health, scientific and research organizations. Following more than a year of concentrated activities, the proposed final text of the policy has been submitted to the American Public Health Association. The complete statements of findings contained in the Policy document are commended to you for detailed study. Below, I summarize briefly and outline only some of the most significant findings.

NEEDS

For the past 40 years key individuals and organizations have seen the needs for focus, and have called for research into aspects of health in the Arctic. Bob Bartlett, in 1948 Alaska's territorial delegate to Congress, called for studies "of conditions as they exist in the Arctic and how they affect all the various aspects of health." This theme was repeated in recommendations of the American Medical Association and American Public Health Association in 1949 and by the National Security Decision Memorandum 144 in 1971.

Despite strong pronouncements and intentions, only relatively weak and limited actions were taken to develop needed research programs during the past 35 to 40 years. Budgets, personnel and facilities were limited extremely and the broad areas of study needs were overwhelming and ambitious: environmental sanitation, biochemistry and nutrition, zoonotic diseases, entomology and insect control; physiology, and the epidemiology of infectious diseases.

In the presence of continuing and increasing needs, several federal research programs in the Arctic were actually dismantled in the 1970s:
--   U.S. Public Health Service's Arctic Health Research Center closed, 1973;
--   U.S. Army's cold weather research Laboratory closed, 1973;
--   U.S. Environmental Protection Agency's Water Research Laboratory closed, 1979.

Now in the 1980s the Polar Research Board of the National Academy of Sciences, the Committee on Polar Biomedical Research, and the American Public Health Association have formulated new initiatives, stressing needs for arctic health research strategies, policies and resources.

FINDINGS SUMMARIZED

1.   In June 1983, President Reagan issued a memorandum through the Interagency Arctic Policy Group affirming his support for the development of a national arctic science policy:

... the United States has unique and critical interests in the arctic region related directly to national defense, resource and energy development, scientific inquiry, and environmental protection. In light of the region's growing importance, it warrants priority attention by the United States.

2.   There continues to be a void in health research in the Arctic. Organizations focusing primarily on health-related research have few personnel, limited funding, and specialized missions. One such organization is the Arctic Investigations Laboratory, of the Centers for Disease Control (CDC), in Anchorage.

3.   Health science in most regions is supported by an "academic infrastructure" which provides facilities and a base of operations for researchers, integrates and applies research knowledge, and trains personnel. This infrastructure is poorly developed in the case of arctic health research. Alaska has no doctoral training programs in psychology, anthropology, or sociology, and no masters degree programs in public health, epidemiology or demography. Nor do U.S. institutions outside Alaska with advanced degree programs in these disciplines offer an emphasis or focus on the Arctic. There is no multi-disciplinary journal of arctic health. This limits communication among the health researchers presently at work in the Arctic.

4.   Historical conditions have resulted in the reduction and fragmentation of health research on the American Arctic. Research opportunism, lack or responsiveness to local concerns and needs, lack of dissemination of findings, noncollaboration among research-

ers, lack of a clear federal commitment to arctic science, and other factors have contributed to uncertain and discontinuous support for research on arctic health.

5. A number of changes have produced an increasing need for more research-based knowledge relevant to health and disease in arctic areas. Increasing economic activity, related especially to natural resource development, has led to an increase in the size of the resident population and has produced dramatic change for residents of existing Native and Euroamerican communities. Large numbers of people are living and working in arctic communities under conditions where health effects are not well known. For example, the deleterious consequences of hard rock and asbestos mining on workers are well known, but not under arctic conditions.

6. The strategic and economic importance of the abundant supplies of oil, gas, coal minerals, and seafood in Alaska has generated an irreversible and increasing demand for the development of these resources. Development of these resources, directly or indirectly, through such activities as the construction of houses, water supplies, waste disposal facilities, other utilities, industrial sites, dams, harbors and piers, artificial islands and pipelines poses significant challenges for health researchers. In other cases, development cannot proceed until basic health science questions are resolved. For example, our understanding of such feared diseases as botulism and paralytic shellfish poisoning has progressed little in past years. Obvious benefits to affected individuals will result from research to improve understanding of the pathogenesis, natural course of disease, specific therapeutic interventions, and preventive strategies. Quite apart from prevention of human suffering, research could have vast economic benefits.

7. Because of the extreme environmental conditions which prevail in the Arctic, people, as well as all living organisms, are under constant environmental pressure. They are subjected to a wide variety of physical strains and mental stresses--low temperatures, battering winds, reduced visibility in icy fogs or whirling snow, prolonged periods of darkness, and transportation hazards. This demanding environment impairs individuals' work performance, and affects social life in remote isolated communities. There are indications that low-frequency atmospheric pressure waves, wind generated noises, shifting photoperiods, and disturbances in circadian rhythms may profoundly influence psychological balance, modify sleep patterns and endocrine function, affect mood and behavior, and cause deep anxieties associated with depression and psychotic disor-

ders. Studies of circadian rhythms and their alterations in the Arctic have enormous implications for clinical medicine, behavioral sciences, and public health.

8. The federal government has unique relationships with and responsibilities to Native Americans who constitute a significant portion of the arctic population. Many Alaskan communities and individuals have been affected socially, as innocent bystanders, during resource development and associated projects, particularly in the last decade. Far-reaching consequences of development in the Arctic are poorly understood. Research is needed not only on social processes in Alaska Native communities, but also on public policy to ascertain developmental options that could minimize negative effects on these communities.

9. Research is needed to evaluate both existing, and new and innovative, approaches to the delivery of health services; to develop appropriate medical technology for arctic conditions; to discover how best to train, recruit, select, and retain health professionals in isolated areas; and to analyze national policies and guidelines to discover which are appropriate for arctic conditions and which need to be adapted.

10. Recognizing its responsibility to protect the environment, the federal government does support environmental studies in the Arctic on the impact of certain types of commercial development, including fisheries, forestry, mining and oil, hydroelectric power development, and community development. Additional research is needed, however, to assure a healthy environment for those affected by such development.

11. Global patterns of atmospheric circulation transport air masses to the Arctic from lower latitudes. These air masses tend to be heavily polluted by industrial or human-related activities, responsible for "arctic haze." As a consequence of this long distance atmospheric transport, mineral dusts, biological materials, micro-organisms, chemicals, and radionuclides are deposited on land where they remain entrapped in the thin, biologically active layer above the frozen ground and enter the trophic chain. Of particular significance for public health are radioactive substances, polychlorinated hydrocarbons, mercury, and other toxic agrochemicals that might reach high concentrations in basic indigenous foods. They may become further concentrated in selected tissues of the human organism. Extensive research is needed to achieve a better understanding of atmospheric pathways, deposition schemes, concentration and uptake processes, and cumulative impacts on sensitive arctic ecosystems.

12. The goal of research into the dynamics of toxic chemicals and radio-nuclides, man-made and natural, in the arctic environment is to determine whether the processes of dispersion and clearance of chemicals and radionuclides in the Arctic are somehow qualitatively different from those in more temperate environments. Particularly among Native people in Alaska, there is an urgent demand for continuous monitoring of radionuclides in the air, water, ice, soil and in plants, animals and man. The essential cohort studies of Eskimo and Indian populations with known exposures to radionuclides from fallout have never been done. Such empirical investigations of population effects from fallout radio-nuclides in these populations can still be carried out but should be initiated as soon as possible.

13. Health policy research could be helpful to federal program management. Topics in this area include research on health manpower; the integration of tradi-tional Native health practices into the Western health-care delivery system; innova-tive alternatives; the impact of health policies; client involvement in policy making; and the social and cultural patterns that affect the delivery, use, and effec-tiveness of health services in arctic communities.

14. Significant mortality and morbid-ity in arctic communities originate in social and behavior processes rather than in organic conditions and infections. Since the leading causes of morbidity and mortali-ty in Alaska are behaviorally based, preven-tion is closely related to modifying behav-ior and changing social conditions. General discussions of social and behavioral aspects of health in the Arctic advance various hypotheses about the etiology of different diseases, and concomitantly, the conditions that generate health. These hypotheses need to be more systematically explored. Pro-grams are needed that deal more effectively with research into the complex problems of murder, suicide, assault, family violence (spouse abuse, child abuse, child neglect), accidental injury and death, alcoholism and drunken behavior, alcohol-related diseases, mental illness, and psychological impair-ments. Such studies could also contribute to the prevention of birth defects that are the result of certain behaviors, such as fetal alcohol syndrome.

15. Studies need to be conducted in the Arctic with particular emphasis on those conditions where solutions may have broad application to other circumpolar arctic nations and to the United States as a whole. Numerous research areas which fulfill these requirements presently are not being inves-tigated or being investigated in inadequate ways. Examples where arctic research discoveries will affect national health policy include vaccine trials currently being conducted by the Arctic Investigations Laboratory, CDC, for the control of hepa-titis B disease and invasive *Haemophilus influenzae* type b disease. Diseases such as these have unusually high incidence and prevalence among arctic residents. Arctic studies will provide the information needed to develop policies for use of these vac-cines for the entire country. Because of the high incidence levels these studies can be conducted most efficiently among arctic occupants. The results can then be applied to the general population, where a larger absolute number of cases of illness occurs at a far lower frequency.

16. In many ways, the American Arctic is similar to developing countries. Innova-tive approaches to the cross-cultural delivery of health services under extremely rural conditions provide an opportunity to test models for the organization of health service. These models might be replicated in rural areas in the United States as well as developing countries. The isolation of communities in the Arctic provides built-in controls over variables, a situation that can be advantageous in the design of re-search on health and social policy.

17. Good research demands that basic epidemiologic studies define the morbidity and mortality rates of arctic populations to compare them to other populations. These studies are currently receiving attention or support. Misconceptions based on past research that was incomplete or scientif-ically tenuous can become accepted as facts, leading to inappropriate priorities and policies. Major problems exist with the data collected on surveillance of disease in the Arctic. Both these and demographic data are too incomplete at present to allow for adequate or credible analysis. In the American Arctic, basic vital statistics such as birth and death registry are far below standards ordinarily accepted for routine data collection and use. Existing statis-tics and data collection methods often do not differentiate population subgroups, thus obscuring trends. Basic data about human diseases collected through surveillance and reporting mechanisms require extensive and well-tested verification procedures to ensure validity.

18. The Arctic Health Science Policy will facilitate a research program that addresses behavioral and social aspects of health. Such a research program can be executed most effectively within a community health perspective because the constella-tions of diseases and conditions as they occur within communities are what concern both residents and health-care providers, and because community conditions contribute largely to both the causes of disease and states of health and to the provision of medical services.

19. The Arctic Health Science Policy recognizes the mores of arctic peoples, the necessity of their involvement as partners in planning research programs, the value of their advice and experience, and a commitment to their health needs. Information that is gathered and results that are synthesized must be reliably returned to the communities and groups that are studied. Thus, this Arctic Health Science Policy provides guidelines that include using local arctic populations to help assess the need for and relevance of proposed studies.

20. Health sciences in the Arctic require multidisciplinary approaches, including but not limited to epidemiology, demography, anthropology, psychology, sociology, economics, history, and the basic and applied biological and medical sciences. Many of the research problems and opportunities in the Arctic do not fit neatly into the goals of existing funding agencies. Officers in agencies facing tight budgets find it difficult to support costly research in the Arctic when the same dollars might be spent on research in less costly areas of the United States and on research on urban populations. Because of higher costs incurred conducting research in the Arctic, emphasis must be placed on exploiting the "opportunities of nature" which are not found outside the Arctic. Unless the United States makes a specific commitment to support health research in the Arctic, these many important opportunities will continue to be neglected.

Frederick P. McGinnis
Department of Human Resources
State of Georgia
878 Peach Tree Street NE
Atlanta, GA 30309
U.S.A.

Circumpolar Health 84:36-39

CIRCUMPOLAR HEALTH: PRESENT AND FUTURE

C. EARL ALBRECHT

All of us at this conference realize full well the value of holding these International Symposia. Here scientists from the circumpolar countries of the world have gathered to share knowledge through presentations, and group and individual discussions because each is concerned about the health and medical problems of their people. Our common purpose is to develop a united front internationally to bring the best health care to everyone living and working in the North.

Most of you, as well as I myself, have worked with the people of the higher latitudes and know the needs and the challenges of unanswered questions. We know the difficulties of cold, darkness, isolation, distance, adaptation, and permafrost. We recognize the economic developments that are taking place, particularly in the last 2 decades, and which have a profound socio-economic effect and are causing cultural and change.

Yet there are many who do not share our belief that the circumpolar regions should be singled out for special consideration. They ask why health-related research should be carried out in the Arctic, since man's physiological and psychological characteristics do not change that much. Such questions could be answered readily by those who have attended any of these 6 health symposia.

Professor Louis Rey recently stated in an address, "The Boreal Lands constitute a world of its own with its distinctive geographical, meteorological and environmental characters and its highly specialized cultures going back into prehistoric times."(1)

Elsewhere, while discussing natural resources, he said: "Enormous deposits of fossil fuels, rare metals, uranium and many fields extend even further northwards, offshore under the continental platform of the coastal seas."(2) Inland are huge forests that offer a wide range of replenishable resources. Fossil fuel deposits are so enormous that Dr. Rey further states, "some specialists claim that more than 50% of the world petroleum reserves lie north of the Arctic Circle."(2) The development of these arctic resources will necessarily involve many thousands of people, probably millions in the U.S.S.R. Wherever people are located our involvement is indicated, for we deal with all aspects of man.

Unfortunately, there is evidence that these facts and predictions are not accepted and consequently some detrimental actions have been taken. For example, the World Health Organization had before it a proposal to set up an arctic health program but it was recently voted down by the member nations because it was of little interest to many of them. In 1967 on the University of Alaska campus in Fairbanks, the Arctic Health Research Center was opened. The memorial plaque dedicated on the wall of the building states: "The far north contains vast untouched reservoirs of strategic materials and of minerals and vegetation that can enrich the world .... These areas are capable of supporting life, perhaps of supporting flourishing civilizations .... Obtaining the basic information necessary for healthful living in low-temperature areas is a major objective of the Arctic Health Research Center. At the same time it can make potentially significant contributions to basic knowledge." Tragically, in 1973 the U.S. federal government chose to fund it no longer, and instead gave the facility to the University of Alaska. Since then the facilities have been put to good use by the University but there is inadequate funding for comprehensive health research. The Naval Arctic Research Laboratory was initiated by the U.S. Office of Naval Research at Point Barrow in 1947. It lost its federal support in 1980 and was closed.

Although these are only a few illustrations they emphasize the need for more national and international bio-medical research. On the positive side, recognition must also be given to the research conducted by 2 Federal agencies, the Centers for Disease Control and the Alaska Area Native Health Service which is concerned with health care delivery to Alaska's Native population.

The International Symposia on Circumpolar Health have permitted scientists to exchange research findings and have demonstrated that a considerable amount of bio-medical research is being undertaken in the circumpolar regions of the world. The Soviets, for example, are active in this type of research and have both a Siberian Branch of the Soviet Academy of Medical Sciences and an Academy Institute of Clinical and Experimental Medicine in Norilsk, with another Laboratory in Irkutsk, a State Medical Institute in Archangel, and a Department of Polar Medicine in the Arctic and Antarctic Research Institute in Leningrad. The Finns, Swedes, Norwegians, Danes, and Icelanders, working cooperatively within the Nordic Council for Arctic Medical Research, located in Oulu, Finland, have conducted much outstanding research. The Canadians are pursuing Arctic bio-medical research at the Northern Medical Research

Unit at the Charles Camsell Hospital in Edmonton, the Northern Medical Unit at the University of Manitoba in Winnipeg and at other universities involved in northern Canada such as Memorial University in St. John's, Newfoundland and McGill University in Montreal.

At this time probably Alaska's greatest need is to have a state-supported research network of some type, possibly within the University of Alaska system or within another existing health organization, to coordinate biomedical research activities. The alternative is a piecemeal approach to research by people associated with various federal, state, university, and private non-Alaskan groups. There are programs at the University of Alaska that might serve as the coordinating body for this research network, such as the WAMI Medical Program, though its main focus is teaching, or the Institute of Arctic Biology on the Fairbanks campus. Because of the number of groups doing human research in Alaska, the Alaska Area Native Health Service, which was responsible for Native health, years ago organized a research committee to coordinate these activities. This committee was not sufficient, however, and the problem of coordination of effort in a coherent program remains.

To meet the need for more arctic bio-medical research, a major step has been taken towards establishing a National Arctic Health Science Policy for the United States.

The Alaska Public Health Association has been working with the American Public Health Association to develop and establish such a national policy. The work has been going on over the last 2 years and is now in the final stages of approval by the American Public Health Association. It should be released as a final document very soon. The Alaska State Medical Association, the American Medical Association and the 2 U.S. Senators from Alaska support the plan. The Alaska State Medical Association's Resolution is significant for it emphasizes the research needs of all the circumpolar regions. Excerpts of this resolution read as follows:

> *Whereas*, An increasing amount of human habitation, occupation, transportation and recreational activity has been occurring under extreme cold weather conditions in connection with recent developments in oil and gas explorations, in the development and utilization of arctic mineral, marine and agricultural resources, and in national defense activities, and
> *Whereas*, The physical, mental and environmental health impacts of such activities are important to national resource development and defense capabilities, and
> *Whereas*, The preventive and therapeutic aspects of such disruptions to human physiologic and homeostatic body mechanisms should have much more coordinated study and research, so be it,
> *Resolved*, that the Association support and endorse further emphasis on the physical, mental, occupational, and environmental aspects of scientific research and development on arctic conditions as they affect human health.

Another exciting and successful development in this connection has been the passage of a National Arctic Research and Policy Act by both the U.S. Senate and House of Representatives. We anticipate that this legislation will be signed by the President and will provide a strong commitment by the U.S. Government to arctic research including arctic health research.

Let me urge every nation in the northern latitudes to encourage its government to support adequate research and studies to find the answers to the problems that still need to be resolved. How best to facilitate such support will of course be decided upon by the respective countries. Our responsibility here at an International Symposium on Circumpolar Health is to strengthen our international bonds.

At the 1981 Symposium held in Copenhagen the International Organizing Committee made an historical decision to take the necessary steps towards establishing an International Union on Circumpolar Health. Based on this action, statutes (constitution) and rules of procedure (by-laws) were drafted and during the past 2 years these documents have been studied by the national representatives.

I am pleased to announce that at this meeting the International Organizing Committee has approved in principle the statutes and rules of procedure. This step should greatly facilitate more international communication and exchange of knowledge useful to all circumpolar scientists, because inevitably through this united effort we can achieve greater results than by independent actions.

But I must share one concern with you. I want to caution all those working in the Arctic not to permit fragmentation, division, duplication, and lack of coordination, because too many groups, institutions, or agencies work independently of each other. If there is no coordination, "man's future" in the arctic environment will be inadequately addressed.

That this lack of coordination is a problem in the United States is one of the pressing reasons that an Arctic Health Science Policy is needed. Each nation or group of nations must address this danger for itself and correct it lest it get out of hand. It is my impression that the Nordic Council is an excellent example of coordination of arctic research activity.

A related matter that needs attention is one in which international groups plan and work independently of others having the same purpose, thus causing duplication and disharmony rather than cooperation. This is not meant to discourage work in the Arctic but rather to urge coordination of effort and avoidance of duplication.

One such example is the International Co-ordinating Council for "Man and the Biosphere Program." At a meeting in Paris Sept. 30 to Oct. 1, 1981, the Canadian delegation proposed "establishment of a network for cooperation among people engaged in problems peculiar to the Circumpolar North." The recommendation was approved by the Co-ordinating Council. Following this an international meeting was called to organize the suggested network. The decisions and actions taken at the meeting are not yet available but it is hoped that our International Union on Circumpolar Health will coordinate and plan its work in harmony with the "Man and the Biosphere" (MAB) programs.

One of our distinguished speakers, Professor Louis Rey, has so aptly stated the many challenges of the future. Here are some of his quotations:

As we can easily understand, the arctic is very demanding and it exerts on all living organisms a constant environmental pressure, which results in a heavy load on both the physiological and psychological performance of individuals. In the arctic zone animals and plants are under constant stress, and, as such, much more vulnerable to outside interference. Man is no exception to this basic rule and, in this difficult area where there is no room for error, he has his full share of physical strain and mental tension. To the obvious thermal constraints should be added the more subtle effects of changing photoperiods and magnetic disturbances.

Still unknown is the action of the natural or induced magnetic fields, which seem to play some role on brain activity and may influence sleep patterns. It has equally been demonstrated that circadian rhythms not only concern physiological variables (like temperature, heart rate, etc.) but that they have a marked effect on psychological sensibility and performance, the sensitivity to external stimuli and even the reaction to drugs, poisons etc. Chronopharmacology in arctic

areas is still a virgin subject but it deserves a lot of attention, since it might lead to important discoveries of high practical value.

In fact, when dealing with man in arctic conditions, we should resist the temptation to make an easy extrapolation using data derived from populations in temperate regions such as New York, Mexico or Paris but not applicable to the human groups living in the arctic environment. What is true for sleep, biological rhythms, or drug sensitivity is equally true in the nutritional field.(3)

Another matter about which I am personally concerned is the future of the aboriginal people in all the circumpolar areas of the earth. The introduction of modern civilization and recent intensive development has made a profound impact on their culture, way of life and traditions. Professor Rey is also concerned, for he states in a recent article:

This is precisely where the acute difficulties lie since this powerful influx of 'modern' civilization has had, without any doubt, both a beneficial and disruptive impact upon the natives and old dwellers and may rupture their traditions. However, every effort should be made to resolve this problem and establish a reasonable working philosophy which will secure a harmonious development of arctic regions with the active support and participation of local populations, and which will keep in balance the socio-economic interests and the ecological requirements while preserving the cultural patrimony. (4)

We as health scientists cannot ignore statistical facts such as that in Alaska the leading causes of death and disability are accidents, suicide, homicide and alcoholism. These may also be present in other circumpolar areas. This situation has implications for much health research and fortunately this Symposium addresses these issue in quite a few presentations. Since it is obvious that these problems are behaviorally based, research is needed in communities rather than in laboratories. In particular, government must take more action to reduce the dangerous per capita levels of consumption of alcohol. Health scientists must participate in the development of control methods because of their knowledge of human behavior and addiction to alcohol.

Whenever people enter extreme environments, the principal objective of medical science is to ensure human survival. Once it has been established that the human population can survive, or even thrive in a particular environment, the medical objective shifts. The emphasis then is on conditions that will facilitate human adjustment, that is, to provide a situation in which a person can expect to be healthy, happy, and effective in family life, work, and community relationships, without the development of crippling emotional symptoms, such as fear, anger, loneliness, envy, or greed. I believe that circumpolar nations will look to us to develop such a biomedical research strategy for the future.

In planning this strategy we must not ignore the impact of change and development that is so traumatic to the "stayers" and "sprinters," as Professor Kaznachev calls the original inhabitants and the newcomers. As persons trained in the health fields we will not overlook this impact.

We cannot mold the environment, nor will the world wait to harvest the vast arctic natural resources. We must meet the challenge so man can live and work better in the future. We as scientists have chosen to work in this environment and with this decision goes a responsibility to improve the living of the men and women who already live and work there as well as to those who will come in the future. Man will migrate in unknown numbers to this challenging environment. And so we must get on with our scientific work.

I have faith and know that there are many enthusiastic, competent, young dedicated scientists out there who will meet this challenge. I know that the six symposia thus far have contributed for we have experienced the value of working together,

---

(Editors' Note: The U.S. National Arctic Health Science Policy was adopted by the American Public Health Association in June 1984. The National Arctic Research and Policy Act of 1984 was signed into law by the President in August 1984.)

and sharing our skills and knowledge to solve these problems in an interdisciplinary manner and with international harmony. We believe the establishment of our International Union will facilitate these objectives even more.

In conclusion, let me propose that all of us contribute to the planning for the next Symposium to be held at Umea, Sweden in 1987. Communicate your ideas with the Nordic Council in Oulu, Finland. Some of you already have this in mind, for in the audience is someone known to me only as Linda, who told me how much she wanted to help with the next Symposium. I hope there are many "Lindas" with equal enthusiasm.

So let us conduct our work and research with the thought uppermost in our minds that we have a responsibility and a share in seeing to it that man's future in an arctic environment will be better than it is today.

REFERENCES

1. Rey L. The role of the arctic regions in the energy challenge. In: Cold Regions Science and Technology. 6. Amsterdam: Elsevier Science Publishers, 1983:6.
2. *Ibid*:7.
3. Rey L. The arctic regions in the light of industrial development--basic facts and environmental issues. In: Cold Regions Science and Technology. 7. Amsterdam: Elsevier Science Publishers, 1983:17-18.
4. *Ibid*:24.

C. Earl Albrecht
Drawer L
Bermuda Run
Advance, NC 27006
U.S.A.

SECTION 2. PHYSIOLOGY AND PATHOLOGY OF COLD CLIMATES

Circumpolar Health 84:41-44

"FUTURE SHOCK" AND THE FITNESS OF THE INUIT

ANDRIS RODE and ROY J. SHEPHARD

The "future shock" of Alvin Toffler is being experienced by many arctic communities at a pace without precedent in southern society, small settlements moving from a neolithic type of economy to what is essentially an urban North American culture in the space of a few decades. This report describes the effect of such future shock upon the physiological status of the Inuit in a region of Canada's Northwest Territories.

In 1970-71, the fitness of arctic communities was studied as part of the Human Adaptability Project of the International Biological Program (1). The Canadian team conducted its studies in Igloolik, a village of some 530 Inuit situated in Canada's eastern Arctic (69°40'N). The resulting reports (2,3,4) described certain unusual physiological characteristics of the traditional Canadian Inuit, including an exceptionally large maximal oxygen intake, particularly when expressed per kg of body mass; a very limited amount of subcutaneous fat; and a superior leg extension strength. These characteristics were attributed to a high level of habitual activity, including frequent walking over rough terrain, ice, and snow; daily carriage of young children by the women; and vigorous forms of hunting, with an average energy cost of 15 to 16 MJ per day.

In support of the importance of the physical activity due to hunting, substantial gradient of both maximum oxygen intake and subcutaneous fat were demonstrated in 1970-71 among those members of the settlement who still followed the traditional pattern of hunting, those who were in transition, and those who had permanent jobs within the settlement (2).

METHODS

The process of acculturation within the Igloolik settlement has progressed rapidly since the original survey of 1970. In 1980-81, we had the opportunity to reassess the working capacity of the Igloolik people, again obtaining cardiorespiratory data on a substantial proportion of the villagers, who by then had increased in numbers to a total of about 720 people. On both occasions, all of our procedures conformed to the standard protocol established for the International Biological Program (5). In 1970-71 we tested a total of 266 subjects aged 9 to 66 and in 1980-81 we used the same methods and equipment to test 344 volunteers aged 9 to 76.

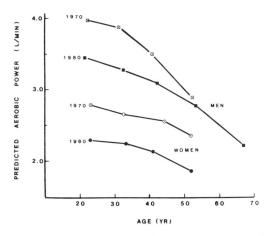

Figure 1. A cross-sectional comparison of aerobic power in Inuit men and women.

RESULTS AND DISCUSSION

A cross-sectional comparison of the men and women tested in 1970-71 with those seen in 1980-81 shows that the predicted maximum oxygen intake has declined in both sexes and at all ages. In women, the decline of the absolute prediction has occurred at all ages but in the men the decrease is most marked in the youngest age groups (Figure 1). The relative prediction shows a similar tendency but because body mass has also increased, the loss of aerobic power is larger than indicated by the absolute prediction in a number of age categories.

All of the sample were well nourished in terms of hemoglobin concentrations both in 1970-71 and 1980-81. In the present survey, readings averaged 15.0 to 15.9 g/dl for the men and 14.0 to 14.7 g/dl for the women.

The rapid increase in height previously described for the Inuit seems now to have halted, at least in Igloolik. The young adults of 1980-81 are insignificantly shorter than those of similar age in 1970-71, and a longitudinal comparison shows that adults of all ages have decreased in height by some 2 cm over the period 1970-71 to 1980-81 (Table 1).

Young adults weigh less than a decade ago, significantly so in the men, and at the same time there has been a significant increase in subcutaneous fat in both sexes. Middle-aged adults are insignificantly heavier than a decade ago, but both sexes show a substantial and significant increase

Table 1. Longitudinal comparison of height in adult Inuit men and women.

| Initial Age 1970-71 (yr) | Height changes in 10 years (cm) | |
	Men	Women
20-29	-1.7***	-2.1***
30-39	-2.2****	-1.8****
40-49	-2.0	-2.1

**** P < 0.005
*** P < 0.01

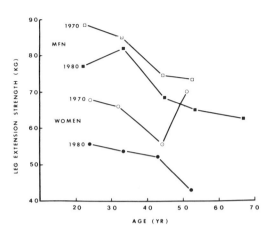

Figure 2. A cross-sectional comparison of leg strength in Inuit men and women.

of subcutaneous fat, implying a loss of lean tissue (Table 2). Current figures for the 40 to 49 year age group (10 mm and 17 mm per fold in men and women, respectively) are much more comparable with southern standards than was the case 10 years ago. The 50 to 59 year age group comparisons are based on rather small samples (6 vs. 10 and 5 vs. 7) but nevertheless suggest that the older members of the community have shown less tendency to accumulate fat than their younger counterparts.

The leg extension strength has decreased by 5 to 14% in the men and 5 to 38% in the women over the past decade (Figure 2). In the men, the change is largest (and statistically significant) in the younger age category, but in the women the largest change is shown by the oldest age category. In contrast, handgrip force has been well preserved and in the 30 to 39 year old men it even shows a significant 14% increase.

The young boys of Igloolik continue to show the high levels of aerobic power demonstrated in 1970-71 and it is not until after age 20 that there is a progressive decline to figures some 10% lower than those observed a decade earlier. The 1980-81 girls have a maximum oxygen intake essentially similar to the 1970-71 survey, but they appear to show a sharper decline of aerobic power co-incident with the pubertal deposition of fat.

Cross-sectional data on skinfold thick-

Table 2. Cross-sectional comparison of the sum of 3 skinfolds (mm) showing means, ± S.D., and (N).

| Age (yr) | Men | | Women | |
	1970-71	1980-81	1970-71	1980-81
20-29	16.6 ±5.2 (30)	20.7** ±9.3 (40)	25.8 ±8.8 (20)	35.6** ±18.1 (24)
30-39	18.6 ±8.0 (27)	24.8* ±15.8 (31)	27.1 ±18.5 (13)	43.2* ±17.3 (23)
40-49	16.1 ±3.3 (9)	29.9** ±22.6 (18)	24.2 ±5.9 (6)	51.6* ±45.6 (15)
50-59	25.2 ±20.1 (6)	25.5 ±16.8 (10)	57.0 ±37.4 (5)	33.1 ±20.7 (7)

** P < 0.025
* P < 0.05

nesses show that over the decade age-matched boys and girls increased the amount of subcutaneous fat by about 1 mm per fold. The average skinfold of the young boys is a little higher than the 4.7 to 4.9 seen in 1970-71, with the main accumulation of fat taking place between 16 and 19 years of age. For the 1980-81 girls, the skinfold totals are substantially greater than in the pre- and postpubertal girls of 1970-71; nevertheless, the average readings for 19 year old boys and girls (9.3 and 11.5 mm per fold, respectively in 1980-81) remain less than in typical southern subjects of similar age.

At any given age both sexes show a substantial decrease of knee extension strength from 1970-71 to 1980-81 (Figure 3). In the boys, the maximum grip strength is closely comparable for the two surveys, but in the younger girls, there appears to be a deterioration of grip strength over the decade. In the girls, these changes seem to be accompanied by a less dramatic pubertal increase of muscle strength.

When we combine our adult sample of men and women into one group aged 20 to 59 years, the effects of acculturation on fitness become even more obvious (Table 3). The cross-sectional comparison of this combined age group shows that between 1970-71 and 1980-81 the men and women showed significant increases in subcutaneous fat of 31 and 40%, respectively. These substantial increases of fat together with insignificant changes in total body mass suggest a loss of lean tissue. This trend is particularly dramatic for the 20 to 29 year old men, who showed a significant 4.5% decrease of body mass together with a significant 38% increase in subcutaneous fat. The 20 to 29 year old women exhibit a similar trend, with a 3.6% decrease in body mass and significant 59.5% increase in subcutaneous fat. Looking at our cross-sectional comparison of 20 to 59 year old men and women, our hypothesis of a loss of muscle tissue is further substantiated by a highly significant 11% and 20% decrease in leg strength in men and women, respectively.

The grip strength in women remained virtually unchanged while that in the men showed a highly significant 8% increase. This apparently anomalous increase in grip strength is due, most likely, to the effort required to handle and control a snowmobile over the rough, hard-packed snow and ice prevalent in the Igloolik area. In 1970 there were 20 snowmobiles in Igloolik compared to the 180 such machines that we counted in 1980-81. Not only has there been a nine-fold increase in the number of snowmobiles over the decade, but today's machines are also considerably larger, heavier, and much faster.

In 10 years, the predicted maximum oxygen intake has decreased substantially in

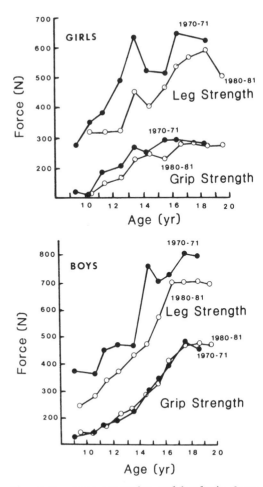

Figure 3. Knee extension and handgrip force for Inuit children, a comparison of cross-sectional data.

both sexes. The men showed a highly significant 12% and 11% decrease in their absolute and relative rates, respectively. The corresponding decreases in women, also highly significant, were 14% and 13%.

The data obtained in many field surveys are compromised by either inadequate sampling or the limitations of available equipment and techniques. In 1980-81 we tested 211 males and 143 females or 75% and 60% of the potential volunteers, respectively. In 1970-71 the proportions were slightly higher. Thus, the secular trend to a deterioration of fitness described here can hardly be attributed to sampling differences.

Further evidence that there has indeed been a decline of personal fitness comes from a consideration of other variables such as body mass, subcutaneous fat, and leg strength. All of these measurements show changes consistent with a deterioration of personal fitness. The only group that has

Table 3. Measures of cardiorespiratory fitness and other variables in men and women aged 20 to 59 years.

Variable	Men 1970	Men 1980	Women 1970	Women 1980
Number ($\underline{N}$)	74	98	44	70
Age (yr)	33.3	33.7	33.1	34.6
Height (cm)	165.3	164.5	155.1	153.2
Weight (kg)	68.0	68.1	57.6	58.8
3 skinfolds (mm)	18.4	24.1***	29.5	41.4**
Leg strength (kg)	84.7	75.7***	65.8	52.5****
Grip strength (kg)	46.8	50.5****	28.3	28.5
Pred. VO_2 max (1/min)	3.73	3.28****	2.57	2.22****
Pred. VO_2 max (ml/kg/min)	54.9	48.6****	44.7	38.7****

**** $P < 0.001$
*** $P < 0.005$
** $P < 0.01$

apparently been spared are the young boys and girls of the village. The similarity of the 1980 data for young people to that of 1970-71 offers further evidence that the loss of fitness in older subjects is a true phenomenon and not a methodological error.

Previous generations of circumpolar residents have enjoyed a low prevalence of cardiovascular risk factors as a tangible reward for a lifetime of vigorous physical effort. Modern technology is progressively robbing mankind of the need for physical effort at work, at home, and even in his leisure activities. The Igloolik community demonstrates the physiological consequences of such inactivity on a vastly accelerated time scale. It will be most important to monitor the future physiological and medical status of the population now that they have adopted the sedentary lifestyle characteristic of our southern communities.

REFERENCES

1. Milan F, ed. The human biology of circumpolar peoples. London: Cambridge University Press, 1979.
2. Rode A, Shephard RJ. Cardiorespiratory fitness of an arctic community. J Appl Physiol 1971; 31:519-526.
3. Rode A, Shephard RJ. Fitness of the Canadian Eskimo--the influence of season. Med Sci Sport 1973; 5:170-173.
4. Rode A and Shephard RJ. Growth, development, and fitness of the Canadian Eskimo. Med Sci Sport 1973; 5:161-169.
5. Weiner JS and Lourie JA. Human biology. A guide to field methods. Oxford: Blackwell Scientific Publications, 1969.

Andris Rode
General Delivery
Igloolik, N.W.T. XOA OLO
Canada

ACCULTURATION AND THE BIOLOGY OF AGING

ROY J. SHEPHARD and ANDRIS RODE

Previous authors have suggested that unusual longevity can emerge in genetic isolates where a high level of physical activity is important to survival (1). There are obvious sources of experimental difficulty in testing this hypothesis in many isolated communities, including poor records of calendar age, and an exaggeration of age among older residents induced by respect for the oldest members of the tribe (2,3). Claims of great longevity have not, to date, withstood critical examination. Nevertheless, we thought it of interest to investigate the course of biological aging in an isolated circumpolar population, testing also the impact of acculturation to a sedentary western lifestyle upon this aging process.

METHODS

The primary data base for our investigation was the Inuit settlement of Igloolik (69°40'N) in the Northwest Territories. Until recently, the population of this region had remained relatively isolated, sustaining a high level of physical activity (4) and a correspondingly high level of physical fitness (5). Moreover, the age of each member of the population had been clearly established and recorded, both in the disc lists and in the parish registers of the Catholic and Anglican churches.

Cross-sectional studies of the aging of aerobic power, body composition and muscle strength were undertaken on the majority of people over the age of 9 years (some 75% of men and 60% of women) in 1970-71 and again in 1980-81. In most instances, the same subjects were tested on the two occasions. Thus a longitudinal assessment of aging was also possible, comparing the two data sets. When first examined, in 1970-71, many of the community still followed an active lifestyle, and 30 to 40% of the food needs of the settlement were met by hunting. By 1980-81, however, most of the population had become sedentary, and full-time hunting was restricted to a much smaller group.

CROSS-SECTIONAL DATA

Cross-sectional data reflect biological aging, societal expectations concerning age roles, and the varying environments encountered by successive cohorts of the population. Older cohorts within the settlement have passed a large part of their lives in a traditional Inuit society, exposed to uncontrolled epidemics of disease, but enjoying also the advantages of a traditional diet and a high level of physical activity. At the same time, the population pyramid is very steep, with few Inuit over the age of 50 years. Cross-sectional analysis thus tends to minimize functional loss, since the oldest cohorts contain only well-endowed individuals who have successfully resisted both disease and starvation.

Aerobic Power

The reported annual loss of aerobic power for circumpolar peoples has varied quite widely from 0.30 to 0.65 ml/kg/min (5). The lowest rates of loss have been cited for male Alaskan Eskimos, male Kautokeino Lapps, and female Skolt Lapps, while the highest rates of loss have been noted among male Skolt Lapps and female Kautokeino Lapps. The erratic picture reflects a narrow age span (25 to 45 or 25 to 55 years) and a limited sample size. Nevertheless, the average rate of loss (0.47 ml/kg/min in the men, 0.41 ml/kg/min in the women) is closely comparable to that established for White subjects in southern settlements (5).

When first tested, the cross-sectional aging curve for the Inuit of Igoolik had a normal overall slope, but somewhat different in shape from that anticipated in a White community: function was relatively well-preserved from 25 to 45 years of age, but deteriorated quickly once the children were able to assume responsibility for hunting (Figure 1). By 1980-81, the cross-sectional curves for the aging of aerobic power had become more like those for the White community, reflecting the reduced physical activity of young adults.

Body Fat

When tested in 1970-71, the male Inuit at Igloolik had extremely thin skinfolds (Figure 1), and there was almost no accumulation of fat from 25 to 55 years of age. Young women were also thin (average skinfold 9.3 mm), but the small group of older Inuit that we tested had a substantial subcutaneous fat (average 24.8 mm). Presumably, younger members of the community were kept thin by an active lifestyle and (in the case of the women) by extended lactation and the carrying of children on their backs. By 1980-81, both sexes showed an accumulation of fat in early adult life, much as in a White community.

Muscle Force

The handgrip force of the Igloolik sample, tested in 1970-71, was lost at least as fast as in a White community, dropping in the men from 510 N at age 25 to 377 N at age

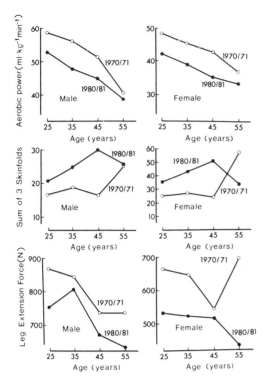

Figure 1.   Cross-sectional data for the aging of predicted maximum oxygen intake, subcutaneous fat thickness and knee extension strength, tested on Inuit > 9 years of age in 1970-71 and 1980-81. Some 75% of male subjects and 60% of female subjects were recruited from the settlement of Igloolik, N.W.T., on each occasion.

55 years, and in the women from 292 N to 267 N. On the other hand, leg extension force was apparently well-preserved over the same age-span, respective values falling from 865 to 754 in the men, and moving from 675 to 681 N in the women. We believe that in this epoch, the leg muscles of both sexes were conserved by the need to carry heavy loads over hard-packed snow. By 1980-81, there was little change in the aging curve for grip force, but leg extension force had diminished (particularly in older individuals). We hypothesize that the weakening of leg strength reflects the newly developed practice of making even short journeys by snowmobile. This, together with greater municipal efforts at snow clearance, have largely obviated the need to walk over rough snow. At the same time, the operations of powerful snowmobiles has helped to preserve grip strength.

LONGITUDINAL DATA

Many authors have argued that a longitudinal study provides the optimal method for examining the rate of aging. This is generally true of White society, but problems arise in applying a longitudinal methodology to indigenous populations that are undergoing rapid cultural change. At Igloolik, all of those tested (except boys aged 9 to 15 years) had become much more sedentary between 1970-71 and 1980-81. The ten year test-retest data thus gave a misleading picture of rapid functional aging, the normal biological deterioration for the decade being boosted by the effects of transition from an active to a sedentary lifestyle.

A second problem with lung function measurements was the passage through the community of a cohort who had been treated for respiratory disease in the 1950s (6); this distorted the shape of both cross-sectional and longitudinal curves for the aging of forced vital capacity and forced expiratory volume.

Longitudinal measurements revealed a 2 cm diminution in stature from 1970-71 to 1980-81, this being shown equally by cohorts that were, initially, aged 20 to 29 years, 30 to 39 years, and 40 to 49 years (7). It is possible that a limited calcium intake (8) accelerated the normal aging of stature, but it would still be surprising if this change was observed between 25 and 35 years of age; a more reasonable explanation seems to be spinal trauma, caused by operation of newly acquired snowmobiles over rough ice and snow (9).

ACCULTURATION

Three assessments were made of the impact of acculturation upon the aging process: first, comparisons were drawn in cross-sectional fashion between those continuing as hunters and those who had accepted permanent employment within the settlement (5); second, correlations were calculated between an empirical index of acculturation developed by Dr. Ross MacArthur (which considered such items as knowledge of the English language, geographic mobility, wage income and domestic equipment) and deterioration of physical fitness (10); and third, comparison was made of cross-sectional data for the entire community in 1970-71 and 1980-81 (Figure 1).

All three assessments yielded the same picture. Acculturation to White society, with the abandonment of traditional hunting pursuits, had led to a deterioration of physical condition, particularly among the younger adults. The loss of physical fitness was equivalent to an acceleration of the aging process, men and women of 25 years now having the maximum oxygen intake that would have been anticipated at 45 years of age in 1970-71.

QUALITY AND QUANTITY OF LIFE

The impact of such physiological deterioration upon the quality and quantity of life as a senior citizen is more debatable. Plainly, aging continues to diminish functional capacity at a similar absolute rate in both fit and unfit subjects, and the unfit groups will sooner reach a situation where they lack the physiological reserves to care for themselves or to withstand intercurrent infection. However, preservation of physical fitness will do little to counter many of the common causes of domestic incapacitation such as blindness or loss of memory. Nor will it influence the liability to some of the common causes of death in the Northwest Territories: accidents, suicides, and neoplasms.

AN INFLUENCE OF GENETIC ISOLATION?

The physiologist usually conceives of aging as a progressive deterioration of biological function, as discussed above. In contrast, the gerontologist views aging as a reduced ability to adapt to environmental stress, and as an increased probability of both cellular and organ death.

At the cellular level, death is a cumulative response to life's insults: exposure to free radicals, viruses and auto-antibodies, intracellular accumulation of debris, and a deterioration in the constancy of the internal environment. In the body as a whole, death or malfunction of key cells impairs general homeostasis, until sudden exertion, infection, or a change in the external environment becomes sufficient to terminate life.

Unusual longevity would in essence require the emergence of an unusually stable genetic material. Resistance of this DNA to environmental insults would reduce errors in transcription of the genetic code, postponing cell death. Less certainly, there would also be a shallower slope for such functions as the aging of maximum oxygen intake and lung volumes. In support of the potential for genetically endowed longevity, monozygous twins show a striking similarity of life-span (11). But arguments for the emergence and persistence of such a genetic variant in an arctic community are less persuasive. Even assuming appearance of a form of DNA that altered the rate of biological aging, or changed the likelihood of cellular death, this variant would influence prospects of survival only in the later part of adult life, at a time when mating and child-rearing had ceased. There would thus be little selective pressure favoring

transmission of this variant to subsequent generations.

Moreover, a relatively early death seems a necessary population adaptation to the harsh arctic habitat. From the viewpoint of the overall community, emergence of a gene for longevity would have had a disastrous impact upon an economy where food reserves were at best marginal.

ENVIRONMENTAL INFLUENCES

To date, many potential environmental influences upon the longevity of arctic communities have been overshadowed by the ravages of communicable disease and violent death.

Despite the favorable influence of a vigorous lifestyle upon the aging of physiological function, evidence from White communities does not suggest that regular exercise appreciably extends life-span (12). Indeed, Rübner (13) found that in animals there was an inverse relationship between energy expenditure per unit of body mass and life-span. Periodic shortages of food may indeed have had a beneficial impact upon the longevity of those surviving the acute famine (14), but the clear air of the Arctic is likely to have increased exposure to natural radiation, and there is no evidence that traditional diet provided any additional supply of anti-oxidants to counter mutagenic free radicals. Likewise, cold exposure seems to shorten life-span (15), partly because of associated socioeconomic disadvantages, and partly because metabolism is stimulated by cold exposure (16).

A further important variable has been a close kinship network. In White societies, "life-events" have a major impact upon mortality, and in the past a closely-knit, non-competitive and mutually supportive Inuit society has helped the individual to withstand such events. One unfortunate consequence of acculturation has been the disruption of such networks, with a parallel increase of mortality from such causes as suicide, alcoholism, and various "accidents".

A final adverse environmental change has been the progressive development of cigarette addiction. This appears likely to cause a substantial shortening of longevity over the next 10 to 20 years.

CONCLUSIONS

Traditional Inuit have enjoyed an advantage of biological age, particularly in the early part of adult life, but the subsequent rate of aging of function has been much as in a White community. The initial advantage of the Inuit reflects a high level of physical activity within traditional communities. Acculturation to a more sedentary lifestyle has brought about a deterioration in biological age of up to 20 years, without any change in the slope of the curve of functional aging. There is no evidence that exposure to the harsh arctic environment has led to the emergence of a genetic isolate with an unusual aging curve. Such a variant would influence survival mainly after the period of child-rearing, and transmission to a subsequent generation would thus be unlikely. Moreover, from the viewpoint of the community, excessive longevity would be a negative adaptation to an environment with limited food resources.

REFERENCES

1. Leaf A. Getting old. Scient Amer 1973; 229:44-54.
2. Mazess RB, Mathisen RW. Lack of unusual longevity in Vilcabamba, Ecuador. Hum Biol 1982; 54:517-524.
3. Mazess RB, Forman SH. Longevity and age exaggeration in Vilcabamba, Ecuador. J Gerontol 1979; 34:94-98.
4. Godin G, Shephard RJ. Activity patterns of the Canadian Eskimo. In: Edholm OG, Gunderson EK, eds. Polar human biology. London: William Heinemann Medical Books, 1973:193-215.
5. Shephard RJ. Human physiological work capacity. London: Cambridge University Press, 1978.
6. Rode A, Shephard RJ. Lung function in a cold environment--a current perspective. In: Fortuine R, ed. Circumpolar Health 84. Seattle: University of Washington Press, 1985 (this volume).
7. Rode A, Shephard RJ. "Future Shock" and the fitness of the Inuit. In: Fortuine R, ed. Circumpolar Health 84. Seattle: University of Washington Press, 1985 (this volume).
8. Jeppesen BB, Harvald B. Low incidence of urinary calculi in Greenland Eskimos as explained by a low calcium/magnesium ratio. In: Fortuine R, ed. Circumpolar Health 84. Seattle: University of Washington Press, 1985 (this volume).
9. Hassi J, Virokannas H, Anttonen H, Jarvenpaa I. Health hazards in snowmobile usage. Paper presented at 6th International Symposium on Circumpolar Health, May 13-18, 1984, Anchorage, Alaska.
10. Shephard RJ. Work physiology and activity patterns. In: F. Milan, ed. The human biology of circumpolar populations. London: Cambridge University Press, 1980: 305-338.
11. Kallman FJ, Sander G. Twin studies on aging and longevity. J Hered 1948; 39:349-357.
12. Shephard RJ. Physical activity and aging. London: Croom Helm, 1978.
13. Rübner M. Das Wachsthumsproblem und die Lebensdauern des Menschen und einiger Säugethiere vom energetischen Standpunkte aus betrachtet. Sber Preuss Akad Wiss, 1908:32-38.
14. Ross MH. Length of life and nutrition in the rat. J Nutrit 1961; 75:197-210.
15. Pearl R. The rate of living. Being an account of some experimental studies on the biology of life duration. New York: AA Knopf, 1928.
16. Johnson HD, Kintner LD, Kibler HH. Effects of 48°F (8.9°C) and 83°F (28.4°C) on longevity and pathology of male rats. J Gerontol 1961; 18:29-36.

Roy J. Shephard
School of Physical and Health Education
320 Huron Street
Toronto, Ontario M5S 1A1
Canada

Circumpolar Health 84:49-52

PHYSICAL FITNESS AND TRAINING PROGRAMS ON AN ANTARCTIC BASE

GRAHAM L. HURST

The men on a scientific station in Antarctica lead a very controlled and restricted lifestyle. This is very true at Faraday because of the geography of the area in which the base is situated. The station is on a small island some 5 km off the west coast of Graham Land Peninsula, at 65°16'S, 65°14'W. This island is only 1,000 m by 700 m and is for the most part covered with a crevassed icecap. Travel from the island is dependent on there being good weather and either stable sea ice for winter sledging or a calm sea for open boating in summer.

The base is a meteorological and geophysical observatory with all the living areas and most of the working areas situated within one building. Thus travel and exercise opportunities are quite limited.

The aims of this study were to investigate the effects on various physiological parameters of a year of life on an Antarctic base, to monitor the physical work capacity of the base members throughout the year and assess the need for any regular training programs to maintain fitness, and to assess two physical training schedules for their acceptability to base personnel and their effectiveness.

METHODS

During the austral winter of 1982 the base complement comprised 10 men: 6 scientists and 4 support staff. All base members took part in the study, which involved having measurements taken each month for a whole year.

The parameters measured included:

Resting Metabolic Rate (RMR)

Expired gas was collected over a 10 minute period using the open-circuit Douglas Bag method. The volume of gas was measured by drawing it through a calibrated dry gas meter and the oxygen concentration was measured with a paramagnetic oxygen analyzer. From the oxygen consumption the RMR was calculated using the formula of Weir (1).

Blood Pressure

Blood pressure was measured with the subject at rest in bed. The first and fifth Korotkoff sounds were taken as the indicators of the systolic and diastolic pressures, which were read from a mercury sphygmomanometer.

Pulse

The pulse rate was measured manually with the subject lying at rest.

Body Weight

Each subject was weighed on a platform balance in the morning prior to breakfast while wearing only underclothing.

Body Fat Percentage

Body fat was estimated using the method recommended by Durnin and Rahaman (2). The skinfold thickness was measured at the biceps, triceps, subscapular, and suprailiac sites using Harpenden calipers. From the mean skinfold thickness the body density was derived. Thence the percentage body fat was calculated, using the Siri equation.

Maximum Oxygen Uptake

Oxygen consumption was measured with each subject cycling at various workloads giving submaximal oxygen uptake. The VO_2max, an index of physical work capacity, was derived using the Astrand and Rhyming monogram and corrected for age (3,4).

Diary cards were used to estimate habitual physical activity (5). Five cards were issued to each subject per month; each card enabled a day's activities to be recorded to the nearest ten minutes. The metabolic cost of nine categories of activity was taken from a range of literature sources and thus the daily energy expenditure was derived.

TRAINING SCHEDULES

Two training schedules were evaluated: isometric quadriceps exercising and dynamic cycling. The progress of 3 groups was investigated:

Group 1: Three men cycled at an estimated 75% of VO_2max for 30 minutes 3 times per week for 14 weeks.

Group 2: Two men undertook an increasing number of maximal voluntary contractions (MVC) of both quadriceps muscles 3 times a week for 17 weeks.

Group 3: A control group of two men undertook no regular exercise training. The progress of all three groups was monitored by measuring VO_2max and MVC each month.

RESULTS

The change of the various physiological parameters throughout the year are shown in Figure 1. The means (± standard errors of the mean) are tabulated (Table 1).

The mean percentage time spent outside was above 19% for two months of the antarctic summer. Thereafter the time outside was

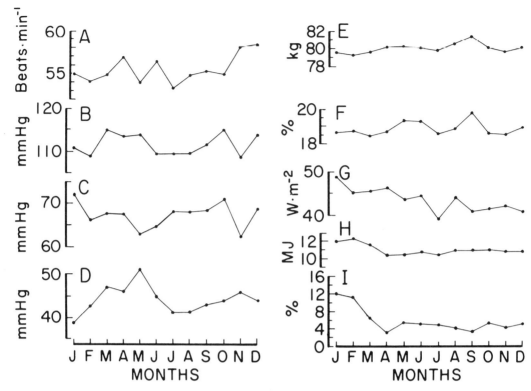

Figure 1. Changes over one year of the measured physiological parameters. A, pulse; B, systolic pressure; C, diastolic pressure; D, pulse pressure; E, body weight; F, body fat %; G, resting metabolic rate per surface area; H, energy expenditure per 70-kg man; and I, % time outside.

about 5% and there was little intermonth variation for the rest of the year. This was surprisingly low compared with previous studies at the British Antarctic Base at Halley Bay: Levack (6) found a mean percentage time outside of about 10% with a similar lack of intermonth variation; Norman showed a marked monthly change with monthly means ranging from 5% to 13%.

The mean daily energy expenditure was

11.1 MJ. Again, this was considerably lower than the findings of both Levack and Norman, who found mean daily energy expenditures of 15.3 and 14.2 MJ, respectively. A similarly low level of 11.5 MJ was reported among the base winterers of the Japanese Antarctic Research Expedition (8).

Figure 2 is a box-and-whisker plot showing change of physical work capacity over the whole year. The mean VO_2max of all

Table 1. Means and standard errors of the means of the physiological parameters for the year.

Variable	Mean	S.E.	Units
A	55.4	± 0.73	beats·min^{-1}
B	111.5	± 0.85	mm Hg
C	67.3	± 0.80	mm Hg
D	44.2	± 0.75	mm Hg
E	80.2	± 0.94	kg
F	18.9	± 0.34	W·m^{-2}
H	11.1	± 0.15	MJ
I	5.9	± 0.15	%

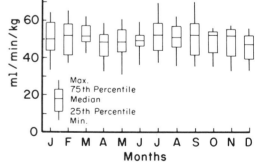

Figure 2. Physical work capacity: Box-and-Whisker plot showing changes of VO_2max over the year.

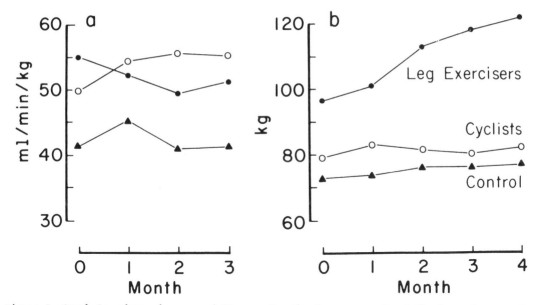

Figure 3. Graph 3a shows changes of VO_2 max for the 3 groups. Graph 3b shows changes of mean leg strength (MVC) for the 3 groups.

base members was 49.5 ml/min/kg. This value was higher than expected in view of the low activity levels and daily energy expenditures. It compares with 43 ml/min/kg at Halley Bay (6) and with 41.7 ml/min/kg among a cross-section of British army recruits (9).

The relationship between the parameters over the whole year was statistically examined. Exploratory analysis of the data was by the method of principal components. These were interpreted as being:

1. General component.
2. "Resting" metabolic state component.
3. "Active" state component.
4. Cardiovascular component.

A comparison was made between the principal components in February and September, which showed activity to be more important in the former and anthropometric parameters to be more important in the latter. This reflects the change in habitual activity patterns and energy expenditure with the season.

The changes of VO_2max and mean MVC for the 2 groups involved on the training programs are shown in Figure 3.

Statistical analysis of the result was by analysis of variance of repeated measurements design, with use being made of the conservative F-test. A level of significance of P=0.1 was used. Group 1: showed no significant changes of either VO_2max or mean MVC; Group 2: showed a significant increase in mean MVC but no VO_2max; Group 3: showed no significant changes of either parameter.

DISCUSSION

The lack of physiological response in those undertaking the cycling training program was surprising. It was most probably due to the nature of the training schedules. The cyclists were expected to exert themselves considerably more than the group undertaking isometric exercises. The former group showed less enthusiasm for their training sessions and probably did not cooperate fully with their efforts. The individual training sessions were not supervised by the author.

CONCLUSIONS

The main conclusions drawn were:
1. The habitual energy expenditure was low compared with previous studies on a British Antarctic Base;
2. The percentage time outside was low for all except the few months of the short summer;
3. Physical fitness was greater than might be expected, being higher than that found at another BAS base and among a cross section of British army recruits;
4. Only the group undertaking a program of isometric training achieved any physiological response. This was considered due to the greater motivation required for continuation of the cycling program.

ACKNOWLEDGMENTS

The author thanks Mr. M. G. Gibson of RGIT School of Mathematics and Computer Studies, Dr. S. Wilcock and Professor J. N.

Norman of RGIT Centre for Offshore Health, the base members of the Faraday Station, and the British Antarctic Survey.

REFERENCES

1. Consolazio CF, Johnson RE, Pecora LJ. Physiological measurements of metabolic functions on man. McGraw Hill, 1963.
2. Durnin JVGA, Rahaman MM. The assessment of the amount of fat in the human body from measurements of skinfold thickness. Br J Nutr 1967; 21:681.
3. Astrand PO, Ryhming I. A nomogram for calculation of aerobic capacity (physical fitness) from pulse rate during submaximal work. J Appl Physiol 1954; 7:218-221.
4. Astrand I. Aerobic work capacity in men and women with special reference to age. Acta Physiol Scand 1960; 49:Suppl 169.
5. Durnin JVGA, Passmore R. Energy, work and leisure. Heinemann Educational Books Ltd., 1967.
6. Levack I. The physical effects of living in Antarctica. University of Aberdeen, MD Thesis, 1980.
7. Norman JN. Cold exposure and patterns of activity on a polar station. BAS Bull 1965; 6:1-13.
8. Ohkubo Y. Basal metabolism and other physiological changes in wintering members of Japanese Antarctic Research Expedition, 1968-1969. Bull Tokyo Med Dent Univ 1972; 19:245-269.
9. Vogel JA, Crowdy JP. Aerobic fitness and body fat of young British males entering the army. Eur J Appl Physiol 1979; 40:73-83.

Graham L. Hurst
Centre for Offshore Health
Robert Gordon's Institute of Technology
Viewfield Road
Aberdeen AB9 2PF
Great Britain

ACCLIMATIZATION TO COLD IN ANTARCTIC SCUBA DIVERS

S.A. BRIDGMAN

Whether man acclimatizes to cold is still a matter of controversy (1,2). Several investigations have been carried out in Antarctica but one central problem is whether the men studied were sufficiently cold stressed (1,3). Previous work has shown that the SCUBA divers at Signy Station are subject to a considerable cold stress while diving (4). The aim of the current work was to investigate the theory that the divers at Signy acclimatize to cold.

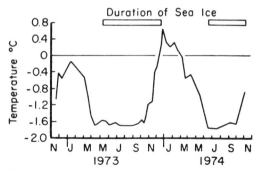

Figure 2. *Typical sea water temperature and sea ice duration at Signy, 1973-4.*

MATERIALS AND METHODS

This study was performed at the British Antarctic Survey's biological station on Signy Island (60°43'S, 45°36'W), in the South Orkney Islands (Figure 1). The shores of these islands are bathed, throughout most of the year, by the very cold Weddell Sea Current, so that the sea temperature rarely rises above 1°C and fast ice forms in the winter (Figure 2). Signy has a typical maritime Antarctic climate (6). Climatic data recorded during this study are summarized in Table 1.

Diving is an invaluable aid to underwater biological research, as it allows scientists direct access to their work. In winter, diving is under the ice and is usually assisted by snowmobile and sledge transport to the dive site, while in summer it is in open water and is usually from boats. Some dives are from the shore in all seasons. For thermal protection, divers wore 7 mm single-lined Neoprene wet-suits, which consisted of a longjohn and a combined jacket and hood, with mittens and booties. There were 209 dives at Signy between December 1981 and November 1982. Most were working dives although a few were for recreation. The number of dives per

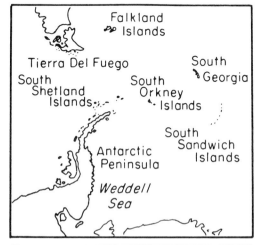

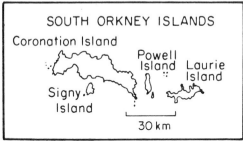

Figure 1. *Map of the Antarctic Peninsula and South Orkney Islands.*

Table 1. *Climatic Data at Signy December 1981 to November 1982.*

Mean annual temperature	-2.8°C
Highest mean monthly temperature	2.3°C (January)
Extreme high temperature*	19.6°C (January)
Coldest mean monthly temperature	-13.4°C (July)
Extreme cold temperature	-28.0°C (August)
Mean annual wind speed	13.2 knots (March)
Extreme maximum gust	73 knots (April)

* New record for Signy, 3.6°C greater than previous highest.

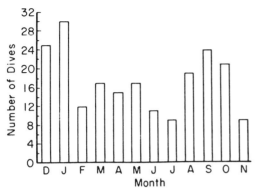

Figure 3. Dives per month, from December 1981 to November 1982.

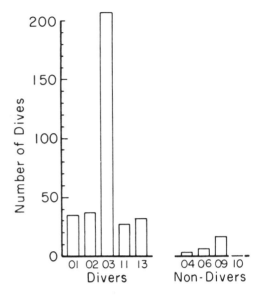

Figure 4. Dives per subject, from December 1981 to November 1982.

month is shown in Figure 3. Table 2 gives further information about these dives.

Nine of the 13 men who overwintered at Signy in 1982 participated in this project. All were Caucasians. Subjects were classified as divers, which included the diving officer and 4 other divers who assisted him when required, and non-divers. The number of dives per subject is shown in Figure 4. Further information about the subjects is given in Tables 3 and 4.

Body Immersion Experiments

Subjects underwent a monthly cold stress of sitting for one hour, immersed to the neck, in a tank of water at 20°C with an estimated average velocity of 0.02 m/sec. Rectal temperature (Tre) and skin temperatures were measured with thermistors. Mean skin temperature (Tsk) was calculated using a modified Hardy and Dubois method (8) and mean body temperature (Tb) was calculated from the following formula from Burton (9);

$$Tb = 0.65Tre + 0.35Tsk$$

Oxygen consumption was estimated by an open circuit method, using polythene Douglas Bags, a paramagnetic oxygen analyzer, and a dry gas meter. Metabolic heat production was calculated from oxygen consumption, using the method of Weir (10).

Thermal comfort, shivering, and pre- and post-immersion urinary epinephrine, norepinephrine, cortisol, and creatinine were also measured.

Local Acclimatization Experiments

Subjects' left index fingers were immersed monthly for 30 minutes in well-stirred iced water. Temperature and assessment of pain were recorded and the time of onset of cold-induced vasodilatation (CIVD) noted.

RESULTS

Some of the results of the body immersion experiments are illustrated in Figures 5 and 6. Figure 7 illustrates time of onset of CIVD in the finger immersion experiments.

In the body immersion experiments, rectal, mean body and mean skin temperatures were analyzed at 0, 20, 40, and 60 minutes of immersion and heat production at 17.5, 37.5 and 57.5 minutes of immersion. In the

Table 2. Further information on dives at Signy December 1981 to November 1982.

	Mean	Range
Duration of dives (min)	30.0	5 to 90
Depth of SCUBA dives (m)	9	2 to 41
Ambient temperature (°C)	-1.87	-27 to +7
Wind speed (knots)	9.6	0 to 33
No. of snorkel dives	34	(out of 209 total)
No. of under ice dives	57	(out of 209 total)

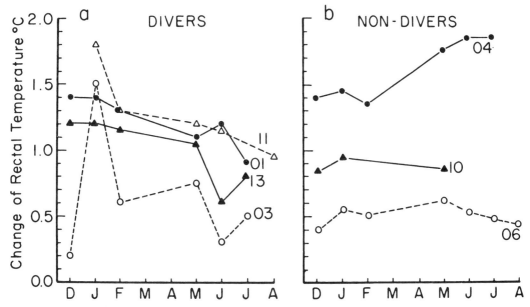

Figure 5. Changes in divers' (A) and non-divers' (B) rectal temperatures after one hour's body immersion in water at 20°C.

finger immersion experiment, mean onset of CIVD was analyzed. Null hypotheses, (Table 5), were tested with analysis of variance techniques, using the conservative F test at the 5% significance level.

As expected, temperatures dropped with time. These were the only statistically significant results, although physiological differences did occur between subjects. Further statistical analyses are being undertaken on these and other results.

DISCUSSION

Preliminary analysis of the data has indicated that there were no significant differences between divers and non-divers, and that there were no seasonal changes in either group, at Signy in 1982, for the variables tested. Several individual or combinations of reasons could explain these findings. For example, it may be that the divers were not diving enough to produce

Table 3. Age, occupation and previous Antarctic experience of all subjects December 1981 to December 1982.

Subject	Age at 1/1/82	Occupation	Previous Antarctic experience
A) Divers			
01	24	Medical Officer	N
02	27	Boatman/Handyman	N
03*	31	Diving Officer/Marine Assistant	N
11	23	Cook	W
13	26	Freshwater Biologist	N
B) Non-divers			
04	24	Limnologist	W
06	25	Terrestrial Biology Assistant	W
09	24	Limnology Assistant/Meteorologist	W
10	23	Diesel Mechanic	N

N=New recruit in 1982; W=Wintered in 1981 also.
* Subject had previous Antarctic diving experience.

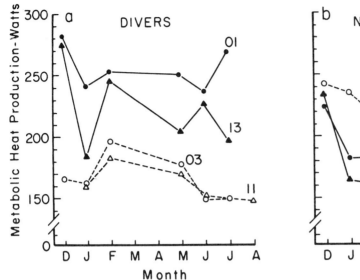 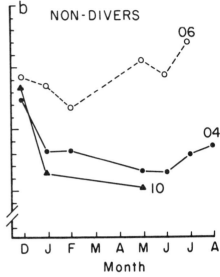

Figure 6.   Divers' (A) and non-divers' (B) mean levels of metabolic heat production after one hour's body immersion in water at 20°C.

Table 4.   Resting metabolic rate (RMR), mean body weight, mean % body fat, and height of all subjects December 1981 to December 1982.

Subject	RMR(W)	Weight (kg)	% Body fat*	Height(m)
A) Divers				
01	67	66.9	14.1	1.69
02	80	74.2	13.7	1.85
03	95	88.9	22.8	1.76
11	96	95.6	21.3	1.90
13	88	75.6	18.5	1.87
B) Non-divers				
04	94	76.3	13.2	1.78
06	83	72.0	20.0	1.73
09	79	72.2	22.4	1.78
10	91	93.9	22.1	1.91

* % Body fat was estimated from Durnin and Rahaman (7).

Table 5.   Hypotheses tested statistically.

1)   No differences exist between groups (divers and non-divers).
2)   No differences exist between months.
3)   No differences exist between times.
4)   No interactions exist between groups and months.
5)   No interactions exist between groups and times.
6)   No interactions exist between months and times.
7)   No interactions exist between groups, months and times.

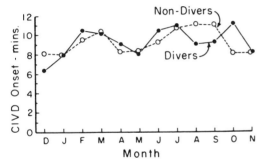

*Figure 7. Mean onset of cold induced vaso-
dilatation in divers compared to
non-divers.*

acclimatization. Alternatively, any acclimatization may have been masked by some
subjects having had previous Antarctic
experience or having acclimatized before
their first experiments. Also the small
subject groups may have led to any acclimatization being statistically insignificant.
On the other hand, physiological acclimatization to cold may not exist.

CONCLUSIONS

No evidence of physiological or local
acclimatization to cold has been found in
the Antarctic divers studied here.

ACKNOWLEDGMENTS

I am indebted to the following:
British Antarctic Survey, for financial
support; M. Gibson (Department of Mathematics, RGIT) for statistical assistance; M.H.
Motherwell SRN for help with data handling;
Dr. S.W. Wilcock and Professor N. Norman
(both at Centre for Offshore Health) for
advice on presentation; Dr. I.M. Light,
(Offshore Survival Centre, RGIT), for help
in setting up this project; Dr. R.M.
Hastings, (Centre for Offshore Health), for
permission to use a figure; last, but not
least, all my stoic subjects.

REFERENCES

1. Edholm OG, Weiner JS. In: Principles
   and practice of human physiology.
   London: Academic Press, 1981:155-156.
2. Goldsmith R. Acclimatization to heat
   and cold in man. In: Baron DN, et al,
   eds. Recent advances in medicine no.
   17. Edinburgh: Churchill Livingstone,
   1977:299-317.
3. Norman JN. Cold exposure and patterns
   of activity at a polar station. Brit
   Antarct Surv Bull 1965; 6:1-13.
4. Light IM. Prevention and management of
   cold exposure in remote locations, Chap
   5. Univ Aberdeen PhD Thesis, 1980.
5. Hastings RM. An investigation into the
   primary productivity of the Antarctic
   macro-alga *Phyllogigas grandifolius*.
   Univ St Andrew's PhD Thesis, 1977.
6. Holdgate MW. Terrestrial ecology in
   the maritime Antarctic. In: Carrick R,
   Holdgate MW, Prevost J, eds. Biologie
   antarctique. Paris: Hermann, 1964:181-
   194.
7. Durnin JVGA, Rahaman MM. The assessment of the amount of fat in the human
   body from measurements of skinfold
   thickness. Br J Nutr 1967; 21:681-689.
8. Hardy JD, Dubois EF. The technic of
   measuring radiation and convection. J
   Nutr 1938; 15:461-475.
9. Burton AC. Human calorimetry 2. The
   average temperature of the tissues of
   the body. J Nutr 1935; 9:261-280.
10. Weir JB deV. New methods for calculat-
    ing metabolic rate with special refer-
    ence to protein metabolism. J Physiol
    1949; 109:1-9.

S.A. Bridgman
British Antarctic Survey and Centre
 for Offshore Health
Robert Gordon's Institute of Technology
Kepplestone Mansion
Viewfield Road
Aberdeen, Scotland
U.K.

Circumpolar Health 84:58-59

HYPOTHERMIC HEMODILUTION HYPOKALEMIA

RAY A. DIETER, JR.

As modern technology advances, variations from normal are encountered with increasing frequency. These changes come about as a result of both natural phenomena and man-made or induced changes from the norm. With the increased variation from the norm, the consequence or variance in other modalities or related areas becomes more pronounced and requires further concern and monitoring. The stimulus of such knowledge and problems encourages the further pursuit of research into areas previously rejected or with which we had little information to work. The recent upsurge of interest in hypothermic drowning and the potential salvage of these individuals has been emphasized in the news headlines over the past two winters. The 4-year-old boy from Chicago who slipped into Lake Michigan and was rescued, transported, resuscitated, and eventually discharged from the hospital is such an example. The use of cardiopulmonary bypass in these individuals is a valuable aid to resuscitation and ultimate survival. With such efforts, however, side effects or complications may occur. One concern revolves about the electrolyte status of the patient and, in particular, the potassium response. This paper presents data on the effects of hypothermic hemodilution on the serum potassium (K+).

MATERIALS AND METHODS

Thirty men who weighed 48 to 98 kilograms (mean 65 kilograms) were studied. Their age varied from 21 to 69 years of age. These patients all underwent cardiopulmonary (C-P) bypass utilizing Ringer's lactate (24 patients) or 5% dextrose in Ringer's lactate (6 patients) as the perfusate. All patients were on digitalis, and one-half of the patients were on diuretics preoperatively. The latter were discontinued 48 to 72 hours prior to surgery. The average perfusate volume utilized per patient was 3,163 cc. All patients had 44.6 mEq of sodium bicarbonate added to the pump initially, and 18 patients received an additional supplement.

Moderate hypothermia to 32.5°C was used. Perfusion times varied between 37 and 263 minutes (the average was 109 minutes). Blood was transfused as necessary in 28 of the 30 patients. Mitral and aortic valve replacement was the usual operation performed. Urine and serum potassium levels were monitored.

RESULTS

Urine studies were completed in 21 patients. Preoperatively, the 24-hour urine volume averaged 1,850 cc in those who had been on diuretics and 1,635 cc in those with cardiac arrhythmias. The diuretic patients had an average 24-hour urine potassium of 67 mEq, and the arrhythmia group averaged 37.4 mEq. During surgery, the diuretic group averaged 19.1 mEq K+, and the nondiuretic group averaged 14.9 mEq K+ excreted. Following surgery, the urine output was substantially decreased in both the diuretic and nondiuretic groups. The diuretic patients excreted nearly double the urine K+, both preoperatively and postoperatively, in comparison to the nondiuretic group (Table 1). Postoperatively, patients with arrhythmias excreted approximately 30% more K+ than did patients with no arrhythmias. The average serum K+ (Table 2) was 4.3 mEq/l preoperatively (range 3.3 to 5.5), 3.8 mEq/l during C-P bypass, 3.9 mEq/l on arrival in intensive care, 3.42 mEq/l (range 2.4 to 4.3) during the next 3 days postoperatively, and 4.0 mEq/l at the end of one week. The preoperative diuretic group had the greatest serum K+ depletion (1.10 mEq/l) as compared to the nondiuretic group (0.78 mEq/l). Patients receiving 4 or fewer transfusions and on diuretics preoperatively showed the greatest postoperative serum K+ depletion. Four of 7 patients developing arrhythmias were in this group, and 6 of 7 developing arrhythmias received 4 or fewer transfusions. The mean tissue K+ was 88.5 mEq/kg preoperatively and 83.6 mEq/kg postoperatively.

Table 1. Urine K+ (mEq) in diuretic and non-diuretic patients.

	Pre-op	OR	18 hr.	PO2	PO3
Diuretic	35.7	14.9	29.0	34.0	38.9
Non-diuretic	67.0	19.1	62.0	73.3	80.6

Table 2. Post-pump serum K+ (mEq per liter) in diuretic and non-diuretic patients.

	Non-diuretic	Diuretic
Immediate	4.11	3.75
3 days	3.55	3.28
Serum K+ depletion	0.78	1.10

DISCUSSION

The serum, urine, and tissue K+ values were determined preoperatively, during surgery, and postsurgery. These values were determined in 30 patients undergoing moderate hypothermia (to 32.5°C) and hemodilution C-P bypass. The patients all underwent cardiac surgical procedures and were monitored throughout their course for the various parameters. When C-P bypass was initially utilized, the priming solution was usually whole blood. Subsequent to wider experience in C-P bypass techniques, wider research in priming solutions for use in the oxygenator, and the need for emergency C-P bypass without blood typing/cross match delays, the use of balanced salt solutions for the oxygenator was advocated (1). Electrolyte monitoring began to show hypokalemia to be a concern postsurgically in these patients, especially in the preoperative diuretic-digitalis groups. Posthemodilution hypothermic C-P bypass patients maintained on the respirator with the consequent respiratory alkalosis seem to be at particular risk (2,3). These patients continue to lose K+ in the urine postsurgically and therefore are at a greater risk.

As noted, our postoperative patients continued to lose K+ and demonstrated a prolonged serum K+ depletion, despite the addition of incremental therapeutic doses of K+ to the patient. Treatment of the postoperative metabolic acidosis with sodium bicarbonate may potentiate the hypokalemia by the development of a metabolic alkalosis(4). Patients receiving blood transfusions had a greater diuresis postoperatively and more available K+ to utilize intracellularly or to diurese. Hypoxic acidosis was avoided by use of the mechanical respirator. This, however, leads to the creation of a respiratory alkalosis and leads to an increased K+ loss. Increased adrenal cortical hormones are secreted after surgery and may further play a role in or potentiate urine K+ loss (5). Hypokalemia, thus resulting, may lead to serious arrhythmias, especially in the patient with total body depletion. Such hypokalemic patients may be particularly susceptible to arrhythmias when receiving digitalis preparations (6). When patients require emergency C-P bypass for supportive or therapeutic purposes, the preoperative condition of the patient is not thoroughly studied nor adequately prepared. Therefore, the variety of conditions which present themselves to the treating physician may be extreme and most challenging. The patient may be essentially normal, except for the one factor now superimposed on him requiring C-P bypass--such as profound hypothermic fresh water drowning, massive pulmonary embolus, or acute valve disruption. Or the patient may be an elderly cardiac on multiple drugs with profound depletion of proteins and electrolytes. Such patients who require treatment with hemodilution hypothermic cardiopulmonary bypass techniques need to have multiple system monitoring. This monitoring should include frequent serum and urine K+ studies and temperature probes (bladder, rectal, and/or esophageal) to avoid temperature drift, resultant changes in circulatory volume, areas of hypoperfusion, and hypokalemia-induced arrhythmias.

SUMMARY

The serum, urine, and tissue K+ levels were monitored in a series of patients undergoing cardiac surgical procedures. Preoperative, operative, and postoperative values were determined while utilizing moderate hypothermia (to 32.5°C) and hemodilution (Ringer's lactate) techniques. These patients demonstrated a progressive serum K+ depletion and an increased incidence of arrhythmias in the diuretic low blood transfusion patient. Further, K+ depletion is partly due to continued K+ loss postoperatively in the urine. Careful K+ monitoring and infusion, where indicated, is recommended following hypothermic hemodilution cardiopulmonary bypass.

REFERENCES

1. Neville WE. In: Ravitch M, ed. Extracorporeal circulation-- current problems in surgery. Year Book Medical Publishers. 1967:67.
2. Dieter, RA Jr, Pifarre R, Neville WE. Serum electrolyte changes following cardiopulmonary bypass using Ringer's lactate hemodilution. J Thorac Cardiovasc Surg (In press).
3. Flemma RJ, Young WG Jr. The metabolic effects of mechanical ventilation and respiratory alkalosis in postoperative patients. Surgery 1964; 56:36.
4. Dieter RA, Neville WE, Pifarre R. Hypokalemia following hemodilution cardiopulmonary bypass. Ann Surg 1970; 171:17-23.
5. Krohn BG, Magidson O, Lewis RR, Tsuji HK, Redington JV, Kay JH. Prevention of metabolic alkalosis following heart surgery. J Thorac Cardiovasc Surg 1968; 56:748.
6. Surawicz B. Role of electrolytes in the etiology and measurements of cardiac arrhythmia. Prog Cardiovasc Dis 1966; 8:364.

Ray A. Dieter, Jr.
454 Pennsylvania Avenue
c/o Glen Ellyn Clinic
Glen Ellyn, Illinois 60137
U.S.A.

Circumpolar Health 84:60-63

LUNG FUNCTION IN A COLD ENVIRONMENT: A CURRENT PERSPECTIVE

ANDRIS RODE and ROY J. SHEPHARD

Some previous authors, particularly Beaudry (1) and Schaefer (2), have noted a relatively poor lung function in the people of arctic communities. Low lung volumes have been associated with enlargement of the pulmonary arteries and a high incidence of electrocardiographic abnormalities which have been ascribed to cold-induced pulmonary damage. Our own research has suggested that "Eskimo lung" is a rarity (3). If there is indeed a cold-induced deterioration of lung function, however, it should now be diminishing since one consequence of acculturation has been a progressive reduction in cold exposure among the indigenous populations. Accordingly, we have carried out cross-sectional and longitudinal determinations of the aging of lung function in the Canadian Inuit community of Igloolik.

METHODS

All measurements of lung function were made by the same observer during the winters of 1970-71 and 1980-81, using a modern 13.5-liter low resistance Stead-Wells spirometer. At the time of the initial survey, many of the population were still making long and frequent hunting trips, but by 1980-81 the majority of the settlement had adopted a more sedentary lifestyle. The proportion of self-reported cigarette smokers among those over the age of 14 years had also increased from 64% of males and 85% of females in 1970-71 to 81% of males and 93% of females in 1980-81. Moreover, the average daily cigarette consumption by the smokers had risen from

11.8 in the men and 7.4 in the women to 20.2 in the men and 12.0 in the women.

On both occasions we tested all of the Igloolik population over the age of 9 years who were willing to complete the tests. We were successful in recruiting a high percentage of those living in the settlement, about 75% of the men and 60% of the women. Medical records allowed us to distinguish those with a prior history of respiratory disease from those with healthy lungs. Only 2 men in the village showed minor right ventricular bundle branch block, and there were no recorded cases of "Eskimo lung". However, about 10% of the adults had a history of chronic respiratory disease (usually primary or secondary tuberculosis).

RESULTS

Looking at the data first in cross-sectional fashion, we fitted the standard type of age and height regression equations to our data, using multiple regression techniques. Figures for men (Table 1) showed a substantial increase in the partial coefficient for aging from 8.3 ml/yr in 1970-71 to 31.4 ml/yr in 1980-81; this change led to an increase in typical predicted lung volumes for the young adult, but a marked decrease in typical predicted volumes for the 60 year old. Results for females show a similar general trend. This pattern of aging seems due entirely to the presence of a diseased cohort within the Igloolik community, and when the equations were recalculated excluding diseased sub-

Table 1. *Equations for the prediction of FVC in Canadian Inuit men as calculated by multiple regression analysis, with typical values for male, height 165 cm.*

	Typical values	
	Age 20	Age 60
All men		
1970 = -7.90 - 0.0083A + 0.0788H	4.93	4.60
1980 = -6.19 - 0.0314A + 0.0738H	5.36	4.11
Healthy men		
1970 = -4.57 - 0.0204A + 0.0617H	5.20	4.39
1980 = -4.78 - 0.0224A + 0.0643H	5.38	4.49
Men with a history of respiratory disease		
1980 = -9.69 - 0.0311A + 0.0940H	5.20	3.95

Table 2. *Equations for the prediction of FEV$_{1.0}$ in Canadian Inuit men as calculated by multiple regression analysis, with typical volumes for male, height 165 cm.*

	Typical values	
	Age 20	Age 60
All men		
1970 = -5.28 - 0.0193A + 0.0584H	3.97	3.20
1980 = -4.28 - 0.0353A + 0.0566H	4.35	2.94
Healthy men		
1970 = -2.88 - 0.0240A + 0.0455H	4.15	3.19
1980 = -4.14 - 0.0269A + 0.0549H	4.38	3.13
Men with a history of respiratory disease		
1980 = -4.95 - 0.0367A + 0.0599H	4.20	2.73

jects, no significant differences of aging coefficients were found between the 1970-71 and 1980-81 surveys.

The same type of picture emerges for cross-sectional analyses of forced expiratory volume (FEV$_{1.0}$) (Table 2). If all members of the community are included in the multiple regression equations, the predicted lung function of the typical 60 year old male shows a decrease from 1970-71 to 1980-81. If diseased subjects are excluded, however, a small improvement in lung function can be seen in the 20 year old subjects, with no deterioration of FEV1.0 in the 60 year old individuals.

When the data are examined in a true longitudinal fashion (Table 3), there is a plainly accelerating curve of aging from those subjects who were initially aged 20 to 29 through those initially aged 30 to 39 to those initially aged 40 to 49 years, this being true of both forced vital capacity (FVC) and FEV$_{1.0}$, and also of both men and women. Such a pattern is at variance with the normal course of aging of lung

function through the middle adult years, but is again readily explicable in terms of the passage through the Igloolik community of a cohort who developed tuberculosis in the 1950s who were subsequently successfully treated, but who still have some residual impairment of lung function.

The lung function of the people of Igloolik continues to develop until the early twenties. Accordingly, it is appropriate to include all young people aged 9 to 19 years in logarithmic equations describing growth of lung function in the community (Table 4). Other factors being equal, one might expect lung volumes to increase as the third power of height (4) although southern communities do not always reach this standard, particularly for girls, because of limited fitness and weakness of the chest muscles. When the Igloolik population was tested in 1970-71, the boys exceeded the theoretical exponent of 3.0 for both FVC and FEV$_{1.0}$, the girls reached an exponent of 3.01 for vital capacity, but had an exponent of only 2.50

Table 3. *Longitudinal data showing loss of lung function (L,BTPS) in Inuit men and women over 10 years (1970-71 to 1980-81).*

Initial age	FVC		FEV$_{1.0}$	
	Men	Women	Men	Women
20-29	-0.13	-0.11	-0.23*	-0.03
30-39	-0.47***	-0.23**	-0.42***	-0.29***
40-49	-0.70***	-0.38**	-0.54***	-0.36***

*** P < 0.01
** P < 0.025
* P < 0.05

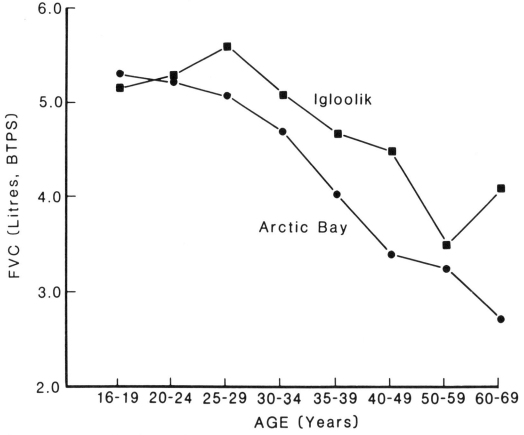

Figure 1. *Cross-sectional comparison of FVC in Inuit men from Igloolik (squares) and Arctic Bay (circles). (At body temperature, pressure, saturated with water vapor, BTPS).*

Table 4. *Cross-sectional comparison of logarithmic equations describing growth of lung function in Inuit children aged 9 to 19 years.*

Forced expiratory volume

Boys	Girls
$1970 = 1.76 \times 10^{-7} \times H^{3.31}$	$1970 = 1.07 \times 10^{-7} \times H^{2.50}$
$1980 = 2.16 \times 10^{-7} \times H^{3.29}$	$1980 = 5.20 \times 10^{-7} \times H^{3.11}$

Forced vital capacity

Boys	Girls
$1970 = 2.55 \times 10^{-7} \times H^{3.28}$	$1970 = 9.72 \times 10^{-7} \times H^{3.01}$
$1980 = 1.30 \times 10^{-7} \times H^{3.43}$	$1980 = 1.36 \times 10^{-7} \times H^{3.41}$

---

for the more effort-dependent $FEV_{1.0}$ measurement. Repetition of the tests in 1980-81 confirmed the impression already mentioned that young adults had a better lung function than in 1970-71. In particular, the exponents and thus predicted volumes were increased for both boys and girls.

DISCUSSION

Schaefer published cross-sectional data for pulmonary volumes measured on male Inuit living in the smaller community of Arctic Bay in 1980 (5). In young men, his findings agree closely with our data, but his cross-sectional curves suggest a faster rate of aging of function than we observed in Igloolik. We illustrate in Figure 1 the FVC data for Igloolik and Arctic Bay: curves for $FEV_{1.0}$ and maximum mid-expiratory flow rate follow a similar general pattern. There are a few miners in Arctic Bay, but we do not believe that either the proportion of miners or the extent of pneumoconiosis among present miners is sufficient to explain this difference of lung function results between the two communities. Arctic Bay is about 400 km north of Igloolik, but both settlements have equally harsh climates. There is thus no intrinsic reason to anticipate greater risk of freezing of the lung in the Arctic Bay region, although caribou hunters at Arctic Bay must travel somewhat farther than their Igloolik counterparts in search of game. Nor is there reason to anticipate a faster development of cigarette smoking at Arctic Bay than at Igloolik. Our data have already shown the marked impact of a diseased cohort upon the apparent aging of lung function, and it is logical to anticipate (as we have previously demonstrated in Igloolik) that a medical team will attract a higher proportion of volunteers with healed lung disease. The important lesson to draw from comparison of results for the two communities is that when examining aging curves for any population, southern or Inuit, subjects with healed respiratory disease must be excluded from the sample if the aging curve is not to be distorted.

A further practical point in the setting of standards for the Inuit population is that our longitudinal data have shown a rapid decrease of adult stature with age (some 2 cm per decade). We are still exploring reasons for this, and we need to consider further whether shortening of the spinal column leads to a parallel restriction of lung function.

Finally, looking ahead to the next decade, it is disturbing to note the ever increasing consumption of cigarettes, particularly by adolescents and young adults. This has not yet apparently had any marked effect upon standard spirometric test scores, but the effects of tobacco smoke are necessarily slow and insidious. A major impact of this adverse lifestyle must thus be anticipated over the next 10 to 20 years.

REFERENCES

1. Beaudry PH. Pulmonary function of the Canadian eastern Arctic Eskimo. Arch Environ Hlth, 1968; 17:524-528.
2. Schaefer O. Knud Rasmussen memorial lecture--Ethnology, demography, and medicine in the Arctic. In: Harvald B and Hart Hansen JP, eds. Circumpolar Health 81. Nordic Council Arct Med Res Rep 1982; 33:187-193.
3. Rode A, Shephard RJ. Pulmonary function of Canadian Eskimos. Scand J Resp Dis 1973; 54:191-205.
4. Astrand PO, Rodahl K. Textbook of work physiology. New York: McGraw-Hill, 1970.
5. Schaefer O, Eaton RDP, Timmermans FJW, Hildes JA. Respiratory function impairment and cardiopulmonary consequences in long-time residents of the Canadian Arctic. Can Med Assoc J 1980; 123:997-1004.

Andris Rode
General Delivery
Igloolik, N.W.T. X0A 0L0
Canada

Circumpolar Health 84:64-65

RURAL-URBAN DIFFERENCES IN LUNG SIZE AND FUNCTION IN ICELAND

JÓHANN AXELSSON, J. G. OSKARSSON, GUDRUN PÉTURSDÓTTIR, ANTHONY B. WAY, N. SIGFÚSSON and M. KARLSSON

INTRODUCTION

The unusual genetic homogeneity of the Icelandic population provides unique opportunities for epidemiological studies, as the inferences which may be made from quantitative findings are often more clearcut than those which would be warranted by studies on more heterogeneous populations.

The results reported here provide an illustration. They represent only a tiny fraction of the findings of our joint project with the Icelandic Heart Association, a project aimed at assessing the relative importance of genetic and environmental factors in chronic disease through comparative studies of various Icelandic subpopulations.

Here, lung size and function are compared in rural and urban dwelling Icelanders. The urban dwellers studied were residents of greater Reykjavik, a thickly inhabited area with a population of approximately 160,000. The rural population included residents of Thingeyjarsyslur in northeast Iceland and Fljótsdalshérad in east Iceland. Both are thinly populated farming areas which include small centers of fishing, light industry, and commerce.

MATERIALS AND METHODS

Between November 1967 and December 1968, the Icelandic Heart Association measured forced vital capacity (FVC) and forced expiratory volume in one second ($FEV_{1.0}$) in 1962 male residents of greater Reykjavik, aged 34 to 60 (1). In 1979-80 we measured these same parameters in 131 individuals of both sexes, aged 31 to 60, residing in Fljótsdalshérad.

From the measurements of FVC and $FEV_{1.0}$, figures for FEV%, that is, $FEV_{1.0}$ expressed as a percentage of FVC, were calculated.

RESULTS

A comparison of the figures obtained for rural and urban dwelling males, aged 31 to 60, revealed that: first, the height-adjusted mean FVC of rural males markedly exceeded that of urban males in all age groups; and second, that again in all age groups and even more markedly, the height-adjusted mean $FEV_{1.0}$ of rural males exceeded that of urban males.

The differences in mean FVC found among rural and urban dwelling males in various age groups are summarized in Table 1. It is evident from this table that the striking rural-urban differences in mean FVC, which ranged from 540 ml in the 56 to 60 age group up to 780 ml in the 41 to 45 age group, cannot be explained by differences in mean height or age.

The differences in mean $FEV_{1.0}$ found among rural and urban-dwelling males in various age groups are reflected in Table 2, which reports calculated FEV%. These values indicate that the mean $FEV_{1.0}$ of rural males exceeds that of urban males to a degree even greater than that observed for FVC.

Table 1. Mean figures for height and FVC in rural and urban dwelling Icelandic males aged 31 to 60 yrs.

Age	Number of Individuals		Mean Height in cm		Mean FVC in liters*		Difference in FVC rural minus urban in liters
	Rural	Urban	Rural	Urban	Rural	Urban	
31-35	22	137	179.2	179.9	5.71(.52)	5.10(.57)	0.16
36-40	22	138	178.1	179.1	5.50(.61)	4.95(.67)	0.55
41-45	19	450	177.5	177.7	5.58(.68)	4.80(.68)	0.78
46-50	12	576	176.6	175.7	5.19(.39)	4.50(.71)	0.69
51-55	20	461	175.6	175.4	5.13(.59)	4.39(.69)	0.74
56-60	19	200	175.5	174.3	4.76(.63)	4.22(.67)	0.54

* Standard deviation in parentheses.

Table 2. Mean figures for FEV% in rural and urban-dwelling Icelandic males aged 31 to 60 years.

AGE	MEAN FEV%	
	Rural	Urban
31-35	87%	81%
36-40	86%	82%
41-45	84%	81%
46-50	81%	80%
51-55	81%	79%
56-60	80%	77%

DISCUSSION

Only males are here compared, because the relevant data for urban Icelandic females have not yet been made available. Indications are, however, that the rural-urban differences here reported for males will prove to be at least as great in females.

Additional findings for males in Thingeyjarsyslur, another thinly populated farming and fishing area in northeastern Iceland are not reflected in our tables, as the male population studied there was younger (aged 7 to 35) than that studied in greater Reykjavik. However, the data collected from Thingeyjarsyslur support indirectly the significance of our findings: no significant differences between the two rural populations have been discovered, which lends strength to the assumption that the Fljótsdalshérad population is a representative rural Icelandic population.

CONCLUSION

We conclude from the reported findings that environmental differences between rural and urban areas have marked effects upon lung size and function. This is a much stronger conclusion that would be warranted by similar findings obtained from a less genetically homogeneous population than the one studied here. In many localities, rural populations differ genetically from urban populations to an extent that would render uncertain the conclusion that observed rural-urban differences are due to environmental factors. But everything we know seems to indicate that the population of greater Reykjavik is not genetically differentiable from rural populations in other parts of Iceland. This is due not only to the unusual genetic homogeneity of the Icelandic population as a whole, but also to the fact that the population of greater Reykjavik consists largely of people who have migrated to the city from rural areas all over Iceland in recent years and of their immediate descendents.

ACKNOWLEDGMENT

We acknowledge the help and cooperation of the Icelandic Anthropological Institute and the Director General of Public Health in Iceland.

REFERENCE

1. Orn Eliasson, et al. Health survey in the Reykjavik area. Stage I, 1967-68. (Unpublished, Preventive Heart Clinic, Reykjavik).

Jóhann Axelsson
University of Iceland
Department of Physiology
Grensasvegur 12
108 Reykjavik
Iceland

Circumpolar Health 84:66-69

ENVIRONMENTAL COLD MAY BE A MAJOR FACTOR IN SOME RESPIRATORY DISORDERS

E. LL. LLOYD

It is generally believed that the very efficient mechanism that the upper respiratory tract has for warming cold inspired air precludes the possibility of cold injury to lung tissues (1). There is evidence, however, that suggests that environmental cold can cause either acute or chronic respiratory problems.

ACUTE EFFECTS

In one interesting experiment with two divers, one developed bronchospasm while the other, at the same thermal load, developed bronchorrhea (2). The divers, who were in a thermoneutral environment (30°C), developed their respiratory problems when breathing cold (0 to 7°C) oxyhelium gas at a depth of 800 feet of sea water. The problem was relieved by breathing warm (23 to 32°C) oxyhelium gas but recurred whenever the cold was re-introduced. Both problems were therefore the direct effect of cold (respiratory heat loss) on the respiratory system.

Bronchospasm (Exercise Asthma)

In some asthmatics airway resistance is increased by exercise-induced hyperventilation, or by voluntary isocapnic hyperventilation at rest. The mechanism in both seems to be through removal of heat and moisture from the respiratory tract. The bronchospasm can be abolished by the inhalation of air humidified and warmed to body temperature (3). Even in normal subjects isocapnic hyperventilation with sub-freezing air can result in a small but significant airflow obstruction (3).

Bronchorrhea

Helium under pressure has a heat transfer capacity similar to that of water and if divers breathe cold oxyhelium under pressure, bronchorrhea may develop (4). Warming and humidifying the gas postpone the bronchorrhea to a later time or greater depth (4). When the divers breathe dry gas, the bronchorrhea is worse than when the gas is humidified (Hayes, P.A. personal communication). This suggests that the bronchorrhea is due to respiratory heat loss and that condensation of water vapor plays no part in its etiology. The fluid layer lining the airways is maintained by active transport of ions across the epithelium with water following as a result of the osmotic gradient produced (3). In the ideal situation the fluid secretion will match the evaporative loss, but if the secretion is greater than the loss, the excess fluid will become clinically evident in the airways (bronchorrhea) and could produce a clinical picture similar to pulmonary edema. Clinical evidence suggests that the stimulus for this secretion is a reflex triggered by cooling and/or drying of the mucosa and that the reflex may sometimes be oversensitive or be triggered inappropriately. With divers breathing oxyhelium, the major portion of the heat is lost through the direct warming of the cold helium, with the evaporative heat loss being a much smaller proportion than under normal conditions. Unfortunately, the respiratory mucosa is unable to differentiate between cooling due to evaporation and cooling due to direct heat loss, and it responds to both with an increased secretion of tracheal fluid. Since the volume secreted is appropriate for the same total respiratory heat loss occurring under normobaric conditions, it is excessive for the particular situation found under hyperbaric conditions and therefore results in bronchorrhea.

In exercise asthma, though the temperature of the airways returns to normal within 5 minutes of stopping the exercise, the respiratory obstruction steadily worsens during the 5 minute period and takes 30 to 60 minutes to abate (5). Similarly, in divers, though the pain and discomfort caused by breathing the very cold gasses stops as soon as the temperature of the breathing mixture is raised, the bronchorrhea persists for 15 to 20 minutes (4). These facts suggest that the bronchospasm and bronchorrhea are both triggered by chemical mediators which are released as soon as the thermal stimulus reaches a significant level, which varies depending on the genetic make-up and/or state of health of the individual. The effects continue, however for some time after the stimulus has been removed, until degradation of the mediators has taken place.

Clinical Syndromes

High Altitude Pulmonary Edema (HAPE)

The risk factors for HAPE are a too rapid ascent to relatively hypoxic altitudes, indulgence in strenuous physical exercise at altitude, and youth (6) (possibly because children are always active?). Because of the lower temperatures (1°C per 150 m) and lower barometric pressures, the water vapor content of the air at high altitude is very low (6). Both hypoxia and exercise markedly increase minute ventilation volumes and will cause a very high respiratory water, and therefore heat, loss. In fact, the respiratory moisture loss at altitude may be sufficient to cause dehydration (6). The typical symmetrical butterfly distribution of pulmonary edema, seen frequently on X-ray in uremia and left ventricular failure, is not seen in HAPE, and basal horizontal lines and pleural effusion are rare. In HAPE the appearance is of a coarse mottling which may occur in any area of either lung, though there are suggestions that it may appear first in the upper and middle lobe areas (6), which have a proportionally higher ventilation/perfusion ratio and could be expected to have a higher respiratory heat loss. By contrast, the lower lobes have a greater volume of pulmonary arterial blood circulating through them and this could be a thermal cushion to reduce the effect of respiratory heat loss on the airways. Similarly, in patients with unilateral pulmonary arteries not only does HAPE develop at a lower altitude but it develops in the lung with the absent pulmonary artery (Houston, C.E. personal communication). The initial pathology in HAPE may be cold-induced bronchorrhea and if this does occur, in view of the relative hypoxia of the environment, a severe secondary hypoxemia is inevitable, producing pulmonary hypertension and the other features.

Freezing the Lungs

In severe exercise in extreme arctic conditions horses can develop "frosting" of the lungs (7) and sled dogs can die showing signs of acute lung edema (7). Similarly, many arctic hunters report having had episodes of "freezing the lungs" which never occurred at rest but only when the hunters engaged in physical activity so demanding that the men would have to pant with open mouths because of air hunger (7). The normal warming and humidifying system of the nasopharynx having been bypassed, the site of respiratory heat loss is moved into the major air passages and beyond. The winter arctic air is very cold and therefore very dry, and the hyperventilation of vigorous exercise might increase the heat loss to the level at which bronchorrhea occurs, providing a possible explanation for "freezing the lungs." It is not stated whether the symptoms occurred during the exercise or in the immediate post-exercise period. The subjective discomfort may have been similar to that experienced by divers (4) and may have given rise to the name for the human condition. If a similar bronchorrhea occurred in overdriven horses, the fluid reaching the pharynx might have frozen, hence "frosting" of the lungs.

CHRONIC EFFECTS

A rise in pulmonary artery pressure (PAP) may be caused by hypoxia (6,8) but it

may also be produced by cold stress (9). The effects of the 2 stresses are additive even though the effector mechanisms are different (9). The rise in PAP is augmented by acidosis (8) and also by hypothermia (10).

Clinical Syndromes

Monge's Disease or High Altitude Pulmonary Hypertension (HAPH)

In HAPH hypoxia is the prime precipitating factor but the temperature also drops with increasing altitude (at 4,500 m the temperature could be 30°C lower than at sea level), and in the tropics there is a further marked drop in temperature at night (6). There is also a very high respiratory heat loss. Vigorous anaerobic exercise will normally cause a metabolic acidosis. The lower the oxygen tension of the air, the lower the intensity at which exercise will be anaerobic. However, the hyperventilation caused by hypoxia causes a severe respiratory alkalosis which is still present on exercise. Because of the homeostatic mechanisms of the body there is likely to be an increase in metabolic acids (fixed acids) which may be at a higher absolute level than during a normal, exercise-induced metabolic acidosis, because of the degree of respiratory alkalosis. Any vigorous exertion at altitude will almost inevitably require anaerobic metabolism and will therefore cause a further accumulation of the metabolic acids. At altitude, therefore, hypoxia, cold stress, and a variable, but consistently raised level of fixed acids might all contribute to the raised PAP. Return to sea level, as well as restoring oxygenation, will reduce the environmental cold stress, the diurnal variation of temperature and the respiratory heat loss. The acid/base status will also revert to normal, and the higher ambient oxygen tension will mean that more vigorous exercise can be undertaken without a metabolic acidosis developing. These factors may explain why oxygen given at altitude does not restore the PAP to normal whereas on returning to sea level there is a steady fall in PAP eventually reaching normality (6).

Eskimo Lung

In the Arctic many middle-aged and elderly Inuit develop progressive pulmonary hypertension with a progressive decrease in maximum mid-expiratory flow. The end result of this so-called Eskimo lung is death from right-sided heart failure (7). The only proven factor in the patients' histories was that all these Inuit had been hunters and trappers when young and the work had involved repeated episodes of hard physical work even during the severe cold of winter.

Similar respiratory problems were noted among elderly white trappers, whose mode of work when young had been similar to that of the Inuit trappers, and among native and immigrant Russian workers engaged for long periods in hard physical work while exposed to extreme temperatures in Siberia (7). The environment for winter hunting in the Arctic will inevitably include severe cold and in these circumstances, even without muscular work, there is a tendency towards acidosis (11) which would augment any rise in PAP due to the cold (9). If the cold exposure is very severe, the oxygen available in the air may be marginally sufficient for the needs of heat production, and vigorous muscular exercise, by taking priority over the needs of heat production, could lead to unexpected and unsuspected lowering of the body temperature (12) in addition to a metabolic acidosis. Both factors would aggravate any rise of PAP. Recurrent episodes of exertion by repeatedly boosting the cold-induced pulmonary hypertension may result in a permanent elevation of the PAP. The high PAP once present may be steadily progressive or may be boosted by subsequent winter hunting expeditions, but whatever the mechanism, Eskimo lung becomes established.

Chronic Bronchitis

It has been noted that the pulmonary vascular pathology in chronic bronchitis and emphysema is identical to that in Monge's disease (HAPH) and both differ from the pathological changes of pulmonary hypertension associated with cardiac shunts or left atrial hypertrophy (13). In the established condition long continued supplementary oxygen may lower the PAP, i.e. improved oxygenation lowers but rarely completely reverses the raised PAP, again similar to HAPH. Hypoxia may be caused by smoking (14), working in or driving through areas of high car density (15), or episodes of sleep apnea (16) but this does not explain the increased incidence of acute exacerbations of chronic bronchitis which occur during the winter as compared with the summer. People in social class 5, especially in large towns, are more likely than those in class 1 to have inadequately heated and damp houses, to work in colder environments, even if indoors, and to be doing work physically hard enough to produce a metabolic acidosis. In the lower social classes there is often a tendency to have the living room heated, sometimes overheated, while the bedroom and bathroom remain totally unheated and therefore, on going to bed, the person is exposed to a sudden marked cold stress which persists until the bed has warmed up and even then, if the bedding is inadequate and the head is still exposed to the cold, there may

be a continuing cold stress. The cold stresses of winter might therefore have more impact on the lower social classes. In the etiology of any individual case of chronic bronchitis it might be worth evaluating the possible contributions from hypoxia (smoking, traffic fumes, or sleep apnea), environmental cold stress, at home or work, and exertion-induced acidosis. By doing this an explanation may be found for the social class difference in urban mortality from chronic bronchitis and the low incidence in farm workers (17).

Sudden Infant Death Syndrome (SIDS)

Pulmonary vascular hyperplasia is reported at necropsy in many cases of SIDS (18), and, as in chronic bronchitis, there is a seasonal variation in the occurrence of SIDS with an increased incidence during the winter months (18). Babies have a low body weight, a large body surface/body weight ratio and their heads, large in proportion to the rest of the body, will be a more significant route for heat loss than in an adult. Therefore an environment which may be comfortable for an adult may in fact be causing cold stress for the baby. In the neonate, exposure to cold may result in an increased metabolic acidosis (19) and sometimes a lower arterial oxygen tension (20), and these effects may persist beyond the immediate neonatal period. In winter therefore the neonate and small baby may be subjected to the same 3 stress factors-- environmental cold, alveolar hypoxia, and metabolic acidosis--which have been shown to be associated with pulmonary hypertension in adult disorders. The social risk factors which have been shown to be associated with an increased risk of SIDS, viz. pre-term delivery or low birth weight, poor weight gain, and the social factors of poverty, an unmarried mother, parent under 20 and social class 5 (18) are all likely to increase the rate of heat loss from the child or lead to inadequate heat in the home. If hypothermia or cold-induced pulmonary hypertension are indeed common causes of SIDS, it is easy to understand the observation that previous near-miss SIDS rarely continues to definite SIDS (21) since the family is likely to keep the environment warmer, even if accidentally, e.g. by having the baby in the same room as the adults for most or all of the 24 hours.

CONCLUSIONS

It may be necessary in the future to include consideration of the thermal environment in epidemiological studies of some respiratory disorders and in the management of patients.

REFERENCES

1. Maclean D, Emslie-Smith D. Accidental hypothermia. Edinburgh: Blackwell, 1977.
2. Hoke B, Jackson DL, Alexander JH, Flynn ET. Respiratory heat loss and pulmonary function during cold-gas breathing at high pressure. In: Lambertsen, CJ, ed. Underwater physiology V. Bethesda: FASEB. 1976:725-740.
3. McFadden ER. Respiratory heat and water exchange: Physiological and clinical implications. J Appl Physiol 1938; 54:331-336.
4. Hayes PA, Padbury EH, Florio JT, Fyfield TP. Respiratory heat transfer in cold water and during rewarming. J Biomechanical Eng 1982; 104:45-49.
5. McFadden ER. An analysis of exercise as a stimulus for the production of airway obstruction. Lung 1981; 159:3-11.
6. Heath D, Williams DR. Man at high altitude. Edinburgh: Churchill Livingstone, 1981.
7. Schaefer O, Eaton RDP, Timmermans FJW, Hildes JA. Respiratory function impairment and cardiopulmonary consequences in long-term residents of the Canadian Arctic. Can Med Assoc J 1980; 123:997-1004.
8. Reeves JT, Wagner WW, McMurty IF, Grover RF. Physiological effects of high altitude on the pulmonary circulation. In: Robertshaw D, ed. Environmental physiology III. Baltimore: University Park Press, 1979:289-310.
9. Bligh J, Chauca D. Effects of hypoxia, cold exposure and fever on pulmonary artery pressure, and their significance for arctic residents. In: Harvald B, Hart Hansen JP, eds. Circumpolar Health 81. Nordic Council for Arct Med Res Rep 1982; 33:606-607.
10. Benumof JL, Wahrenbrock EA. Dependency of hypoxic pulmonary vasoconstriction on temperature. J Appl Physiol 1977; 42:56-58.
11. Alexander G. Cold thermogenesis. In: Robertshaw D, ed. Environmental physiology III. Baltimore: University Park Press, 1979:43-155.
12. Hirvonen J. Accidental hypothermia. Nordic Council for Arct Med Res Rep 1982; 30:15-19.
13. Heath D, Brewer D, Hicken P. Cor pulmonale in emphysema. Springfield: Charles C Thomas, 1968.
14. Calverley PMA, Leggett RJ, McElderry L, Flenley DC. Cigarette smoking and secondary polycythemia in hypoxic cor pulmonale. Am Rev Respir Dis 1982; 125:507-510.
15. Wright GR, Shephard RJ. Physiological effects of carbon monoxide. In: Robertshaw D, ed. Environmental physiology III. Baltimore: University Park Press, 1979:311-368.
16. Lancet. Sleep apnoea syndrome. Lancet 1979; 1:25-26.
17. DHSS prevention and health: Everybody's business. London: HMSO, 1976.
18. Powell J, Machin D, Kershaw CR. Unexpected sudden infant deaths in Gosport--some comparisons between service and civilian families. J Roy Nav Med Serv 1983; 69:141-150.
19. Gandy GM, Adamson SK, Cunningham N, Silverman WA, James LS. Thermal environment and acid base homeostasis in human infants during the first few hours of life. J Clin Invest 1964; 43:751-758.
20. Stephenson JM, Du JN, Oliver TK. The effect of cooling on blood gas tensions in newborn infants. J Paediat 1970; 76:848-852.
21. Stanton AN. "Near-miss" cot deaths and home monitoring. Br Med J 1982; 2:1441-1442.

E. LL. Lloyd
Princess Margaret Rose Orthopaedic Hospital
Fairmilehead
Edinburgh, EH10, 7ED, Scotland
U.K.

Circumpolar Health 84:70-73

SEASONAL VARIATIONS OF BLOOD PRESSURE, BASAL METABOLISM, AND SKIN TEMPERATURE IN OUTDOOR WORKERS IN NORTHERN FINLAND

JUHANI LEPPÄLUOTO, JUHANI HASSI and RAUNO PÄÄKKÖNEN

There are several reports in the literature on seasonal acclimatization responses in man. In the cold season, elevated oxygen consumption in the basal state, or after stimulation with experimental cold (3), has been observed. Muscle shivering begins later in winter (3) than in summer, and the skin temperature in response to a cold test falls more in winter than in summer, indicating an increase in insulation by vasoconstrictor tone during the cold season (3,4). Others report rises in blood pressure levels in winter under resting conditions (5-8) or after a cold pressor test (9). According to a recent observation, the urinary secretions of catecholamines and sodium also appear to be greater in winter than in summer (6).

Although the aim of acclimatization is to enhance chances of survival, some responses may turn out to decrease these chances. For example, increased incidence and mortality rates for heart and vascular diseases have been observed in winter in several countries with temperate and subarctic climate (10-12). Therefore, in our search for causal mechanisms for diseases which change in incidence seasonally, we have measured the levels of some acclimatization responses of outdoor workers from northern Finland exposed to moderately warm summer and cold winter. Since increased blood pressure is a significant risk factor for cardiovascular disease, special attention was paid to it.

METHODS

Seven healthy male outdoor workers from Rovaniemi Tele District (68°N) participated in this study after giving informed consent. The physical characteristics of the subjects are presented in Table 1. Meteorological data were obtained from the Meteorological Institute, Helsinki, Finland and are presented in Table 2. The subjects fasted overnight, arrived at the Department of

Table 1. Physical characteristics of the subjects, with $\bar{x} \pm S.E.$

Subject no.	Age yr	Height cm	Weight kg	Body fat %
1	31	178	72.5	21.4
2	42	181	83.5	17.1
3	41	170	82.9	31.6
4	52	172	73.5	21.8
5	41	172	76.0	25.4
6	44	175	77.0	26.6
7	22	168	73.8	22.3
	39±3.7	175±1.9	77±1.73	23.7±1.78

Physiology in Oulu between 8 and 9 a.m., and were reviewed and weighed and then rested approximately 1 hour before the experiments at 9 to 11 a.m. They were not allowed to smoke on the day of the experiment. Each subject sat in shorts for 30 min at 28±1°C and was thereafter moved to a climate chamber with a temperature of +10±1°C. The relative humidity was 20 to 40% and wind speed less than 0.2 m/s in the chamber. Skin (chest, arm, thigh, and leg) and rectal temperatures were measured by a YSI Series 400 Thermistor according to the method of Ramanathan (12). Oxygen consumption and carbon dioxide production was registered by paramagnetic and infrared detection for 5 min at the end of their stay at +28°C and +10°C by Fenyves (Dr. Fenyves et Gut CH4051, Basel) after calibration with a known oxygen/carbon dioxide mixture. Blood pressure was measured with a sphygomanometer after a 25 min stay in a sitting position at +28°C and 10°C. The measurement was repeated 3 times and the median value was recorded. Radial pulse was taken before the blood pressure recording. All the blood

Table 2. Mean temperature and wind velocity in Sodankylä.

January 1981		April 1981		August 1981	
Mean daily temperature (Min, Max)	Mean wind velocity	Mean daily temperature (Min, Max)	Mean wind velocity	Mean daily temperature (Min, Max)	Mean wind velocity
-12.7°C	3.5 m/s	-0.3°C	3.7 m/s	+10.4°C	4.0 m/s
(-30.2, 2.0)		(-11, 2.5)		(6.2, 16.2)	

pressure measurements were carried out by one of us (JL). The experiments occurred in January 1981, April 1981, and August 1981.

Statistical analyses were performed with paired t-test or with analysis of variance and the Tukey-Kramer test.

RESULTS

The mean monthly temperatures during the experiments are presented in Table 2. The mean systolic blood pressure under basal conditions (30 min at +28°C) ranged from 145 to 123 mmHg and diastolic blood pressure from 82 to 76 mmHg during the experiments (Table 3). The systolic blood pressure was significantly lower in summer than in winter, the mean difference being 22 mmHg. The mean pulse under basal conditions was 66 to 72 beats/min. The rate pressure product was lower in August than in January, but the decrease was non-significant (Table 3).

Table 3. Seasonal variation of blood pressure, pulse, and rate pressure product in outdoor workers.

	28°C	10°C
Systolic		
Diastolic		
January	145±3 / 78±5	145±5 / 84±4
April	147±5 / 82±3	143±5 / 82±4
August	123±4** / 76±2	132±4 / 81±4
Pulse		
January	66±5	54±3
April	72±5	67±3*
August	69±4	62±1
Rate pressure product		
January	0.96	0.78
April	1.06	0.96
August	0.85	0.82

Mean and S.E. are given. Systolic and diastolic blood pressure (mmHg), pulse per min, and rate pressure product 0.0001 x systolic blood pressure x pulse).

* P<0.05 from the January values (Tukey-Kramer test).
** P<0.01.

Table 4. Seasonal variation of oxygen consumption and RQ values in outdoor workers.

	28°C	10°C
O_2 consumption ml/min		
January	406±54.6	468±55.8
April	297±30.3*	318±30.7
August	312±18.8	344±15.1
RQ		
January	0.83±0.02	0.79±0.02
April	0.78±0.03	0.74±0.02
August	0.75±0.03	0.77±0.04

Mean and S.E. are given.
* P<0.05 from January values.

There was a seasonal variation in basal oxygen consumption and carbon dioxide production in outdoor workers, so that significantly lower values were detected in April in oxygen consumption and in August both in oxygen consumption and carbon dioxide production (Table 4).

Effect of Cold Exposure

During the cold exposure (30 min at +10°C), there was a significant increase in blood pressure only in the summer experiments (Table 3). Pulse rates were generally lower at the end of the cold exposure, the decreases being significant in the spring experiment. The rate pressure product at +10°C was always smaller than at +28°C, but did not reach statistical significance. Increased oxygen consumption (p<0.05) was observed in all experiments after the cold exposure. The RQ values were similar throughout the whole experiment since the changes in oxygen consumption and carbon dioxide production were in the same direction.

Mean Skin and Rectal Temperatures

There were no statistically significant changes in the mean core (rectal) temperature between the seasons at 28°C or the end of the 30-min cold test (Table 5). The mean skin temperatures under basal conditions were also similar during all the seasons when the experiments were being carried out. In response to cold, mean skin temperature decreased by 5.7-6.6°C and there was no significant seasonal variation, although during the January tests the mean skin temperature levels tended to be lower than in August. No general differences between the seasons were found in different body regions, such as the chest, arm, thigh, or leg (data not shown).

DISCUSSION

During the present series of experiments, the seasonal changes in daily temperatures were maximally 46°C and therefore there are great demands for physiological adaptation mechanisms in these areas. The most important finding of this study was that the basal systolic blood pressure was distinctly higher in winter than in summer in outdoor workers. The difference in systolic blood pressure between winter and summer levels was as high as 22 mmHg. In a recent study in England concerning mostly indoor workers, the greatest seasonal difference in systolic blood pressure was 7 mmHg and similar differences have been observed in earlier studies (5,8). Our finding of elevated blood pressure in winter is also in agreement with the results of the standard cold pressure test in which greater systolic blood pressure responses were obtained in summer than in winter in Norwegian fishermen and control subjects (9). Our subjects participated in the experiments for the first time in January, which might have had an increasing effect on the blood pressure. It has been assumed that systolic blood pressure, when measured for the first time, is about 5 mmHg higher than in later measurements (14). On the other hand, the April blood pressure values of our male subjects were still high.

There are also changes in dietary habits between summer and winter in Finland,

Table 5. Seasonal variation of the rectal temperature and mean skin temperature.

	28°C	10°C
Mean skin		
January	33.8±0.26	27.2±0.44
April	34.0±0.09	28.3±0.26
August	33.8±0.22	28.0±0.44
Rectal		
January	37.2±0.10	37.2±0.18
April	37.7±0.08	37.0±0.09
August	37.1±0.11	37.1±0.10

Mean and S.E. are given. In all cases the decrease from 28°C to 10°C in the mean skin temperature was highly significant (P<0.01).

so that more vegetables and cereal products are eaten in summer. For example, a recent study from Finland shows that when the diet is changed to cereal products, lower blood pressure values are observed (4). However, similar RQ values in this study throughout the seasons indicate that no great relative changes in the carbohydrate or fat contents of the diet occurred between the months.

Considering the data, we conclude that the observed difference in blood pressure is due to environmental factors, mostly cold, although further studies are needed to examine the effects of other factors, such as diet or unspecific stressors, on blood pressure.

The increased blood pressure values registered in winter are most probably related to increased sympathetic activity and peripheral vasoconstriction caused by cold. Other contributory factors might be increased salt or catecholamine secretion, which have been shown to be higher in winter than in summer (6). The seasonal changes in rate pressure products were here generally similar to those of systolic blood pressure but smaller, more variable, and hence non-significant.

The results of this study showed that oxygen consumption was lower in spring or summer than in winter. In a review about the acclimatization of man to cold, Goldsmith concludes that measurements of basal metabolic rates in cold climates have resulted in variable results (4). The reason for the discrepancies is not obvious, but may be related to the geographical heterogeneity of the studies. It appears rational that oxygen consumption and metabolic rate are high in the cold season when environmental cold stimuli may lead to increased thermogenesis, as found in our study.

Two reports of the previous literature concerning skin temperature responses to cold test show that there are no seasonal variations in the responses (3,9). Our present results also showed that there were no detectable seasonal changes in skin temperature responses to our cold test. This may indicate that the clothing used had protected the surface of the skin effectively from cold. In fact, these outdoor workers have special clothing which they wear on cold days. If the assumption is made that the seasonal changes of blood pressure and oxygen we observed in this study are due to the changes in environmental temperature, it is possible that cooling occurred via the facial skin and/or the respiratory system. The cooling of facial skin or respiratory airways is impossible to avoid when working outdoors in winter.

Whatever the mechanism for the increased blood pressure in winter, it is well known that even a modest increase in blood pressure is associated with an increased occurrence of cardiovascular and stroke mortality (15-17). In corollary to this, increased incidence and mortality rate of heart diseases and stroke are seen in winter in this country (8,11).

The present series of experiments demonstrates that cold acclimatization is clearly manifested in the blood pressure and metabolic rate in outdoor work in circumpolar areas. This should be taken into account when the levels of these parameters are followed seasonally for scientific studies or medical check-ups for therapy.

REFERENCES

1. Yoshimura M, Yukiyoshi K, Yoshioka T et al. Climatic adaptation of basal metabolism. Fed Proc 1966; 25:1169-1176.
2. Yoshimura M, Yoshimura H. Cold tolerance and critical temperature of the Japanese. Int J Biometeor 1969; 13:163-172.
3. Davis TRA, Johnston DR. Seasonal acclimatization to cold in man. J Appl Physiol 1961; 16:231-234.
4. Goldsmith R. Acclimatization to cold in man--fact or fiction? In: Monteith JL, Mount LE, eds. Heat loss from animals and man. London: Butterworths, 1974:311-319.
5. Brennan PJ, Greenberg G, Miall WE, Thompson SG. Seasonal variation in arterial blood pressure. Br Med J 1982; 285:919-923.
6. Hata T, Ogihara T, Maruyma A, Mikami H, Nakamaru M, Naka T, Kumahara Y, Nugent CA. The seasonal variation of blood pressure in patients with essential hypertension. Clin Exper Hyper Theory and Practice 1982; A4:341-354.
7. Nagata H, Isumiyama T, Kamata K et al. An increase of plasma triiodothyroine concentration in man in a cold environment. J Clin Endocrinol Metab 1976; 43:1153-1156.
8. Rose G. Seasonal variation in blood pressure in man. Nature 1961; 189:235-239.
9. LeBlanc J. Man in the cold. Springfield: Charles C Thomas, 1975.
10. Anderson TW, Le Riche WH. Cold weather and myocardial infarction. Lancet 1970; 1:2981-2986.
11. Näyhä S. Short and medium-term variations in mortality in Finland. Scand J Soc Med 1980; suppl 21.
12. Sotaniemi E, Vuopala U, Huhti E, Takkunen J. Effect of temperature on hospital admissions for myocardial infarction in a subarctic area. Br Med J 1970; 4:150-151.
13. Ramanathan NL. A new weighting system for mean surface temperature of the human body. J Appl Physiol 1964; 19:531-533.
14. Aromaa A. Kohonnut verenpaine ja sen kansanterveydelliner merkitys Suomessa. (Epidemiology and public health impact of high blood pressure in Finland). Vammalan Kirjapaino Oy, Vammala 1981. (English summary).
15. Kannel SB, Wolf PA, Vester J, McNamara P. Epidemiological assessment of the role of blood pressure in stroke. The Framingham study. JAMA 1970; 214:189-198.
16. Keys A. Coronary heart disease in seven countries. Circ 1970; 41, 42:suppl I:1-211.
17. Morris JN, Kagan A, Pattison DC, Gardner MJ, Raffle PAB. Incidence and prediction of ischaemic heart-disease in London busmen. Lancet 1966; 2:553-559.

Juhani Leppäluoto
Nordic Council for Arctic Medical Research
Department of Physiology
University of Oulu
Oulu
Finland

Circumpolar Health 84:74-77

WORK STRESS OF NORWEGIAN COAL MINERS IN SPITSBERGEN

NILS O. ALM and K. RODAHL

INTRODUCTION

The Spitsbergen Archipelago lies between 74° and 81°N, but the climate is not as cold as one would expect at these latitudes. The mean winter temperature is not much lower in Spitsbergen than in the mountain districts in Norway, and the wind conditions are hardly worse than along the Norwegian west coast or in northern Norway.

Still, Spitsbergen is part of the High Arctic. Glaciers cover two-thirds of the land. The vegetation is sparse, even along the coast, and the climate is very dry, the annual precipitation being normally between 200 and 400 mm.

The coal deposits are found mainly in the central area of West Spitsbergen. Geologically, almost all the coal resources date back to the Tertiary period, 50 to 60 million years ago. The thickness of the coal seams varies from a few centimeters up to 5 m.

The geological conditions, namely the almost horizontal sedimentary layers, the thickness of the coal seams, and the considerable strength of the roof, together with the arctic temperature, i.e., the extension of the permafrost zone, are determining factors for the mining methods, and secondarily for the work environment and the possible health hazards of the miners.

In the mine in Longyearbyen, the thickness of the coal seam varies between 70 and 110 cm. The mine entrance is approximately 200 m above sea level and the mine is in the permafrost zone. The production method is longwall mining along a coal face 150 to 200 m long.

The narrow passages and the minimal height at the working sites along the coal face force the workers to creep or crawl several hundred meters. The work is performed in lying, half-sitting, or squatting positions for the 2 periods of approximately 3 hours each in the shift period. These extreme working positions, however, are tolerated amazingly well by the workers.

The permafrost causes a nearly constant temperature of 2 to 4°C below zero in the mine all the year round. This seems to be accepted by the workers as a rather comfortable temperature for heavy physical labor, but it has always been regarded as difficult to keep the feet warm in this sitting or lying position.

The below-zero temperature provides a convenient dry environment at the working sites in the mine, but at the same time it prohibits the use of water to remove the dust produced when drilling in coal and stone. Those who are working along the coal face are heavily exposed to coal dust with low siliceous content, while workers in the main transport tunnels and entries are exposed to mixed dust with a considerable content of siliceous dust.

Workers operating heavy mining machinery are exposed to noise to a certain extent, but the mine workers as a group are definitely less exposed to noise than workers in mechanical workshops. Those workers engaged in removing the steel friction supports and remounting them nearer the coal face, however, are exposed to noise from hammering steel against steel, especially harmful for the hearing.

The uniqueness of the Longyearbyen coal mines, as far as the miners are concerned, is the combination of the awkward working position necessitated by the narrow coal seam, the low temperature, and the dry and dusty atmosphere in the mine, together with the isolation of the arctic mining community.

Table 1. Subjects and their physical work capacity.

Subject	Job	Age years	Height cm	Weight kg	Physical work capacity	
					Max O_2 l/min	ml/kg/min
O.O.	Driller	23	199	91	2.9	32
N.G.	Assistant cutter	21	177	78	4.2	54
J.C.S.	Timberman (foreman)	29	182	91	3.5	38
B.L.	Timberman	26	182	85	4.1	48

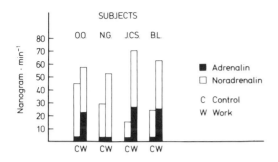

Figure 1. Urinary catecholamines for coal miners, Longyearbyen.

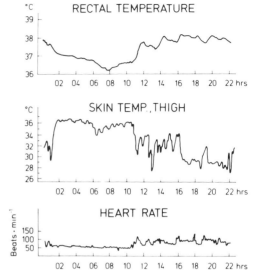

Figure 2. Physiological responses of driller O.O., Svalbard, 14 March 1979.

Although the work stress of coal miners has been studied elsewhere (3-8), none, as far as we know, have been made of the work stress of coal miners working under conditions such as those encountered at the Longyearbyen mines. The purpose of this study was therefore to make a physiological assessment of the work stress of coal miners operating in low coal seams in very restricted surroundings under arctic conditions.

MATERIAL AND METHODS

Four miners 21 to 29 years of age, engaged in actual mining operations in one of the typical low seam mines at Longyearbyen, volunteered to serve as subjects for the study. The body size and physical work capacity are listed in Table 1.

The miners were studied for 24-hour periods, both during work in the mine and during time off and sleep. The study included assessment of maximal oxygen uptake based on the recording of heart rate during submaximal cycle ergometer exercise (9), assessment of work load based on the continuous recording of heart rate with the aid of shielded miniature portable magnetic tape recorders (Oxford Medilog), assessment of thermal stress based on continuous recording of rectal and skin temperature (thigh) by same Medilog recorder, and the assessment of general stress response on the basis of the analysis of urinary catecholamine eliminations (2).

RESULTS

The estimated work load for the 4 subjects ranged on the average from 1.1 to 1.6 l oxygen/min, corresponding to 30 to 40% of their maximal oxygen uptake (Table 2).

Adrenaline excretion reached levels up to 25 nanograms/min, and noradrenaline

Table 2. Estimated work load of subjects from Longyearbyen mines.

Subject	Work Load		
	Mean work pulse	Estimated mean oxygen uptake l/min	Estimated % of VO_2 max
O.O.	120 (100-150)	1.2	40
N.G.	110 (80-140)	1.5	35
J.C.S.	105 (85-130)	1.1	30
B.L.	105 (80-135)	1.6	40

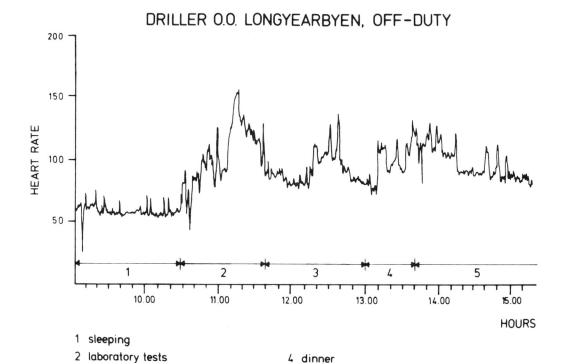

DRILLER O.O. LONGYEARBYEN, OFF-DUTY

1 sleeping
2 laboratory tests
3 various leisure activities
4 dinner
5 changing, proceeding to the mine

Figure 3. Continuous heart rate recording for driller O.O., Longyearbyen, while off duty.

values ranged from 50 to 70 nanograms/min during work (Figure 1).

The rectal temperature ranged from 37.5 to 38.5°C during work. Despite high rectal temperatures, the skin temperature of the thigh fell in two of the subjects to about 28°C (Figure 2). In the two remaining subjects, the skin temperature remained around 33°C.

An example of the detailed analysis of the recorded work pulse, paired with the activity record, is presented in Figures 3 and 4. The example is in general quite typical for all 4 subjects, and may therefore be considered representative. On the whole, the level of physical strain in terms of heart response is about the same during leisure activity as during the work in the mine.

In the example shown in Figure 4, the subject works about 5.5 hours in the mine, interrupted by a half-hour break. During work he maintains a fairly steady work pace for extended periods, especially during the first half of the work shift.

It is evident from the record that this type of mining operation may impose some rather unique types of stress on the miner, as is the case when he at the start of the work shift crawls along the narrow passage, pulling a box containing 50 kg dynamite tied to his leg, causing his heart rate to rise to close to 165.

DISCUSSION

Although this study only involves 4 subjects, the uniformity in their response on the whole indicates that the results may be considered fairly representative for this type of mining operation.

Compared to other occupations in which the same methods of assessment have been used, it is reasonable to conclude that the miners operating these low seam coal mines in Spitsbergen are subject to considerable physical work stress.

Physical work loads of this magnitude (30 to 40% of VO_2max) exceed work loads commonly encountered in most industries, where the work load seldom exceeds 25% of VO_2max. The work load of these coal miners is comparable to that of coastal fishermen, in whom the levels of urinary catecholamine excretion equalled those observed for the present coal miners.

It also appears that at least some of the coal miners may be subject to some degree of cold stress of the lower extremities while operating the low coal seam mines, necessitating crawling and working in a stooped or lying position in an ambient temperature slightly below freezing.

The long-term health effect of these working conditions should be subject to further studies.

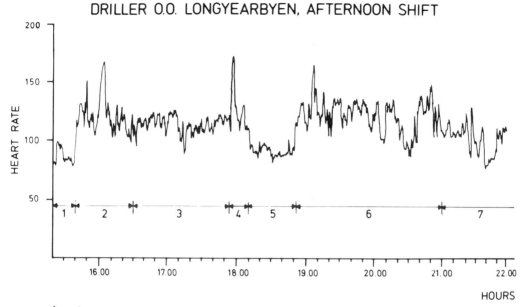

DRILLER O.O. LONGYEARBYEN, AFTERNOON SHIFT

1 rest room
2 crawling while dragging box containing 50 kg dynamite tied to leg
3 drilling and loading
4 crawling out

5 coffee break
6 back in the mine
7 leaving the mine

Figure 4. Continuous heart rate for driller O.O., Longyearbyen, afternoon shift at mine.

REFERENCES

1. Althouse R, Hurrell JJ Jr. An analysis of job stress in coal mining. NIOSH Research Report. US Department of Health, Education and Welfare. Cincinnati, Ohio. May 1977.
2. Anderson B, Houmøller S, Karlson C-G, Svensson S. Analysis of urinary catecholamines: An improved autoanalyzer fluorescence method. Clin Chem Acta 1974; 51:13.
3. Bobo M, Bethea NJ, Ayoub MM, Intaranont K. Energy expenditure and aerobic fitness of male low seam coal miners. Hum Factors 1983; 25(1):43.
4. Chakraborty MK, Sensarma SK, Sarkar DN. Blood lactic acid in determining the heaviness of different mining work. Indian J Physiol Pharmacol 1974; Oct-Dec:341.

5. Hieber AR, Smidt U. Ergometrische Untersuchungen an Bergleuten und Hüttenarbeitern zur Differenzierung der Ursachen einer Belastungsdyspnoe. Praxis Pneumalogie 1982; 36.
6. Oleinikov VA. Physiological aspects of the work of miners on working faces. Hum Physiol 1975; 4(5):677.
7. Ross MH. The Appalachian coal miner: His way of living, working, and relating to others. Ann New York Acad Sci 1972; 200:184.
8. Vaida I, Pafnote M. Physical work load in modern mining. Rev Roum Morphol Embryol Physiol 1979; 16(2):133.
9. Åstrand PO, Rodahl K. Textbook of work physiology. New York: McGraw-Hill, 1977.

Nils O. Alm
Kysthospitalet
3290 Stavern
Norway

Circumpolar Health 84:78-82

EFFECT OF COLD EXPOSURE ON EXERCISE TOLERANCE AND EXERCISE EKG IN PATIENTS WITH ANGINA OF EFFORT

CHRISTER BACKMAN and HÅKAN LINDERHOLM

Many patients with angina of effort due to coronary heart disease discover that an exertion that can be performed comfortably in a warm environment causes angina in the cold (1,2). A cold wind can also provoke an attack of angina pectoris. Other patients do not state that their symptoms are influenced by cold (2,3). Earlier reports (4,5) have shown that some patients who perform a standardized exercise test both at room temperature and in a cold room achieve a lower work capacity in the cold. Further, more pronounced ST depressions have been observed in the exercise EKG in the cold, and also a faster increase in the rating of subjective exertion (4). Other patients do not show such reactions. It has also been reported that nitroglycerin can abolish these reactions (6). It is therefore of interest to examine whether there is an association between the deterioration of work capacity and the more marked ST depressions in the cold, and also whether the results of an exercise test at room temperature can predict the outcome of an exercise test in the cold.

MATERIALS AND METHODS

Fifty patients with angina pectoris, 43 men and 7 women 24 to 64 years of age (mean 50 years), were examined. They represent an unselected sample of individuals, most of whom were being evaluated pre-operatively for coronary bypass surgery. None were chosen because of any particular difficulties in cold weather. All had EKG changes with SI depressions typical for coronary insufficiency during or after at least one of the exercise tests. Twenty-four had had a previous myocardial infarction according to history or EKG. Most of the patients were on beta blockers.

The exercise tests were performed on a bicycle ergometer with individually chosen stepwise increments of work load every sixth minute (7). The test was interrupted when the patients were unable to continue or if angina pectoris, EKG changes, or any other signs contraindicating its continuation occurred. Thus, the exercise was close to the maximum. Heart rate, respiratory frequency, blood pressure, and the subjective rating of exertion (8) were recorded at the end of each work load.

The bicycle ergometer tests were performed under the following conditions:
1) in the sitting position in a room at a temperature of approximately +23°C (RT);
2) in the sitting position at a temperature about -15°C (CR); and

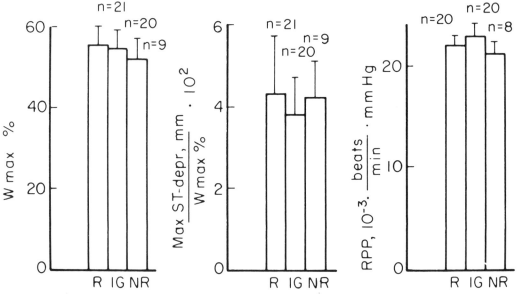

Figure 1. *Maximum work capacity in percent of the predicted normal value (Wmax%), maximum ST-depr/Wmax%, and the largest rate pressure product (RPP) measured in the sitting position at room temperature in the three groups $\bar{x} \pm S.E.M.$*
R = responders, IG = intermediate group, NR = nonresponders.

3) in the supine position at room
temperature.

Equal work loads were used for each
patient under the different conditions. In
the cold room the patients were dressed in
warm clothes, gloves, and a cap covering the
head except for the face. Before the
cycling the patients had stayed in the cold
room for about 2 minutes.

The maximum work performed (Wmax) was
the heaviest work load at which the patient
worked for 6 minutes. If the patient worked
for less than 6 minutes at the highest work
load the proportion of the last increment in
work load that corresponded to the completed
period of that load was added to the previous load (9). The maximum work capacity was
also calculated as a percentage of the
predicted normal value (Wmax%). The prediction was based on data from examinations of
93 healthy male and female subjects (Linderholm, unpublished observations). The rate
pressure product (RPP), i.e., heart rate
times systolic blood pressure, was calculated for the maximum work load and used as
an expression of heart work load (10).

ST depressions were measured at rest
and during exercise in the chest leads with
the largest ST depression 0.04 to 0.06 sec
from the ST-junction on the highest work
load and on comparable loads under different
conditions. In the results, ST depression
(ST-depr, mm) is defined as the ST depression
during exercise minus the ST depression at
rest.

RESULTS

The patients were divided into 3 groups
with regard to their reaction to cold.
Twenty-one patients were "responders." They
worked less and had more pronounced ST
depression on equal work load in the cold
than at room temperature. Nine patients
were "nonresponders," i.e., they had the
same or higher work capacity and the same or
less pronounced ST depression in the cold
room. The rest, 20 patients, constituted an
"intermediate group." In that group, 9 had
more pronounced ST depression and lower work
capacity in the cold.

At room temperature in the sitting
position there were no statistically significant differences between the 3 groups with
respect to maximum work capacity, measured
as a percentage of normal value, Wmax%. The
ST depression divided by Wmax% at room
temperature was also similar in the 3
groups, as was the RPP close to the termination of the test (Figure 1).

Figure 2 shows the difference between
maximum work capacity, Diff Wmax%, measured
in the sitting position at room temperature,
and in the cold room as well as at room
temperature in the sitting and supine
positions. In the cold the responders

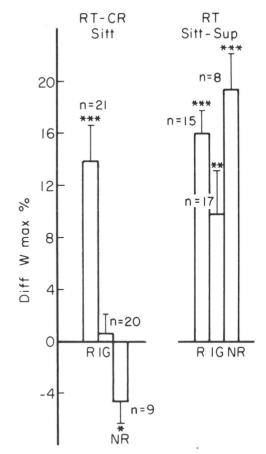

Figure 2. *The difference between Wmax%
(Diff Wmax%) measured in the
sitting position at room temperature (RT) and in a cold room at
-15°C (CR) as well as that measured at room temperature in the
sitting (Sitt) and supine (Sup)
position ($\bar{x} \pm S.E.M.$). * = 0.01
< p < 0.05; ** = 0.001 < p <
0.01; *** = p < 0.001 where p is
the probability that the differences are caused by random factors. Other symbols as in Figure
1.*

decreased their physical performance by an
average of 25%, the intermediate group by
2%, while the responders increased it by 9%.
In the supine position all groups reacted
similarly, as did the responders in the
cold.

The differences between ST depressions
on an equal work load under identical
conditions are shown in Figure 3. The
responders had a significantly more pronounced ST depression on equal work load in
the cold than the other 2 groups. In the
supine position all 3 groups had more

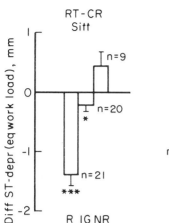
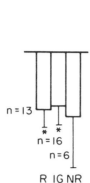

Figure 3. *The difference between ST depression on equal work load (Diff
ST-depr, eq work load) measured
at room temperature (RT) and in a
cold room (CR) in the sitting
position as well as in the
sitting (Sitt) and supine (Sup)
position at room temperature ($\bar{x}$ ±
S.E.M.). Symbols as in Figures 1
and 2.*

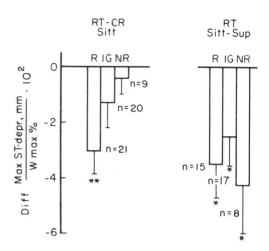

Figure 4. *The difference between maximum ST
depression divided by Wmax% in
the sitting position at room
temperature (RT) and in a cold
room (CR) as well as at room
temperature in the sitting (Sitt)
and supine (Sup) position ($\bar{x}$ ±
S.E.M.). Symbols as in Figures 1
and 2.*

pronounced ST depressions on equal work load
than in the sitting position.

The difference between maximum ST
depression divided by Wmax% at room temperature and in the cold room was significantly
more pronounced among the responders than
the nonresponders (Figure 4). In the supine
position ST-depr/Wmax% was significantly
greater than in the sitting position in all
3 groups. However, there were no statistically significant differences with regard to
the maximum ST depressions at maximum work
load between any of the patient groups and
under any of the different conditions of
examination (RT, CR, Sitt, Sup).

The heart rate in the cold room was
higher than at room temperature on all the
corresponding work loads in the responder
group (p < 0.05 to 0.001), while in the
intermediate group the pulse rate in the
cold room was lower than at room temperature
(p < 0.05). The nonresponders showed no
significant differences. Systolic blood
pressure during the different corresponding
work loads was not significantly different
between the cold room and at room temperature in any of the groups.

Figure 5 shows that on the average the
responders and patients in the intermediate
group worked up to a lower RPP, while the
nonresponders worked to a higher product in
the cold room. All patients interrupted the
exercise test at a mean lower RPP in the
supine position than at room temperature.
The differences between the groups were not
statistically significant.

Figure 6 shows the relation between on
one hand the difference between work capacity at room temperature and in the cold, and
on the other the difference between ST
depression on equal work load under these 2
conditions. There is a statistically
significant covariation between these
variables. Thus, most of the patients whose
work capacity decreased in the cold also had
the most pronounced ST depressions at equal
work loads.

DISCUSSION

The 3 different groups of patients,
"responders," "intermediate group," and
"nonresponders," did not differ with regard
to their physical work capacity, ST depression, and RPP at room temperature. Thus, it
is not possible to predict the reaction to
cold from the value of these variables
recorded at room temperature.

In the whole group of patients, however, there is an association between the
deterioration of exercise tolerance and an
increase in ST depression at comparable work
load in the cold, i.e., the greater the
deterioration of the physical work capacity
in the cold as compared with room temperature, the more pronounced the depression of
the ST segment at an equal work load in the
cold.

The reaction to cold might be explained
by various mechanisms such as reflex coronary vasospasm as the result of cold stimulus to the skin (2,11,12). This explanation

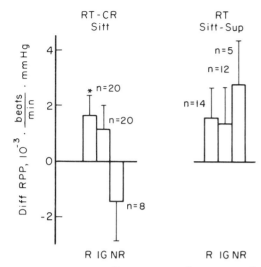

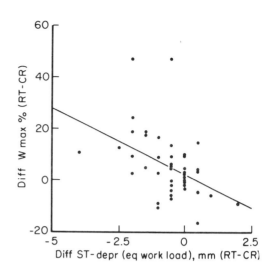

Figure 5. The difference between the largest rate pressure product (RPP) measured in the sitting position at room temperature (RT) and in a cold room (CR) as well as at room temperature in the sitting (Sitt) and supine (Sup) position ($\bar{x} \pm S.E.M.$). Symbols as in Figures 1 and 2.

Figure 6. The relation between the difference in SI depression on equal work load (RT-CR) and the difference in Wmax%(RT-CR) in the whole group of patients, N = 50. Diff Wmax% (RT-CR) = 2.2 - 5.1 · Diff ST-depr (equal work load)(RT-CR); r = 0.43.

is favored by recent findings (13) that coronary blood is diminished during a cold pressure test, and more often in coronary artery disease than if normal coronary arteries are present. Reflex constriction of cutaneous and other arteries might lead to an increased vascular resistance and increased blood pressure (1,14) and thus increased afterload with concomitant increase in left ventricular work (15). However, the responders had a lower RPP when they interrupted the exercise in the cold than at room temperature, which does not speak in favor of this hypothesis.

The responders reacted to cold in much the same way as all 3 groups in the supine position with regard to physical work capacity, EKG changes, and RPP determinations. Cold may influence hemodynamics in a similar way as a change from an upright to a supine body position, by causing a redistribution of blood from contracting peripheral vessels to the central blood pool (16,17). Cold causes increased secretion of catecholamines, which may also be a mechanism which moves blood centrally (18,19). Cold has also been shown to increase the carbon monoxide diffusion capacity (20), an indication of increased pulmonary capillary blood volume. Both cold and a supine position (21) might thus result in an increase in the central blood volume and in the diastolic volume of the heart. According to La Place's law this should increase myocardial

demand to oxygen for the same cardiac output (22).

The reason why some patients do not react to cold might be adaptation to cold (23). This suggestion is supported by the fact that the responders on the average had a higher heart rate during exercise in the cold room compared with room temperature than the other two groups. The difference between responders and the intermediate group was statistically significant (p < 0.001).

REFERENCES

1. Epstein SE, Stampfer M, Beiser GD, Goldstein R, Braunwald E. Effects of a reduction in environmental temperature on the circulatory response to exercise in man. N Engl J Med 1969; 280:7-11.
2. Freedberg AS, Spiegl ED, Riseman JEF. Effect of external heat and cold on patients with angina pectoris: Evidence for the existence of a reflex factor. Am Heart J 1944; 27:611-622.
3. Riseman JEF, Stern B. A standard exercise tolerance test for patients with angina pectoris. Am J Med Sci 1934; 188:646-659.
4. Backman C, Holm S, Linderholm H. Reaction to cold in patients with coronary insufficiency. Upsala J Med Sci 1979; 84:181-187.

5. Lassvik C, Areskog N-H. Effects of various environmental temperatures on effort angina. Upsala J Med Sci 1979; 84:173-180.
6. Backman C, Holm S, Linderholm H. Effect of cold in patients with coronary insufficiency. Scientific and technical progress and circumpolar health. Fourth International Symposium on Circumpolar Health, Novosibirsk, 1978; 2.
7. Sjöstrand T, ed. Clinical physiology. Stockholm: Svenska Bokförlaget, 1967.
8. Borg G, Linderholm H. Exercise performance and perceived exertion in patients with coronary insufficiency, arterial hypertension and vasoregulatory asthenia. Acta Med Scand 1970; 187:17-26.
9. Strandell T. Heart rate and work load at maximal working intensity in old men. Acta Med Scand 1964; suppl 414.
10. Robinson B. Relation of heart rate and systolic blood pressure to the onset of pain in angina pectoris. Circulation 1967; 35:1073-1083.
11. Mudge GH Jr, Grossman W, Mills RM Jr, Lesch M, Braunwald E. Reflex increase in coronary vascular resistance in patients with ischemic heart disease. N Engl J Med 1976; 295:333-337.
12. Neill WA, Duncan DA, Kloster F et al. Response of coronary circulation to cutaneous cold. Am J Med 1974; 56:471-476.
13. Emanuelsson M. Hemodynamic and myocardial metabolic changes in experimentally induced angina pectoris. Göteborg 1983. Dissertation.
14. Hayward JM, Holmes WF, Gooden BA. Cardiovascular responses in man to stream of cold air. Cardiovasc Res 1976; 10:691-696.
15. Leon DF, Amidi M, Leonard JJ. Left heart work and temperature responses to cold exposure in man. Am J Cardiol 1979; 26:38-45.
16. Glaser EM, Berridge FR, Prior KM. Effects of heat and cold on the distribution of blood within the human body. Clin Sci 1950; 9:181-187.
17. Linderholm H. The cold environment and coronary insufficiency. Nordic Council for Arct Med Res Rep 1977; 8:48.
18. Caldini P, Permutt S, Waddell JA, Rilley RL. Effect of epinephrine on pressure, flow and volume relationships in the systemic circulation of dogs. Circ Res 1974; 34:606-623.
19. Brunner M, Shoukas AA, MacAnespie CL. The effects of carotid sinus baroreceptor reflex in blood flow and volume redistribution in the total systemic vascular bed of the dog. Circ Res 1981; 48:274-285.
20. Wise RA, Wigley F, Newball HH, Stevens MB. The effect of cold exposure on diffusing capacity in patients with Raynaud's phenomenon. Chest 1982; 81:695-698.
21. Bygdeman S, Wahren J. Influence of body position on the anginal threshold during leg exercise. Eur J Clin Invest 1974; 2:201-206.
22. Rolett EL, Yurchag PM, Hood WB Jr, Gorlin R. Pressure volume correlates of left ventricular oxygen consumption in the hypervolemic dog. Circ Res 1965; 17:499-518.
23. Le Blanc J, Dulac S, Côté J, Girard B. Autonomic nervous system and adaptation to cold in man. J Appl Physiol 1975; 39:181-186.

Christer Backman
Department of Clinical Physiology
University Hospital
S-901 85 Umeå
Sweden

Circumpolar Health 84:83-84

THERMAL BIOFEEDBACK TRAINING WITH FROSTBITE PATIENTS

BRUNO M. KAPPES and WILLIAM J. MILLS

Thermal biofeedback training as an aid in the self-regulation of blood flow to the extremities has shown favorable results in the amelioration of certain specific vascular disorders (e.g. Raynaud's syndrome). The potential usefulness of thermal self-regulation with patients with varying degrees of cold insult or cold injury has demonstrated early promising results. Typical cold injuries are often accompanied by an array of vasospastic and vasoconstrictive complications, depending on the severity of the injury and the method of treatment received. Frostbite patients seem to be logical candidates for thermal biofeedback, specifically since a patient's vascular control of his/her extremities may be irregular or non-existent. The most favorable prospect is that for some cases a 1° to 2°C temperature change may mean the difference between surgery or the viable use of one's digits. Thermal biofeedback seems equally applicable during post-hospital recovery for those with labile vasomotor activity, Raynaud's syndrome or acute hypersensitivity to pain and cold. The following report is intended to discuss and highlight the issues and procedures associated with this particular patient population.

MATERIALS AND METHODS

Two patients who had sustained a recent freezing injury are described in this report. Although several patients have received thermal training to date, these patients seem to represent typical training results. Patient A was a 24-year-old mountain climber who was injured while attempting the summit of Mt. McKinley at an altitude of 17,200 feet, the summit being 20,300 feet. Temperatures in the region reached -30°F. The injury involved was superficial for the hands and left foot; however, superficial to deep injury occurred to all digits of the right foot. Technetium studies indicated adequate profusion throughout the foot and toes.

Patient B was a 20-year-old mountain climber who suffered deep frostbite injury to the right foot while descending the south buttress of Mt. McKinley. Technetium scan showed a lack of profusion of the first and second toe. The patient at discharge was diagnosed as likely to experience tissue loss to the second and first toes.

Both patients received a basic frostbite treatment regime developed by Dr. Mills, which consisted of the following abbreviated protocol. First, skin temperatures of the extremities were measured before, midway through and after tubbing upon admission. Second, patients were required to receive daily whirlpool for 20 minutes at a day at 35°C twice a day with Betadine or pHisoHex. Patients were placed on a high calorie and high protein diet. Dibenzyline was prescribed for vasodilation while digital and Berger's exercises were required on a regular basis to enhance circulation and prevent venous stasis.

Patients received taped instructions on four different types of relaxation exercises and were required to practice one or more of them twice a day prior to biofeedback. These included Progressive, Antogenic, Breathing and Guided Imagery. Patients practiced thermal biofeedback twice a day for 20 to 25 minute periods. Practice was only allowed 1 to 2 hours after whirlpool or meals (or before those activities) but not directly after. Two separate thermistors were placed on two different sites. Site A was located in an area close to the injury where circulation was evident. Site B was placed on or close to the injury or on the line of demarcation where there was questionable blood flow. Patients were instructed to practice exclusively on Site A so as to receive the maximum amount of reinforcement possible with hopes of encouraging greater blood flow to the injured area. Both sites were recorded and results are shown in Figures 1 and 2.

Technetium 9⁹ m scans were used to measure profusion in the blood vessels and a Doppler Ultrasound Instrument was used to test for arterial pulsations. A Digitec thermometer model no. 5820 with Yellow Springs thermistors was used to measure skin temperature of the extremities on admission and a Cyborg P642 thermal trainer was used for biofeedback training.

RESULTS AND DISCUSSION

The results demonstrated some promising effects of increased blood circulation to both patients' foot temperatures. However, there was some irregularity in the amount and frequency of temperature increases. Patients A and B both displayed an initial drop in the beginning sessions, which is typical for most persons learning these new responses (e.g. trying too hard). Patient A seemed to demonstrate early success by increasing his temperature of site A concomitantly with increases in site B. Recall that patients did not receive any feedback on site B and therefore these increases seem to represent a generalization of blood flow resulting from training on site A. This was clearly evident in Patient A. However, the

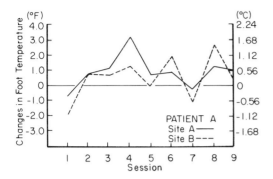

Figure 1. *Changes in foot temperatures by site over sessions for Patient A.*

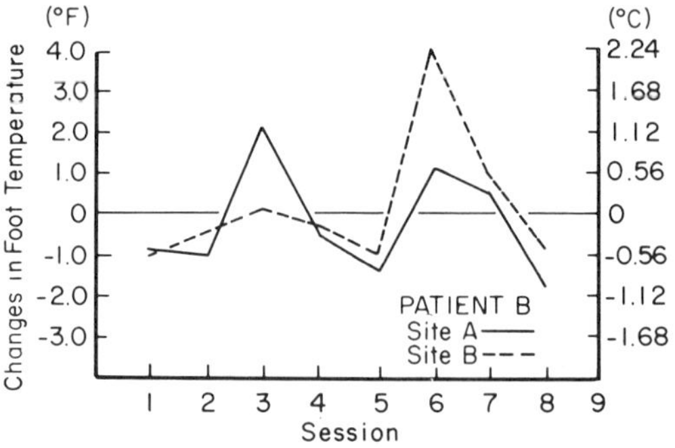

Figure 2. *Changes in foot temperatures by site over sessions for Patient B.*

patterns for Patient B were not as striking and appear irregular and somewhat lower than Patient A. This is not surprising since the severity of the injury was greater for Patient B. Both patients were extremely cooperative and found their biofeedback allowed them to take an active role in their recovery.

The problems in isolating the exclusive effects of biofeedback are too numerous to mention here; however, a few of the difficulties are summarized below. First, thermistor placements are extremely awkward considering each injury has its own unique severity and associated complications. Second, the type and sterility of thermistors are important in preventing bacterial infection. Infra-red cameras are currently under consideration. Third, the effects of vasodilators or pain medication confound the influence of self-regulatory abilities. Fourth, the emotional and psychological problems associated with body image at the thought of losing a limb or the possibility of being handicapped are quite devastating on one's concentration. Fifth, the effects of phantom pain after surgery or paralysis, pain, and sensitivity to cold all contribute to important issues requiring counseling and support to ensure the effectiveness of the biofeedback. Since mountain climbing in Alaska often attracts international climbers, language difficulties add further to an already problematic situation.

Although it is premature to determine the specific effects of thermal biofeedback for frostbite patient populations, it nevertheless makes sense to encourage its use. Most cold injury treatment methods are concerned with techniques known to increase blood circulation. Since blood flow to the injured extremity may mean the difference between dead tissue and live tissue, it certainly deserves our consideration.

Bruno M. Kappes
Psychology Department
University of Alaska
Anchorage, AK 99508
U.S.A.

INCREASED TENDENCY TO COLD-INDUCED VASOSPASM IN THE FINGERS (RAYNAUD'S PHENOMENON) IN COPPER SMELTER WORKERS EXPOSED TO ARSENIC

HÅKAN LINDERHOLM and B. LAGERKVIST

Raynaud's phenomenon (1) and even gangrene (black foot disease) (2,3) have been reported after long-term heavy exposure to arsenic in drinking water (arsenic intake about 2 mg/day). Peripheral vascular disease has not previously been observed among smelter workers. Some smelter workers in northern Sweden exposed to arsenic dust below accepted Swedish occupational limits, however, complained of cold hands and feet and white fingers in a cold environment.

The aim of this study, which is part of a larger one dealing with the toxicity of arsenic (4), was to examine if changes in the peripheral circulation of workers exposed to arsenic dust could be detected with physiological methods, and whether such changes could explain an abnormal sensitivity to cold.

MATERIALS AND METHODS

Forty-seven male workers who had been exposed to arsenic dust for 8 to 40 years (mean 23 years) at the copper smelter Rönnskärsverken in northern Sweden were examined. The arsenic content of the air had been below the accepted Swedish occupational standard which until 1975 was 500 $\mu g/m^3$ and since 1975, 50 $\mu g/m^3$. All workers with illness unrelated to arsenic in which the nervous or vascular systems were involved were excluded.

Controls were 48 male workers from a mechanical industrial enterprise in the same county not exposed to arsenic. No major differences between arsenic workers and controls were found on clinical examination, except nasal septum perforation in 10 arsenic workers. Twenty-eight arsenic workers and 28 controls were exposed to vibrating hand tools. The subjects considered not to be exposed to vibrating hand tools fulfilled the following criteria (5):
- No exposure or exceptionally short and sporadic exposure to vibrating hand tools during the last 2 years;
- Less than 1 year's full-time work with vibrating hand tools more than 10 years ago;
- Less than one-half year's full-time work with vibrating hand tools between 2 and 4 years earlier.

Workers who had used vibrating hand tools to a greater extent were considered to have been exposed to vibration.

Complaints of cold hands and feet and of white fingers (Raynaud's phenomenon) were recorded in the clinical history of all subjects, in addition to further factors which might impair peripheral circulation

such as trauma, diabetes, peripheral vascular disease, drug use, and environmental factors such as use of vibrating hand tools.

Systolic blood pressure and pulse curves in fingers were recorded at a skin temperature of 36°C (6) and simultaneously in the arm with the cuff method. Systolic blood pressure in the fingers at local cooling (FSP) was measured according to Nielsen et al. (7). FSP was measured simultaneously in 2 fingers of the same hand after 5 minutes of arterial occlusion, 1 finger being cooled to 15 and to 10°C.

FSP at 15 and 10°C was expressed as a percentage of the pressure at 30°C corrected for blood pressure changes in the reference finger according to the following equation.

$$FSP\% = \frac{100 \cdot (FSP_{15 \text{ or } 10°C})}{FSP_{30°C} - (FSP_{ref,30°C} - FSP_{ref,15 \text{ or } 10°C})}$$

where FSP_{ref} is the FSP of the reference finger.

Normal limits for the finger systolic pressure at 15°C and 10°C expressed as FSP% were obtained from measurements in 20 control subjects with no exposure to vibrating hand tools. The lower normal limit for FSP% at 15°C was 67% and at 10°C (see Figure 1). Subjects with FSP% values lower than one or both of these limits were regarded as having a vasospastic reaction in the finger to local cooling. Three control subjects who had a vasospastic reaction were not included in the calculation of normal limits.

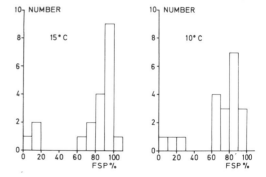

Figure 1. Finger systolic pressures (FSP) at 15°C and 10°C expressed in percent of the pressure at 30°C in 20 controls with no exposure to vibration. Lower normal levels ($\bar{x}$ - 2 S.D.), 67% at 15°C and 59% at 10°C.

RESULTS

The presence of Raynaud's phenomenon (white fingers) in the arsenic workers and the control group according to history is shown in Table 1. Raynaud's phenomenon was more common in the arsenic workers than in the control group and usually occurred in a cold environment.

Distal blood pressure and finger pulse curves indicated a slight arterial obstruction only in 1 arsenic worker with an arm-finger blood pressure difference of 40 mmHg.

The FSP% at 10°C was on an average lower in the arsenic workers, 52%, than in the control group, 62%, (p < 0.01). A vasospastic reaction in the fingers after cooling was more common among arsenic workers than among controls (Table 2), particularly if all subjects exposed to vibrating hand tools were excluded.

The urinary concentration of arsenic in early morning urine samples was 71 (10 - 340) μg/l in the arsenic workers and 7 (5 - 20) μg/l in controls.

DISCUSSION

The particle size of the airborne dust at the smelter of the present study has been reported to be about 5 μm (8). A rough estimate of the daily absorption of arsenic from the air with a concentration of less than 50 μg As/m^3 air, mainly arsenic trioxide, resulted in a total absorption of about 60% of the arsenic in the inhaled air or less than 300 μg/day. This corresponded fairly well to an average mean excretion of arsenic in urine of the smelter workers of 105 μg/day. A daily intake of arsenic of 105 μg/day for 47 weeks of work in a year would give a total absorption of 25 mg/year over the last 7 years and previously about 250 mg/year when the occupational exposure limit was 10 times higher. The mean duration of exposure was 23 years which gives a mean total ab- sorption of about 4 g. This is less than the total dose of about 20 g, which subjects who developed black foot disease ingested with drinking water (3,9).

The moderate exposure to arsenic of the arsenic workers was associated with an increased prevalence of vasospastic reaction in the fingers after local cooling and complaints of white fingers compared to controls. It seems reasonable to assume that the differences between arsenic workers and controls, which were statistically significant, are due to exposure to the arsenic.

Exposure to vibrating hand tools (10, 11,12) is known to cause a vasospastic reaction. In our study concomitant exposure to arsenic and vibrating hand tools did not cause an increase of vasospastic reactivity compared to exposure to arsenic alone nor was it possible to demonstrate any significant effect of exposure to vibration alone. This may be due to the relatively small and heterogeneous exposure to vibrating hand tools. Factors other than arsenic and vibrating hand tools which may possibly cause vasospastic disease were present to about the same extent in arsenic workers as in controls.

The copper smelter workers more often than controls complained of cold hands and white fingers in cold weather. The complaints did not affect their ability to work indoors but forced them to wear warm gloves in a cold environment when other people managed to work with uncovered hands.

Table 1. Number of workers exposed to arsenic (As-workers) and controls with a history of Raynaud's phenomenon (white fingers).

Group	White fingers +	-	P
All workers			
As-workers N=47	10	37	
			< 0.05
Controls N=48	2	46	
No exposure to vibration			
As-workers N=19	3	16	
			> 0.10
Controls N=20	0	20	
Exposure to vibration			
As-workers N=28	7	21	
			> 0.10
Controls N=28	2	26	

Table 2. Number of As-workers and controls with and without a vasospastic reaction in the fingers after cooling.

Group	Vasospastic reaction +	-	P
All workers			
As-workers N=47	28	19	
			< 0.05
Controls N=48	17	31	
No exposure to vibration			
As-workers N=19	14	5	
			< 0.01
Controls N=20	4	16	
Exposure to vibration			
As-workers N=28	14	14	
			> 0.20
Controls N=28	13	15	

CONCLUSION

Increased vasospastic reactivity to cold and increased prevalence of Raynaud's phenomenon were found among smelter workers and were probably caused by long-term exposure to moderate levels of inorganic arsenic in airborne dust. These workers had difficulties working with uncovered hands in a cold environment. These changes may be related to earlier findings of peripheral gangrene, or "black foot disease," after heavy exposure to arsenic.

REFERENCES

1. Borgoño JM, Vicent P, Venturino H, Infante A. Arsenic in the drinking water of the city of Antofagasta: Epidemiological and clinical study before and after the installation of a treatment plant. Environ Health Perspect 1977; 19:103-105.
2. Astrup P. Blackfoot disease. Ugesk Laeger 1968; 130:1807-1815.
3. Tseng W-P. Effects and dose-response relationships of skin cancer and blackfoot disease with arsenic. Environ Health Perspect 1977; 19:109-119.
4. Lagerkvist B, Linderholm H, Blom S, Thorulf P, Nordberg G. Systemeffekter av arsenik. The Coal-Health-Environment Project. Report no 78. The Swedish State Power Board, Vällingby, Sweden, 1983. English summary.
5. Lidström I-M. Lokala vibrationers inverkan på övre extremiteterna. Arbete och Hälsa, 8. The Work Health Protection Board and the Dept. of Hygiene, Umeå University, 1974. English summary.
6. Strandness DE, Bell JW. Peripheral vascular disease: Diagnosis and objective evaluation using a mercury strain gauge. Ann Surg 1965; suppl 4:3-35.
7. Nielsen SL, Sørenson CJ, Olsen N. Thermostatted measurement of systolic blood pressure on cooled fingers. Scand J Clin Lab Invest 1980; 40:683-687.
8. Leffler P, Gerhardsson L, Brune D, Nordberg G. Lung retention of antimony and arsenic in hamsters after intratracheal installation of industrial dust. 1983. Unpublished.
9. Pershagen G, Vahter M. Arsenic. A toxicological and epidemiological appraisal. The National (Swedish) Environmental Protection Board PM 1128.
10. Gemne G. Pathophysiology and multifactorial etiology of acquired vasospastic disease (Raynaud syndrome) in vibration-exposed workers. Scand J Work Environ Health 1982; 8:243-249.
11. Taylor W, Pelmear P. Raynaud's phenomenon of occupational origin, an epidemiological survey. Acta Chir Scand 1976; suppl 465:27-32.
12. Thulesius O. Primary and secondary Raynaud phenomena. Acta Chir Scand 1976; suppl 465:5-6.

Håkan Linderholm
Department of Clinical Physiology
University Hospital
S-901 85 Umeå
Sweden

Circumpolar Health 84:88-91

MERCURY SURVEILLANCE IN SEVERAL CREE INDIAN COMMUNITIES OF THE JAMES BAY REGION, QUEBEC

CHARLES DUMONT and RUSSELL WILKINS

INTRODUCTION

"Mad as a hatter." This well-known English expression reminds us that the adverse health effects of occupational exposure to mercury have been recognized for well over a century. Since 1956, when the tragic consequences of acute methylmercury poisoning among fish-eaters living near a source of industrial pollution in southern Japan began to be reported, "Minamata disease" has been linked to ingestion of mercury through food sources. Outbreaks of acute methylmercury poisoning have also occurred in Iraq and Guatemala among populations exposed to extremely high concentrations of mercury from diets which included bread made from mercury-treated seed grain.

In Canada, mercury exposure exceeding by several times the World Health Organization (WHO) standards (which are 20 parts per billion in blood and 6 parts per million in hair) has occurred among native peoples in northern Ontario, Quebec, and the Northwest Territories[1]. The concentrations reported, however, were usually well below the levels proven to produce clinical symptoms in susceptible individuals (approximately 10 times the WHO standards).

Nevertheless, chronic exposure to moderate concentrations of mercury (above the WHO standards but below acutely toxic levels) through dietary sources has recently been linked to a somewhat greater risk of relatively mild neurological disturbances[2,3]. These symptoms include a tendency to reduced peripheral vision, trembling of the hands, numbness of the limbs, and lack of coordination in muscle and eye movements. As such symptoms may also be associated with conditions and factors unrelated to mercury exposure, positive diagnosis of borderline mercury poisoning is difficult if not impossible. Moreover, insofar as prolonged exposure to relatively low levels of mercury is concerned, it has not yet been possible to determine if there exists a critical threshold, or whether any exposure is eventually likely to be harmful, at least to some extent.

Inorganic mercury occurs naturally in the rocks of northern Quebec. Mining and smelting activities also result in the release of mercury into the region's air and waterways. Until 1978, a chlor-alkali process paper plant at Lebel-sur-Quévillon regularly dumped mercury into the waters of the Bell-Nottaway river system on the southern fringe of the region.

Under favorable conditions, inorganic mercury is changed (methylated) by bacteria into organic mercury (especially methylmercury), which can be readily incorporated into the living tissues of plants and animals. Although the concentration of mercury in the water may be very small, as it works its way up through the food chain, the concentration increases at each step. Another problem is that when the water in a lake becomes more acidic (as tends to happen after a dam is built or when the catchment area of the lake receives acid rainfall), mercury is released more rapidly into the water to begin its way up the food chain.

After a person eats mercury-contaminated food, the mercury spreads throughout the body but concentrates most heavily in the liver, kidney and brain. If no more mercury-contaminated food is eaten, the body can eventually rid itself of most if not all of the mercury. On the average, about half of the mercury is eliminated in about 70 days, but this "half-life" period varies from 30 to 180 days [4]. Mercury levels tend to build up, however, any time mercury-contaminated food is taken in at a rate faster than the body can eliminate it, such as when contaminated food forms an important part of the regular diet of Native hunters and trappers.

The purpose of the mercury surveillance program among the James Bay Cree of Quebec was to identify individuals presumed to be "at risk" of suffering adverse health effects from high levels of mercury exposure, and to provide them with nutritional counselling which would allow them to reduce their level of exposure.

For the purposes of the surveillance program, the "at risk" level was taken as three times or more the WHO standards. This appeared to offer some margin of safety without requiring the total abandonment of traditional bush life which strict adherence to the WHO standards would have seemed to imply. All parties involved were concerned not to impose a "cure" which might entail consequences as bad as or worse than the disease itself, especially among persons exposed to levels only moderately above the WHO standards.

MATERIALS AND METHODS

Within the 8,000 population of the eight James Bay Cree communities in northern Quebec, two sub-populations were identified as targets for the mercury surveillance program: all persons aged 35 and over (about 2,000 individuals), and all pregnant women and their babies (about 200 births a year). In 1983, approximately 40 percent of the target population was tested.

Umbilical cord blood samples were taken at three northern Quebec hospitals (Chisasibi, Val d'Or and Chibougamau). Hair samples were usually taken at the nursing stations in each community. Laboratory analyses were carried out on the first, second, and third cm of hair nearest to the scalp. Assuming an average growth rate of one cm per month, the three centimeters were indicative of mercury exposure in each of the three months preceeding the taking of the hair strands. In the case of a blood sample, the test results indicated the current level of exposure at the time the sample was taken.

Except in the case of pregnant women, for whom samples were taken during the course of pregnancy as well as at the birth of their child, only one set of tests was done per person each year. Thus, in discussing the test results for a given year based on the centimeter yielding the highest reading in each sample of hair, we are essentially referring to maximum values for individuals. The same is not necessarily true of results for two or more years, as the same individuals were likely to have been tested more than once.

From the summer of 1982, when the present surveillance program began, to the end of the first quarter of 1984, over 1,300 hair and blood samples were taken, yielding nearly 5,000 separate laboratory test results. These were compiled by age, sex, and community of residence. For each community, lists of results for each individual tested as well as summary statistics for all communities were sent to the nursing stations and the Chisasibi hospital. Summary statistics were presented to the Cree Regional Board of Health and Social Services of James Bay.

RESULTS

As seen in Table 1, about half of all persons tested showed concentrations exceeding the WHO standards, and one in twelve showed concentrations exceeding three times the WHO standards. The highest exposures measured were 15 to 20 times the standards.

Table 2 shows the breakdown of the test results by age, sex, and community of affiliation. Men were somewhat more likely than women to have high concentrations. The oldest (65+ years) and youngest (<1 year) were more likely to be in the "at risk" category than were young (15 to 34) or middle-aged adults (35 to 64). (Tests on persons aged 15 to 34 were limited to pregnant women and new mothers). Infants were much more likely to show high test results than were their mothers. The

Table 1. *Mercury concentration in hair or blood compared to WHO standards*, James Bay Cree of Quebec, 1982 to March 1984.*

Exposure/ Standard	Test Results	
	N	%
≥ 0.0	1,337	100.0
≥ 1.0	650	48.6
≥ 2.0	270	20.2
≥ 3.0	99	7.4
≥ 4.0	57	4.3
≥ 5.0	28	2.1
≥10.0	3	0.2

*   The WHO standards are 20 ppb in blood, and 6 ppm in hair.

communities of Great Whale, Waswanipi and Wemindji (Paint Hills) showed the highest percentage of persons exposed to concentrations of mercury exceeding three times the WHO standards.

DISCUSSION AND CONCLUSIONS

As shown in Table 3, compared to results of the earlier federal testing program for 1977 and 1978,(1) the percentage of persons tested found to be "at risk" had declined substantially in Mistassini, but increased in Great Whale and Waswanipi. Note however, that because the persons tested were not selected at random (or even in the same non-random fashion over the years), the observed increase may not be representative of concentrations in the entire target populations. Other problems affecting the comparability of test results over time are due to the marked seasonal variation in mercury exposure, together with the fact that tests frequently did not cover exposure over the same months of each year.

With those cautionary notes in mind, it is still possible to draw certain conclusions from the first two years of this surveillance program. First, a substantial portion (7%) of the population tested was found to have excessively high concentrations of mercury in their bodies (3 times or more the WHO standards). Older adults and infants were most likely to be highly exposed. Great Whale, Waswanipi, and Mistassini were the communities where high exposure was most likely to occur. Since 1978, the situation appears to have improved in Mistassini, but deteriorated in Great Whale and Waswanipi.

As persons with abnormally high concentrations of mercury in their bodies are presumed to be at greater risk of neurologic disturbance because of their exposure, the

Table 2.   Summary of mercury test results among the James Bay Cree of Quebec, by age, sex, community, and level of exposure, 1982 to March 1984.

Category	Persons tested N	Exposure compared to WHO standards	
		% ≥ 1.0	% ≥ 3.0
Total	1,337	41.2	7.4
Age			
<1	168	34.5	11.3
1-14	2	100.0	
15-34	198	15.2	1.5
35-64	767	45.1	6.6
65+	202	56.9	12.9
Sex			
Male	548	47.4	9.5
Female	735	36.5	6.0
Unstated	54	42.6	5.6
Community			
Great Whale	109	50.5	28.4
Chisasibi	188	20.7	3.7
Wemindji	302	52.3	6.0
Eastmain	90	21.1	
Rupert	171	29.8	2.3
Nemaska	11	63.6	
Waswanipi	88	39.8	12.5
Mistassini	370	50.0	7.6
elsewhere	8	25.0	

Table 3.   Comparison of mercury test results for 1977-1978 and 1982-1983-1984.

Community	Number of Tests		% > 3.0 x WHO standards	
	1977-78	1982-83-84	1977-78	1982-83-84
Great Whale	919	109	18.7	28.4
Chisasibi	1,890	188	7.6	3.7
Wemindji	509	302	4.5	6.0
Eastmain	308	90	3.6	
Rupert	274	171	1.8	2.3
Nemaska	0	11		
Waswanipi	314	88	5.7	12.5
Mistassini	762	370	19.0	7.6
elsewhere		8		
Total	4976	1337	10.4	7.4

surveillance program should be continued, if only to bring these facts to the attention of the individuals concerned. Continued surveillance of the target population is called for in all communities, and nutritional counselling for all highly exposed individuals is important. Pregnant women and their babies should continue to be the most important priority of the program, both in terms of testing, and in terms of nutritional education. Tests should be carried out on women giving birth in Montreal and Moose Factory as well as in the three northern Quebec hospitals. Great Whale and Waswanipi, where mercury exposure appears to have increased, are the two communities where implementation of the above suggestions are of most importance.

Nutritional guidelines for Native peoples should be updated to reflect current environmental conditions. They should also be revised to take account of possible contamination from wild foods other than fish. It may be necessary to make particular recommendations concerning the very high concentrations of mercury found in the internal organs of some fish and game animals.

Current concentrations of mercury content in the wild foods of each area should be determined. Tests should be conducted on all possible sources of exposure, including fowl, small and large game, as well as fish of various species. Determination of the mercury content in the internal organs and parts of the body other than the flesh should be considered, so as to take account of the actual eating habits of Native persons.

ACKNOWLEDGMENTS

This mercury surveillance program was sponsored by the Quebec Ministry of Social Affairs and the Cree Regional Board of Health and Social Services of James Bay. Since 1982, analysis of hair and blood samples has been performed by the Quebec Public Health Laboratory. Until 1982, the Medical Services Branch of Health and Welfare Canada was responsible for the testing.

REFERENCES

1. Health and Welfare Canada. Methylmercury in Canada. Exposure of Indian and Inuit residents to methylmercury in the Canadian environment. A review of the Medical Services Branch, Department of National Health and Welfare, mercury program findings to Dec 31, 1978. Written by Brian Wheatley. Ottawa: Medical Services Branch, Health and Welfare Canada, Dec 1979.
2. McKeowen-Eyssen GE, Ruedy J. Methylmercury exposure in northern Quebec. I. Neurologic findings in adults. Amer J Epidemiol 1983; 118(4):461-469.
3. McKeowen-Eyssen GE, Ruedy J, Neims A. Methylmercury exposure in northern Quebec. II. Neurologic findings in children. Amer J Epidemiol 1983; 118(4):470-479.
4. National Research Council of Canada (NRCC). Effects of mercury in the Canadian environment. Executive Report. Compiled by J.F. Jaworski. Subcommittee on heavy metals and certain other elements. NRCC associate committee on scientific criteria for environmental quality. Ottawa, 1980.

Charles Dumont
Department of Community Health
Montreal General Hospital
1597 Pine Avenue West
Montreal, Quebec H3G 1B3
Canada

Circumpolar Health 84:92-95

ENDOGENOUS AND EXOGENOUS SOURCES OF NITRATE/NITRITE AND NITROSAMINES IN CANADIAN INUIT WITH A TRADITIONAL OR WESTERN LIFESTYLE

HANS F. STICH and A. PAUL HORNBY

INTRODUCTION

Environmental and lifestyle factors seem to be involved in the etiology of about 80 to 85% of human cancers, which should therefore be preventable. Shifts in cancer patterns among immigrants support this assumption: for example, Japanese immigrants to the United States or Canada (reduced incidence of stomach carcinomas), Chinese immigrants to Singapore (reduced incidence of hepatomas), English immigrants to New Zealand and Australia (reduced incidence of bronchogenic cancer), and Indian immigrants to Canada (reduced incidence of oral cancers). More recently, the idea seems to find general acceptance that the prevention of cancer can be achieved either by removal of the carcinogenic agents from man's environment or the addition of anti-carcinogenic compounds to the diet. The removal of carcinogens from man's environment would appear to be the simplest approach. Indeed, a significant reduction of many occupational cancers has been achieved by reducing exposure to the carcinogens in the workplace. However, the average citizen is exposed to many small doses of carcinogens over a prolonged period of time. In such a situation, it becomes more difficult to trace the carcinogens responsible, and cancer prevention by the administration of chemo-preventive agents would appear to be the more promising approach.

Canadian Inuit, Alaskan and Greenland Eskimos, and Natives of Siberia show elevated frequencies of cancers at particular sites, including the nasopharynx, salivary glands, and esophagus (1-4). The particular cancer patterns of arctic inhabitants are changing drastically, seemingly due to changing lifestyle and dietary habits (1). The proposed approach in cancer prevention is based on the assumption that population groups with a limited intake of anti-carcinogenic compounds should be highly responsive to the correction of the dietary deficiencies. However, there are certain limitations to identifying etiological factors of particular cancers. The great time lapse between cancer induction and the actual appearance of a detectable tumor makes the tracing of causative factors difficult. Thus, conditions which prevailed in the Arctic about 10 to 25 years ago would be responsible for most cancers seen today. To tackle this problem, 2 approaches can be taken. Firstly, one must seek to examine population groups which are still close to past dietary and behavioral patterns. Secondly, one must define the lifestyle factors which have changed over the last 2 decades and which may be responsible for the shift of cancer frequencies. We have therefore selected 3 Inuit settlements (Spence Bay, Pelly Bay, and Gjoa Haven) which still adhere, at least most of the year, to a more traditional dietary pattern; Cambridge Bay, where the residents live part of the year on a traditional diet and at other times on a more westernized diet; and Inuvik, as a place where the residents consume to a large degree "westernized" food products.

N-nitroso compounds have been repeatedly implicated in the etiology of carcinomas of the esophagus, nasopharynx, stomach, and oral cavity (5). It would be beyond the scope of this paper to discuss all the pros and cons of the involvement of nitroso compounds in the etiology of human cancers. We will point only to 2 observations which are pertinent to our research projects.

The first is that population groups in South China, the Philippines, and Indonesia, who are at elevated risk for nasopharyngeal cancers, consume relatively large quantities of fermented fish juice which seems to contain several carcinogenic and mutagenic nitroso compounds. The Inuit of the Northwest Territories do not use any fish juice but frequently ingest arctic char, whale flippers, and muskox or caribou meat which is kept under soil or pebbles until rotten. This delicacy is appropriately called "stink meat," and may contain numerous nitroso compounds formed during fermentation. The other observation is that secondary amines are relatively abundant in fish and whale meat (6), both common dietary items of the Inuit. Thus, the northern groups may consume large amounts of precursors which could conceivably be nitrosated within the acid gastric juice into carcinogenic and mutagenic nitroso compounds. Among the Inuit, this endogenous nitrosation could be particularly favored because of the alleged low intake of dietary inhibitors, which are found predominantly in fruits and vegetables (7).

METHODS AND RESULTS

To yield information on the possible involvement of nitrosamines in the development of cancer among the Inuit, we examined the salivary nitrite levels since they may influence the endogenous formation of nitroso compounds. The results are shown in Figure 1. For comparison, the nitrite levels of two population groups at elevated risk for oral cancer and esophageal carcinomas, respectively, have been added. The

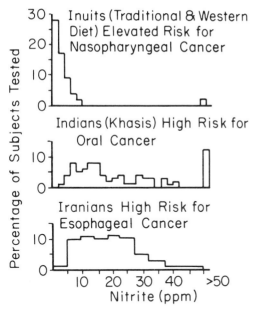

Figure 1. *Nitrite levels in the saliva of 3 groups at elevated risk for cancer: Inuit (Pelly Bay, Gjoa Haven, Inuvik, Yellowknife), Khasis of the northeastern hill regions of India (Meghalaya) and Iranians (Zaboli) (16).*

salivary nitrite levels of Inuit consuming a mainly traditional diet (Pelly Bay and Gjoa Haven) and of those ingesting a traditional and "westernized" diet are presented in Figure 2. A slight but significant increase of salivary nitrite levels can be seen in individuals on a mixed dietary pattern.

Urinary levels of N-nitrosoproline (NPRO) were chosen as an indicator for endogenously formed or ingested, preformed N-nitroso compounds (8,9). NPRO was selected since it is not metabolized within the

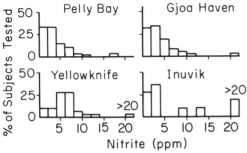

Figure 2. *Nitrite levels in the saliva of Inuit on a traditional diet (Pelly Bay, Gjoa Haven) and a mixed consumption of traditional and "western" food products (Yellowknife, Inuvik).*

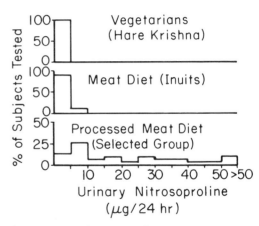

Figure 3. *N-nitrosoproline (NPRO) levels of Inuit, vegetarians, and volunteers consuming a "European" diet of nitrite-preserved sausages and ham.*

human body, and virtually all ingested or endogenously formed NPRO is excreted in the urine. The results are shown in Figure 3, which also includes NPRO levels of strict vegetarians and persons consuming nitrate-preserved meat products. Despite the relatively large intake of proline-rich fish and meat products, the NPRO levels among Inuit are relatively low. This observation is of particular interest considering the very small amount of ingested vegetables and fruits. The Inuit of the western arctic regions, however, consume exceptionally large quantities of tea, which contains phenolics that are excellent trappers of nitrite (7,11). Once the Inuit start to consume "western" food products as part of the traditional meat diet, the NPRO levels in the urine significantly increase (Figure 4).

Another approach to gain insight into the role of preformed N-nitroso compounds consists of ingesting known quantities of a particular food product and estimating the amount of NPRO excreted over a 24-hr period (10). Table 1 shows urinary NPRO levels after consumption of fish and mammalian meats collected in the settlements of the Northwest Territories. These food products are the main staples of an Inuit diet in the villages previously mentioned. For comparative reasons, a few "western-type" nitrate-preserved meat products were eaten by a group of volunteers and the excreted NPRO measured. None of the Inuit meat and fish samples led to a high increase in urinary NPRO levels.

DISCUSSION

An elevated cancer risk could conceivably be due to high levels of carcinogens in man's environment (e.g., most

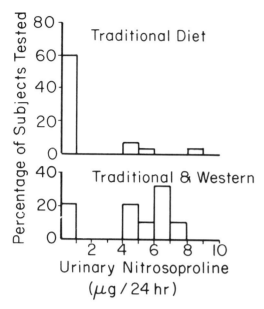

Figure 4. N-nitrosoproline levels of Inuit on a traditional diet (Pelly Bay) and a mixed consumption of traditional and "western" food products (Inuvik).

occupational cancers), a lack of anti-carcinogenic agents in the diet, and a strong activity of tumor promoters. The results revealed relatively low levels of nitrite in the saliva of Inuit consuming a traditional fish/meat diet virtually devoid of vegetables and fruits. NPRO levels in the urine were also low. Thus neither an intensive endogenous nitrosation nor a large intake of preformed NPRO occurred in the examined Inuit population groups. In this regard, the arctic population groups who are at elevated risk for nasopharyngeal and esophageal cancers differ from those in northern China, who are at high risk for esophageal cancer and who show high levels of urinary NPRO (9).

Chewing tobacco could be a source of preformed nitrosamines (12). In the past, the chewing of tobacco was apparently widespread, but has declined over the last few decades. More recently, however, the use of commercially available chewing tobacco has reached epidemic proportions among children and young adults of several settlements in the Northwest Territories (13). The seriousness of this new health hazard can be seen from damage to the mucosa of the lower groove, including an increase in the frequency of micronucleated cells (Table 2), which indicates cytogenetic damage in the tissues which give rise to oral carcinomas (14). An elevated frequency of micronucleated cells was also observed in the oral mucosa of tobacco chewers among Indians of Bihar and Orissa (India) and was considered to be among the first signs of preneoplastic changes (15). If the experience on tobacco users in India is applicable to tobacco users in the arctic regions, then one should expect to find in the near future a considerable increase in oral leukoplakias and carcinomas among Inuit chewers.

ACKNOWLEDGMENTS

This study was supported by Health and Welfare Canada. We wish to acknowledge the communities of Sachs Harbour, Paulatuk, Holman, Spence Bay, Pelly Bay, Gjoa Haven, and Cambridge Bay and the nursing stations of these settlements for their invaluable cooperation. In addition, we thank COPE and the N.W.T. Medical Services Branch for their generous assistance.

Table 1. Urinary levels of nitrosoproline (NPRO) following ingestion of typical Inuit fish and meats.

Food Product	Amount ingested (g)	NPRO excreted over 24 hr (µg)
Inuit dietary items:		
Muskox	100	0.38
Caribou	150	1.10
Arctic char	100	3.15
Goose	100	1.62
Muck tuk	100	7.05
Nitrate-preserved food items:		
Processed canned ham	170	38.50
Dutch salted meat	100	78.50
Chinese sausage	120	26.00
Salami	100	15.90

Table 2. Frequency of micronucleated oral mucosa cells of heavy tobacco chewers in Gjoa Haven, Northwest Territories.

Site sampled within the oral cavity	No. of chews/day	Micronucleated Cells (%)	
		Individual cases	Average*
Mucosa of site of tobacco	>10	0.6, 0.7, 1.7, 1.7, 2.0, 2.1 2.2, 2.3, 2.6, 2.6, 3.1, 3.8	2.11
Buccal mucosa at opposite side	>10	0.6, 0.2, 0.0, 1.0, 0.0, 0.7 0.0, 0.0, 1.0, 1.2, 1.2, 0.5	0.53

* The average frequency of micronucleated mucosa cells of non-chewers was 0.47%.

REFERENCES

1. Schaefer O, Hildes JA, Medd LM, Cameron DG. The changing pattern of neoplastic diseases in Canadian Eskimos. In: Shephard RJ, Itoh S, eds. Proceedings of the Third International Symposium on Circumpolar Health. Toronto: University of Toronto Press, 1976:130-134.
2. Lanier AP, Blot WJ, Bender TR, Fraumeni JF, Jr. Cancer in Alaskan Indians, Eskimos and Aleuts. J Natl Cancer Inst 1980; 65:1157-1159.
3. Nielsen NH, Mikkelsen F, Hansen JPH. Nasopharyngeal cancer in Greenland. Acta Path Microbiol Scand Sect A 1977; 85:850-858.
4. Kolicheva NI. Epidemiology of esophageal cancers in the USSR. In: Levin DL, ed. Cancer epidemiology in the USA and USSR. NIH Publ. No. 80-2044, 1980: 191-198.
5. IARC Scientific Publications Nos 3, 9, 14, 18, 19 and 31. Lyon: International Agency for Research on Cancer, 1972-1980.
6. Ishidate M, Tanimura A, Ito Y, Sakai A, Sakuta H, Kawamura T, Sakai K, Miyazawa F, Wada H. Secondary amines, nitrates and nitrosamines in Japanese foods. In: Nakahara W, Takayama S, Sugimura T, Odashima S, eds. Topics in chemical carcinogenesis. Baltimore: University Park Press, 1972:313-321.
7. Stich HF, Rosin MP. Naturally occurring phenolics as antimutagenic and anticarcinogenic agents. In: Friedman M, ed. Nutritional and toxicological aspects of food safety. New York: Plenum Press, 1984. In press.
8. Ohshima H, Bartsch H. Quantitative estimation of endogenous nitrosation in humans by monitoring N-nitrosoproline excreted in the urine. Cancer Res 1981; 41:3658-3662.
9. Bartsch H, Ohshima H, Munoz N, Pignatelli B, Friesen M, O'Neill I, Crespi M, Lu SH. Assessment of endogenous nitrosation in humans in relation to the risk of cancer of the digestive tract. In: Hayes AW, Schnell RC, Miya TS, eds. Developments in the science and practice of toxicology. Amsterdam: Elsevier Science Publishers, 1983:299-309.
10. Stich HF, Hornby AP, Dunn BP. The effect of dietary factors on nitrosoproline levels in human urine. Int J Cancer 1984. In press.
11. Stich HF, Ohshima H, Pignatelli B, Michelon J, Bartsch H. Inhibitory effect of betel nut extracts on endogenous nitrosation in man. J Natl Cancer Inst 1983; 70:1047-1050.
12. Hoffmann D, Adams JD. Carcinogenic tobacco-specific N-nitrosamines snuff and in the saliva of snuff dippers. Cancer Res 1981; 41:4305.
13. Milar WJ. Use of chewing tobacco and snuff by students in the Northwest Territories 1982. Chron Diseases in Canada 1984; 4:54-56.
14. Stich HF, Rosin MP. Micronuclei in exfoliated human cells as an internal dosimeter for exposures to carcinogens. In: Stich HF, ed. Carcinogens and mutagens in the environment. Vol II, Naturally occurring compounds: Endogenous formation and modulation. Boca Raton, Florida: CRC Press, 1982:17-25.
15. Stich HF, Curtis JR, Parida BB. Application of the micronucleus test to exfoliated cells of high cancer risk groups: tobacco chewers. Int J Cancer 1982; 3U:553-559.
16. Castegnaro M. Nitrite in saliva--possible relevance to in vivo formation of N-nitroso compounds. IARC Annual Report, Lyon, 1978:47-51.

Hans F. Stich
Environmental Carcinogenic Unit
British Columbia Cancer Research Centre
601 West 10th Avenue
Vancouver, British Columbia V5Z 1L3
Canada

Circumpolar Health 84:96-102

ALLERGENIC AIRBORNE POLLEN AND SPORE RESEARCH IN ALASKA AND ADJACENT CANADA

JAMES H. ANDERSON

INTRODUCTION

Many people in Alaska and adjacent Canada suffer from the seasonal allergy commonly known as hay fever caused by antigenic proteins in airborne pollen and spores. Although these aeroallergens may be rare in the far northern and western tundra zones, within the rest of this vast region they are abundantly produced in the spring and summer by most of the dominant components of the vegetation. These include several wind-pollinated tree and shrub species, a variety of grasses and other herbs, and many spore-producing fungi. As the non-Native population of Alaska, Yukon, and northwestern British Columbia continues inevitably to grow, victims of pollen and spore allergies will probably become more numerous.

A palynology laboratory, devoted to the study of modern and fossil pollen grains and spores, is being developed in the University of Alaska at Fairbanks. Aeropalynology, in addition to paleopalynology, has been chosen as a component of the laboratory's research program, partly for the purpose of acquiring knowledge of interest to physicians and hay fever victims. Research objectives are: 1) to determine the composition of the aeroflora taxonomically and numerically; 2) to determine relationships between the aeroflora and the vegetation; 3) to determine the dynamics of the aeroflora, including within-season and year-to-year variations; 4) to determine meteorologic or other environmental controls of aeroflora dynamics; and 5) to develop a predictive capability for allergenically significant aeropalynological events. An additional objective has been to determine the extent of pollen and spore allergies by conducting surveys of physicians in several cities. In Fairbanks a survey of hay fever victims has also been conducted, in an attempt to determine any quantifiable relationships between allergy symptoms and aerial concentrations of pollen and spores.

METHODS

The Alaskan aeroflora was sampled briefly by Durham (1) in 1939. The present writer began examining it in 1978 using 3 gravimetric samplers at the University in Fairbanks. This sampling was resumed in 1981, when the palynology laboratory was started, with sampling in Fairbanks and Palmer. In 1982 the program was upgraded through the acquisition of Burkard volumetric samplers made possible by a grant from the Alaska Council on Science and Techno-

logy. Since then the sampling program has been expanded to Juneau, Anchorage, and Whitehorse. Sampling will be continued for a total of at least 10 consecutive years in the key locations of Fairbanks, Anchorage, and Juneau. This is because year-to-year variations in aeroflora dynamics appear to be considerable, requiring a long-term data base for statistical analyses and the testing of hypotheses regarding controls over aeroflora dynamics. Future plans also include basic aeroflora surveys, with 2 or 3 years' sampling, in other population and tourist centers such as Ketchikan, Homer, and Dawson.

In Anchorage a Burkard volumetric sampler was used on the roof of Providence Hospital in 1982 and 1983. It was moved in 1984 to the roof of a lower building on the University campus just across the street. Burkard samplers in Juneau and Whitehorse were also installed on the hospitals of those cities. In Palmer the Burkard and a gravimetric sampler were used at the Agricultural Experiment Station near the hospital.

Progress in analyzing the numerous daily samples and the data has been slow owing to a lack of funding and technical assistants. In spite of this, a fair amount of new information is already available (see references). The rest of this brief paper will do 2 things: summarize results of the Anchorage physicians' survey, which have not been presented before, and show a few aspects of the results from aeroflora sampling in Fairbanks, Anchorage, and Juneau.

RESULTS AND DISCUSSION

In January 1984 survey forms were sent to 83 physicians in the Anchorage area selected for the possibility that they treated pollen and spore allergy patients. These forms included an explanatory letter, a summary of an earlier physicians' survey in Fairbanks, a questionnaire containing 10 easily answered items, plus a stamped and addressed return envelope. Even with the convenience of the latter, only 34 of the questionnaires were returned, but of these, 24, or 29% of those sent out, contained useful information.

The first question was: Approximately how many patients do you treat in a year for hay fever or other allergies or asthma caused by, or probably caused by airborne pollen or spores? Answers ranged from 5 to 175 for individual physicians and to 600 on 1 questionnaire returned collectively by 4 physicians in an allergy and pediatric clinic. The average per physician was 66,

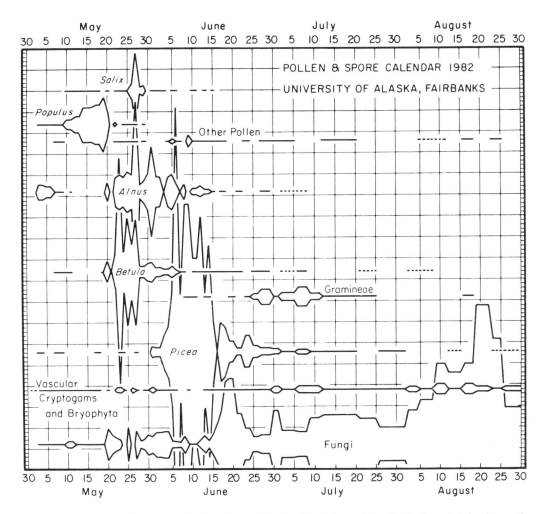

Figure 1. Pollen and spore calendar for 1982 at the University of Alaska, Fairbanks. The vertical scale indicates numbers of pollen grains and spores per square centimeters of sticky sample per day. Such data are an indication of atmospheric abundances.

and the total was 1,572. This is a substantial number of hay fever sufferers, but it is certainly a deficient estimate for Anchorage, whose population is now well over 200,000. This conclusion is based on the assumption that at least a few of the 49 physicians who did not return questionnaires, including Alaska's most well-known allergist, also see pollen and spore allergy patients. It is further substantiated by the responses to question 6.

Question 6 was: How many people in the Anchorage area would you guess have mild pollen or spore allergies and do not seek medical attention for them? Three of the 24 responding physicians checked very few, 8 checked quite a few, and 12, or 50%, checked many.

In Fairbanks, where the return from the physicians' survey was more substantial, 1,162 persons were indicated as having pollen/spore allergies severe enough to require medical attention (2). This was about 2.2% of the population. Furthermore, 6% of the cases were considered severe, 38% intermediate, and the rest mild.

The distribution in severity categories was similar in Anchorage. Question 3 was: What numbers or percentages of your pollen/spore allergy patients are in the following severity categories? The physicians indicated, on average, that 4.3% were severe, defined in the questionnaire as totally disrupting to normal activity. They indicated that an average of 23.6% of their pollen/spore allergy cases were of interme-

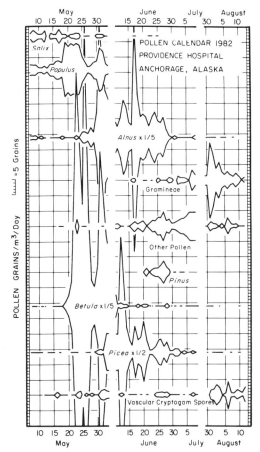

May   June   July   August
 10 15 20 25 30   15 20 25 30 5   30   5   10

POLLEN CALENDAR 1982
PROVIDENCE HOSPITAL
ANCHORAGE, ALASKA

Salix

Populus

Alnus x 1/5

Gramineae

Other Pollen

Pinus

Betula x 1/5

Picea x 1/2

Vascular Cryptogam Spores

POLLEN GRAINS / m³/Day

= 5 Grains

 10 15 20 25 30   15 20 25 30 5   30   5   10
May   June   July   August

Figure 2. Pollen calendar for 1983 at Providence Hospital in Anchorage. Gaps in sampling are June 3-10 and July 7-29.

diate severity, defined as quite distracting, but with determination the sufferer can carry on. The rest, 72.1% on average, were low-severity cases defined as annoying, but normal activities were reasonably comfortable for otherwise healthy persons.

Question 5 was: What are, or what do you suspect are the allergenic pollen and spore types in the Anchorage area? Fifteen of the 24 physicians responded to this question, indicating that the most important types were, in order of decreasing frequency of mention, grass, birch, cottonwood and aspen, fireweed, willow, and spruce. Several general terms were given, such as trees, weeds, and assorted, and a few additional items, including molds, were mentioned at least once. Nine of the physicians or 38% of the 24 otherwise responding, apparently did not know the allergenic pollen and spore types at all.

To the extent the physicians were knowledgeable of aeroallergens, this knowl-

edge presumably came mostly from the results of skin testing rather than from direct information on the composition of the aeroflora. In response to question 4 of the survey, the physicians indicated that on average 22% of their patients had been skin tested by them. Even so, the physicians' knowledge agrees with data now being obtained in aeroflora sampling, with the exceptions of grass, which is in general poorly represented in the Alaskan aeroflora, and fireweed, whose pollen, while highly allergenic, is big and bulky and not windtransportable.

Question 7 was: Do you know of any articles or information on airborne pollen and spores in the Anchorage area? All 24 of the physicians answered no or left the question blank. This response, in conjunction with the limited array of specific responses to the preceding question, supports the contention that aeropalynology research will be useful by providing definite knowledge of what pollen and spore types are and are not present in the atmosphere. Such knowledge may promote greater efficiency in skin testing by circumscribing the set of critical types. Four other items in the survey questionnaire were not as important as the above and will not be treated here.

Turning to aeroflora sampling results, Figure 1 is a pollen and spore calendar for Fairbanks for the 1982 season. For each of 9 pollen and spore categories, it provides information on several parameters: 1) daily abundance, which tends to fluctuate greatly, 2) onset date, the first day of significant atmospheric abundance, 3) termination date, the last day of significant abundance, 4) season length, 5) peak abundance and its date, and 6) annual production, which may be estimated from the area within the graph of a pollen type and may be determined precisely by adding the daily pollen counts. From the allergy standpoint, annual production may be called pollen season severity. This is one of the most interesting and important parameters in aeropalynology research, particularly because it appears to vary greatly from year to year.

The 1982 Fairbanks work along with 3 other years' gravimetric sampling are dealt with in detail elsewhere (3-5). The results of volumetric sampling at the University and at Bassett Army Hospital across town from the University will be reported as soon as possible.

Figure 2 is the pollen and spore calendar for Anchorage in 1982. Here the data are volumetric, and atmospheric abundances are concentrations, or average numbers of grains per cubic meter of air per day. The pollen types in Anchorage are generally similar to Fairbanks and include, starting at the top, several species of willow (*Salix*), balsam poplar and aspen (*Populus*),

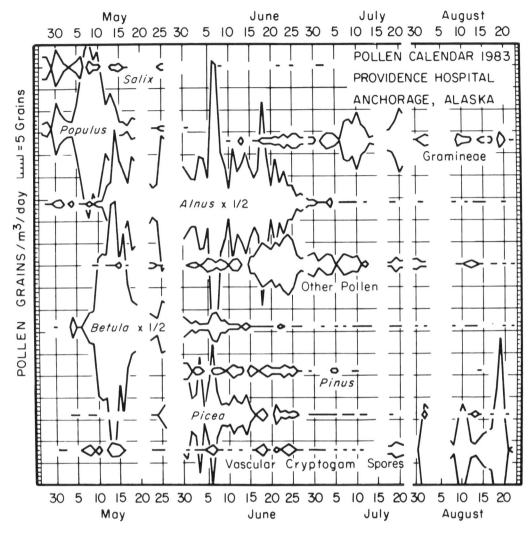

May   June   July   August
30 5 10 15 20 25 30 5 10 15 20 25 30 5 10 15 20 30 5 10 15 20

POLLEN CALENDAR 1983
PROVIDENCE HOSPITAL
ANCHORAGE, ALASKA

Salix

Populus

Gramineae

Alnus x 1/2

Other Pollen

Betula x 1/2

Pinus

Picea

Vascular Cryptogam Spores

30 5 10 15 20 25 30 5 10 15 20 25 30 5 10 15 20 30 5 10 15 20
May   June   July   August

POLLEN GRAINS / m³/ day   ⊔⊔⊔ = 5 Grains

Figure 3. Pollen calendar for 1983 at Providence Hospital in Anchorage. Gaps in sampling are May 19-22 and 26-30, June 28, July 14-17 and 21-29, and August 2-7 and 16.

2 or 3 species of alder (*Alnus*), and several species of grass (Gramineae). The "other pollen" category comprises several weedy herbs and certain less important woody plants. Lodgepole pine (*Pinus contorta*) is a species introduced in the Anchorage area for horticulture. The genus *Betula* is represented mostly by paper birch, whose pollen is by far the most serious aeroallergen in the Fairbanks and Anchorage areas. The genus *Picea* is represented by white and black spruce, and "vascular cryptogam" spores include those produced by horsetails and ferns. It is noted that alder, birch, and spruce pollen occurred in extremely high concentrations on some days in 1982, and the data had therefore to be reduced by one-

fifth or one-half so the graphs of these genera would fit on the calendar.

Figure 3 is the 1983 Anchorage pollen calendar. This calendar is similar to the preceding one in terms of the pollen categories represented, but a close comparative study of the 2 calendars would reveal major differences between them in the several within-season and year-to-year aeroflora parameters listed above with the Fairbanks calendar. These and other aspects of the aeropalynology research in Anchorage are treated more thoroughly elsewhere (6). There is room here to mention only one of the most important of these differences, that of annual production in birch. In 1982 this totaled 5,583 pollen grains per cubic

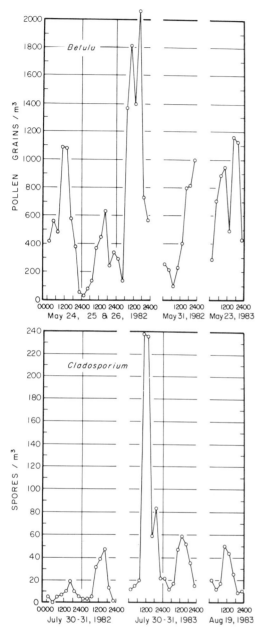

Figures 4a and 4b. Circadian fluctuations in atmospheric concentrations of birch pollen and Cladosporium spores. Data are 3-hour averages on the 5 days of highest average concentration in 1982 and 1983.

meter of air, and in 1983 it was 981 grains, only 17% of the 1982 value. The related parameter peak concentration was in 1983 only 13% of the 1982 value. Hay fever victims, therefore, should have been considerably more comfortable in 1983 than in 1982.

The big difference in annual production by birch, the chief component of pollen season severity, along with similar differences in the other pollen types in Anchorage, and in Fairbanks and Juneau, has led to this hypothesis: The major broadleaf deciduous trees and shrubs in Alaska produce pollen with a biennial cyclicity that is primarily genetically controlled but that may be suppressed and reset in a year of abnormally unfavorable weather. If this hypothesis turns out to be valid, and if the weather preceding and during birch flowering is more or less normal, 1984 should be another bad hay fever year in Anchorage. This hypothesis is examined in detail elsewhere using 4 years' palynological and meteorological data from Fairbanks (5).

Figures 4a and 4b show that another major form of variation in the aeroflora is circadian fluctuations in concentrations. Birch and *Cladosporium* are shown here as only 2 of several possible illustrations of such variation. In birch, concentrations tend to be low in the late night and morning hours, and quite high by comparison in the afternoon and evening hours. In *Cladosporium* the pattern is slightly different, with distinct high concentrations occurring only from noon to 6 p.m. This kind of information should be helpful to hay fever sufferers.

Figure 5 is the 1982 spore calendar for Anchorage. Bryophyta and Hepatophyta comprise the mosses and liverworts, respectively, and the other 6 categories illustrated here represent broad groups of fungi. The identification of fungus spores at lower taxonomic levels is a problem in aeropalynology research, but it has been possible tentatively to determine that most of the fungus genera commonly mentioned in the allergy literature from other areas, such as *Alternaria* and *Helminthosporium*, are rare in the Alaskan aeroflora. Of these genera, only the ubiquitous plant mold *Cladosporium*, illustrated here at the bottom, is of real importance.

Figure 6 provides an introduction to the pollen component of the aeroflora in Juneau. The environment here is botanically quite different from Fairbanks and Anchorage, and this is reflected in the aerial samples. The most immediately noticeable differences from the earlier pollen calendars are the appearance of Alaskan yellow cedar pollen (*Chamaecyparis*) and western and mountain hemlock pollen (*Tsuga*). In addition, pine pollen is important in the Juneau aeroflora, even though the species involved (lodgepole pine), while native to the region, is restricted in its distribution.

In contrast with Fairbanks and Anchorage, birch pollen is almost negligible in Juneau, a fact undoubtedly of interest to persons sensitive to it. Nevertheless, some

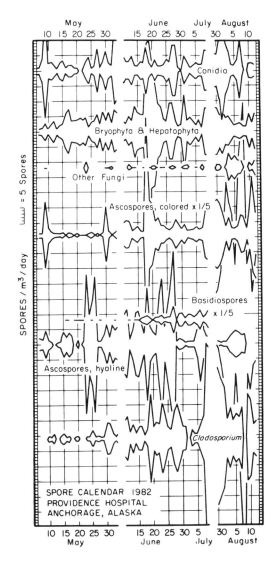

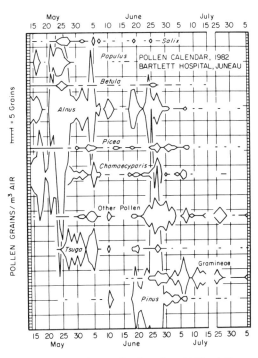

Figure 6. *Pollen calendar for 1982 at Bartlett Memorial Hospital in Juneau. A sampling gap is July 15-23.*

The occurrence of hay fever in a certain portion of the Juneau area population was indicated by a physicians' survey there. This was also indicated by a survey in Whitehorse, Yukon Territory. It appears that in Whitehorse, several patients are sensitive to pine pollen, a condition almost unknown elsewhere.

REFERENCES

1. Durham OC. Atmospheric allergens in Alaska. J Allergy 1941; 12:307-309.
2. Anderson JH. Report of a survey of physicians pertaining to proposed aeropalynological research in the Fairbanks area, Alaska. Fairbanks: Institute of Arctic Biology, University of Alaska, 1980.
3. Anderson JH. Aeropalynology research in Alaska--Review and outlook. 34th Alaska Science Conference, Whitehorse, Yukon, September 28 to October 1, 1983.
4. Anderson JH. A survey of allergenic airborne pollen and spores in the Fairbanks area, Alaska. Ann Allergy 1984; 52:26-31.
5. Anderson JH. Annual variations in the aeroflora at Fairbanks, Alaska. Research Report. Fairbanks: Institute of Arctic Biology, University of Alaska, 1984.

Figure 5. *Spore calendar for 1982 at Providence Hospital in Anchorage. Note that data are reduced by one-fifth for the extremely abundant colored ascospores and basidiospores, the latter of which reached a 24-hour average of 716 spores per cubic meter of air on August 8.*

of the other types, especially alder, grass, and probably *Chamaecyparis*, plus some of the many fungus spores not illustrated here, do present an allergy risk. Allergenic and other components of the Juneau aeroflora in 1982 are treated in a separate report (7), and this material will be published when the 1983 results have been incorporated.

6. Anderson JH. Aeropalynology in Anchorage, Alaska. Research report on the first two years' sampling at Providence Hospital for allergenic and other airborne pollen and spores. Fairbanks: Institute of Arctic Biology, University of Alaska, 1984.

7. Anderson JH. Aeropalynology in Juneau, Alaska. Results of the first season's use of a volumetric sampler for allergenic and other airborne pollen and spores. Research report. Fairbanks: Institute of Arctic Biology, University of Alaska, 1983.

James H. Anderson
Institute of Arctic Biology
University of Alaska
Fairbanks, Alaska 99701
U.S.A.

Circumpolar Health 84:103-104

THE EYE IN HIGH ALTITUDE: COMPARISON BETWEEN ARCTIC POPULATIONS
AND 392 ADULTS IN THE TITICACA REGION OF PERU

HENRIK FORSIUS and W. LOSNO

INTRODUCTION

People can live at very high altitudes, up to 5,000 m in tropical mountains. Already at 4,000 m one finds dilated retinal blood vessels. When strong physical stress is added, as in mountain climbing, the dilatation of capillaries easily causes superficial retinal hemorrhages (1).

Snow blindness is known from snow-covered mountains all over the world, including the high South American Andes.

The prevalence of pterygium at high altitude has already been studied in the Andes in South America. In 1979 Goldsmith et al. (2) reported a low prevalence of pterygium from an altiplano in north Chile. On the other hand, Buck et al. (3) found an age-corrected prevalence of 8.1% in the Titicaca region at 4,000 m altitude.

METHODS

We studied 388 adults in south Peru at 4,000 m altitude in 2 populations (Puno and Iliave). The area around Lake Titicaca is sunny most of the year and the humidity is low. There has been practically no rain in recent years and thus the ground is naked in most places. The color of the earth is dark brown or black, which reflects very little of the sunlight, especially the ultraviolet light. The temperature on winter nights goes below the freezing point but in daytime it is comparatively warm though not hot (Meteorological Bureau, Puno).

RESULTS

The mean refraction was a little on the myopic side (Table 1). As seen from the table, no increase in the prevalence of myopia is to be seen in the younger generation. For males the highest mean value of refraction is in the age group 40 to 49 and females between 50 and 59 years. In many populations (e.g. in the Arctic) young people show an increase up to 50 to 70% of the population in myopia over the older age groups (4).

Corneal thickness was measured on 19 males, with a mean of 0.523 mm, and on 16 females with a mean of 0.516 mm. The values for corneal thickness are a little lower than those for Caucasian populations but comparable to values measured in some arctic populations (5).

Pterygium was extremely common in this area (Table 2). These values are extremely high and comparable to prevalences from tropical islands. Compared to arctic populations such as Eskimos and Lapps, values are high (6). Pterygium is rare in central Europe, for example 1% in Copenhagen (7). In most statistics males have a higher prevalence of pterygium than females. In the Lake Titicaca study population, however, the females had more pterygium, although the difference is not statistically significant ($p > 0.05$)

Climatic keratopathy was rare, only 3.78% in males and 1.46% in females. In this respect the subjects differ distinctly from arctic populations, in which keratopathy was more common than pterygium (6).

Pinguecula was usually prominent in the Indians in Peru, and often dilated blood vessels could be seen on the highly elevated pinguecula. In males with climatic keratopathy, pinguecula was more pronounced than in people without keratopathy ($p < 0.05$). In females there was also a difference but it was not significant. In both sexes with pterygium, the pinguecula was more marked ($p < 0.01$) than in the controls.

Table 1. Mean refraction in adults, Puno district, Lake Titicaca region.

Age in years	20-29	30-39	40-49	50-59	60+
Males					
dx	-0.625	-0.078	-0.672	-0.174	-0.059
sin	-0.550	-0.070	-0.615	-0.258	-0.430
Females					
dx	-0.194	-0.102	-0.195	-0.598	-0.068
sin	-0.076	-0.113	-0.082	-0.454	-0.186

Table 2. Pterygium in adults, Lake Titicaca region.

Age in years	20-29		30-39		40-49		50-59		60+		Total (all age groups included)	
	N	%	N	%	N	%	N	%	N	%	N	%
Males*	0	0	8	18.18	10	27.03	15	36.59	11	25.58	44	21.46
Females	3	9.37	12	24.49	1	3.57	7	18.42	8	22.22	31	16.94

* 205 males and 183 females were investigated.

DISCUSSION

Pinguecula, pterygium, and climatic keratopathy are caused by the environment and most probably by ultraviolet light. Compared to regions at sea level, the amount of UV-light in the air is much higher in high altitude as the air resorbs much of the sun's UV-rays. Climatic keratopathy was thus also expected to be high in this region but was nearly absent. This can only be explained by the supposition that the ultraviolet rays which cause remarkable changes to the cornea in arctic regions are caused by UV-light reflected from the snow. In the Puno district the ground reflects very little of the UV-light, in any event not enough to cause keratopathy. The UV-light in the sky in Peru seems to be strong enough to cause pterygium and a marked pinguecula.

REFERENCES

1. Kramar PO, Drinkwater BL, Folinsbee LJ, Bedi JF. Ocular functions and incidence of acute mountain sickness in women at altitude. Aviat Space Environ Med 1983; 54:116-120.
2. Goldsmith RI, Rothhammer F, Schull WJ. The multinational Andean genetic and health program: III. Ophthalmic disease and disability among the Aymara. Bull Pan Am Health Organ 1979; 13:58.
3. Buck AA, Sasaki TT, Anderson RI. Health and disease in four Peruvian villages. Contrasts in epidemiology. Baltimore: The Johns Hopkins Press, 1968.
4. Morgan RW, Speakman JS, Grimshaw SE. Inuit myopia: an environmentally induced "epidemic"? Canad Med Assoc J 1975; 112:575-577.
5. Forsius H, Eriksson AW. Investigations in ophthalmology and population genetics in Iceland. Nordic Council Arct Med Res Rep No 26, 1980:40-47.
6. Forsius H. Pterygium and band-shaped climatic keratopathy in arctic versus tropical populations. Scientific and technical progress and circumpolar health. Vol II, 237. Novosibirsk: USSR Academy of Medical Sciences Siberian Branch, 1978.
7. Norn M. Spheroid degeneration, keratopathy, pinguecula, and pterygium in Japan (Kyoto). Acta Ophthal 1984; 62:54-60.

Henrik Forsius
Department of Ophthalmology
University of Oulu
SF-90220 Oulu
Finland

Circumpolar Health 84:105-109

HADDON'S STRATEGY FOR PREVENTION: APPLICATION TO NATIVE HOUSE FIRES

B. FRIESEN

Mortality rates from injuries are significantly elevated in Canadian Native peoples. Menno and Boldt in a prospective study of mortality on 35 reserves in Alberta documented 32.4% of Native deaths were due to injuries, as compared to 8.6% in the population as a whole (1). This gives a proportional mortality ratio (PMR) of 3.8 for deaths due to injuries among Alberta Indians. Similar elevations have been documented in other provinces and territories in Canada. The causes of such elevations are complex, involving in major part socioeconomic and cultural factors.

Fire-related deaths contribute substantially to the elevated mortality rates (1). For the period 1971 to 1981 fires accounted for 11% of the fatalities due to injury among Canadian Indians, or 775 deaths. The percentage of Indian deaths due to fire was uniform across Canada (Table 1). It was thought to be useful to review the experience of Manitoba Indians in order to identify prevention strategies.

METHODS

Data were reviewed from the Medical Services Branch, Health and Welfare Canada; Fire Commissioner, Province of Manitoba; and the Chief Medical Examiner of Manitoba. The files of the Chief Medical Examiner were complete for all cases of fatalities. Sex specific mortality ratios (MR) for Indian fire deaths were determined as a ratio of observed versus expected deaths. Statistical significance was determined using χ^2 analysis with 95% confidence intervals. The relative percentage of the fatalities and populations that were age 14 or less was determined.

All fire fatalities involving Indians were reviewed from the period 1976 to 1982. Indian fatalities were identified by residence on or near an Indian reserve with a

Table 1. Percentage of Indian deaths from injury due to fire by region of Canada 1971 to 1981.

Region	Fire-related deaths	Deaths from all injuries	%
N.W.T.	33	287	12
Yukon*	7	108	7
Pacific	127	1,708	10
Alberta	151	1,085	14
Saskatchewan	115	1,173	10
Manitoba	96	907	11
Ontario	126	1,190	11
Quebec	50	375	13
Atlantic	21	193	11
All Canada	775	7,026	11

* Data for the Yukon were not available for 1971, so only the period from 1972 to 1981 is represented.

name common to that reserve. Information was abstracted on the time, location, and probable cause of the fire, whether people survived, the factors that allowed or prevented escape, the age and sex of the fatalities, and whether alcohol or smoking were involved. The involvement of alcohol was documented by the measurement of blood alcohol in body fluids or on the basis of statements in the police report.

RESULTS

There are approximately 49,000 Indians in Manitoba. Ninety-six Indian deaths occurred during the period 1971 to 1981. Based on Manitoba rates of fire fatality, 21 fire deaths could be expected in this population. This difference is statistically significant and gives a mortality ratio (MR) = 4.3 (P<0.005) (Table 2). The mortal-

Table 2. Mortality from fire for Manitoba Indians 1971 to 1981.

Sex	Number of fire fatalities Observed	Expected	Mortality ratio (O/E)*	Confidence intervals**
Male	60	14.5	4.1	3.1-5.1
Female	36	7.0	5.2	3.4-7.0
Both sexes	96	21.5	4.5	3.5-5.5

*   Probability < 0.005.
** 95% confidence interval.

Table 3.   Morbidity from burns* for Manitoba Indians 1981 to 1982 fiscal year.

Age group	Separations observed	Separations expected	Ratio (O/E)
1	6	1.8	3.4
1-4	31	5.6	5.6
5-14	17	3.8	4.8
15-64	31	8.5	3.6
65	5	0.4	11.7
Total	90	20.1	4.5**

* ICD code 940-949.
** $P < 0.005$.

ity ratio for females was greater than for males, (5.2 versus 4.1).

Indians also had greater morbidity from fire injuries than other Manitobans. The number of hospitalizations for burns, based on data from the Manitoba Health Services Commission, was greater than expected (Table 3). Indians had 4.5 times as many hospitalizations for burns as other Manitobans. All age groups were affected, with rates in the one to four year and the 65+ year groups being especially high.

Age-specific fatality rates were not determined; however, proportional mortality is shown in Table 4. Forty-six percent of the Indian fatalities involved children under 15 (44% of population), as opposed to 28% for Manitobans under 15 (24% of population). Thus the increase in the crude fatality rate for Indians cannot be due solely to their age distribution but must also reflect increased age-specific rates.

The five-year average fatality rates for Indians and Manitobans show a downward trend for Indians, both males and females, and for Manitoban females. Manitoban males show little change in five-year mean rates but the three-year mean rates do demonstrate a 25% reduction since 1978.

The review identified 29 fires during the period 1976 to 1982. Fifty-nine Indians died as a result of the fires. The number of fatalities per fire ranged from one to seven. In 17 (59%) of the fires, one or more people managed to escape.

The causes identified for the fires are shown in Table 5. Potential years of life lost (PYLL) were calculated from the difference between their age at death and age 65. In the fires reviewed, some 2,484 potential years of life were lost. Just under a quarter of the PYLL were in fires caused by candles even though they accounted for just 17% of the fires. Conversely, almost a quarter of the fires and fatalities were caused by smoking but less than 16% of the PYLL were due to fires caused by smoking.

Fires due to smoking occurred throughout the year while fires due to wood stoves and space heaters were most common in the winter months. The majority of fires caused by candles were in the spring or summer when the hours of daylight are long. Candles may burn through the night as night lights for small children (and would therefore account for the large PYLL). The majority of the fires occurred between 10 p.m. and 7 a.m.

Table 4.   Comparison of the percentage of fire fatalities under age 15 by sex for Indians* and Manitobans 1978 to 1981.

| | Indian | | Manitoban | |
	Male	Female	Male	Female
Percentage of fire fatalities	26.2	20.1	26.2	31.0
Percentage of population	43.7	44.1	24.4	23.2

* All Indians in Canada.

Alcohol was directly involved in the cause of 10 fires with the loss of 27 lives and indirectly involved in causing 4 other fires in which 10 lives were lost. Thus in 14 (49%) of the fires and 37 (63%) of the fatalities alcohol was associated with the cause of the fire. In 22 (76%) of the fires alcohol was determined to have impaired people's ability to escape, with the resultant loss of 44 lives.

The various factors under host, agent, and physical and socioeconomic environment that were associated with fatal fires are outlined in Table 6.

DISCUSSION AND CONCLUSIONS

The factors associated with fire mortality and morbidity rates are complex. Jarvis and Boldt (1) in their study found that 90% of the adult victims of house fires were under the influence of alcohol. In our review alcohol was associated with 76% of the fatalities. (Deaths of children who were under the supervision of an intoxicated adult were defined as being associated with alcohol in this study).

A descriptive study such as this can identify factors associated with fatal house fires (Table 6). Hypotheses regarding causation can be made but cannot be tested. It is not possible to determine the amount of risk or attributable risk associated with any factor. As a result it is difficult, if not impossible, for planning to take place.

Haddon, who has been active in the field of injury epidemiology since the 1960s, recognized this as a common problem and has developed two planning strategies for dealing with it (2,3). The one that will be discussed here is a matrix which recognizes three phases in the occurrence of an injury: pre-event, event, and post-event. There are 4 categories of factors involved in an injury at each phase: factors related to the host (person), the agent (hazard), the physical environment, and the socioeconomic environment. Haddon has used this matrix to outline strategies for the prevention of automobile injuries (Table 7). This

Table 5. The number of fires, fatalities, and potential years of life lost (PYLL) by cause of fire in Manitoba Indians.

Cause		No. fires (%)	No. fatalities (%)	PYLL (%)
Wood stoves:				
Chimney fire		1	2	126
Ignition combustibles		2	8	394
Other		2	4	214
	Total	5 (17.2)	14 (23.7)	734 (29.5)
Candles		5 (17.1)	10 (16.9)	591 (23.8)
Smoking in bed (Mattress fire definite)		5 (17.2)	12 (20.3)	323 (13.0)
Smoking (possible cause)		2 (6.9)	3 (5.1)	63 (2.5)
Electrical appliance (Stove, TV)		3 (10.3)	3 (5.1)	64 (2.6)
Electrical wiring (Lighting)		2 (6.9)	6 (10.2)	331 (13.3)
Electrical heater		2 (6.9)	4 (6.8)	219 (8.8)
Oil or space heater		2 (6.9)	2 (3.4)	71 (2.8)
Playing with fire		*1 (3.4)	2 (3.4)	61 (2.5)
Suicide		1 (3.4)	2 (3.4)	25 (1.0)
Unknown		1 (3.4)	1 (1.7)	25 (1.0)
	Total	29	59	2,484

* 1 fire assigned to woodstoves may have been due to children playing. 3 deaths resulted with PYLL 185.

Table 6.   Factors associated with the occurrence of fatal house fires among Indians during 1976 to 1982.

	Host	Agent	Physical environment	Socioeconomic environment
1.	Smoking	Candles	Highly combustible building material	Disconnection of electricity for non-payment
2.	Drinking	Oil burners	Exits blocked	Community acceptance of drinking
3.	Inadequate	Electric kitchen stoves		Absence of fire department
4.	Children playing with fire	Wood stoves	Malfunctioning extinguishers	Community standard for supervision of children
5.	Children hiding under beds during fires		Flammable clothing	Building codes
6.	Suicide intent	Hazardous wiring	Flammable mattresses	Absence of community mental health program
7.	Disability	Portable electric heaters	No water	

matrix has also been used by Baker and Dietz in outlining approaches for preventing drowning (4).

If this matrix is applied to the problem of fire-related injuries it is possible to identify the opportunities for prevention within each phase.

Pre-Event Phase

Prevention strategies may be aimed at modifying risk factors in the host's behavior by reducing drinking or smoking. Activities could also seek to eliminate the hazard present by substituting safer forms of heating and lighting than wood stoves or candles. The physical environment could be made safer by the removal of flammable substances. Action under the socioeconomic environment could include a referendum prohibiting alcohol or changes to building codes to require safer means of heating and lighting.

Event Phase

Activities could be aimed at increasing the host's resistance by having him or her seek the safest place during a fire. The hazard presented by the agent is reduced by having oil burners go out if tipped over. The physical environment is modified to provide warning and protection through smoke detectors and fire extinguishers. Societal

action to pass building codes specifying flame-resistant materials also reduces risk.

Post-Event Phase

The provision of information on the immediate treatment of burns by running them under cold water would allow action to reduce the severity of the burn. The effects of the agent, in the cause of fire, heat and carbon monoxide, are reduced by identifying people who have been exposed.

The program to put stickers on children's windows so that firefighters check those rooms first is an example. The physical environment should be modified to allow access by fire-fighting equipment and to provide a source of water. The societal response after fire would be the provision of fire departments and burn care units.

Haddon's matrix thus provides a means by which strategies can be outlined. It does not prioritize the prevention strategies that should be adopted. Each activity must still be evaluated to ensure that it is effective. For example, if alcohol is involved in 50% of the fatal fires but there is no effective intervention program for reducing alcohol use, it would be a poor choice as the major thrust of a fire prevention campaign. In addition to determining effectiveness of a program it is also important to consider whether it is active or passive. An active prevention program

Table 7. Haddon's model for approach to prevention of injuries.*

Factors	Pre-event	Phases Event	Post-event
Host	1	5	9
Agent	2	6	10
Environment	3	7	11
Socioeconomic environment	4	8	12

1. Reduce drinking or drug use of individual drivers.
2. Improve vehicle handling.
3. Improve road conditions, install traffic lights.
4. Lower speed limits, increase penalties for drunken driving.
5. Increase people's resistance to injury.
6. Improve vehicle's "crashworthiness," i.e. its ability to protect occupants in a crash.
7. Have break-away poles on road signs to minimize the hazards they present.
8. Pass federal/provincial standards covering vehicle "crashworthiness," i.e. seat belt laws.
9. Treat injuries received in crash.
10. Prevent post-crash fires.
11. Remove crash debris from road; mark accident site.
12. Improve emergency medical care service.

* Adopted from Haddon "Approaches to Prevention of Injuries" presentation at American Medical Association Conference on Prevention of Disabling Injuries, Miami, Florida, May 1983.

requires an individual to take action one or more times, for example, seatbelts, whereas passive prevention measures do not require any action by an individual in order to be protected. Generally, passive measures are much more successful than active in reducing injuries. This has been demonstrated by Project Burn Prevention, which was a public education program aimed at increasing public awareness about burn hazards and reducing the incidence and severity of burns. It was carried out in Massachusetts and the conclusion was that education for personal responsibility was not sufficient. Product modification and environmental re-design must be instituted through education and legislation for successful control of burn injuries (5).

Although fire fatality rates in Indians have been declining they are still significantly greater than in other Canadians. There exists a number of opportunities for reducing fire fatalities by making changes in their physical and socioeconomic environments. These changes will require a cooperative approach between Indian people, health care providers, and various provincial and federal agencies.

ACKNOWLEDGMENTS

I would like to acknowledge the cooperation and assistance I received in undertaking this study from the offices of the Chief Medical Examiner and the Fire Commissioner, and the Royal Canadian Mounted Police.

REFERENCES

1. Jarvis GK, Boldt M. Death styles among Canada's Indians. Soc Sci Med 1982; 16:1345-1352.
2. Haddon W. Advances in the epidemiology of injuries as a basis for public policy. Am J Epidemiol 1980; 95:411-421.
3. Haddon W. Reducing damage from hazards of all kinds. Foresight 1981; 6:16-21.
4. Dietz EP, Baker SP. Drowning epidemiology and prevention. Am J Public Health 1974; 64:303-312.
5. McLoughlin E, Vince CJ, Lean AM, Crawford JD. Project burn prevention. Outcome and implications. Am J Public Health 1982; 72:241-247.

B. Friesen
Northern Medical Unit
University of Manitoba
61 Emily Street
Winnipeg, Manitoba R3E 1Y9
Canada

Circumpolar Health 84:110-112

INCIDENCE AND ETIOLOGY OF JAW FRACTURES IN GREENLAND

JENS JØRGEN THORN and PEDER KERN HANSEN

INTRODUCTION

The incidence of mandibular fractures in Greenland has been previously reported as extremely high. The etiological pattern was different in many respects from what was observed in other western countries (1). That study covered only cases from the municipality of Nuuk/Godthåb and was retrospective. The purpose of the present prospective investigation was to record the incidence and etiological patterns of jaw fractures throughout Greenland.

METHODS

All cases of fractures of the mandible or the maxilla were examined by the local dentists and physicians during one and a half year period (July 1, 1981 to December 31, 1982), and all were verified by radiographs. Fractures of only the alveolar process were excluded. Information was obtained on personal characteristics, type of fracture, time, place, type of accident and whether alcohol was involved. The simplicity of the data recording made calibration unneccessary. In the statistical analysis the chi-square test was used, with a level of significance at 0.05.

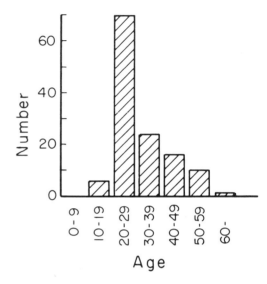

Figure 1. *129 persons with jaw fractures in Greenland (July 1, 1981-December 31, 1982). Distribution by age groups.*

Table 1. *Nationality, sex, place, etiology, type of fracture, and alcohol involvement of 129 persons with jaw fractures in Greenland recorded from July 1, 1981 to December 31, 1982. Etiology was unknown for 5 persons and intoxication with alcohol unknown or uncertain in 15 cases.*

		Number of persons n = 129	%
Nationality	Greenlanders	123	95
	Danes/others	6	5
Sex	Women	47	36
	Men	82	64
Place of accident	Towns	120	93
	Settlements	9	7
Etiology	Violence	112	90
	Traffic	2	2
	Work	2	2
	Miscellaneous	8	6
Fracture	Mandible	125	97
	Maxilla	3	2
	Mandible and maxilla	1	1
Alcohol	Intoxicated	90	79
	Sober	24	21

RESULTS

During the time of observation 129 persons sustained jaw fractures in Greenland. On January 1, 1982, the size of the population was 51,435 (2). The incidence was thus 17 per 10,000 population per year.

Other results are shown in Table 1 and Figures 1-4.

DISCUSSION

The incidence of jaw fractures in Greenland (17 per 10,000 per year) exceeded by at least 4 times the incidence reported in Sweden, Norway, and Finland (respectively 4.1 and 1 per 10,000 per year) (3-5).

Greenlanders made up 95% of the patient group but only 82% of the whole population (2). As this difference was statistically significant, events resulting in jaw fractures were proven to take place mainly in the Greenlandic part of society.

More than half of the patients were in the age group of 20 to 29 years (Figure 1). This age group is commonly reported as the largest in studies of this kind, but never to this extent (4-10).

Female patients constituted 36%, a figure which is in accordance with the previous report from Godthåb (1). The proportion of women is high in populations where violence plays an important etiological role (6,7) and this proportion seems to be increasing (6). The figures from Greenland are the highest yet reported.

One-fourth of the cases occurred in Godthåb, the capital of Greenland, where approximately one-fifth of the population lives (Figure 2); this difference was not statistically significant. The incidence of jaw fractures in all of Greenland is close to the previously reported incidence of mandibular fractures in Godthåb (19 per 10,000 per year) (1). Various municipalities in the south (Narssaq, Julianehåb) had the same frequency of cases as Godthåb; some (Frederikshåb, Scoresbysund) had even more (Figure 3).

Twenty percent of the population lives in settlements and only 7% of the accidents occurred there, a statistically significant difference. Jaw fractures in Greenland are closely related to interpersonal violence (Table 1), which is a typically urban phenomenon in Greenland, as well as in other societies (11).

The etiological pattern of jaw fractures reported from different communities shows great variability depending on the selection of material, socioeconomic factors, and traffic (7). This study covers all parts of Greenland, thus reflecting the infrastructure and social conditions of the entire society. Traffic is very sparse in Greenland and accounts for only 2% of cases. Violence is an important cause of jaw fracture in most communities and seems to play an ever increasing role (7,8,12), but nowhere is the figure as high as in Greenland (Table 1). This specific etiology explains the distribution of fractures of

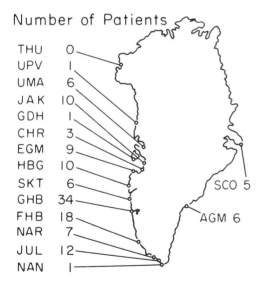

Figure 2. Distribution of cases of jaw fractures (N=129) by municipalities in Greenland in the period July 1, 1981 to December 31, 1982.

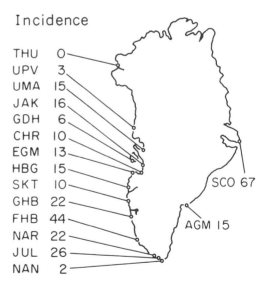

Figure 3. Incidence (number per 10,000 population) of jaw fractures in Greenland municipalities.

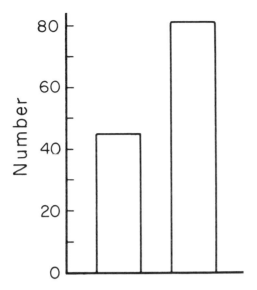

Figure 4. Distribution of cases of jaw fractures (N=129) in Greenland in the 2 periods of equal size before and after alcohol was deregulated (I: July 1, 1981 to March 31, 1982; II: April 1 to December 31, 1982).

the upper and lower jaw. Mandibular fractures are a typical outcome of interpersonal violence, whereas fractures of the maxilla more often are seen in victims of traffic accidents.

Another striking figure is the many patients with alcohol intoxication at the time of the accident. This association is well known from other reports but not to such a great extent (5-7,9). Alcohol was deregulated in Greenland April 1, 1982, and in the following 9 months the occurrence of jaw fractures nearly doubled (Figure 4). Since then the number of patients has decreased, but the level is still higher than before deregulation.

CONCLUSION

The incidence of jaw fractures in Greenland is the highest ever reported. The percentage of women, of patients in the age group of 20 to 29, of assault and battery and involvement of alcohol is also the highest reported. Jaw fractures most often occurred in the towns and mostly in the Greenlandic part of the society. Etiological patterns of jaw fractures change from one subculture to another depending on social conditions. The figures from Greenland demonstrate this principle.

ACKNOWLEDGMENT

This study was supported by the Commission for Scientific Research in Greenland.

REFERENCES

1. Thorn JJ, Hansen PK, Møgeltoft M. Mandibelfrakturer i Grønland. I. Årsager og frakturtyper. Tandlaegebladet 1981; 85:725-731.
2. Danmarks statistik. Grønlands befolkning. Kalatdlit nunane inuit. 1 januar 1982. Statistikservice fra Danmarks Statistik. Copenhagen, 1982.
3. Lundin K, Ridell A, Sandberg N, Ohmann A. One thousand maxillo-facial and related fractures at the ENT-clinic in Gothenburg. Acta Otolaryng 1973; 96:420-422.
4. Torjussen W, Brydøy B, Grønås HE, Korsrud FR. Mandibulafrakturer: Et 4-årsmateriale. T Norske Laegeforen 1976; 96:420-422.
5. Lamberg MA. Site, type and causes of mandibular fractures in 704 inpatients. Proc Finn Dent Soc 1978; 71:162-175.
6. James RB, Frederickson C, Kent JN. Prospective study of mandibular fractures. J Oral Surg 1981; 39:275-281.
7. Voss R. The aetiology of jaw fractures in Norwegian patients. J Maxillofacial Surg 1982; 10:146-148.
8. Hedin M, Ridell A, Söremark R. Käkfraktur i Sverige 1966-1967. Swed Dent J 1971; 64:49-62.
9. Heimdahl A, Nordenram A. The first 100 patients with jaw fractures at the Department of oral surg, Dental School, Huddinge. Swed Dent J 1977; 1:177-182.
10. Müller W. Häufigkeit und Art der Spätfolgen bei 2733 Frakturen des Gesichtschadels. Fortschr Kiefer Gesichtschir 1962; 12:220-224.
11. Gold R. Urban violence and contemporary defensive cities. J Amer Institute Planners 1970; 36:146-159.
12. Brook IM, Wood N. Aetiology and incidence of facial fractures in adults. Int J Oral Surg 1983; 12:293-298.

Jens Jørgen Thorn
Department of Oral Medicine and Oral Surgery
Rigshospitalet
Tagensvej 20
2200 Copenhagen N
Denmark

SECTION 3. DEMOGRAPHY, MORBIDITY AND MORTALITY

Circumpolar Health 84:115-119

STUDY OF A COHORT OF YUKON-KUSKOKWIM DELTA ESKIMO CHILDREN: AN OVERVIEW OF ACCOMPLISHMENTS AND PLANS FOR THE FUTURE

THOMAS R. BENDER, CHRISTOPHER J. WILLIAMS and DAVID B. HALL

INTRODUCTION

One of the most serious health problems involving American Indians and Alaska Natives, particularly Eskimos, has been disease and death in infants during the first year of life. Examination of the figures available for the 1950s reveals the severity of the problem. For all races of the U.S. in 1954, the mortality rate for neonates was 19.1 deaths per 1,000 live births, and for post-neonates the rate was 7.5 deaths per 1,000 live births (1). For the U.S. Indian population in 1953 through 1955 the neonatal and postneonatal mortality rates were 22.8 and 43.8 respectively (2). For Eskimos living in the Yukon-Kuskokwim Delta region of southwest Alaska in 1956 through 1958, the corresponding rates were 50.1 and 93.4 (3).

Because of the high mortality rate among Eskimo infants and other evidence that suggested that morbidity was also severe, an infant morbidity and mortality study was initiated in the Yukon-Kuskokwim Delta Region in 1960 (Figure 1). The project, which took place in the region shown on the map, was planned and conducted by Dr. James E. Maynard and the staff of the Epidemiology Program of the Arctic Health Research Center, in cooperation with the Alaska Area Native Health Service.

The purpose of the study was to document precisely, within a set time period, the actual number of Eskimo infants born and dying within selected remote villages of this region of Alaska, and to investigate carefully the causes of death and non-fatal diseases occurring in the first and second years of life (3).

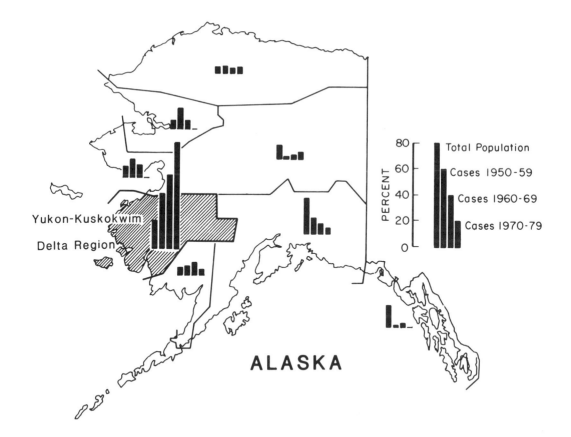

Figure 1. Proportion of bronchiectasis cases in Alaska, from each service unit by 10-year birth cohorts. The Yukon-Kuskokwim Delta region is shaded.

Table 1.   1961-1962 Yukon-Kuskokwim cohort vital statistics.

	Total	Yukon	Coast	Kuskokwim
Population (April 1, 1960)	6,080	2,308	1,928	1,844
Total pregnancies	696	277	219	200
Stillbirths	53	23	12	18
% of total	7.6	8.3	5.5	9.0
Live births	643	254	207	182
Premature live births	50	17	15	18
% of live births	8.7	7.6	8.1	10.7
Infant mortality				
Number	66	26	15	25
Rate	102.6	102.4	72.5	137.4
Neonatal mortality				
Number	30	11	10	9
Rate	46.7	43.3	48.3	49.5
Post-neonatal mortality				
Number	36	15	5	16
Rate	56.0	59.1	24.2	87.9

METHODS AND STRATEGY

Twenty-seven villages on the Yukon-Kuskokwim Delta were selected because they had been participating in the Bethel tuberculosis prophylaxis program. When the villages were visited between October 1, 1960, and January 2, 1961, all women of childbearing age who were residents were asked to enter the study. The recruitment of new participants was continued until December 1962. During routine visits to the villages, the investigators gathered data on those women who entered the third trimester of pregnancy in order to evaluate the health, nutrition, and hygiene of the mother during her pregnancy. They also gathered considerable information on the subsequent delivery of the infant and the growth, illnesses, and development of the child after birth.

The total population of the region at the time was just over 6,000 Eskimos (Table 1) (4), who lived in small villages along the Yukon River, the Bering Sea Coast, and the Kuskokwim River. There were 696 total pregnancies during the study period, 7.6% of which terminated as stillbirths. Of the live births, 8.7% were premature. The eventual enrollment of infants reached 643 live-born children, of whom 577 survived beyond infancy. Follow-up, originally scheduled for the first 12 months of life, was extended to include the first 24 months. Thus a comprehensive set of important and useful data was established for a large cohort of Alaskan Eskimo children living in traditional Yupik-speaking villages.

It was soon recognized that this set of baseline data was unique and that further study of the health and development of this group would allow full use of the valuable data set which had been established. As a consequence, a number of special follow-up studies, in addition to careful reviews of the medical records, were carried out over the years, as the children grew up through the 1960s, 1970s, and early 1980s.

For example, in 1965 pure tone and audiometric testing was undertaken in 24 of the 27 original study villages in order to investigate the relationship between otitis media and hearing loss. In 1966, a revised Stanford-Binet psychometric test was administered to 305 children from 21 of the study villages. Between 1969 and 1970, investigators were able to contact 77% of the surviving members of the original cohort and gather comprehensive data on medical illness, physical growth, bone age, hemoglobin, and psychological status. The psychological examinations performed included WISC psychometric tests, the Draw-a-Person-Percentile test, and the Bender-Gestalt test. In

Table 2. Infant mortality rates in 1961-1962 Yukon-Kuskokwim cohort, 1960 American Indians, and 1960 United States residents.

	Yukon-Kuskokwim	United States	U.S. Indians
Neonatal mortality (≤28 days old)	46.7*	19.2	22.3
Post-neonatal mortality (1-11 months old)	56.0	7.2	34.7
Infant mortality (<12 months old)	102.6	26.4	57.0

*rates per 1,000 live births

addition, audiograms were obtained on 91% of the children.

Although the Arctic Health Research Center was closed in 1974, the study was not terminated. A 15-year follow-up of the cohort was implemented in 1976 by the Alaska Investigations Division of the Centers for Disease Control (CDC) and the Alaska Area Native Health Service. As before, the data collection was extensive. Families were interviewed and medical charts were reviewed. Hemoglobin was again measured, serum was tested for evidence of infection with hepatitis B virus, and red blood cells were tested for genetic markers. Psychological exams were performed including the WAIS psychometric test, the Draw-a-Person test, a map test, and the Bender-Gestalt test.

A questionnaire was also administered to the cohort children in order to evaluate their nutritional knowledge and to explore their use of alcohol and tobacco. Most recently, in 1982, members of the cohort living in 10 villages (281 individuals) had their vision uniformly tested to describe the prevalence of refractive errors and to investigate the causes of poor vision.

RESULTS

The crude birth rate found at the beginning of the study was 53 per 1,000 population, a rate more than double that found in most areas of the U.S. in the 1960s.

The overall infant mortality rate for Eskimos in this study was found to be 102.6 per 1,000 live births, a rate four times that for the U.S., and twice that of American Indians (Table 2). Two patterns were discernible when infant mortality in this group was compared to that for the U.S. and for non-Alaskan American Indians. First of all, in comparison to that seen for the other groups, both components of the infant mortality rate for Eskimo infants were quite high: 46.7 deaths per 1,000 live births in neonates and 56.0 deaths per 1,000 live births in post-neonates.

Secondly, within the Eskimo cohort, the post-neonatal mortality rate (56.0 per 1,000 live births) was slightly higher than the neonatal mortality rate (46.7 per 1,000 live births). This pattern was in a direction similar to that seen for American Indians, but contrasts sharply to that for the U.S., where the post-neonatal rate was considerably lower (7.2) than the rate for neonates (19.2).

There was no variation in the neonatal mortality rate by region; however, the post-neonatal mortality ranged from a low along the coast of 24.2 per 1,000 live births to a high along the Kuskokwim River of 87.9 per 1,000 live births (Table 1).

Of the deaths that occurred among Eskimo infants in the neonatal period, 57% were attributed to prematurity. Other causes of death at this age were asphyxia, respiratory infection, hyaline membrane disease, neonatal Hirschsprung's disease, and congenital anomaly. Thirty-six Eskimo infants died in the post-neonatal period, all with infectious disease as the cause of death. The specific causes were pneumonia, pertussis, gastroenteritis, measles, meningitis, influenza, and upper respiratory infection.

There was considerable morbidity, especially from infectious respiratory disease, among the 577 children who survived the first year of life, and these diseases often led to long-term sequelae (5). Maynard reported that 76% of the surviving children experienced at least one episode of otorrhea, with an average of 4.3 episodes per child prior to the age of 10 years (6). Although high attack rates of otitis media have been documented elsewhere among northern Indian, Eskimo, and even English children, the rates have not been as high as those found for this cohort. The first year of life was the year of highest risk for onset of otorrhea, and there was an increased probability of secondary episodes after the initial episode (7). Early otitis media was associated with an increased frequency of respiratory illness and a significant reduction in verbal skills (8). Documenting this and other relationships between disabilities and infant diseases, particularly those preventable by hospital delivery or by immunization, has enabled us better to set priorities for public health measures and preventive medicine programs. Recently, the neonatal mortality rate for this part of Alaska was calculated as 12 deaths per 1,000 live births, and the post-neonatal mortality rate was 5 per 1,000.

Most infectious disease was identified in the cohort study on the basis of reported symptoms, and often there was no laboratory or hospital confirmation of the diagnosis. With this in mind we wanted to determine whether an epidemic of an infectious disease detected in the cohort data could be followed spatially and temporally. Such a study was carried out for pertussis and is reported elsewhere in this volume by Ireland et al. (17).

We believe that such a technique for documenting epidemics can be put to good use in the study of predisposing factors for chronic disease, such as bronchiectasis. Bronchiectasis has been a continuing problem in the Bethel area, even as it becomes a memory in other parts of the United States and, indeed, in much of Alaska. Joseph Wilson has been maintaining a registry of bronchiectasis cases in Alaska Natives since the 1950s. Throughout the last 30 years (Figure 1), the Yukon-Kuskokwim Delta has had a disproportionate share of cases: of the Alaska Native children born in the 1970s, 80% of the bronchiectasis diagnosed in Alaska occurred in children from this region, including 14 members of the 1960-1962 cohort. We are in the process of investigating the role of diseases in infancy, such as pneumonia and measles, in the subsequent development of this chronic and disabling form of lung disease.

Plans for the Future

Work in progress will continue to benefit from the careful, detailed data collection efforts of several generations of researchers. In addition to the descriptive epidemiology of myopia (9) which was presented at this meeting, the actual causes of this newly acquired condition, nearsightedness, will be explored. Further work on the relationship between genetics and disease is planned. In addition, measles and pneumonia epidemics will be studied to evaluate their relationships to subsequent long-term illness. Psychometric data will be used to explore the effects of infant morbidity and nutrition on intellectual development. In each situation, longitudinal analysis will allow us to test hypotheses which could usually not be investigated. Now that the members of this cohort are entering young adulthood, their continued cooperation will allow further information to be gathered, possibly even important information about the health of their own neonates and their new generation of families.

Results of studies of this cohort of Eskimos have been presented at previous symposia on circumpolar health. In 1974, at the third symposium in Yellowknife, the results of a study of the relationship between anemia, illness, and intellectual development were presented (10, 11). In 1981, at the fifth symposium in Copenhagen, 2 papers were presented: Nobmann reported the results of a health and nutrition questionnaire which had been completed by the study participants when they were 16 to 18 years of age (12), and Scott reported the results of an analysis of the association between genetic isozyme markers and disease (13).

At this 1984 symposium, some 6 poster presentations reported the findings of several lines of investigation using the cohort data. The results of psychological testing by Nachmann and Doak were presented (14), as were the results of an alcohol and tobacco use questionnaire, designed by Anne Lanier and distributed in conjunction with the health and nutrition questionnaire (15). Three other presentations examine infant morbidity and its serious sequelae (16-18). Finally, the descriptive study of myopia was presented (9).

These projects illustrate the power of this data set as a research tool. Collaborative use of the data on this cohort for comparative and etiologic investigations of specific Native health problems will continue.

REFERENCES

1. National Vital Statistics Division, Monthly vital statistics report. Vol 10: No. 12, 1962.
2. DHEW, Division of Indian Health, Indian Health Highlights, Fourth ed, 1960.
3. Maynard JE, Hammes L. Arctic Health Research Center infant morbidity and mortality study: Interim report. Technical report, PHS, 1962.
4. Maynard JE, Hammes L. Arctic Health Research Center infant morbidity and mortality study: Interim report. Technical report, PHS, 1964.
5. Maynard JE, Hammes L. A study of growth, morbidity and mortality among Eskimo infants of western Alaska. Bull WHO 1970; 42:613.

6. Maynard JE. Otitis media in Alaskan Eskimo children: An epidemiologic review with observations on control. Alaska Med 1969; 11:93.
7. Reed D, Struve S, Maynard JE. Otitis media and hearing deficiency among Eskimo children: A cohort study. Amer J Public Health 1967; 57:1657.
8. Kaplan G, Fleshman J, Bender T, Baum C, Clark P. Long term effects of otitis media: A ten-year cohort study of Alaskan Eskimo children. Pediat 1970; 52:577.
9. Wallace LM, Alward WA, Hall DB, Bender TR, Demske J. The refractive errors of young adult Yupik Eskimos. Paper presented at Sixth Int Symp Circumpolar Health, Anchorage, 1984.
10. Burks JM, Baum C, Fleshman JK, Bender TR, Vieira TA. Associations of anemia and illness in infancy with subsequent intellectual development of children. Paper presented at Third Int Symp Circumpolar Health, Yellowknife, 1974.
11. Burks JM, Baum C, Fleshman JK, Bender TR, Vieira TA. Associations of nutrition and illness in infancy with subsequent growth of a cohort of children. Paper presented at Third Int Symp Circumpolar Health, Yellowknife, 1974.
12. Nobmann E. Health and nutrition attitudes, knowledge and practices of southwest Alaskan Eskimo adolescents. In: Harvald B, Hart Hansen JP, eds. Circumpolar Health 81. Nordic Council for Arct Med Res Rep 1982; 33:40.
13. Scott EM, Wright R. Genetic polymorphism and disease in Eskimos. In: Harvald B, Hart Hansen JP, eds. Circumpolar Health 81. Nordic Council for Arct Med Res Rep 1982; 33:154.
14. Doak B, Nachmann B. The psychometric component of the infant mortality and morbidity cohort study. Paper presented at Sixth Int Symp Circumpolar Health, Anchorage, 1984.
15. Lanier A, Hall D, Malatsi L. Tobacco and alcohol use among teenagers in a cohort of Southwest Alaskan Eskimos. Paper presented at Sixth Int Symp Circumpolar Health, Anchorage, 1984.
16. Heyward W, Hall D. Hepatitis B and lower respiratory infections: Evidence of an association. Paper presented at Sixth Int Symp Circumpolar Health, Anchorage, 1984.
17. Ireland B, Knutson L, Alward W, Hall D. Pertussis: A study of incidence and mortality in a Yukon-Kuskokwim Delta epidemic. In: Fortuine R, ed. Circumpolar Health 84. Seattle: University of Washington Press, 1985 (this volume).
18. Hall D, Wilson J, Alward W, Ireland B. Bronchiectasis: An epidemiologic study of pre-disposing factors. Paper presented at Sixth Int Symp Circumpolar Health, Anchorage, 1984.

Thomas R. Bender
Arctic Investigations Laboratory
Centers for Disease Control
225 Eagle Street
Anchorage, Alaska 99501
U.S.A.

Circumpolar Health 84:120-124

VILLAGE HEALTH CARE: A SUMMARY OF PATIENT ENCOUNTERS FROM ALASKAN VILLAGE CLINICS

PENELOPE M. CORDES

INTRODUCTION

Community Health Aides are village residents who provide primary health care in 171 predominantly Native villages in Alaska. Health aides administer a full range of routine acute and preventive care as well as emergency treatment. What cannot be treated at the village level is referred to physicians at regional hospitals in the state's nine service units of the Indian Health Service. Basic training provided at centers in Bethel, Nome, and Anchorage consists of three sessions totalling 10 weeks of didactic and practical instruction completed over a one or two year period after initial hire. Health aides become Certified Health Practitioners upon completion of a 2 week preceptorship at one of the regional hospitals, 600 hours of directed field experience in their village clinic, demonstrated mastery of a defined set of skills, and successful completion of a certification examination administered by the training centers. Approximately one-half of the health aides presently employed have been certified. Although the health aide program is funded by the federal government and some legislative grants from the State of Alaska, health aides are employed and supervised by 12 Alaska Native non-profit corporations which provide health and social services to over 70,000 shareholders of the Alaska Native regional corporations established by the Alaska Native Claims Settlement Act of 1971.

METHODS

Despite some regional differences in the administration of the program by the non-profit corporations, health aides statewide employ a uniform mechanism for recording patient encounters in the village clinics. This mechanism is the Daily Medical Log in which are recorded for each patient: age, sex, health problem or health promotion activity, treatment prescribed, whether or not a physician was consulted via radio or telephone, and whether or not the patient was referred to the regional hospital or the Alaska Native Medical Center in Anchorage. Using data from these Daily Medical Logs, this paper will describe the nature of the village clinic visits, present a synchronic comparison of village clinic and hospital outpatient department data for 2 regions, and suggest some diachronic trends in village level care in one region of the state.

The following data on village patient encounters are derived from Daily Medical

Logs recorded by Community Health Aides during a 6 month period in 1983 in 5 villages--2 in the Kotzebue Service Unit where the health aide program is administered by the Maniilaq Health Corporation and three villages in the Yukon-Kuskokwim Health Corporation.

RESULTS

Physician Support and Medications Prescribed

Health aides in the sample villages, which range in size from 350 to 650 residents, recorded a total of 6,677 patient encounters in the 6 month period. Of these, only 194 patients, or 3% of the clinic load, were referred directly to the regional hospital for treatment. Including patients for whom health aides arranged appointments at regional hospital outpatient clinics, this figure is increased to 5.3%. Thus only a small percentage of the health problems that are seen at the village level would be represented in data obtained from regional hospital inpatient and outpatient visits, which are currently the primary source of data on rural Alaska Native morbidity.

Physician backup for health aides is provided by daily radio or telephone communication with the regional hospital. Alternatively, health aides practice under medical standing orders following procedures outlined in the health aides' manual (1). In this sample of village clinic encounters, physicians were consulted concerning 1,268 patients, or 19.5% of the cases, whereas health aides functioned under medical standing orders for the remaining 80% of the cases. For 51% of the total patient encounters no medications aside from over-the-counter preparations, such as aspirin or antacids, were prescribed. Antibiotics were prescribed in 32% (2,104) of the cases typically for strep throat, otitis media, respiratory problems, urinary tract infection, impetigo, infected cuts, gonorrhea, and in 40 cases for dental problems. In prescribing antibiotics, health aides were acting in consultation with physicians in 34% of the cases; otherwise they were operating under medical standing orders for 66% of the cases in which antibiotics were prescribed.

Leading Causes of Village Clinic Visits

In order to assess the leading causes of visits to village clinics, multiple presenting complaints were tallied. For example, if a patient presented symptoms of

Table 1. Leading causes of village clinic visits.

Diagnosis	No. of cases	% of total
Total upper respiratory problems	1,893	29.2
Pharyngitis, Tonsillitis	942	14.5
Strep throat	393	6.1
Common cold	299	4.6
Other upper respiratory	259	4.0
Total ear problems	882	13.5
Otitis Media	720	11.0
Other ear problems	162	2.5
Total accidents and injuries	546	8.1
Lacerations, open wounds	279	4.0
Dislocations, sprains, strains	134	2.1
Burns	58	0.9
Superficial contusions	46	0.7
Fracture or possible fracture	29	0.4
Well child care	366	5.7
Total skin disorders		
Infected wounds	134	2.1
Rashes, skin allergies, eczema	112	1.7
Impetigo	100	1.5
Prenatal care	241	3.7
Blood pressure screening	128	2.0
Acute bronchitis	97	1.5
Urinary tract infection	86	1.3
Sexually transmitted diseases	82	1.3

N = 7,836 cumulative health problems/health promotion activities.

otitis media and strep throat during one visit, both were counted. This method yields a cumulative total of over 7,800 health problems or health promotion activities handled by the health aides in the five villages for the period under consideration.

The category of "upper respiratory problems" (including pharyngitis, tonsillitis, strep throat, common cold and other upper respiratory disorders) is the leading cause of clinic visits, comprising 29.2% of patient encounters. This figure does not include the 821 recorded throat cultures performed by the health aides (Table 1).

The second most prevalent health problem is otitis media and other ear disorders, which constitute 13.5% of the clinic load.

In the category of "accidents and injuries" (which includes lacerations, dislocations, sprains, fractures, superficial contusions, and burns) are 546 patients or 8% of the total. Lest this figure overstate the extent of accidents and injuries treated by health aides, it should be noted that this figure includes at least 25% follow-up visits and many of the cases involve less severe injuries than would be encountered at the hospital outpatient department. For example, fracture or possible fractures make up only 5% of these injuries.

The fourth most frequent cause of clinic visit, at 5.7% of the total, is "well child care" including visits for immunizations. This is followed by patient encounters for skin problems (5.3%) and then prenatal care, which makes up 3.7% of the clinic load (241 patient visits).

Perhaps as significant as the health problems that are presented most often are

Table 2. Leading causes of visits, regional hospital outpatient department and village clinics.

Diagnostic category		Percentage of total visits			
		Kotzebue		Yukon-Kuskokwim	
		OPD	Village	OPD	Village
	N* =	22,414	2,367	56,143	4,310
Respiratory system** diseases		14.0	28.0	13.6	36.3
Genito-urinary and gyn.		12.0	13.3	12.4	8.0
Well child, physicals,*** and diagnostic tests		11.2	20.0	9.4	7.7
Ear and nose problems		8.3	11.6	8.8	14.3
Accidents and injuries		11.8	7.4	7.6	9.2
Diseases of the skin		5.7	6.5	5.8	6.3

Source: Indian Health Service Inpatient/Outpatient Reporting System, APC Report 1C.
*   No. of cases for hospital OPD based on 12 months; no. of cases for village clinics based on 6 months.
**   Includes upper respiratory problems, influenza, strep throat, tuberculosis, bronchitis, and pneumonia. Does not include throat cultures administered.
*** Does not include visits for monthly verification of WIC Program eligibility.

those problems which are infrequently recorded in the Daily Medical Logs. Among those worth mentioning for their absence are frostbite (12 cases), village delivery (5 cases), labor or false labor (9 cases), and accidental poisoning (5 cases). Alcohol-related problems are rarely noted in the daily medical logs unless it is an injury immediately related to drinking or unless a patient's inebriation prevents the health aide from providing treatment for a problem.

Comparing village clinic encounters in the 2 service units several differences were noted: 1) the Yukon-Kuskokwim villages had a slightly higher incidence of otitis media (11.3% of all visits) than the Kotzebue region villages (9.8%); 2) more significantly, the number of visits for pharyngitis and strep throat in the Yukon-Kuskokwim villages (12.4% of total encounters); and 3) although the number of cases is small, there is a considerably higher percentage of visits for treatment of venereal disease in the Kotzebue villages (2.15% of all visits versus 0.7% of Yukon-Kuskokwim clinic encounters). This difference may be due to the fact that the Kotzebue region health aides in this sample have the equipment and training to test for sexually transmitted diseases,

whereas only one of the Yukon-Kuskokwim village clinics in this study is so equipped. Of those patients tested for sexually transmitted diseases, 92% were treated with antibiotics.

Leading Causes of Outpatient Visits

The primary source of morbidity statistics for the rural Alaska Native population is the Indian Health Service reporting system which compiles inpatient and outpatient figures from the regional hospitals and the Alaska Native Medical Center in Anchorage. For purposes of comparing the leading causes of village clinic encounters with patient visits at the hospital outpatient departments, data from the Daily Medical Logs and corresponding outpatient department data compiled by Indian Health Service have been grouped into diagnostic categories primarily according to body system. Data on total visits for outpatient services in FY 1982 for the Yukon-Kuskokwim and Kotzebue services in FY 1982 for the Yukon-Kuskokwim and Kotzebue Service Unit hospitals, compared to the Daily Medical Log data from their respective villages in this study reveal very similar data from their

Table 3. Yukon-Kuskokwim village visits 1975.

Diagnostic category	Curative visits			Curative and preventive		
	No.	Rate per 100	Percent of total	No.	Rate per 100	Percent of total
Population	10,470					
Respiratory	16,855	160.93	36.14	16,855	160.98	24.61
Ear and nose	8,537	81.53	18.30	9,006	86.01	13.15
Skin	7,965	76.07	17.08	7,965	76.07	11.63
Gastrointestinal	3,230	30.85	6.92	3,230	30.85	4.71
Musculoskeletal	1,560	14.89	3.34	1,591	15.19	2.32
Accidents and injuries	2,354	22.48	5.04	2,924	27.92	4.27
Genito-urinary and gyn.	1,532	14.63	3.28	3,048	29.11	4.45
Eye	1,235	11.79	2.64	2,873	27.44	4.19
Circulatory sys. and blood	1,401	13.38	3.00	4,903	46.82	7.16
Mental health	340	3.24	0.72	461	4.40	0.67
Misc. comm. disease	237	2.26	0.50	730	6.97	1.06
Neurology						
All other symptoms	1,380	13.18	2.95	1,380	13.18	2.01
Well child, physicals, tests				13,510	129.03	19.72
Total patient contacts	46,626		99.99	68,476		99.99

Source: Yukon-Kuskokwim Health Corporation Monthly Summaries of Health Problem/Health Promotion Activities by Village of Residence.

respective villages in this study, reveal very similar patterns for leading causes of visit. For both hospitals and for the corresponding village clinics, the leading causes of visits are: "respiratory problems", "ear diseases", "genito-urinary and gyn. problems", "accidents and injuries", and "diseases of the skin" (Table 2). What differs significantly between hospital outpatient departments and village clinics is the magnitude of the first leading cause of visit--respiratory problems. For the Yukon-Kuskokwim and Kotzebue Service Unit hospital outpatient departments, respiratory problems including strep throat comprise 13.6% and 14% of the total patient encounters respectively. At the village level, patient visits for these respiratory problems comprise 36.3% of the Yukon-Kuskokwim village patient load and 28% of the patient encounters for the Kotzebue region villages. Villages in both regions also treat a higher relative percentage of ear problems (14.3% and 11.6%) than is seen at the regional outpatient departments, where ear problems comprise less than 9% of all visits.

Another significant difference between hospital and village level care is that 32% of the health aide's documented clinical activities are preventive and health sur-

veillance measures, whereas only approximately 14% of the services provided at the regional outpatient departments would fall into that category.

Village Clinic Patient Encounters Over Time

A diachronic analysis of village clinic encounters is difficult because the data have not been systematically compiled over a number of years. Available data from the Yukon-Kuskokwim Health Corporation, however, permit some comparison over the period from 1975 to 1980 (Tables 3 and 4). During this 5 year period the village population in the region increased by about 2,000. Although the patient load in the region's clinics increased commensurately, the number of visits for respiratory problems remained constant, the number of patient encounters for ear problems and skin infections noticeably decreased, and only half as many visits for accidents and injuries were reported in 1980 as in 1975. On the other hand, preventive and health surveillance activities increased greatly over these 5 years as indicated by the figures on blood pressure screening, hemoglobin checks, Snellens, immunizations, physical exams, and well child and prenatal care.

Table 4. Yukon-Kuskokwim village visits 1980.

| Diagnostic category | Curative visits | | | Curative and preventive | | |
	No.	Rate per 100	Percent of total	No.	Rate per 100	Percent of total
Population	12,323					
Respiratory	16,894	137.09	42.19	16,894	137.09	22.92
Ear and nose	5,692	46.19	14.21	6,693	54.31	9.08
Skin	4,843	39.30	12.09	4,843	39.30	6.57
Gastrointestinal	3,392	27.52	8.47	3,392	27.52	4.60
Musculoskeletal	1,717	13.93	4.28	1,717	13.93	2.33
Accidents and injuries	1,564	12.69	3.90	1,564	12.69	2.12
Genito-urinary and gyn.	1,550	12.57	3.87	3,540	28.72	4.80
Eye	1,323	10.73	3.30	3,754	30.46	5.09
Circulatory sys. and blood	1,258	10.20	3.14	7,388	59.95	10.02
Mental health	287	2.32	0.71	368	2.98	0.49
Misc. comm. disease	273	2.21	0.68	1,474	11.96	2.00
Neurology	132	1.07	0.32	132	1.07	0.17
All other symptoms	1,114	9.04	2.78	1,114	9.04	1.51
Well child, physicals, etc.				20,805	168.83	28.23
Total patient contacts	40,039		99.99	73,678		99.99

Source: Yukon-Kuskokwim Health Corporation Monthly Summaries of Health Problem/Health Promotion Activities by Village of Residence.

CONCLUSION

The data on village clinic encounters presented here are suggestive of the contribution that Community Health Aides are making in the prevention, detection, and early treatment of such problems as otitis media, strep throat, upper respiratory problems and, in the villages where they are equipped to do so, sexually transmitted disease. This early intervention translates into a decrease in these problems and their complications being seen at the regional hospitals. The data on village clinic encounters, particularly regarding respiratory problems, also suggest that the current system of data collection on Alaska Native morbidity, relying as it does on hospital level data, may in fact underrepresent the prevalence of some health problems in rural Alaska, thus arguing for further collection and analysis of village level data.

ACKNOWLEDGMENTS

Support for the research on which this paper is based has been provided by NIMH, National Research Service Award No. 1F31MH08912-01, and by Stanford University.

REFERENCES

1. Whitaker JC. Guidelines for primary health care in rural Alaska. US Dept of Health, Education and Welfare. Washington: US Govt Printing Office, 1976.

Penelope M. Cordes
6731 Crooked Tree Drive
Anchorage, Alaska 99516
U.S.A.

Circumpolar Health 84:125-128

NORTHWEST TERRITORIES PERINATAL AND INFANT MORBIDITY AND MORTALITY STUDY: FOLLOW-UP 1982 I. UTILIZATION, MORBIDITY AND MORTALITY

B.D. POSTL, JAMES B. CARSON, D. SPADY and OTTO SCHAEFER

The Perinatal and Infant Morbidity and Mortality Study (PIMM) of 1973-1974 collected many data and provided important information relating to morbidity, mortality, service utilization, and sociodemographics of infants in the Northwest Territories. Perinatal and infant mortality and morbidity rates were much higher for Indian/Inuit infants than for the Caucasian population, or for that of Canada as a whole (1).

The expansion of these data into childhood was felt to be of importance and was a recommendation of the initial study.

METHODS

A pilot study for this follow-up was undertaken in the Keewatin District of the Northwest Territories in 1980 (2) which provided a standard collection tool for this study.

The non-Caucasian cohort (1973-74) was chosen for follow-up. Caucasians were excluded due to the expected high rate of attrition secondary to movement out of the Northwest Territories and because their health status was not unlike that of Caucasians in southern Canada (1,2).

Data were collected January to July of 1982 in all communities of the Northwest Territories. The collection was geographically divided into the Keewatin/Baffin Island regions (by B. P. and J. C.) and the Mackenzie/Inuvik regions (by D. S. and O. S.). A total of nine investigators were involved, with six seeing in excess of 80% of the study group.

Data were collected retrospectively using nursing station records for three data types, including basic sociodemographic, family and home life, nursing station visits, height and weight records, and hospitalizations. Data were collected from the first birthday until the time of the study visit to that community.

All nursing station visits were reviewed and recorded as one of fifteen systems-related diagnostic codes with status recorded as infectious or non-infectious. Criteria for interpretation and recording were developed and utilized.

All hospitalizations were recorded with up to four separate diagnoses entered using ICDA-9 codes.

Height and weight measurements were recorded by date of measurement.

Data relating to sociodemographics, family and home life, and physical exam were collected in a cross-sectional manner at the time of the community visit.

Physical examination measurements included height, weight, blood pressure, skinfold thicknesses, otoscopic examination, dental examination, hemoglobin, tympanometry, and spirometry.

RESULTS AND DISCUSSION

The initial PIMM cohort included 1,179 study infants. There were 49 deaths and 362 excluded Caucasians, leaving 768 children in our study group.

Of the 768 children, we examined 584, for an overall response rate of 76%. The rates for Inuit, Indian, and mixed/other groups were 85%, 60%, and 80%, respectively (Table 1). There were seven post-infancy deaths in our study group. The six Inuit deaths included two from gastroenteritis, one each from pneumonia, meningitis, congenital heart disease, and a severe burn. The single Indian death was due to a head injury.

The Inuit post-infancy death rate was 190 per 100,000 per year (Figure 1). This compares to an American age-specific standard of approximately 50 per 100,000 per year (3). The infant mortality rate for Inuit of the PIMM cohort was 72 per 1,000 live births (1). The single Indian childhood death is considered to provide too small a numerator for meaningful rate calculation.

Table 1. *Cohort follow-up in the PIMM study.*

Inuit	353/412	85%
Indian	151/255	60%
Mixed/other	80/101	80%
Total	584/768	76%

Table 2. *Meningitis rates for Inuit children per 100,000 per year.*

	Infancy	Post-Infancy	Total
Inuit	4,600 (20)	322 (10)	794*
Reference	210	20	

* 7% of Inuit children had meningitis at some time in their first 8-1/2 yr.

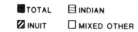

MORTALITY RATES /YR

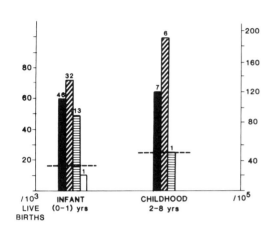

Figure 1. Mortality rates for infants and children in the PIMM study.

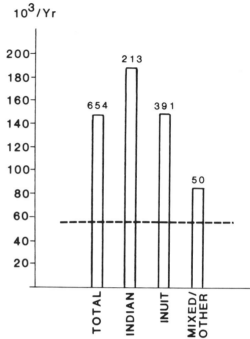

Figure 2. Rates of hospitalization for infants and children in the PIMM study.

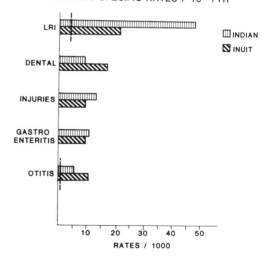

Figure 3. Disease-specific rates for hospitalization of Indian and Inuit children in the PIMM study.

There were 654 hospitalizations involving 318 children. Fifty-five percent of all children had one or more hospitalizations during childhood (Figure 2). Indian children showed a predominant hospitalization rate of 188 per 1,000 per year with Inuit and mixed/other groups demonstrating rates of 148 and 83 per 1,000 per year, respectively.

The five most common reasons for hospitalization were lower respiratory tract infections, dental, injuries, gastroenteritis, and otitis (Figure 3). Indian children were predominant for all but dental service and otitis. Indian children were admitted to hospital at a yearly rate of 46 per 1,000 with lower respiratory tract infections, compared to an age-specific Manitoba Health Services Commission rate of 4 per 1,000.

There were 10 cases of meningitis in Inuit children post-infancy or 323 per 100,000 per year (Table 2). If combined with the 20 Inuit cases of meningitis during infancy, 7% of Inuit children born in 1973-74 had meningitis some time in their first 8.5 years. This markedly increased incidence of meningitis has been previously documented (4).

Well child visits accounted for 23% of nursing station visits, with upper respiratory infections or otitis comprising an additional 30% (Figure 4).

Race and disease-specific rates showed Inuit children averaging in excess of one well child visit per year and almost four illness visits (Figure 5). These rates were significantly higher for Inuit children and

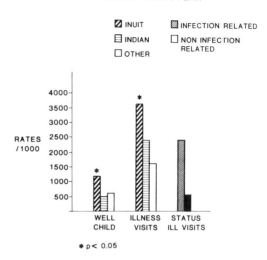

UTILIZATION : NURSING STATION VISITS
% FREQUENCIES

Figure 4. *Reasons for nursing station visits by children in the PIMM study.*

UTILIZATION : NURSING STATION VISITS
RATES / 1000 /YEAR

* p< 0.05

Figure 5. *Utilization rates by cultural groups and nature of nursing station visits.*

showed no difference by sex or zone. The frequency of well child visits compared well with or exceeded the recommendations of the Canadian Task Force on Periodic Health Examinations (5). Eighty percent of illness visits in all groups were of an infectious nature.

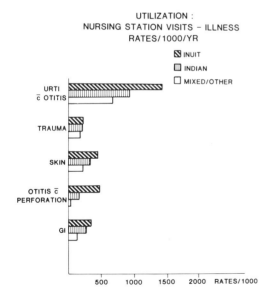

Figure 6. *Illness-specific rates of nursing station visits by Inuit, Indian, and other children in this study.*

Disease-specific rates show an Inuit predominance (Figure 6). Upper respiratory infections and otitis with or without perforation contributed 1,900 visits per 1,000 Inuit children per year.

Sociodemographic factors were statistically examined for their effects on patterns of mortality, morbidity, and utilization. There were surprisingly few factors that had any effect on utilization, morbidity, or mortality. Of those breast-fed in the first year of life, there were significantly fewer hospitalizations in childhood. This protective effect has previously been shown for Indian children in Manitoba (6). Use of alcohol by parents resulted in significantly fewer nursing station well child visits but not illness visits or hospitalizations.

Of those infants whose mothers smoked in the first year of life, there were significantly more nursing station illness visits.

About 25% of all Inuit, and 15% of all Indian children were adopted, without effect on utilization services, morbidity, or mortality.

Fifty percent of Inuit children had one or more deceased sibling without effect upon utilization, morbidity, or mortality.

CONCLUSIONS

1. Mortality of Inuit children of the Northwest Territories remains far in excess of Canadian standards.
2. Hospitalization rates for Inuit and especially Indian children greatly exceeds southern rates.

3. Meningitis has affected an astonishingly high rate of the Inuit childhood population.
4. Utilization of nursing stations is high, well visits are especially well attended by Inuit children.
5. Morbidity rates are predominantly from infectious causes and involve the respiratory tract.
6. Expected correlations between socio-demographic data and morbidity are weak.

REFERENCES

1. Spady DW, Covill FC, Hobart CW et al. Between two worlds: The report of the Northwest Territories Perinatal and Infant Mortality and Morbidity Study. Occasional Publication 16, Boreal Institute for Northern Studies. Univ Alberta. March, 1982.

2. Postl B. Six year follow-up of Keewatin Inuit children born 1973-74. In: Harvald B, Hart Hansen JP, eds. Circumpolar Health 81. Nordic Council Arct Med Res Rep 1982; 33:175-179.

3. Wallace HM, Gold EM, Oglesby AC. Maternal and child health practices, 2nd edition. New York: Wiley, 1982.

4. Wotton K, Stiver G, Hildes JA. Meningitis in the Central Arctic: A 4 year experience. Canad Med Assoc J 1981; 124:887-890.

5. Canadian task force on periodic health examinations: The periodic health exam. Canad Med Assoc J 1979; 121: 1193.

6. Ellestad-Sayed J, Coodin FJ, Tilling LA. Breastfeeding protects against infection in Indian infants. Canad Med Assoc J 1979; 120:295-298.

B. D. Postl
Northern Medical Unit
University of Manitoba
61 Emily Street
Winnipeg, Manitoba   R3E 1Y9
Canada

Circumpolar Health 84:129-133

NORTHWEST TERRITORIES PERINATAL AND INFANT MORBIDITY AND MORTALITY STUDY: FOLLOW-UP 1982 II. PHYSICAL EXAMINATION

B.D. POSTL, JAMES B. CARSON, D. SPADY and OTTO SCHAEFER

The follow-up of the NWT birth cohort of 1972-73 was described in part I of this report entitled Utilization, Morbidity and Mortality. We report here the measures of physical growth and function.

METHODS

The physical examinations reported here each required approximately 20 minutes, and were undertaken in the nursing stations, using an interpreter as necessary.

Heights (cm) and weights (kg) were retrospectively recorded from nursing station records at all episodes at which they were entered into the nursing record. Height and weight were also measured cross-sectionally at the time of examination.

Skinfold thicknesses (mm) were measured at subscapular, triceps, and suprailiac sites, using Lange skinfold calipers. Mid-arm circumference (cm) was measured at a point mid-way between the acromion and the olecranon.

Dental status was determined by gross visual count as diseased, missing, or filled.

Hemoglobin was measured using a hemoglobimeter (Buffalo Medical Specialties).

Blood pressure was measured (systolic and diastolic) on the child in a sitting position, using a V-lok Baumanometer sphygmomanometer with cuff size equal to two-thirds of the left upper arm.

Tympanometry was performed on all children who underwent examination (American Optical). Amplitude, impedance, ' curve shape, and acoustic reflex were determined.

Spirometry was performed using a McKesson portable spirometer. These values were standardized to a water-bell spirometer.

RESULTS AND DISCUSSION

The mean heights and weights for both Indian and Inuit groups showed mean weights above the 50th percentile (Figures 1-4). Relative weights showed some decrease by five years of age with means approaching the 50th percentile for NCHS standards. The use of American standard growth curves has been valid in cross-cultural measurements (1,2). The increased weight/height ratio for Inuit children has been previously described (3).

Skinfold thicknesses and mid-arm circumference showed Indian and Inuit groups having similar measurements, with females

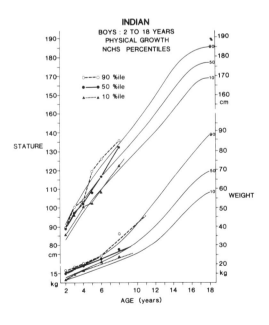

Figure 1. Growth rates of Indian boys, ages 2 to 18, in relation to NCHS percentiles.

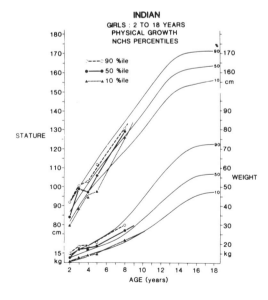

Figure 2. Growth rates of Indian girls, ages 2 to 18, in relation to NCHS percentiles.

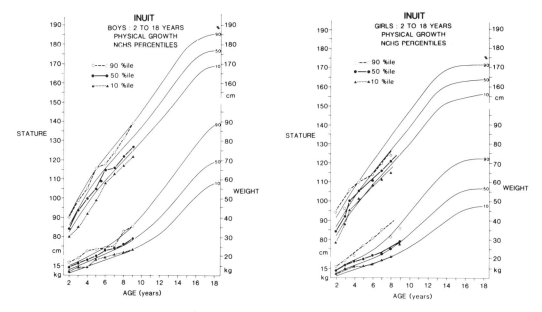

Figure 3. *Growth rates of Inuit boys, ages 2 to 18, in relation to NCHS percentiles.*

Figure 4. *Growth rates of Inuit girls, ages 2 to 18, in relation to NCHS percentiles.*

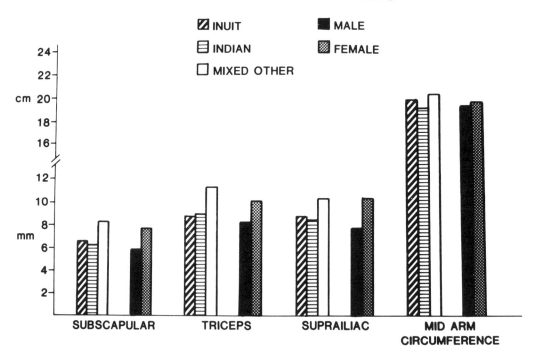

Figure 5. *Skinfold thickness and mid-arm circumferences in Inuit, Indian, and other groups of children.*

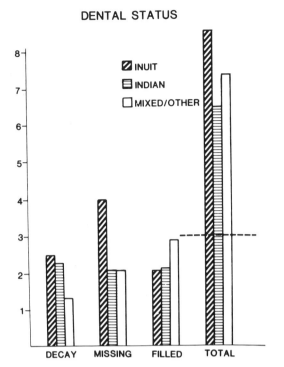

DENTAL STATUS

INUIT
INDIAN
MIXED/OTHER

DECAY MISSING FILLED TOTAL

HEMOGLOBIN LEVELS

INUIT
INDIAN
MIXED/OTHER

gm

Figure 6. Dental status in Inuit, Indian, and other children in this study, as represented by decayed, missing, and filled teeth (DMFT) standard.

Figure 7. Hemoglobin levels (g per 100 ml) in Inuit, Indian, and other children in this study.

showing an increase in all measurements (Figure 5). These figures are similar to those found in the U.S. Health and Nutrition Examination Survey (4) and suggest an adequate level of nutrition. With an increase in weight/height ratio, these figures also suggest that increased lean body mass is a predominant feature.

Dental status (Figure 6) was of significant concern. Using a gross visual model of the DMFT (decayed, missing, or filled teeth) (5), all groups showed a remarkable mean of 7 teeth or greater. A mean of 3 teeth is usually considered dental health.

Mean hemoglobin levels (Figure 7) were 12 g per 100 ml or greater for all groups and both sexes. These values were within the low-risk category of the Nutrition Canada interpretive standard (6).

Blood pressure measurements (Figure 8) approximated those found in larger American studies (7), with mean systolic measurements being less than 50th percentile for all groups and both sexes.

Otoscopic examination (Figure 9) showed 40% of children to be normal. Over 50% of children, however, had evidence of scarring or perforation, both likely to have an adverse effect on hearing.

Tympanometry (Figures 10, 11) revealed Inuit children with significantly decreased impedance. Both amplitude and impedance were significantly decreased in cases where history indicated more than two episodes of otorrhea during childhood.

Spirometric findings are reported elsewhere in this Symposium (8).

We were unable to identify any sociodemographic or health index that adversely affected growth or nutrition measurements.

CONCLUSIONS

1. Indian and Inuit children are well grown at eight and one-half years. There is evidence of increased lean body mass.
2. Anemia is not a problem in this age group in these populations.
3. Dental status lags far behind that in the south and requires major efforts.
4. Ear infections leading to hearing loss continue to be a major cause of morbidity.

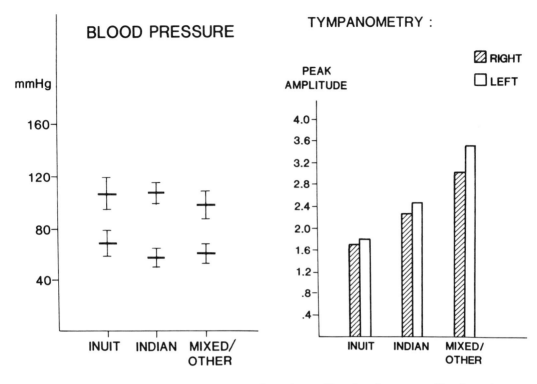

Figure 8. Blood pressure measurements of
          Inuit, Indian, and other children
          in this study.

Figure 10. Impedance results from tympano-
           metric examinations of children.

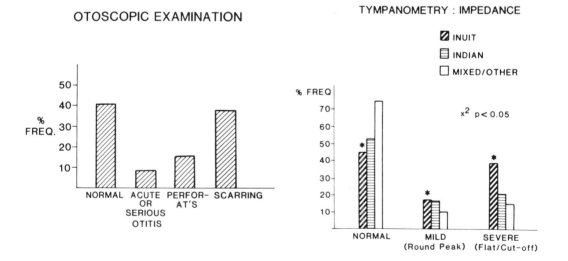

Figure 9. Results of otoscopic examinations
          on children in this study.

Figure 11. Amplitude results from tympano-
           metric examinations.

5. There were no significant effects on growth by sociodemographic factors nor by events in the first year of life.

REFERENCES

1. Greulich WW. Science 1958; 127:515.
2. Leary MD. The use of percentile charts in the nutritional assessment of children from primitive communities. African Med J 1969; 43:1165.
3. Heller CA, Scott EM, Hammes CM. Amer J Dis Child 1967; 113:338.
4. National Center for Health Statistics: First health examination survey: Anthropometric and clinical findings. Rockville, Maryland, 1972.
5. Klein A, Palmer CE. The dental problem of elementary school children. Millbank Fund Quart 1938; 16:267.
6. Nutrition Canada, Department of Health and Welfare: Nutrition Survey, 1973.
7. Task Force on Blood Pressure Control in Children. National Heart, Lung, and Blood Institute. Peds (Supp), 1977: 59-803.
8. Carson J, Postl B, Spady D, Schaefer O. Lower respiratory tract infections among Canadian Inuit children. In: Fortuine R, ed. Circumpolar Health 84. Seattle: University of Washington Press, 1985 (this volume).

B. D. Postl
Northern Medical Unit
University of Manitoba
Winnipeg, Manitoba R3E 1Y9
Canada

Circumpolar Health 84:134-138

VARIATION AND CONVERGENCE BETWEEN SELF-PERCEIVED AND CLINICALLY MEASURED HEALTH STATUS VARIABLES OF THE INUIT IN NORTHERN QUEBEC

PETER M. FOGGIN, ROGER BELLEAU, BERNARD DUVAL and JEAN-PIERRE THOUEZ

INTRODUCTION

The health status of a Native population such as the Inuit of northern Quebec needs to be better understood (1) since classic indicators (e.g. infant mortality) still suggest that general health levels are often lower than those for Canadians as a whole (2-4). Change in lifestyle and in the physical and social environment have probably also had considerable impact, both positive and negative, in health levels (5-6) among the Inuit and other Native populations in Canada.

Although the subject of this study is the health status and risk factors of the Inuit and Cree population of northern Quebec, the focus of this paper is primarily methodological. The question is how to obtain one or several indexes of general health status, based on several symptomologies of epidemiologically suggested tracer diseases (7,8). The goal of this analysis, then, is first, to learn the extent to which clinically measured data (9) can be compared to subjectively obtained (by Inuit interviewers) self-evaluative socio-medical data (10-13), and second, to obtain some kind of relatively stable indexes of health status for this particular Inuit population.

After a series of factor analyses (14), on all health status variable categories, it became apparent for two reasons that certain variables could and should be grouped together. First, they would line up with almost identical factor loadings on the same statistically independent factors. Second, because of the problem of large numbers of zeros in the dichotomous response data, it was deemed advisable to add certain related variables together in order to create preliminary indexes. This eliminated a large proportion of the zeros (negative responses) in the basic data matrix that would subsequently be factor analysed.

Three factor matrixes will be presented and discussed: a factor analysis of the self-evaluative socio-medical data, another of the clinically obtained health status data, and finally a combined analysis of these two data matrixes taken together.

METHODS

A total of 195 Inuit adults (aged 15 years and over) were selected from a sample of adults (72% of total sample cases) on the basis of having been involved specifically in two separate data-gathering procedures carried out at the end of 1982. The source population was three Inuit villages of

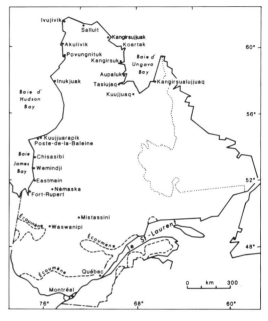

Figure 1. Inuit and Cree communities of northern Quebec.

northern Quebec: 57 cases were from Kangirsuk (Payne Bay), 51 from Koartak, and 87 from Salluit (Figure 1). These three villages represent the initial phase of the on-going PLASANNOUQ (PLANIFICATION/SANTÉ-NOUVEAU-QUÉBEC--or in English NEW QUEBEC HEALTH PLANNING PROJECT) study. These cases represent 22% of the population of Kang-

Table 1. PLASSANNOUQ health status variables.

Subjective self-evaluated variables:

. health care service utilization
. use of medication
. past illness and symptoms

Functional variables (self-evaluated):

. physical impairments/handicaps
. prevented from functioning "normally"

Epidemiological variables (clinically measured):

. pulmonary function and history
. ear and dental health

Variables	I (General medication index)	II (Nursing station usage index)	III (Chest disease index)	IV ("Normal' handicaps index)	V ("Serious' functional health index)	VI ("Serious' handicap index)	VII (Mild functional impairment index)
1- Clinic visit		.90					
2- Visit : 'seriousness'		.89					
3- Medication-use	.85						
4- Medication-type	.91						
5- Medication ('seriousness')	.92						
6- Medication ('constant')							
7- Home remedies					.80		
8- Home remedies ('seriousness')							
9- Too sick for work or activity (w./a.)						.84	
10- Too sick for w./a. ('seriousness')					.82		
11- Breathlessness							
12- Chest pains			.90				
13- Physical impairment						.82	
14- Physical impairment (kind)				.57			
15- Glasses				.67			
16- Dental problems							.48
17- Hearing problems				.65			
18- Serious disease					.88		
19- Serious disease (kind)							
Eigen value:	3.76	1.75	1.69	1.40	1.33	1.11	1.03
% total variance:	19.80	9.20	8.90	7.40	7.00	5.90	5.50

(63.7%)

Figure 2. Self-evaluative indexes of health status.

Variables	I (General chest symptoms index)	II (Spirometry index)	III (Bronchitis/T.B. treatment index)	IV (Ear infection index)	V (Ear damage index)	VI (Frequent pneumonia index)
1- Coughing	.86					
2- Phlegm	.86					
3- Wheezing	.66					
4- Breathlessness	.60					
5- Chest problems	.57					
6- Bronchitis			.73			
7- Pneumonia			.48			
8- Tuberculosis (prophylaxis)			.82			
9- Bronchitis (chronic)	.65					
10- Heart problems						-.44
11- Ear infections				.93		
12- Ear perforations					.92	
13- Frequent pneumonia (last 5 years)						.83
14- Age		-.59				
15- F.V.C. Best *		.91				
16- F.E.V. Best *		.92				
17- F.E.F. Best *		.67				
Eigen value:	4.99	2.12	1.34	1.13	1.07	1.00
% total variance	29.40	12.50	7.90	6.70	6.30	5.90

* spirometry

(68.7%)

Figure 3. Standardized epidemiological indexes of health status.

irsuk, 30% of the population of Koartak, and 16% of the Salluit population.

The first procedure was based on the household (family) with one respondent per family answering questions on behalf of all household-members. Approximately 30 households were randomly selected per community, 92 in all. A sociomedical questionnaire was used, one purpose of which was to obtain information on self-perceived and self-evaluated health status. Whenever a question about health, disease, or health care utilization was answered in the affirmative, the identity of the subject was determined, resulting in the 195 cases.

The second information-gathering procedure was clinical, involving spirometric measurements, an epidemiological lung health questionnaire, and a brief medical examination by a doctor during which emphasis was placed on tracer disease factors (otoscopy, blood pressure, etc.). Each person of the same sample of households aged 15 or over was examined. The 195 cases from this second sample were matched with the 195 cases from the household adult data file for which self-perceived, self-evaluative data existed. Both procedures were carried out over a 2-week period in each village by a six-person team consisting of a medical doctor, a field coordinator, and 4 local assistants (Table 1).

RESULTS AND DISCUSSION

The first series of health status indexes is based on the self-evaluative data obtained in the sample households (Figure 2). Nineteen additive ("preliminary index") information categories were used (see the description of "variables" in Figure 2) and seven factors were retained through principal components analysis using the Kaiser Varimax rotation to enhance the clarity (specificity) of the factor loading values. (This particular factor analytic model was used in all the index creation analyses). These are in descending order of statistical power and importance: the general medication index (S^2=19.8%), the nursing station utilization index (S^2=8.9%), the "normal" handicaps index (S^2=7.0%), the "serious" functional index (S^2=7.0%), the "serious" handicap index (S^2=5.9%), and finally the "mild functional impairment" index (S^2=5.5%). The highest factor loadings associating each variable with corresponding factors are underlined. It can be noted from Figure 2 that there is a clear demarcation between factor identification variables and variables not associated with a given factor. For example, the top 3 loadings of Factor I are 0.92, 0.91, and 0.85 after which the next three highest are 0.40, 0.25, and 0.24. Observation-based factor scores are calculated relating each factor to all the observations and in so doing each case is assigned a relative weight in relation to each factor (component). In this way it is possible to evaluate how important each factor analytic index is in relation to each of the observed cases (14).

To compare how the three Inuit villages related separately to each of the first two

Variables	Factors (components)						
	I	II	III	IV	V	VI	VII
1- Clinic visit				.84			
2- Visit seriousness				.87			
3- Medication - use		.86					
4- Medication-type		.87					
5- Medication-seriousness		.91					
6- Medication - constant		.38				.53	
7- Home remedies (H.R.)							
8- H.R.							
9- Too sick for activity				.37		.59	.16
10- Too sick-seriousness							
11- Breathlessness							
12- Chest pains							.86
13- Physical impairment							
14- Physical impairment-kind							
15- Glasses							
16- Dental problems							
17- Hearing problems							
18- Serious disease (S.D.)							.86
19- Serious disease-kind					.32	.34	
1- Coughing	.83						
2- Phlegm	.84						
3- Wheezing	.71						
4- Breathlessness	.56						
5- Chest problems	.55				.35		
6- Bronchitis					.69		
7- Pneumonia					.46		
8- T.B. (prophylaxis)					.73		
9- Bronchitis-chronic	.65						
10- Heart problems						.68	
11- Ear infections							
12- Ear perforations							
13- Frequent pneumonia							
14- Age				.47			.47
15- F.V.C. Best				.89			
16- F.E.V. Best				.91			
17- F.E.F. Best				.67			
Eigen value	6.12	3.06	2.40	2.12	1.74	1.69	1.41
% total variance	17.00	8.50	6.70	5.90	4.80	4.70	3.90

Column index labels: I — General chest symptoms index; II — General medication index; III — Bronchitis / T.B. treatment index; IV — Pulmonary function / Spirometry index; V — Nursing station usage index; VI — Heart disease index; VII — 'Serious' disease index. (51.60 %)

Figure 4. Combined self-evaluative and epidemiological indexes of health status.

factors, the factor scores were arranged from highest to lowest for each village. Only the first two factors were considered to be sufficiently variable to warrant drawing conclusions at the village level (Figure 5). Each box represents the lower and upper end of the spectrum of standardized values (Z-scores). (The factor scores showed a standardized Z-score type of distribution because the basic data matrix to which the factors are recombined was standardized at the outset). In a normal distribution one would expect about 16% in each box (more than 1.0 standard deviation above or below the mean). This factor score summary for the first two self-evaluative factor indexes gives us some feeling for the variation between villages. All three villages seem to be skewed toward a high manifestation of positive values on the general medication index, Koartak being the highest and Salluit the lowest. What can this index tell us about the health level of these local populations (15)? It seems that the trend may be related to the second

	Low ⟵	⟶ High	
Factor I	0.00 %	13.70 %	Payne Bay (n = 51)
General medication	1.70 %	17.60 %	Koartak (n = 57)
Index	2.30 %	3.00 %	Salluit (n = 87)
Factor II	3.90 %	19.60 %	Payne Bay (n = 51)
Nursing station	10.50 %	17.50 %	Koartak (n = 57)
Usage index	5.70 %	11.40 %	Salluit (n = 87)

(More than 1.0 standard deviation below X̄)   (More than 1.0 standard deviation above X̄)

Percent of total number of cases (factor scores) per village

In a 'normal' distribution one would expect about 16% in each of the above boxes

Figure 5. Variation in self-evaluative indexes by village.

factorial index: nursing station usage (Figure 5), whereas Koartak and Kangirsuk manifest similar positive ratings (17.5% and 19.5%) with Salluit skewing at a lower level (11.4%). The population:nurse ratio is higher in Salluit than in the other two communities, however.

With the second analytic procedure, a different series of epidemiological health status indexes is obtained (Figure 3). As usual, factors reflecting the nature of the basic data matrix emerge from a multivariate principal components analysis. The factors (or components) obtained are a general chest symptoms index ($S^2=29.4\%$) a pulmonary function/spirometry index ($S^2=12.5\%$), an index associating bronchitis with a preoccupation with tuberculosis prophylactic treatment ($S^2=7.9\%$), an ear infection index ($S^2=6.7\%$), an index of ear damage ($S^2=6.3\%$), and finally an index related to frequent attacks of pneumonia ($S^2=5.9\%$). As in the self-evaluative indexes the factor loadings show a clear distinction in each case between factor-related variables and those which have no real association whatever (Figure 3). When the factor scores relating these factor indexes to individual cases are calculated and ranked for each village, an interesting health geography picture emerges (Figure 6). On the chest symptoms index, Kangirsuk (Payne Bay) shows a "normal" (in statistical terms) distribution (17.6% and 17.7% in the upper and lower extremes). The other two villages depart markedly from this situation. Koartak shows very much lower values on the chest symptoms index (31.6% as opposed to 12.3%) while Salluit shows a completely opposite trend (5.7% on the low end versus 20.7% on the high end). This pattern indicates that on the chest symptoms index value spectrum, Salluit shows the highest levels of chest respiratory symp-

Low ← → High

Factor I	17.60 %	17.70 %	Payne Bay (n=51)
General chest symptoms	31.60 %	12.30 %	Koartak (n=57)
Index	5.70 %	20.70 %	Salluit (n=87)
Factor II	13.80 %	3.90 %	Payne Bay (n=51)
Spirometry / Pulmonary function	12.20 %	8.80 %	Koartak (n=57)
Index	8.00 %	16.10 %	Salluit (n=87)

More than 1.0 standard deviation below X̄ (More than 1.0 standard deviation above X̄)

Figure 6. Variation in epidemiological indexes by village. (See Figure 5 for further explanation of scores).

Low ← → High

Factor I	15.70 %	15.70 %	Payne Bay (n=51)
General chest symptoms	22.80 %	8.80 %	Koartak (n=57)
Index	6.90 %	21.80 %	Salluit (n=87)
Factor II	0.00 %	11.70 %	Payne Bay (n=51)
General medication	3.50 %	17.50 %	Koartak (n=57)
Index	2.30 %	11.50 %	Salluit (n=87)

(More than 1.0 standard deviation below X̄) (More than 1.0 standard deviation above X̄)

Figure 7. Variation by village in combined self-evaluative and epidemiological indexes. (See Figure 5 for further explanation of scores.)

toms, Koartak the lowest and Kangirsuk a sort of "average" position. Clearly there is some geographical variation involved with this particular health status index. The spirometry index shows a surprising correlation between the forced vital capacity (FVC) and forced expiratory volume (FEV). To a lesser degree (factor loading - 0.67), forced expiratory flow (FEF) is also related to this second epidemiological health status index. The FEF is, however, the least precise of these measurements. Interestingly, age is negatively associated with this factor so that we can conclude that the higher the age the lower the FVC/FEV/FEF results will be. Because of the bipolar nature of this age-spirometry component the factor scores on this index vary in the opposite direction from the factor scores of other indexes. Consequently, high negative factor scores (corresponding roughly to standardized Z-scores) should be interpreted as high pulmonary function performance (Figure 6, Factor II). In the light of this definition it can be seen once again that in the case of Salluit the pulmonary function factor as measured by spirometry tests is low (i.e. high positive factor scores indicate low performance in this case only), whereas the opposite is the case for Koartak and especially for Kangirsuk (Payne Bay).

Finally, the two data matrixes (self-evaluative and epidemiological) were taken and analyzed together in a combined principal components analysis. In Figure 4 the highest factor loadings are shown for each of the seven factors that were retained. Only in the case of Factor VI (heart disease index) was there a real combination of variables flowing from the two combined data matrixes (self-evaluative: constant medication and too sick for activity; epidemiological: heart problems and age).

There seems rather to be a general and intractable cleavage between the two types of health status data. However, an inter- esting type of alternance seems to emerge: Factor I (S^2=17.0%) is the general chest symptom index from the epidemiological data, Factor II (S^2=8.5%) is the general medication index from the self-evaluative data, Factor III (spirometry), and Factor IV (Nursing station usage) alternating once again as to the body of basic data being reflected. The encouraging observation is that, at least in the case of the first five factors, there is a health status index stability that seems to be demonstrated. The first two factor indexes of the epidemiology analysis (Figure 3) are all found in the first five factors (components) of the combined multivariate analysis (Figure 4).

Examination of the variation by village of the first two factors of the combined analysis (chest symptoms index and the general medication index--Figure 7) shows that the percentages in the extreme positive and negative ends of the two factor score distributions are relatively similar to the corresponding factor indexes in the two separate data analyses (Figures 5 and 6). The village positions are identical and the value trends are very similar (e.g. 6.9% and 21.8% for Salluit in Figure 7 as compared to 5.7% and 20.7% in Figure 6). This observation also tends to confirm a marked stability in at least five of the health status factor indexes.

CONCLUSIONS

At least five relatively stable statistically independent health status indexes emerge from this preliminary multivariate data analysis: general chest symptoms; general medication; pulmonary function/ spirometry; nursing station usage; bronchitis/tuberculosis treatment. Because the data base is still fragmentary (data were available from only 3 of the 13 Inuit villages involved in the overall on-going study) the present results must be considered tentative. These preliminary observations are promising, however, in that we have learned which independent underlying health status factors can be gleaned from the mass of interrelated and intercorrelated information coming of the the PLASANNOUQ survey. There is convergence between the two data matrixes only at the level of heart disease symptoms (Figure 4, Factor VI). For the rest, the two types of data measured over the same array of individuals yield statistically independent health status indexes (Figure 4, Factors I to V). It should be possible to conclude from this observation that each measurement process is assessing different, if complementary, information. It also appears that, in the case of the more statistically powerful factors (components), there is a decided spatial variation in health levels (on a village to village basis) for the relevant health status indexes. This tends to confirm one of the underlying hypotheses of the overall study, namely that there is significant geographic variation in health status among the Inuit of northern Quebec.

ACKNOWLEDGMENTS

We thank Pierre Philie, Field Research Coordinator; Dr. Normand Tremblay, Field Research Doctor; and Mary Weetaluktuk, Kativik Health Board.

REFERENCES

1. Labbé J. La santé des Inuits du Nouveau-Québec, Etudes Inuits 1981; 5:63-81.
2. Duval B, Therrien F. Natalité, mortalité et morbidité chez les Inuit du Québec arctique, Recherches Amérindiennes au Québec, 1983; Vol. XII, No. 1.
3. Schaefer O. Changing morbidity and mortality patterns of the Canadian Inuit. Chronic Diseases in Canada 1981; 2:12-14.
4. Robitaille N. La population Inuit du Canada: variations régionales en 1981. Paper presented at University of Montreal, April 1984.
5. Wenzel G. Inuit health and the health care system: Change and status quo. Inuit Studies 1981; 5:7-16.
6. McKeown T. Les déterminants de l'état de santé des populations depuis trois siècles: le comportement, l'environement et la médecine. In: Bozzini L, Renaud M, Gaucher D, Leambias-Wolff J, eds. Médecine et société; les années 80. Montréal: Editions Coopératives Albert St-Martin, 1982; 143-175.
7. Berg L. Health status indicators. Chicago: Hospital Research and Educational Trust, 1973.
8. Bergner M, Bobbitt RA, Pollard WE, Martini DP, Gilson BS. The sickness impact profile: Conceptual formulation and methodology for the development of a health status measure. Int Health Serv 1976; 6:417.
9. Ferris G. Epidemiology standardization project. American Thoracic Society, 1978.
10. Collishaw N. Canada health survey: Health problems. A content proposal, Ottawa: Health and Welfare Canada, 1976.
11. Anderson DO, Kohn R, White K, et al. Health care: an international study, Geneva: WHO, 1976.
12. Brodman K, Ersmann AJ, Wolff HG. Cornell Medical Index: Health Questionnaire. New York: Cornell University Medical College, 1974.
13. Elison J, Siegman A. Socio-medical health indicators. New York: Baywood Publishing, 1979.
14. Rummel BJ. Applied factor analysis. Evanston: Northwestern Univ Press, 1970.
15. Wilson W. Do health indicators indicate health? Amer J Public Health 1981; 71:461-463.

Peter M. Foggin
Département de Géographie
Université de Montréal
C.P. 6128 succursale A
Montréal Québec H3C 3J7
Canada

Circumpolar Health 84:139-142

MORTALITY OF LABRADOR INNU AND INUIT, 1971-1982

KATHRYN A. WOTTON

INTRODUCTION

Few peoples have experienced such drastic changes in their ways of living and dying as have the Indians and Inuit in the Canadian North in the last generation. Many of the facts and figures about the health of Canada's Native people have been displayed often and widely. One group of Native people for whom the statistics have not been available is the Innu and Inuit of northern Labrador.

When Newfoundland joined Canada in 1949, the special status of its Native inhabitants was not recognized. Because of this historical quirk, Native statistics in Newfoundland continue to be pooled with those of the rest of the province where their relatively small numbers are rapidly diluted and hence easier to overlook.

To determine some basic parameters of health for the Native people in northern Labrador it was necessary therefore to go first to the communities for a list of deaths over the past 12 years and then search out details and verification from hospitals, nursing stations, vital statistics, and community members. Although the process was tedious and time-consuming, there is reason to believe that the list of vital events obtained was fairly complete. Since the population is small and the rates therefore subject to chance fluctuation that could be large, 10- and 12-year averages have been used, centered on 1976. Although the problem of population size exists, it does not invalidate analysis of the population or comparison between populations. Although rates from small localities must be interpreted with caution, they often allow a more intimate assessment of the factors involved.

The 2,500 Native people of northern Labrador live in six remote isolated coastal communities north of Melville Inlet. The area lies between 53°N and 60°N latitude with the cold Labrador Stream bringing an arctic and subarctic climate to the region. Five of the communities are Inuit and Settler, one is Nauscaupi Indian. The Settler designation is a uniquely Labradorian one. Settler families are of mixed Inuit and white origin, tracing their lineage back six or seven generations to a white man who married and settled on the Labrador coast. Both Settler and Inuit are represented by the Labrador Inuit Association in their land claims. The Nauscaupi are part of a larger group straddling the Quebec-Labrador border and are represented by the Nauscaupi Montagnais Innu Association.

Of the six communities, Nain, the farthest north, is the largest, with a population of 1,000, of whom over half are Inuit. The proportion of a community that is Inuit decreases as one proceeds southward. Many of the Inuit families formerly resided in Hebron and Nutak, north of Nain, but were relocated in the 1950s. Half the population is under 15 years of age. The average income is $7,000 per worker. Most of the work is seasonal and related to fishing in summer. Half of the protein and caloric intake of northern residents is still from country food. In contrast to the situation elsewhere in the North, the Inuit of Labrador have been greatly metamorphosed by Moravian mission influences that extend back over 200 years. The Nauscaupi of Davis Inlet have sustained most of the changes associated with the modern world in the short period since 1968, when their community was built and they started to spend more time off the barrenlands away from their traditional life as nomadic caribou hunters. Despite these historical differences, both Inuit and Indian traditional values have been very severely strained by the revolutionary pace of change over the past 20 years.

RESULTS

The 10-year mean crude death rate for northern Labrador was 9.97 per 1,000 population compared to a rate of 7.2 for all of Canada (Table 1). Because of the youth of this population, compared to that of Canada as a whole, a more accurate comparison is provided by age standardization, increasing the crude death rate by approximately 80% to 17.9 per 1,000. The Native group used for comparison is that of Sioux Lookout Zone, where the rates are known for the same time period.

In every age group in northern Labrador, mortality is higher than the rate for Canadians as a whole and also higher than the rate for Native people as a whole (Table 2). The difference is especially striking below age 45. Differences range from almost 4 times the national rate in the age group 15 to 24 years, to 5.5 times the national rate in the age group 0 to 4 years. The age-specific averages do not include Rigolet, as the age breakdown of this community was not available for 1976.

Children contributed most heavily to the overall mortality on the northern Labrador coast. Almost one-quarter of all deaths (53 of 220) occurred in those under 5 years of age, as opposed to only 3% of deaths in Canada as a whole. One of the

Table 1.   Crude mortality rate.

	CMR	Age standardized MR
Labrador	9.97	17.9
Native people	6.4	11.5
Canada	7.2	7.2

Table 3.   Infant mortality rate.

	IMR	Neonatal death rate	Post neonatal death rate
Labrador	60	21.4	38.6
Native people	36.7	15.1	21.7
Canada	13.9	9.4	4.5

most important indices of the quality of health care and level of socioeconomic development is the infant mortality rate. In high mortality populations, infant mortality is the largest single age category of mortality. Of a total of 700 live births occurring between 1971 and 1980 there were 15 neonatal deaths, 27 postneonatal deaths and 42 infant deaths. The 10 year average has been used to allow comparisons with both the national rate and the Native rate for the same time period.

The infant mortality rate for northern Labrador was 60 per 1,000 live births (Table 3), or more than four times that for Canada as a whole. Even compared to other Native groups it was much higher. Sioux Lookout Zone had an infant mortality rate per 1,000 for the same time period of 25.5.

The postneonatal rate in Canada was half that of the neonatal rate. In northern Labrador the postneonatal rate exceeded the neonatal rate and was in fact 8 to 9 times the national rate.

Of the neonatal deaths more than half (8 of 15) were a result of prematurity. Infections featured more prominently in the postneonatal deaths, with pneumonia, gastroenteritis, laryngotracheobronchitis and meningitis accounting for almost 60% of deaths (16 of 27). Sudden infant death syndrome (SIDS) was diagnosed in 5 infant deaths at autopsy.

Overall, the most common cause of death in northern Labrador over the 12-year period was "accidents, poisonings, and violence," which accounted for 90 of 262 deaths or 34%. If one excludes infant deaths, then 85 of 213 or 40% of the remaining deaths were accidental. The toll was particularly high in children over 1 year where 20 of 24 deaths or 80% were accidental, compared to 9% for the rest of Canada. For young adults 15-24 years old, 95% of deaths were accidental (21 of 22).

The proportion of deaths due to accidents is not only particularly high in younger age groups but it also increases as one proceeds northward. Equally disturbing is the indication that violence as a cause of death appears to be on the increase (Table 4). The problem with averaging deaths over a 12-year period is that one loses temporal trends. Change is proceeding rapidly in the Canadian North. The direction of that change and the accelerating pace of the change can, however, be appreciated by comparing the first 10 years, 1971 to 1980, to the last two years, 1981 to 1982. Accidents as a percentage of total deaths for the north coast and Nain respectively has risen from 31% and 37% (1971-80) to 50% and 68% (1981-82).

To appreciate the magnitude of violence as a factor contributing to death in northern Labrador, one can compare it to rates

Table 2.   Age-specific mortality rate per 100,000 people.

Age Group	N. Labrador	Canada	Sioux Lookout Zone
0 - 4	(55) 1,637	296	1,066
5 - 14	(11) 158	37	63
15 - 24	(19) 411	106	399
25 - 44	(36) 638	144	548
45 - 64	(53) 1,963	856	1,098
>65	(53) 8,030	5,091	5,110

Table 4. Trend in adult accidental deaths.

	1971-80	1981-82
Labrador	31%	50%
Nain	37%	68%

Table 5. Death rates per 100,000 people.

	APV	Fire	Drowning	Suicide
Labrador	330	66.9	129.3	65.5
Indian	239	23.6	21.5	24.3
Canada	72	3.5	3.2	14.3

elsewhere. The national rate of accidental deaths was 72 per 100,000 (Table 5). Both Indian and Inuit rates are higher and a cause for much concern at 239 and 160 respectively. Northern Labrador over the past 10 years has had an average of 330 violent deaths per 100,000 population, almost five times the national rate.

Almost 60% of all lethal accidents were due to either fires or drownings. Fifteen fire deaths and 29 drownings gave rates of 67 and 129 per 100,000. National rates for fires and drowning were 3.5; Native rates were approximately 25.

Suicide was not recorded in Labrador prior to 1979 despite meticulous record-keeping by the Moravians. In the five years since the first recorded suicide there have been a total of eight suicides. Considering the five years from 1979 to 1983, the rate is 65.6 per 100,000 population, compared to a national rate of 14.3, an Indian rate of 24.3, and an Inuit rate of 25.5 (Table 6). Overall, Native rates are twice as high as national rates and a cause for great concern. Northern Labrador has twice the Native rates and almost five times the national rate.

In the Northwest Territories, the Native rate of suicide was close to or below the overall Canadian rate up until 1971. Since then it has been diverging dramatically. The greatest discrepancy between Canadian and Native rates had been in the age group 15 to 24 years where Native rates exceed the national rates by a factor of 7. The age group 15 to 24 years accounted for all but one of the recent suicides in northern Labrador yielding an age-specific rate of 295 per 100,000 population, 15 times the national rate.

Although greatly eclipsed by violent deaths, deaths from infectious causes contributed a sizeable burden upon Native Labradorians, accounting for one-fifth of all deaths (Table 7). National and Native rates per 1,000 are not comparable because meningitis and pneumonia are included under other categories. Correcting the Labrador figure to exclude meningitis and pneumonia, however, would still leave infections accounting for 7.6% of all deaths, and a rate 12 times the national rate.

Cancer resulted in 39 deaths over the 12-year period, or 15% of all deaths. The crude cancer rates per 100,000 population are almost equal to those of Canada as a whole. Again as the population is young, age standardization would increase the Labrador rates considerably. Since only one of the cancer deaths from the northern coast was an Indian, it is possible to calculate the Inuit rate for 1971 to 1982 as 161 per 100,000. In the Northwest Territories at the beginning of this time period, the Inuit rate of cancer was 100 per 100,000 population. The extraordinary male to female ratio of 8:1 noted in Inuit malignancies by Schaefer [1] was not demonstrated in Labrador where both sexes seem equally at risk (20:19). Lung cancer accounted for 11 deaths or 28% of malignancies. The primary site of three of the carcinomas was not known.

Tuberculosis has been reduced but not totally eliminated as a lethal disease in Labrador. In the past 12 years there were only 2 deaths from tuberculosis on the whole

Table 6. Suicide.

	Rate per 100,000	Age-specific rate 15-24
Labrador	65.5	295
Indian	24.3	130
Canada	14.3	20

Table 7. Causes of death per 100,000.

	APV	Infection	Cancer
Labrador	330	193	145
Native people	239	96	59
Canada	72	43	154

north coast. This is a remarkable change from the 46 deaths recorded in a single community between 1920 and 1959. Chronic obstructive lung disease was cited in 7 Inuit deaths, 4 of them males. These deaths may well reflect a high incidence of "Eskimo Lung," a condition noted in Inuit men who engaged in long term winter hunting activity (2).

A final observation deals with what appears to be a relatively high incidence of berry aneurysm in northern Labrador. A relatively unusual event, berry aneurysm was diagnosed in 3 Inuit deaths, while at least 4 living Labrador Inuit have had the diagnosis made in the past 5 years following a subarachnoid hemorrhage. Although not previously recorded, it may well be an explanation for the not uncommon and therefore puzzling finding in the past of strokes in a people known to have little atherosclerosis and few hypertensives. A frequent occurrence of berry aneurysm was also noted by the author in the Keewatin District, N.W.T.

CONCLUSIONS

The mortality figures collected on the north coast of Labrador reflect many phenomena previously noted for both Indian and Inuit. They also reveal a condition of ill health that parallels and even appears to exceed that of Native people elsewhere in Canada. To decrease the hazards associated with being born Native in Labrador today, major improvements in environmental and socioeconomic conditions are needed. Not only must there be more meaningful input by indigenous people in the delivery of their health services but they must also be assisted in achieving real control over the decisions which affect their lives, their land, their culture, and their health.

REFERENCES

1. Schaefer O. The changing pattern of neoplastic disease in Canadian Eskimos. Canad Med Assoc J 1975; 112:1399.
2. Schaefer O, Eaton RDP, Timmermans FJW, Hildes JA. Respiratory functions: impairment and cardio pulmonary consequences in long term residents of the Canadian Arctic. Canad Med Assoc J 123:997-1004.

Kathryn A. Wotton
AMREF
Box 30125
Nairobi
Kenya

"COUNTRY FOOD" USE IN MAKKOVIK, LABRADOR JULY 1980 TO JUNE 1981

MARY G. ALTON MACKEY and ROBIN D. ORR

INTRODUCTION

For generations the people of the Labrador coast have relied upon the harvesting of wildlife on the land and in the sea for much of their food supply. Each season brings a variety of animal species to the region, to feed, breed, or rest while on migration, and the people orient their hunting activities and consumption of game to these seasonal changes. Community economies, in the present as in the past, are marked by the relative abundance or scarcity of game. While imported foodstuffs have recently become more available in coastal communities, access to "country food" or "wild food" (the term residents use for game which they obtain themselves) continues to be important not only to the economy but also to the health and social well-being of families.

Although Labrador residents have traditionally harvested game (including fish and birds) for food, quantitative estimates of the consumption and dietary value of country food have been unavailable.

METHODS

This study was designed to investigate the supply of country food to Makkovik, Labrador during one food cycle from July 2, 1980 to June 30, 1981. It is part of a larger study of imported and country food use in selected coastal Labrador communities. The country food use by household was tabulated weekly on a calendar by the fieldworker in consultation with the representative of the household.

Estimates of the weight of each species (i.e., fish, birds, seal, etc.) harvested for family consumption were recorded in avoirdupois weights, with the exception of birds and rabbits which were occasionally noted by number of animals caught. These numbers were converted to pound values on the basis of figures calculated from data received from officials of the Provincial Department of Wildlife on edible (bone in) weights for different species. In general, household country food records refer to game which was hunted, fished, or gathered (and usually consumed) during the recording week. However, some households reported country food that was harvested in earlier seasons, as they consumed it. Some families reported their consumption of caribou throughout the year, although the most intensive caribou hunts are undertaken in early spring. Household weekly reports were consolidated at the end of the study period and data from all households were coded each week and keypunched for computer analysis.

To ensure the quality and accuracy of data collection, the following measures were instituted. Prior to the research, a special training workshop, including a supervised practicum, was conducted for all survey personnel. Regular household participation in data collection was encouraged by community informational meetings. Each household was visited by the fieldworker and one of the principal investigators or the research assistant; the purpose and methods of the research were carefully outlined and household cooperation invited. Each participating household was visited by the fieldworker to assist in the record-keeping requested for the project. During the study, one of the principal investigators or the research assistant visited the community every six weeks to monitor adherence to recording procedures, to advise and encourage the local fieldworkers, and to spot-check the accuracy of data collected.

The data from this study refer to a one-year food cycle, lasting from July 1980 to June 1981, and reflect the biological, economic, climatic, and social conditions that prevailed during the research period.

RESULTS AND DISCUSSION

Labrador coastal residents concentrate their harvesting activities on species that are most readily available in any season. People prefer to consume game when it is "fresh"--soon after it has been hunted, fished, or gathered--and thus people's diets reflect the seasonal availability of different species on the Labrador coast.

Native and Settler inhabitants of the Labrador coast recognize six seasons in a year: summer, early fall, late fall, winter, early spring, and late spring. Each season is characterized by the availability of certain species of wildlife and by climatic conditions that are important to hunting activities.

Summer (July and August)

Makkovik households depend mainly in summer on their harvests of Atlantic cod, salmon, and arctic char or trout. The volume of Atlantic cod, 2,812 pounds (1,278 kg) was the largest of the three species fished in summer 1980 (Table 1). Fishing prevails over other harvesting activities with fish comprising 85% of the total yield of country food reported in the season. The total fish harvest included 6,181 pounds

Table 1.   Seasonal volumes of species harvested at Makkovik July 2, 1980–June 30, 1981.[1]

	Summer		Early fall		Late fall	
Fish						
Atlantic cod	2,812	(1,278)	2,296	(1,043)	974	(443)
Rock cod	59	(27)	17	(8)	12	(5)
Salmon	1,500	(682)	380	(173)	52	(24)
Char/trout	1,668	(758)	182	(83)	175	(79)
Other[2]	142	(65)	311	(141)	41	(19)
Total fish	6,181	(2,810)	3,185	(1,448)	1,254	(570)
Shellfish	53	(24)	1	--	50	(23)
Seals						
Jar	40	(18)	144	(66)	1,046	(475)
Harp	10	(5)	--	--	79	(36)
Ranger	232	(105)	141	(64)	12	(5)
Other[3]	--	--	9	(4)	46	(21)
Total seals	282	(128)	294	(134)	1,183	(537)
Dolphins/porpoises	316	(144)	174	(79)	--	--
Land mammals						
Caribou	588	(267)	118	(54)	313	(142)
Rabbit	--	--	15	(7)	72	(33)
Other[4]	5	(2)	--	--	--	--
Total land mammals	593	(269)	133	(61)	385	(175)
Birds						
Canada geese	--	--	1,587	(721)	30	(14)
Black duck	69	(31)	144	(66)	803	(365)
Eider duck	15	(7)	884	(402)	2,677	(1,217)
Scoters	76	(35)	471	(214)	36	(16)
Guillemots	--	--	423	(192)	90	(41)
Partridge	--	--	81	(37)	571	(259)
Other[5]	6	(3)	341	(155)	129	(59)
Total birds	166	(76)	3,931	(1,787)	4,336	(1,971)

[1]All data collected in pounds converted to kilograms.
[2]Other fish include herring, capelin, smelt, flounder, mackerel, turbot, halibut, white-fish, redfish, sculpin, and squid.
[3]Other seals include square flipper, ranger, and gray seals.

(2,810 kg) and exceeds the volume of fish harvested in any other season.

Seals, dolphins/porpoise, and birds are also hunted during summer to provide variety in household diets (Table 1). More than half of the total annual catch of ranger seals and dolphins/porpoise was made in July and August, bringing 232 pounds (105 kg) of ranger seal and 316 pounds (144 kg) of dolphin to people's country food larders (Table 1). In addition, 588 pounds (267 kg) of caribou were consumed, although not harvested during summer. Two percent of the total caribou reported was recorded in the summer, a time when it was unlikely that caribou were harvested but may have been gifts. A small amount of shellfish, 53 pounds (24 kg) was also gathered in the summer (Table 1). Shellfish was not a significant food source for Makkovik households.

Early Fall (September and October)

Cod fishing continues into early fall, as long as weather conditions permit, and

Table 1. (Continued)

Winter		Early spring		Late spring		Totals	
132	(60)	77	(35)	10	(4)	6,300	(2,863)
1,980	(900)	1,221	(555)	77	(35)	3,366	(1,530)
83	(38)	49	(22)	201	(91)	2,265	(1,030)
72	(33)	443	(201)	3,687	(1,676)	6,227	(2,830)
55	(25)	4	(2)	152	(69)	705	(321)
2,322	(1,056)	1,794	(815)	4,127	(1,876)	18,863	(8,575)
--	--	12	(6)	24	(11)	140	(64)
3,372	(1,533)	913	(415)	394	(179)	5,909	(2,686)
289	(131)	89	(40)	65	(30)	532	(242)
6	(3)	--	--	76	(34)	467	(211)
8	(4)	--	--	2	(1)	65	(30)
3,675	(1,671)	1,002	(455)	537	(244)	6,973	(3,169)
--	--	5	(2)	--	--	495	(225)
764	(347)	22,283	(10,129)	46	(21)	24,112	(10,960)
55	(25)	2	(1)	--	--	143	(65)
5	(2)	--	--	--	--	10	(4)
824	(374)	22,285	(10,130)	46	(21)	24,265	(11,029)
10	(4)	20	(9)	12	(9)	1,659	(753)
96	(44)	33	(15)	15	(7)	1,160	(523)
299	(136)	240	(109)	57	(26)	4,172	(1,897)
--	--	2	(1)	--	--	585	(265)
--	--	--	--	--	--	513	(233)
2,052	(933)	437	(199)	11	(5)	3,153	(1,433)
5	(2)	15	(7)	--	--	496	(226)
2,462	(1,119)	747	(340)	95	(43)	11,737	(5,336)

[4]Other land mammals include black bear, beaver, porcupine, and lynx.
[5]Other birds include mergansers, goldeneye, harlequin ducks, turr, wigeons, tinkers, bull birds, and wobby (shorebirds).
(Appendix to Table 1 lists species cited.)

harvests are almost as large as those made during summer. The catch of Atlantic cod, 2,295 pounds (1,043 kg), and other fish species produced a total of 3,185 pounds (1,448 kg) of fish for household use (Table 1). While fishing contributes significantly to household resources, the major early fall harvesting activity is the hunting of migratory birds. Several species are abundant but the most important are Canada geese, eider ducks, scoters, guillemots, and black ducks. The harvest of migratory birds in early fall 1980 amounted to 3,931 pounds (1,787 kg) with the volume of Canada geese (1,587 pounds, 721 kg) exceeding the catch of all species. Migratory birds comprise 52%, and fish 42% of the total yield of country food produced in the season. The hunting of migratory birds extends into late fall when the largest seasonal harvests are made.

Other species hunted in early fall are seals, which provide a total of 294 pounds (134 kg), and dolphins, which provide 174 pounds (79 kg), of food for household use. In addition, 118 pounds (54 kg) of caribou

Appendix to Table 1.   List of species cited:

FISH
Atlantic cod   Gadus morhua
Rock cod   Gadus ogac
Salmon   Salmo salar
Arctic char   Salvelinus alpinus
Brook trout   Salvelinus fontinalis
Capelin   Mallotus villosus
Smelt   Osmerus sp.
Herring   Clupea harengus
Sculpin (Family)   Cottidae
Whitefish   Coregonus clupeaformis
Turbot   Reinhardtius hippoglossoides
Redfish   Sebastes sp.
Halibut   Hippoglossus hippoglossus
Flounder (winter)   Pseudopleuronectes americanus
Mackerel   Scomber scombrus
Squid   Illex illecebrosus

SHELLFISH
Shrimp   Pandalus borealis
Scallop   Chlamys islandicus
Clam   Mya arenaria
Mussel   Mytilus edulis

SEALS
Jar (ringed)   Phoca hispida
Harp   Phoca groenlandica
Ranger (harbor)   Phoca vitulina
Gray   Halichoerus grypus
Square flipper (bearded)   Erignathus barbatus
Dolphin (white-beaked)   Lagenorhynchus albirostris
         (white-sided)   Lagenorhynchus acutus

LAND MAMMALS
Caribou   Rangifer tarandus
Black bear   Ursus americanus
Rabbit (arctic hare)   Lepus arcticus
        (snowshoe or varying hare)   Lepus americanus
Beaver   Castor canadensis
Lynx   Lynx
Porcupine   Erethizon dorsatum

BIRDS
Partridge (willow ptarmigan)   Lagopus lagopus
          (rock ptarmigan)   Lagopus mutus
          (spruce grouse)   Canachites canadensis
Canada goose   Branta canadensis
Black duck   Anas rubripes
Eider duck (common)   Somateria mollissima
           (king)   Somateria spectabilis
Scoters (common)   Oidemia nigra
        (white-winged)   Melanitta fusca
        (surf)   Melanitta perspicillata
Guillemot   Cepphus grylle
Turrs (tinkers, murre)
      (thick-billed)   Uria lomvia
      (common)   Uria aalge
      (razorbill)   Alca torda

Appendix to Table 1. (Continued)

Bullbird (dovekie)	*Alle alle*
Goldeneye (common)	*Bucephala clangula*
(Barrow's)	*Bucephala islandica*
Merganser (common)	*Mergus merganser*
(red-breasted)	*Mergus serrator*
(hooded)	*Lophodytes cucullatus*
Teal (blue-winged)	*Anas discors*
(green-winged)	*Anas carolinensis*
Harlequin duck	*Histrionicus histrionicus*
Loon (common)	*Gavia immer*
(wobby, red-throated)	*Gavia stellata*
Oldsquaw	*Clangula hyemalis*
Wigeon (American)	*Anas americana*
Sandpiper (Families)	*Scolopacidae*
	Charadriidae
Snowy owl	*Nyctea scandiaca*

harvested in spring and an incidental catch of 15 pounds (7 kg) of rabbit were consumed.

Late Fall (November and December)

Three species comprise most of the country food harvested by Makkovik residents in late fall: eider ducks, jar seals, and cod (Table 1).

Harvests of migratory birds peak during this season, with a total of 4,336 pounds (1,971 kg) of wildfowl harvested in 1980 (Table 1). Eider ducks contributed 2,677 pounds (1,217 kg), or 61% of the total catch. Seal hunting produced 1,183 pounds (537 kg) of meat of which 1,046 pounds (475 kg), or 88% of the total catch, consisted of jar seals (Table 1). Cod predominated over other species fished in late fall, with 974 pounds (443 kg) of cod harvested in a total yield of 1,254 pounds (570 kg) of all fish species. In addition, 313 pounds (142 kg) of caribou and 71 pounds (32 kg) of rabbit were consumed.

Winter (January, February, and March)

Seal hunting is the major winter harvesting activity at Makkovik. The catch of seals reported in winter 1981, amounting to 3,675 pounds (1,671 kg), exceeds the volume of seals recorded in any other season (Table 1). Jar seals were the main species hunted, contributing 3,372 pounds (1,533 kg) or 91% of the total harvest.

Fishing for rock cod is also an important winter activity: 1,980 pounds (900 kg) of rock cod were produced in a harvest of 2,322 pounds (1,056 kg) of all fish species. Some migratory birds are hunted, particularly eider ducks, but the main bird harvested in winter is partridge. The volume of partridge caught in winter is the largest harvest of the year. In 1981, 2,052 pounds

(933 kg) of partridge were reported from a total yield of 2,462 pounds (1,119 kg) of birds. Some caribou (764 pounds, 347 kg) and rabbit (55 pounds, 25 kg) were also consumed.

Early Spring (April and May)

Most of the caribou meat consumed during the year by Makkovik households is taken in early spring hunts. The total volume of caribou reported by residents during the survey year amounts to 24,112 pounds (10,960 kg), of which 22,283 pounds (10,129 kg) was harvested in early spring (Table 1), and 18,001 pounds (8,182 kg) was hunted in a 3-week period, from April 1 to April 22, 1981. During the last decade Makkovik hunters have taken most of their caribou in the interior barrens north, west, and south of Nain where herds are large and easily accessible.

Other important species harvested in early spring are rock cod, jar seals, partridge, and eider duck. The rock cod harvest amounted to 1,221 pounds (553 kg) of a total volume of 1,794 pounds (815 kg) of all fish species caught in the season. Most of the 1,002 pounds (455 kg) of seal reported consisted of jar seals (913 pounds, 415 kg). Partridge comprised more than half (437 pounds, 199 kg) of the total volume of birds harvested, amounting to 747 pounds (340 kg), but eider ducks (240 pounds, 109 kg) also contributed significantly to household diets.

Late Spring (June)

As ice begins to break up in late spring, arctic char migrate from ponds to the heads of bays. Here they are plentiful and easily fished, and the largest seasonal harvest of the year is taken. In late

Table 2. Features of household production of country food in Makkovik, July 2, 1980-June 30, 1981.

Volume	Income			No. of households	Size of family	
	< $13,000	$13-24,000	≥ $25,000		1-4	≥ 5
< 1,000 lbs	17	15	5	37	27	10
≥ 1,000 lbs.	4	18	4	26	8	18
Total	21	33	9	63	35	28

spring 1981, the catch of arctic char amounted to 3,687 pounds (1,676 kg) with a total harvest of 4,127 pounds (1,876 kg) of all species of fish (Table 1).

Char fishing is the main harvesting activity in late spring but other wildlife species are also sought. Seal hunting contributed 537 pounds (244 kg) of meat, most of which consisted of jar seals (394 pounds, 179 kg), to household resources. Occasional catches of various migratory birds were also made and a small volume of caribou, 46 pounds (21 kg), was consumed (Table 1).

Household Production of Country Food

Harvests of 1,000 pounds or more (455 kg or more) of country food were made by 26 households in the community (41% of 63 participating households). Of these, four households had fully employed heads whose income was $25,000 or greater (see above); 18 householders were fishermen, plant workers, or fully employed with incomes between $13,000 and $24,000; and four households had incomes less than $13,000 from fishing, work at the fish plant, or part-time employment.

Most of the 26 households that produced 1,000 pounds or more of country food during the study year contained five or more people: 18 households had from five to ten residents and eight households had three to four residents. While the majority of the 37 households that produced less than 1,000 pounds (455 kg) of country food during the study year had from one to four residents, 10 households contained five or more people: three households had five residents, two households had six, seven, and eight residents each, and one household had nine residents. These 10 households that produced the lowest volumes of country food and had large families did not necessarily have the lowest incomes in the community; five had incomes of $12,000 or less a year, four earned between $13,000 and $24,000, and one had an income higher than $25,000. The other 27 of the 37 households that produced less than 1,000 pounds (455 kg) of country food during the study year were almost equally distributed in earning incomes of $12,000 or less (12 households), and $13,000 to $24,000 (11 households); four households earned incomes of $25,000 or more (Table 2).

The per capita consumption of country food in the 26 households with large harvests, and large families, was almost twice the rate of the 37 households with small harvests, and small families: 269 pounds (112 kg) per capita as compared to 141 pounds (64 kg) per capita, respectively (Table 3).

Table 3. Volume and per capita rates of household production of country food in Makkovik, July 2, 1980-June 30, 1981.

Volume	No. of households	Population	Total harvest	Per capita consumption
< 1,000 lbs	37	138	19,495	141
≥ 1,000 lbs or more	26	160	42,978	269
Total	63	298	62,473	

Table 4. Per capita consumption rates of country food in participating households at Makkovik, July 2, 1980–June 30, 1981.

Lbs. per capita	No. of households	No. of individuals in households
≤ 50	5	22
50–99	8	33
100–149	9	59
150–199	6	32
200–258	13	59
259–299	6	28
300–349	3	19
359–399	3	11
400–499	4	16
450–449	4	11
≥500	2	16
	63	296

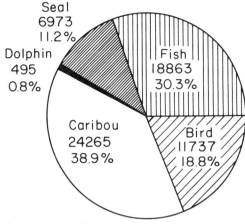

Figure 1. Food consumption in Makkovik, Labrador over one annual cycle. Values given for each major harvested species group are in pounds.

Per Capita Consumption of Country Food

The average per capita consumption of country food, based on the total community harvest and population, is 210 pounds (95 kg); however, this average rate increases to 225 pounds (102 kg) when the relation between the number of people in a household and the volume of country food produced by that household is calculated.

Statistics Canada figures in 1980–81 indicate a national per capita consumption rate of 258 pounds (117 kg) for meat, poultry, and fish (1). Table 4 shows the range of per capita consumption of country food among participating households in the study.

People in 13 Makkovik households representing 20% of the population in participating households consumed a volume of country meat, fish, and birds close to the national average, from 200–258 pounds (91–117 kg), members of 22 households, representing 31% of the population consumed a higher per capita rate than the national average; and people in 28 households representing 49% of the population had a lower per capita consumption rate than the national per capita average consumption of all meat, fish, and poultry. Five households with 7% of the population had a per capita rate of less than 50 pounds (23 kg). The highest per capita consumption of country food, over 500 pounds (227 kg), occurred in two households. Thus members of slightly more than half of the households participating in the study had a per capita consump-

tion rate of country food that was the level of, or higher than, the national average while less than half of the households in the community had lower per capita consumption rates.

SUMMARY

During the study year from July 1980 to June 1981, Makkovik households harvested a total of 62,473 pounds (28,397 kg) of country mammals, fish, and birds and 1,831 pounds (832 kg) of berries from their environment. Caribou contributed the largest volume of country food, 24,112 pounds (10,960 kg). Fish harvests amounted to 18,863 pounds (8,574 kg) and wildfowl harvests amounted to 11,737 pounds (5,335 kg). The volume of seals harvested during the study year was 6,973 pounds (3,170 kg) (Figure 1). This volume appears to be an underestimate of the expected level of harvest by the community. Other marine mammals such as dolphin and other land mammals such as rabbit did not contribute significantly to the local economy during the study year.

Forty-one percent of participating households harvest 1,000 or more pounds (455 or more kg). These households represented 54% of the population and provided two-thirds of the total volume of country food harvest.

Residents in 35 of the 63 households representing 51% of the population consumed a per capita volume of country meat, fish, and birds close to or above the national average for meat, fish, and poultry. Five households with 7% of the population harvested less than 50 pounds (23 kg) per person and two households harvested over 500 pounds (227 kg) per capita.

The data reported in this study record one country food cycle, July 1980-June 1981, only. Because of both the short-term and long-term variations in the availability of many boreal and arctic species, general inferences from the recorded information are risky. Hunting and gathering of food are important for most families' in Makkovik. Their society had a central hunting tradition and food preferences and habits are important to their cultural heritage. Food is an integral part of a way of life in Makkovik and foods have meaning which not only relates to their eating but to the procurement, distribution, and preparation as well.

REFERENCES

1. Statistics Canada: Apparent per capita food consumption in Canada. Cat. No. 32-226, 1982.

Mary G. Alton Mackey
School of Food Science
Box 285
Macdonald College of McGill University
21,111 Lakeshore Rd.
Ste-Anne de Bellevue, Quebec H9X 1C0
Canada

REGIONAL VARIATION IN MORTALITY FROM INFECTIOUS DISEASE IN GREENLAND

PETER BJERREGAARD

INTRODUCTION

An association has been shown to exist between low socioeconomic status and a high level of disease in arctic communities (1-3). Unpublished data from Upernavik, Northwest Greenland, suggest that the association is especially pronounced with infectious diseases, and diseases leading to admission to hospital. The purpose of the present study was to investigate whether the demonstration of this association could be extended to the whole of Greenland.

Mortality due to infectious diseases in the Inuit population of the 16 public health districts in Greenland was compared with socioeconomic conditions. These comprised housing density, measured as available room per person, and income.

MATERIAL AND METHODS

The investigation was based on official statistics of the Chief Medical Officer in Greenland, the Ministry for Greenland, the Danish National Board of Health, and the Central Bureau of Statistics.

The official term "persons born in Greenland" was replaced by "Inuit," and persons born outside Greenland were called Danes.

Although information on causes of death does not distinguish between Inuit and Danes, 95% of deaths occurred in Inuit, and approximate mortality rates of Inuit were calculated with all deaths as numerator and the Inuit population as denominator. Information on socioeconomic variables comprised Inuit only.

The chi-square test was used for statistical evaluation. Ammassalik was considered atypical and has been excluded from the statistical calculations and the calculations of 4 values.

RESULTS

From 1971 to 1980, 3,210 deaths were recorded in Greenland. The cause of death was infectious disease in 529 cases (16%). There was no difference in mortality rate due to infectious diseases between the first and second half of the period. Table 1 shows the distribution on specific causes.

The districts of Greenland can be grouped according to a number of socioeconomic variables; average housing density and income were considered variables of major importance.

The public health districts of Greenland were divided in three groups according to housing conditions of the Inuit popula-

Table 1. Deaths due to infectious diseases. Greenland 1971-80.

International classification. List B.	Number	%
B 32 Pneumonia	226	43
B 33 Bronchitis, emphysema pulmonum, and asthma	115	22
B 31 Influenza	57	11
B 05-06 Tuberculosis	50	10
B 11, 24 Meningitis and (meningococcal infection)	24	5
B 04 Enteritis	11	2
B 14 Morbilli	6	1
Rest of B 01-18	40	8
Total	529	102

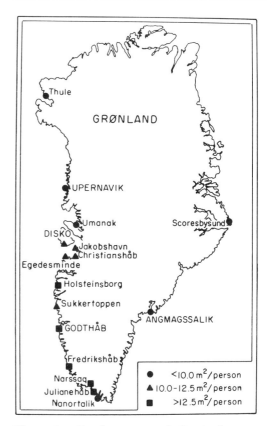

Figure 1. Housing space of the Inuit population of Greenland, averages for 1970 and 1976. Reproduced with the permission of Geodaetisk Institut (A.262/84).

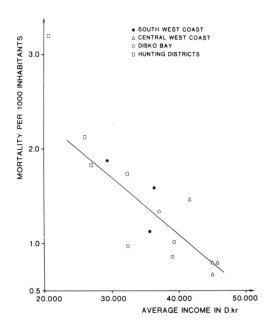

Figure 2. Housing density and mortality due to infectious diseases in public health districts of Greenland Inuit, 1971-80.

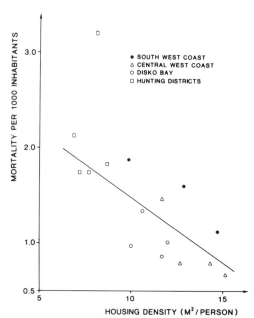
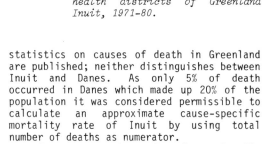

Figure 3. Income and mortality due to infectious diseases in public health districts of Greenland Inuit, 1971-80.

tion (Figure 1). The average space per inhabitant ranged from 8 to 17 m² (1976); for comparison it should be noted that the average for Denmark was 43 m² (1980). The districts on the middle West Coast (the so-called districts of open water) together with two districts of South Greenland had the best housing conditions. Districts of Disko Bay had intermediate housing conditions, and the hunting districts had the poorest housing conditions.

Mortality due to infectious diseases varied between 0.66 in Nuuk (Godthåb) and 2.12 in Upernavik with Ammassalik having an extreme mortality of 3.20. A linear association (r = -0.78) existed between housing density and mortality due to infectious diseases (Figure 2). In districts with less than 10.0 m² housing space was 0.94; a ratio of 2.0 (p < 0.0005).

A linear association (r = -0.83) also existed between average income and mortality due to infectious diseases (Figure 3).

DISCUSSION

This investigation was based on official statistics the validity of which could not be controlled. Two slightly differing statistics on causes of death in Greenland are published; neither distinguishes between Inuit and Danes. As only 5% of death occurred in Danes which made up 20% of the population it was considered permissible to calculate an approximate cause-specific mortality rate of Inuit by using total number of deaths as numerator.

Autopsy was only performed occasionally and many deaths occurred without previous treatment by a medical officer. The reliability of the registered causes of death is therefore reduced.

Conditions of life are different in towns and settlements of Greenland. As causes of death were not published separately for towns and settlements the influence of these differences on the mortality rate could not be examined.

Regional differences of health similar to those of the present study have been found with hepatitis B (4) and infant mortality (5), but could not be demonstrated for registered cases of respiratory infections (6).

An investigation based on the original death certificates, parish registers, and other sources is in progress to overcome the obvious limitations of official statistics.

REFERENCES

1. Berg O, Adler-Nissen J. Housing and sickness in South Greenland: A socio-medical investigation. In: Shephard RJ, Itoh S eds. Proceedings of the Third International Symposium on Circumpolar Health. Toronto: University of Toronto Press, 1976:627-635.
2. Bjerregaard P. Housing standards, social group, and respiratory infections in children of Upernavik, Greenland. Scand J Soc Med 1983; 11:107-111.
3. Hobart CW. Socio-economic correlates of mortality and morbidity among Inuit infants. In: Shephard RJ, Itoh S eds. Proceedings of the Third International Symposium on Circumpolar Health. Toronto: University of Toronto Press, 1976:452-461.

4. Skinhøj P, McNair A, Andersen ST. Hepatitis and hepatitis B - antigen in Greenland. Amer J Epidemiol 1974; 99:50-57.
5. Jørgensen P, Møller J, Zachau-Christiansen B. Live born in Greenland, birth weight, neonatal and infant mortality during 1975-1979. In: Harvald B, Hart Hansen JP, eds. Circumpolar Health 81. Nordic Council Arct Med Res Rep 1982; 33:166-168.
6. The State of Health in Greenland. Annual report from the Chief Medical Officer in Greenland. Godthåb.

Peter Bjerregaard
Department of Epidemiology
State Serum Institute
Amager Boulevard 80
DK-2300, Copenhagen S
Denmark

Circumpolar Health 84:154-158

CAUSES OF DEATH, AGE OF DEATH, AND CHANGES IN MORTALITY IN THE TWENTIETH CENTURY IN AMMASSALIK (EAST GREENLAND)

JOËLLE ROBERT-LAMBLIN

INTRODUCTION

Ammassalik's population was made known to Europeans one century ago (1884) by the Dane Gustav Holm. Due to the difficult access to this region, this small group of 413 Eskimos had remained isolated and untouched by European colonization. Subsequently, the principal stages of Danish colonization having direct relationship to health improvement for the east coast of Greenland, are:

- 1894: first settlement of a trading post and administration
- 1906: first Greenlandic midwife
- 1932: first Danish nurse
- 1944: first permanent Danish physician and small hospital

Since the beginning of colonization in 1894 the Ammassalimiut population has gone through an exceptional demographic expansion, reaching up to 3 or 4% annual rate of growth; this demographic explosion was due both to a lowering of the death rate and a rise in birth rate.

A detailed study of mortality, through its causes and fluctuations, is particularly interesting as a means to understand this small society's adaptation to a severe environment and to measure the importance of changes brought on by Western culture since its first impact on this region.

METHODS

I was able to analyze abundant and accurate demographic data, within its own sociological and economic context, observed during lengthy anthropological field work. Demographic data were collected from parish registers, from administrative and medical documents, in archives of the Centre de Recherches Anthropologiques (directed by Prof. R. Gessain, Musée de l'Homme, Paris) and through personal inquiries during field work. For the more detailed analysis of mortality according to sex, age, season, and causes of deaths, I chose to start with 1917, because from then on a more complete

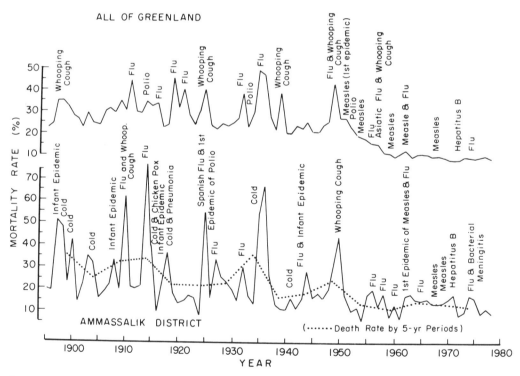

Figure 1. Epidemics and mortality: Greenlandic population, throughout the country and in Ammassalik district (.... death rate by five-year periods).

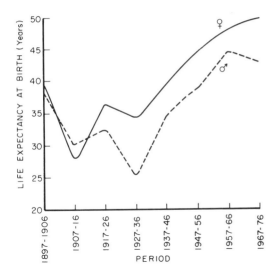

Figure 2. *Evolution of life expectancy (at birth) in Ammassalimiut population.*

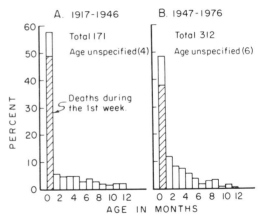

Figure 3. *Distribution (in percentage) of infant deaths according to age at death in Ammassalimiut population. A. 1917-1946 (total = 171 infant deaths, 4 age unspecified). B. 1947-1976 (total = 312 infant deaths, 6 age unspecified).*

and reliable recording of mortality is available.

Anthropological field work conducted in this region between 1967 and 1979 allowed me to follow transformations within the Ammassalimiut ethnic group, in material life as well as in social, religious, and economic activities (1). These more recent observations were added to all past records obtained from visitors, administrators, or scientific researchers, such as G. Holm, K. Rasmussen, W. Thalbitzer, J. Petersen, E. Mikkelsen, A. Høygaard, and R. Gessain.

RESULTS AND DISCUSSION

Evolution of Death Rate

One of the most striking effects of Danish colonization on the Ammassalimiut population appears to be the sizeable reduction in death rate. The disappearance of famines, improved conditions of hygiene, and the development of medical assistance lowered the death rate from more than 30 per 1,000 at the end of last century to 20 per 1,000 in the middle of the 1900s; today it is around 11 per 1,000. However, the decrease in death rate has by no means been regular. Before the 1950s, the annual rate oscillated between 8 and 77 per 1,000 (Figure 1). Severe epidemics of the common cold, influenza, whooping cough, measles, poliomyelitis, chickenpox, etc. gave periods of very high mortality, for a few years the number of deaths being higher than the number of births (as in 1910, 1915 and 1936). Thus, starting with a high rate such as found in developing countries, mortality

in this region is now closer to the European average. One must, however, keep in mind that the East Greenlandic population has a particular age structure (almost 50% being below the age of 15) and that despite a sizeable decrease in death rate, life expectancy in this population remains far from that of contemporary Western populations (Figure 2).

Infant Mortality

The decrease in infant mortality has been most spectacular (Table 1); it started at the beginning of the century, even before the presence of a permanent nurse, or a Danish doctor. It was essentially due to improved hygiene during delivery and post-natal care, thanks to an innovation: the presence of one, then several, Greenlandic midwives trained in Western Greenland or Denmark.

In the past the women of Ammassalik gave birth alone or were helped by an older woman of the family, with an almost total lack of hygiene. The cord was usually cut with a mussel shell, and to help cicatrization the newborn's umbilicus was covered with a poultice of fresh seal fat. In case of a long and difficult delivery, the older woman assistant would help by inserting her hands rubbed with seal oil. In such conditions, it is easy to understand the magnitude of risks which faced mother and child during and after childbirth.

At the beginning of the century, more than one Ammassalimiut child out of four died before one year of age; in 1962-66 the rate had dropped to 1 out of 7, and in

Table 1.   *Evolution of infant mortality rate in the Ammassalimiut population. Total 1897-1976:   4,214 births; 577 infant deaths.*

Years	Rate per 1,000	Years	Rate per 1,000
1897-1901	284	1937-41	70
1902-06	225	1942-46	157
1907-11	143	1947-51	181
1912-16	128	1952-56	120
1917-21	123	1957-61	114
1922-26	146	1962-66	146
1927-31	140	1967-71	109
1932-36	192	1972-76	84

1972-76, to 1 out of 12. In more recent times, the effort of health authorities to reduce infant mortality has been particularly oriented towards vaccinations, distribution of powdered milk to pregnant women and nursing mothers (since 1945), development of prenatal care, and encouragement to give birth in the hospital. Nevertheless, infant mortality--although showing an important decrease from 300 per 1,000 at the end of the last century to 84 per 1,000 in 1972-76--still remains twice as high as that for the whole population of Greenland, and much higher than rates for European countries.

Figure 3 clearly shows that the decisive period for a young Ammassalimiut is the first month of life, since about half of the infant deaths occur during that month. By dividing the period between 1917 and 1976 into two parts, before and after the arrival of the first permanent physician in 1947, we notice a sizeable decrease in infant mortality during the first month for the second period (this decrease being particularly noticeable for the first week of life) and we can observe for the same period an increased mortality between 2 and 6 months. These infant deaths should be attributed to a deteriorating social environment. The disappearance of the traditional anorak (amaut) allowing the mother to carry the child with her during outside activities, the disintegration of patriarchal families, and alcohol abuse entailing a deterioration of family life, led to the loss of familial surroundings providing effective security and supervision for the infants.

The most frequent causes of infant mortality today are congenital malformations and prematurity (from 1967 to 1976, in the Ammassalik district, 1 infant death out of 3 happened during birth or during the first day of life), lung disorders, diarrhea, and smothering in bed. A greater fragility can

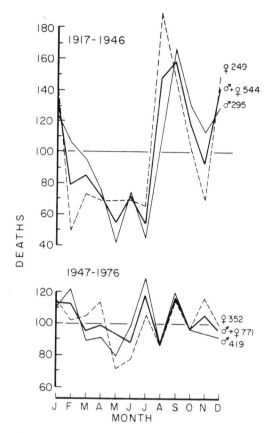

Figure 4. *Seasonal variations in mortality among the Ammassalimiut population, in 1917-1946 and 1947-1976.*

be noted for the males since for the whole period 1917 to 1976, there were 113 male infant deaths per 100 female infant deaths. For the same period, the sex ratio at birth was 102 males per 100 females.

Seasons and Mortality

If we consider mortality throughout the different periods of the year, it appears that an important change occurred between the two main periods covering 1917-1946 and 1947-1976 (Figure 4). During the first period, the population had remained more traditional in its lifestyle; the post-war second period corresponds to a time of greater acculturation.

In the more traditional period, mortality showed contrasting fluctuations: December and January and more particularly August and September were at that time periods of high mortality. April to July, in contrast, showed the lowest death rate. Two factors can explain these fluctuations: the calendar for hunting, fishing and gathering, and

Table 2. Causes of death among the Ammassalimiut in 1897-1916 and 1959-1978.

Mortality	1897-1916		1959-1978					
	No. of deaths	%	Males		Females		Total	
			No. of deaths	%	No. of deaths	%	No. of deaths	%
Infant mortality	95	30.5	111	37.0	78	32.5	189	35.0
Mortality beyond 1 year:								
Disease	166	53.4	89	29.7	115	47.9	204	37.8
Accident	35	11.3	64	21.3	25	10.4	89	16.5
Homicide, suicide	6	1.9	16	5.3	7	2.9	23	4.3
Old age	5	1.6	4	1.3			4	0.7
Unknown cause	4	1.3	16	5.3	15	6.3	31	5.7
Total	311	100	300	100	240	100	540	100

contacts between this isolated population and outsiders. During the favorable period for hunting and gathering (between April and July), the population's nutritional state was generally good. On the contrary, during the months of December and January when hunting was difficult and gathering almost nil, food could be very scarce if the reserves put aside during the summer were insufficient. The peak of August and September was essentially due to contacts with Westerners, through ships' crews visiting the area, most often bringing diseases developing into lethal epidemics.

The more recent period, 1947-1976, shows a totally different yearly distribution of deaths, indicating that the population is less dependent on hunting and fishing resources, food supplies such as canned goods and groceries being available at all times of the year in small shops throughout the district. On the other hand, diseases brought on by foreigners are either better tolerated by the population, or better attended.

Age at Death

After one year, the risk of dying very young decreases. For this part of the world, childhood after that age is not a difficult period, unlike other regions such as Africa.

Figure 2 shows the evolution of life expectancy during the 20th century, emphasizing the very important repercussions of epidemics at the beginning of the century. It is striking, however, that for the most recent period under study, life expectancy remains low, despite the development of medical assistance, which played an important part in prevention (through vaccination) and brought on better means to fight diseases, such as penicillin and other antibiotics. Today, medical assistance is quite remarkable; for this population of less than 2,500 Greenlanders and 200 Danes, the public health service has a staff of around 60, including two doctors, one dentist, several Danish and Greenlandic nurses, and Greenlandic midwives or midwife-helpers in each village. Medical treatment and transportation to the district hospital or outside (by boat, helicopter, or plane) are totally free of charge.

Despite all these efforts, the chances of reaching old age in that region are still low and even in 1976, only 3% of the local population was over 60. One is led to conclude that climatic, social, and economic factors are opposed to a real increase in life expectancy in Ammassalik. The continuing high infant mortality, numerous violent deaths, a low average standard of living, a poor nutritional state despite the disappearance of famines, and alcohol abuse are all major obstacles to such an increase. For the period 1967-1976, the figures for life expectancy at birth among Ammassalik's population were 42.8 years for males and 48.7 for females, and at one year 47.7 for males and 51.7 for females. These rates were close to those found for certain areas of Alaska, but they remained much lower than those for Greenland's west coast. This shows that there is still a marked difference in the standard of living and development between East and West Greenland, differences which could decrease in forth-coming years.

Causes of Death

This little isolated group lacked immunity to infectious agents previously unknown to them and Figure 1 shows how great were the damages brought on by diseases introduced from the outside world. The worst epidemics were whooping cough and influenza in 1910, influenza in 1914-15, Spanish influenza and poliomyelitis in 1925, the common cold, degenerating in broncho-pneumonia in 1935-36, and whooping cough in 1949-50. Since 1950 epidemics have not been as lethal; for example, the first measles epidemic in Ammassalik, in 1962, affected 1,804 persons out of a total of 2,110 (Greenlanders and Danes), but caused only 12 deaths.

Pulmonary tuberculosis was an important cause of death from the late 1930s and up to the 1960s, when it decreased drastically after an intensive public health campaign.

Since epidemics and tuberculosis are under control, mortality from violence and accidents has become very important (Table 2). The harshness of the arctic climate is the cause of very specific risks; for example, the sea choked with ice and danger-ous for navigation, the ice pack giving way under the weight of man or sledge, snow storms or wind storms at sea catching up with hunters away from the village, risks of avalanche, and very low temperature of the sea causing hypothermia in case of falling in. Men are most exposed to these dangers since they must leave the village to hunt or to fish. The most frequent accidents are due to the dangers of navigation.

The other victims of environmental risk factors are children and teenagers who are left very free in their games and activi-ties. They are also exposed to guns acci-dentally fired, ingestion of toxic sub-stances, or to fires due to playing with matches.

In the 1960s a new cause of mortality has appeared and is becoming increasingly important: that is, violent deaths due to alcohol abuse, such as unintentional homi-cides, drowning or freezing to death of drunken individuals, or suicides of teenag-ers and young adults in the depressive phase of alcoholic intoxication.

The suicide rate has been sharply increasing since the 1960s: from 19.7/100,000 in 1961-65, to 27.0/100,000 in 1966-70, to 52.7 in 1971-75, and finally to 124.9/100,000 in 1976-80. For this last period, suicides represent 11.4% of all deaths. Male suicide rates are four times higher than those of females, the age group most affected, for both sexes, being 20-24.

This dramatic rise of alcohol abuse leading to situations of open conflict and violent actions, and this growing tendency to self-destruction in young adults is the sign of a deep psychological and social perturbation among the Ammassalimiut in recent times.

SUMMARY

The study of mortality and its evolu-tion through time are good markers for the level of physical and mental health of a given population.

In Ammassalik, social and economic changes appear clearly through these demo-graphic phenomena, and with positive and negative aspects. Beneficial aspects of westernization can be seen in the suppres-sion of famines, in improved hygiene, in the remarkable development of medical assistance and social welfare for the needy and elder-ly. On the negative side one can note the introduction of contagious diseases with fatal consequences and the appearance and increase of social and psychological prob-lems which are seriously disturbing today's Greenlandic society.

REFERENCES

1. Robert-Lamblin J. Ammassalik (Groen-land oriental), fin ou persistance d'un isolat? Etude anthropodémographique du changement. Thèse de Doctorat d'Etat. Paris-Sorbonne, 1983:1-513.

Joëlle Robert-Lamblin
Laboratoire d'Anthropologie
Musée de l'Homme
Place du Trocadéro
75116 Paris
France

Circumpolar Health 84:159-161

TRENDS IN GREENLANDIC INUIT TEENAGER PREGNANCY RATES

PEDER KERN HANSEN and SØREN FRIIS SMITH

Teenage pregnancy constitutes a special social, psychological, and obstetric group at risk (1,2,3); moreover, subarctic (4) and Inuit teenagers (5) have posed particular obstetrical problems. In most industrialized countries, family planning and modern contraceptives have reduced the general fertility, including age-specific teenage fertility (2,6). A decline in teenage fertility has been reported from other subarctic areas during the last decade (7). We have found it valuable to study the trends of fertility in Greenland Inuit, as these data will create an important baseline for intervention and further investigations.

SOURCES AND METHODS

Figures and calculations are based on data from the Office of the Chief Medical Officer in Greenland (8), the Ministry of Greenland (9,10), the Danish Central Bureau of Statistics (11), and the Nordic Statistical Secretariat (12).

In the statistical analysis the chi-square test was used, with a level of significance of 0.05.

RESULTS

The increase in fertility rate from 1948 until the mid-1960's took place in all age groups. The dramatic decrease in general fertility rate began some years ago and was more pronounced than the decrease in teenage fertility rate (Figure 1). From 1960 to 1970 and from 1970 to 1980, teenage fertility was reduced by 9 per 100, to 32 per 100, and the general fertility by 44 per 100, to 34 per 100. Concomitantly the proportion of children of teenage mothers

INCIDENCE OF TEEN-AGE MOTHERS / 100 LIVEBORNS

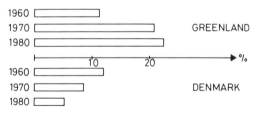

Figure 2. Proportion of liveborn children of teenage mothers compared to all liveborns.

increased from 11.3 per 100, to 22.1 per 100 of all live born from 1960 to 1970. The increment is statistically significant from 1960 to 1970 but not from 1970 to 1980 (Figure 2). During the same intervals, the Danish teenage proportion of children decreased significantly from 12 to 5 per 100 live born.

The number of legal abortions increased steadily since 1966 and in 1982 32% of all pregnancies were terminated by abortion (Figure 3). From 1978 to 1982 the number of legal teenage abortions increased significantly compared to the total number of teenagers (Figure 4) and constituted in 1982 42% of all pregnancies in this age group. However, the proportion of teenage pregnancies terminated by abortion decreased slightly but insignificantly from 45 per 100 in 1978 to 42 per 100 pregnancies (spontaneous abortions omitted) in 1982. In contrast to Greenland, the rate of the teenage abortions in Denmark declined significantly from 24.3 per 1,000 in 1978 to 18.2 in 1982.

DISCUSSION

The Greenlandic population was stable in the 19th century, with only a minor population increase from 1850 to 1900 (13). The fertility rate of teenagers in the first part of this century was, according to Bertelsen (14), 325 per 1,000 married women and only 3 per 1,000 unmarried (14). Bertelsen in another report argued that premarital coitus was not uncommon and the resulting children were accepted in society. This seems in contradiction with the low fertility rate of unmarried teenagers, which could be caused by under-registration. However, the teenage fertility rate at the beginning of more exact registration in 1948 was also rather low. Nevertheless, Greenlandic politicians in 1951 discussed the problems of young, unmarried mothers who gave away their children (16).

THE GENERAL AND THE TEEN-AGE FERTILITY OF GREENLANDERS
1948-1982

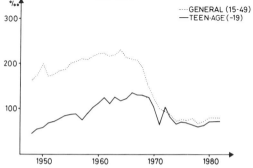

Figure 1. Liveborn children per 1,000 women in the age groups 15-19 and 15-49.

NUMBER OF ABORTIONS IN GREENLAND
1966-1982

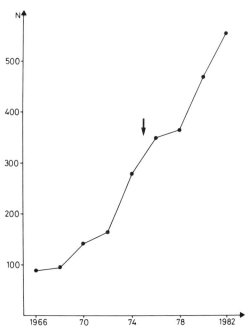

Figure 3. Abortions in Greenland 1966-1982. Arrow indicates legalization of abortions (1975).

Natural fertility, trends in birth rates in the 1950s and 1960s, and the later decline of fertility in the course of economic development and modernization have been thoroughly scrutinized by H. O. Hansen (13). The remarkable decline in birth rates at the end of the 1960s was facilitated by the introduction of modern reliable contraceptives in 1966-67 (8,17). As seen from Figure 1, teenagers obviously did not readily use the effective contraceptives or were not encouraged to use them, as the teenage fertility rate declined later and to a less pronounced degree than did the general fertility rate. The increasingly larger proportion of teenage mothers (Figure 2) is mostly due to the reduced fertility of the other age groups.

Maternal and child health is elsewhere promoted by reduction in teenage fertility rate (2). Yet there are no investigations nor are there social or obstetrical statistics concerning the problem in Greenland. An earlier report could not identify teenagers as an obstetrical high risk group (18). The impressively high teenage fertility rate requires further investigation, however, since general problems of teenage motherhood (1) also are most likely to be encountered in Greenland.

In light of the recent increasing teenage fertility rate in Greenland, the Danish decline may be explained partly by cultural differences and partly by the long-standing Danish tradition of sex education (6). Fifteen years ago, sex education was found to be very poor in Greenland (19) and the increased number of abortions probably reflects that it still is. The necessity for sex education in the schools and health facilities in Greenland has been urged before (20), but the abortion rate is still extreme and the nearly exponential growth of the total amount of abortions (Figure 3) calls for increased efforts in public family planning.

CONCLUSIONS

In the course of economic development, the birth rate of Greenland declined, facilitated by the introduction of modern contraceptives. The teenage fertility rate was not reduced at the same rate, has increased, and is high compared to other countries. Since the abortion rate is also increased, it is found necessary to improve family planning policies and sex education, especially among the very young. More sophisticated prophylactic strategies must await research on determinants concerning teenage pregnancy and childbirth among Greenlandic Inuit teenagers.

ACKNOWLEDGMENT

This study was supported by the Commission for Scientific Research in Greenland.

LEGAL TEEN-AGE ABORTIONS 1978-1982

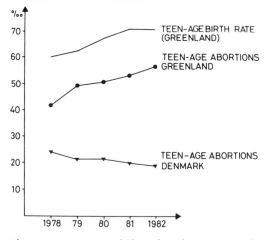

Figure 4. Age-specific abortion rates in Greenland, Denmark, and Iceland 1978-82. For comparison is inserted the teenage-specific fertility rate in Greenland.

REFERENCES

1. Phipps-Jonas S. Teenage pregnancy and motherhood: A review of the literature. Amer J Orthopsychiat 1980; 50:403-431.
2. Maine D. Family planning: Its impact on the health of women and children. The center for population and family health. New York: Columbia Univ, 1981.
3. Smith SF. Biological and social characteristics of pregnant girls aged 14-19 years. Ugeskr Laeger 1982; 144:1412-1416.
4. Johnson MA, Owers J, Horwood SP. The pregnant teenager in the subarctic. In: Harvald B, Hart Hansen JP, eds. Circumpolar health 81. Nordic Council Arct Med Res Rep 1982; 33:338-342.
5. Murdock AI. Factors associated with high-risk pregnancies in Canadian Inuit. Canad Med Assoc J 1979; 120:291-294.
6. Kozakiewicz M. Highlights on changes in adolescent behaviour as observed by the Europe regional social science group 1980 for a broad, complex approach to adolescent sexuality. In: Adolescent sexuality. The Danish Family Planning Association. Copenhagen, 1983:9-19.
7. Maltau JM, Grünfeld B. The fertility decline in Finnmark and Troms counties during the period 1970-1981. Nordic Council Arct Med Res Rep 1983; 36:7-9.
8. The state of health in Greenland. Annual report from the chief medical officer in Greenland for the year (1965-1982). Godthåb, 1965-1982.
9. Den grønlandske befolknings fødselshyppighed. Meddelelser fra statistisk afdeling 3. Ministeriet for Grønland. Copenhagen, 1961.
10. Grønland. Annual report on Greenland from 1968. Ministry of Greenland.
11. Statistisk årbog. (Statistical Yearbook) Annual. Central Bureau of Statistics. Copenhagen.
12. Yearbook of Nordic Statistics. Annual. Nordic Council. Stockholm.
13. Hansen HO. From natural to controlled fertility: Studies in fertility as a factor in the process of economic and social development in Greenland c. 1851-1975. In: Leridon H, Menken J eds. Natural fertility. Liège: IUSSP Ordina Editions, 1979:495-547.
14. Bertelsen A. Grønlandsk medicinsk statistik og nosografi I. (English abstract). Meddelelser om Grønland. 1935; 117:1. Copenhagen.
15. Bertelsen A. Om fødslerne i Grønland og de sexuelle forhold sammensteds. Bibliotek for Laeger 1907; 99:527-572.
16. Ministeriet for Grønland. Beretninger vedrørende Grønland, 1951-2. Copenhagen, 1952; 3:192-193.
17. Berg O. IUDs and the birth rate in Greenland. Stud Fam Plan 1972; 3:12-14.
18. Hansen PK. Decline of perinatal mortality in the district of Godthåb. In: Harvald B, Hart Hansen JP eds. Circumpolar health 81. Nordic Council Arct Med Res Rep 1982; 33:172-175.
19. Olsen GA. Sexual behaviour among the youth of Greenland - sociomedical aspects. Institute for Social Medicine. Publication No 4. Copenhagen, 1974.
20. Misfeldt J. Family planning in medical districts in Greenland. Ugeskr Laeger 1979; 139:1501-1504.

Peder Kern Hansen
Department of Obstetrics and Gynecology
Hvidovre Hospital
DK 2650 Hvidovre
Denmark

Circumpolar Health 84:162-165

INFANT FEEDING PRACTICES ON MANITOBA INDIAN RESERVES

GAIL MARCHESSAULT

INTRODUCTION

In 1981, the Community Task Force on Maternal and Child Health identified Native Indian mothers and children as a high-risk population group (1). Infant feeding practices have an impact on the health of babies, as has been amply demonstrated for the general population. The effect seems to be greater for Native babies.

Schaefer and Spady, commenting on information collected for 1,179 Inuit, Indian, and non-Native children born during 1973-1974 in the Northwest Territories, concluded that "within each ethnic group of all factors examined infant morbidity appeared related most consistently, and often also most significantly, to mode of infant nutrition" (2). After a 5-year health promotion campaign the study was repeated. They reported that the incidence of breast-feeding at 6 months had increased in all three ethnic populations. The average number of days away from home due to illness decreased. Of the Native mothers who selected bottle-feeding, the use of proprietary formulas doubled, there was a delay in solid food supplementation, a decrease in sweet consumption, and an increase in the use of native meat and fish (2). Macauley reported that bottle-fed babies suffered 5 times as many episodes of infectious illnesses in their first year of life as babies who were exclusively breast-fed for 3 months (3). Ellestad-Sayed, studying infants on Manitoba Indian reserves, reported that the fully bottle-fed infants were hospitalized 10 times more often and spent 10 times as many days in hospital during the first year of life as fully breast-fed infants (4). The Manitoba Pediatric Society reported that only 36% and 39% of mothers on Indian reserves were breast-feeding in 1978 and 1979 compared to 62% and 66% in Winnipeg and 55% and 47% in rural Manitoba (5). Although these statistics seem to indicate that the incidence of

breast-feeding in the Indian population differed from that of the general population, the sample size was made up of only 25 and 23 infants, respectively. Myre's national survey done in 1982 gives Manitoba (prairie provinces) an incidence of 76% of mothers breast-feeding at birth, which is higher than the national average of 69.4% (6). An infant feeding practices pilot survey, done in the summer of 1981 on 50 infants from 6 Manitoba Indian reserves, gave an 82% incidence of breast-feeding at birth (7). Mothers were asked whether previously raised children had been breast-fed. Although more mothers were currently breast-feeding, a trend towards the increasing use of a bottle to supplement breast-feeding was observed. This trend may be associated with a quicker demise of breast-feeding. Solid foods were introduced earlier than the recommended 4-6 months for 35% of the babies. Even with only 50 mothers, the percentage of babies with reported illnesses was greatest for bottle-fed babies (55%), middling for the babies who received both breast and bottle (50%), and least for the breast-fed babies (29%).

Forty-two percent of the mothers said that relatives had influenced their decision regarding how to feed their babies, 26% of the mothers indicating that the baby's father had influenced their decision and 25% and 22% of the mothers mentioning the doctor and the nurse as influential in infant feeding decisions.

METHODS AND MATERIALS

A more comprehensive infant feeding practices survey was begun in January of 1982. The survey instrument used was patterned on Dr. Schaefer's questionnaire and was administered by nurses at regular well-baby clinics. The survey was to monitor all babies born on Manitoba Indian reserves during 1982 and follow them until they were 1 year of age. The objectives

Table 1. Distribution of fully breast-fed babies at hospital discharge, and duration of breast-feeding.

	South zone		North zone		Region	
	No.	%	No.	%	No.	%
Yes	146	53	62	62	208	55
No	132	47	38	38	170	45
Mean duration of breast-feeding	6.2 months		5.5 months		6 months	

Table 2. Factors influencing mother's choice to breast-feed.

- Baby's health	104
- Easier/convenient	45
- Cheaper	21
- Advice from others	20
- Wanted to try	10
- Best	9
- Breast-fed other children	8
- Other	15
- No response	59

Table 3. Factors influencing mother's choice not to breast-feed.

- Psycho-social	33
- Maternal/infant factors	32
- Doesn't know	18
- Returning to work/school	17
- Bottle feeding easier	17
- Previous unsuccessful attempts	7
- Other	4
- No response	31

were to document the incidence and duration of breast-feeding, the reasons for choice of infant feeding method, the patterns of formula feeding, the age of introduction of solids, the use of sweets, the use of vitamin and mineral supplements, and the effect of breast-feeding on infant morbidity.

The results presented here are preliminary. Further analysis will be provided by Headquarters, Medical Services Branch, Health and Welfare Canada.

Out of a potential 1,092, 393 (36%) questionnaires were returned. The Manitoba region has 56 reserves, divided into 2 zones. The north zone, which consists of 19 reserves, had a 25% response rate, whereas the south zone, which represents 37 reserves, had a 44% response rate. In total 33, or 59% of Manitoba reserves, participated in the survey. This is not a random sample. The responses are representative of those who participated. The percentages that are reported are calculated upon the number of responses received for each question. Reasons for non-participation were a high staff turnover at the field and supervisory levels, compounded by the 2-year duration of the survey. Other factors were the mobility of families and the refusal of 2 reserves for their band members to participate.

A slight majority of the babies in the sample were male, with the male/female ratio 55/45. Ninety-five percent of the babies were of Indian ethnicity, 4.6% were Métis, and 0.5% were of other backgrounds. There were 5 sets of twins among the respondents.

RESULTS

When asked "Was this baby fully breast-fed at hospital discharge?" 55% of the mothers responded "Yes" and 45% of the mothers responded "No." Slightly more mothers breast-fed initially from the north zone than the south zone. The mean duration of breast-feeding was approximately 6 months--slightly longer in the south zone than in the north zone. This average is based only on the mothers who breast-fed and only until 12 months of age. Some mothers continued to breast-feed past this age (Table 1).

The most common reason given by the mothers for choosing to breast-feed was the baby's health, followed by ease, convenience, and economy. The influence of others was fairly significant, other reasons given being that the mother wanted to try it, that it was best, that the mother had breast-fed other children, for mother's sake, for bonding, and for personal reasons (Table 2).

The most common reasons given for not choosing to breast-feed fell under the category of psychosocial reasons and included responses such as the mother was shy, scared, single, or didn't want to. The "don't know" response might also fall under the psychosocial reasons. Maternal and infant factors included nipple problems, maternal or infant illness, adoption, prematurity, and twins. Returning to work or school, a perception that bottle-feeding was easier, previous unsuccessful attempts to breast-feed, medical advice, and success

Table 4. Breast- and bottle-feeding as a function of infant age.

Age	Exclusively breast-fed %	Breast- and bottle-fed %	Exclusively bottle-fed %
Birth	55	62	39
0.5 months	29	57	44
2 months	23	47	54
4 months	19	37	64
6 months	14	29	70

Table 5. *Factors influencing mother to stop breast-feeding.*

- No milk	32
- Maternal dissatisfaction	23
- Maternal illness	15
- Lifestyle factors	11
- Infant not tolerating breast	9
- Biting	7
- Separation	7
- Others' advice	3
- No response	109

Table 6. *Types of formula used in bottle-feeding.*

- Commercial formula	210
- Evaporated milk formula	205
- Whole milk	32
- Whole milk formula	20
- 2% milk	15
- Skim milk	2
- Other	22

at bottle-feeding other children were other responses given (Table 3).

Among Indian mothers, 62% initiated breast-feeding. The incidence of breast-feeding decreases to 29% by 6 months. The incidence of exclusive breast-feeding drops to 29% by 2 weeks and is only 14% at 6 months (Table 4). This drop is of concern because the mixed-feeders seem to be at higher risk of morbidity than those who are exclusively breast-fed. Lack of milk or baby not being satisfied was the number one reason that mothers gave for discontinuing breast-feeding. This could relate to a lack of information regarding growth spurts. Maternal dissatisfaction included frustration, breast-feeding was too difficult, the mother didn't like it, the mother wished to

leave the baby for longer periods of time, or the mother found breast-feeding to be inconvenient. Lifestyle factors included returning to school or work, another pregnancy, dieting, and birth control. Many of the stated reasons for discontinuing breast-feeding might have been averted with education and support (Table 5).

Evaporated milk formulas were used only slightly less often than commercial formulas. Whole milk was introduced very early and 17 mothers were using 2% or skim milk (Table 6).

Two-thirds of the mothers who were using formula were doing so incorrectly. The responses to this question indicate a receptiveness to teaching, as improvement was noticeable with subsequent visits (Table 7).

Table 7. *Methods for mixing formula.*

	South zone		North zone		Region	
	No.	%	No.	%	No.	%
Correct	51	37	16	28	67	34
Incorrect	87	63	41	72	128	66

Table 8. *Infant age at introduction of solids into diet.*

	South zone %	North zone %	Region %
Birth	0.8		0.7
0.5 months	0.4		0.4
2 months	40.0	9.0	34.0
4 months	31.0	36.0	32.0
6 months	3.5	32.0	26.0
9 months		16.0	6.0
12 months		9.0	1.4
Mean	3.6 months	5.8 months	4.1 months

Table 9. Extras in Manitoba infant diets.

	Sugar water		Pop, Tang Kool-Aid		Chocolate Candy		Tea	
	No.	%	No.	%	No.	%	No.	%
Use	125	45	145	50	152	51	128	45
Non-use	154	55	147	50	145	49	155	55

The mean age of introduction of solids falls within the recommendation of 4 to 6 months in both zones: 3.6 months in the south zone, 5.8 months in the north zone, and 4.1 months for the region. Nevertheless, 35% of the mothers introduced solid foods prior to 4 months and at least 7% of the mothers delayed the introduction of solids until the infant was past 6 months. Some infants receive solids from birth. Others are not receiving solids even at age 1. There is a tendency for solids to be introduced earlier in the south zone and later in the north zone (Table 8).

The reported use of sugar water, pop, Tang and Koolaid, chocolate and candy, and tea was approximately 50% (Table 9). The effect of sweets is well known. The effect of tea is less well known; but, advice for pregnant women is to limit consumption of caffeine-containing beverages. Any need for caution for the prenatal would be increased for the infant.

Analysis of the information collected on morbidity has not yet been completed.

DISCUSSION

Manitoba region is committed to using the results of this survey to influence favorably the health of babies living on reserves. These preliminary results highlight the need to promote, support, and educate breast-feeding mothers past the initiation phase of breast-feeding, to reach relatives and fathers as well as potential mothers, to increase community support and acceptance of breast-feeding exclusively until 4 to 6 months, to educate mothers regarding appropriate commercial milks for the first year and how to make infant formula correctly, to educate mothers regarding when to introduce solids and in what order, and to promote the avoidance of sweets and tea for infants.

ACKNOWLEDGMENTS

I thank the regional and zone nursing officers, Dr. Murdock, Dr. Sevenhuysen, Louise Dilling, and members of the Health Programs Committee for their assistance in designing the questionnaire. I also thank the community health nurses who collected the information.

REFERENCES

1. Community Task Force on Maternal and Child Health. The Manitoba native Indian mother and child. Discussion paper on a high risk population group. 412 McDermot Ave, Winnipeg, Man., 1981.
2. Schaefer O, Spady DW. Changing trends in infant feeding patterns in the Northwest Territories 1973-1979. Northern Medical Research Unit, Medical Services Branch, Health and Welfare Canada.
3. Macaulay AC. Infant feeding and illness on an Indian reservation. Canad Fam Phys 1981; 27:963.
4. Ellestad-Sayed J, Coodin FJ, Dilling LA, Haworth JC. Breast-feeding protects against infection in Indian infants. Canad Med Assoc J 1979; 120:295.
5. Manitoba Pediatric Society. Breast-feeding promotion in Manitoba. Canad Med Assoc J 1982; 126:639.
6. Myres AW. National survey of infant feeding patterns: A synopsis. Health Protection Directorate, Health and Welfare Canada, 1983.
7. Marchessault G. Infant feeding practices on six Manitoba Indian reserves. Medical Services Branch, Health and Welfare Canada, 1982.

Gail Marchessault
Medical Services Branch
Health and Welfare Canada
500-303 Main Street
Winnipeg, Manitoba R3C OH4
Canada

Circumpolar Health 84:166-169

MORTALITY AMONG THE JAMES BAY CREE, QUEBEC, 1975-1982

ELIZABETH ROBINSON

INTRODUCTION

This communication will present mortality data for the period 1975-1982 for a population of 8,000 Cree Indians living east of James Bay between the 49th and 55th N. parallel in the Province of Quebec, Canada.

In 1975, Cree leaders signed the James Bay Agreement (1) and the Cree Board of Health and Social Services was set up in 1978 under the jurisdiction of the Quebec Ministry of Social Affairs to administer health care in the eight Cree communities. Our department's role is to be a consultant to the Cree board in the areas of needs analysis, priority setting, and program planning and evaluation. The study of Cree mortality was undertaken as a first step in the process of setting priorities for this population, and in order to see how the Crees compare with other Native and non-Native populations in terms of mortality.

The Cree population is based in eight communities. Five of the eight communities are on the James Bay coast and are practically inaccessible except by airplane; the three other communities are inland, and of these, the two largest are accessible to northern Quebec mining towns by road.

The traditional activities of hunting and trapping are still important both as sources of food and of income; 50% of the population benefits from an income security program for hunters (2).

Each community has a clinic with at least two nurses working full time, and doctors make regular, usually monthly, visits. One Cree community, Chisasibi, has a 32-bed hospital; patients are referred to Val d'Or, Moose Factory, Chibougamau, or Montreal for surgery or other consultations.

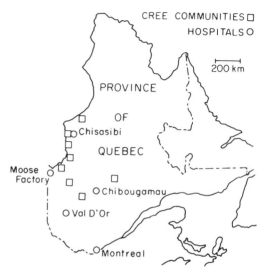

Figure 1. Location of Cree communities and referral hospitals.

METHODS

The list of deaths and births was compiled from several sources: hospital and clinic registers; Quebec Vital Statistics Registry, which provided death and birth certificates; church records; and the list of beneficiaries of the James Bay Agreement.

For this study, the population was defined as Cree beneficiaries of the James Bay Agreement living in category 1, 2, or 3 lands (according to definitions in the James Bay Agreement) (1). This includes the Native population of the eight communities plus some Cree people living nearby these

Table 1. Age distribution of deaths among James Bay Cree and for Quebec generally.

Age group	James Bay Cree 1975-1982		Quebec 1975-1981
	no.	%	%
0-4	85	27.4	2.9
0-1	65	21.0	2.4
1-4	20	6.5	0.5
5-14	16	5.2	1.0
15-24	23	7.4	3.1
25-44	27	8.7	6.4
45-64	48	15.4	25.5
65 plus	111	35.8	61.1
all ages	310	100.0	100.0

Table 2. Life expectancy at birth, 1975-1981.

	Total	Male	Female
Cree - all	71.8	69.8	73.2
Coastal	73.9	70.5	77.7
Interior	68.7	68.9	67.7
Quebec (3)	73.9	69.9	78.2

communities either in the bush or in northern towns. The denominator used for the rates was an estimation of this population as it was for December 31, 1978. This estimation was obtained from the beneficiary list by removing births and adding deaths occurring after December 31, 1978; the total population at this time numbered 7,290 persons.

Information on causes of death was obtained principally from death certificates, and also from hospital and clinic records.

RESULTS

The Cree population is young; both the birth rate (30.1 per 1,000 population) and the fertility rate (139.0 per 1,000 females, aged 15 to 49) are twice Quebec levels (15.4 and 57.6 respectively) (3). Persons aged 65 and over represent only 4.2% of the population compared to 9.7% for Canada in 1981 (4).

The following data on mortality are based on 310 deaths from 1975 to 1982 (271 from 1975 to 1981). The age distribution of deaths (see Table 1) is very different for the Crees from that for Quebec as a whole (3). Many more Cree deaths occur in children, partly due to the fact that there are relatively more children in the population and partly due to higher rates in Cree infants and children.

Life expectancy at birth is shown in Table 2. Cree life expectancy, while lower than that of Quebec, generally is still considerably higher than that of the poorest districts of Montreal.

Indirect age standardization using Canadian rates for 1978 (6,7) indicates that 200 deaths would have been expected in the period 1975 to 1981 in the Cree population

Table 3. Causes of infant mortality, James Bay Cree, 1975-1982.

ICD-9 category		Neonatal	Post-neonatal	Total
I	Infectious	0	8	8
	gastroenteritis	0	7	7
	meningococcemia	0	1	1
VI	Nervous/sense organs	0	10	10
	meningitis	0	5	5
	leukodystrophy	0	4	4
	other	0	1	1
VII	Circulatory	1	0	1
VIII	Respiratory	0	12	12
	pneumonia		11	11
	other		1	1
XII	Skin/subcutaneous	0	1	1
XIV	Congenital	6	5	11
XV	Perinatal	4	1	5
XVI	Ill defined	2	13	15
	SIDS	0	1	1
	unknown	2	12	14
XVII	Injuries/poisoning	1	1	2
	Total	14	51	65

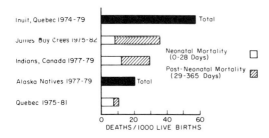

Figure 2. Infant mortality comparisons.

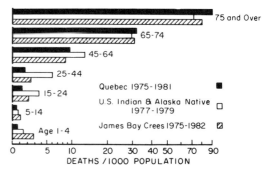

Figure 3. Comparative age-specific death rates.

of 7,290 persons if the death rates for each age group of Crees had been similar to those for Canada. In fact, 271 Cree deaths were observed during this period making the overall Cree death rate 1.4 times the Canadian rate.

Infant mortality decreased from 49.7 deaths per 1,000 live births for the 3-year period 1975 to 1977, to 22.2 for 1981 to 1983. Over the 8-year period 1975 to 1982, infant mortality averaged 37.0 per 1,000 live births, compared with 10.8 per 1,000 (3) for the Quebec population from 1975 to 1981. Cree neonatal mortality (0 to 28 days) was 8.0 per 1,000, close to Quebec's 7.5, while postneonatal mortality (29 to 365 days) at 29.0 per 1,000 was more than 8 times the Quebec rate.

Cree infant mortality was higher than that of Canadian Indians and Alaska Natives (8,9) but does not appear to be as high as that of the Quebec Inuit population (10) (Figure 2). Within the Cree population, infant mortality from 1975 to 1982 was different in the 5 coastal villages, where it was 27.4 deaths per 1,000 live births, from in the 3 inland villages, where it was 49.2 deaths per 1,000 live births.

Causes of infant mortality are shown in Table 2. Twenty-four children died in the post-neonatal period of gastroenteritis, meningitis/meningococcemia, or pneumonia; many of the deaths from these causes are potentially preventable.

In Figure 3, age-specific death rates among Crees are compared with rates in Quebec (1975-1981) (3) and for American Indians and Alaska Natives (1977-1979) (9). Cree death rates are higher than Quebec rates up to age 44, and they are especially high in children under 15. For adults 15 to 44, Cree death rates are not as high as those in American Indian and Alaska Natives, whose rates are 3 times those of the U.S. population in these age groups.

Proportionate mortality and standardized mortality ratios are shown in Table 4. Cree death rates for tumors and heart disease are lower than those for Canada, while rates for respiratory and infectious diseases, and injuries and poisoning are higher. The age-adjusted rate of drownings (including all deaths in ICDA-9 categories

Table 4. Causes of death, James Bay Cree, 1975-1982.

ICD-9 category		% of deaths	SMR*
I	Infectious	4.8	
II	Tumors	11.0	0.72
VI	Nervous/sense organs	5.8	
VII	Circulatory	21.9	0.77
VIII	Respiratory	11.6	2.6
IX	Digestive	2.3	
X	Genito-urinary	2.6	
XIV	Congenital malformations	4.5	
XV	Perinatal	1.6	
XVI	Ill-defined/unknown	9.4	
XVII	Injuries and poisonings	20.3	2.0
	Others	4.2	

* Standardized mortality ratio = observed deaths in Cree population/expected deaths based on Canadian rates for 1978 (6,7).

E830, E832, and E910) for Crees is 12 times the Canadian rate. Almost 10% of Cree deaths are due to drowning, and nearly half of all deaths due to injuries and poisonings are drownings. Nevertheless, deaths in the category injuries and poisoning (which include car accidents, drownings, fires, suicide, drug overdose, homicide, etc.) appear to be less common in Crees than in other Native groups. While the injury and poisoning death rate for Crees is twice that of Canada, in American Indian and Alaska Natives it is 2.5 to 3 times the U.S rate (9), and in Indians in northwestern Ontario it is 4.5 times the Canadian rate (11). Injuries and poisonings caused 35.7% of deaths in Canadian registered Indians in 1978 and 1979 (8) but only 20.3% of Cree deaths for 1975 to 1982.

CONCLUSIONS

What are the implications of these findings? Maternal and child health, particularly in the postneonatal period of the first year of life, are priorities because of the young age of the population and the higher death rates in children. Preventive strategies for respiratory illness and injuries should be examined. In general, Crees seem to be relatively healthy compared to other Native populations, and this is especially true for young and middle-aged adult males.

It will be interesting to follow Cree death rates over the next few years; infant and child mortality will probably continue to decline, but will reductions in deaths due to drowning be possible? Will death rates for heart disease and cancer become similar to those in the general population? Finally, will the Crees be able to continue to enjoy relative freedom from the tragically high accident and suicide rates seen in other Native populations?

ACKNOWLEDGMENTS

I thank Andrée Jobin, Richard Letarte, Paul Brassard, and the many people working for the Cree Board of Health and Social Services who helped me to obtain these data; Russell Wilkins and other colleagues in the Community Health Department, Montreal General Hospital; and the Département de Médecine sociale et préventive, Université de Montréal, where I was a M.Sc. student while beginning work on this study. This work was supported in part by a grant from the Ministry of Social Affairs, Quebec.

REFERENCES

1. The James Bay and Northern Quebec Agreement. Editeur officiel du Québec, 1976.
2. LaRusic I. Income security for subsistence hunters. Indian and Northern Affairs Canada, 1982.
3. Wilkins R. Personal communication.
4. Canada Census. Statistics Canada. Catalogue no. 82-901. 1981.
5. Wilkins R. L'inégalité sociale face à la mortalité à Montréal, 1975-1977. Cahiers québécois de démographie 1980; 9:157-183.
6. Causes of death: by province according to sex and age, by detailed ICD categories, for 1978, 1979. Statistics Canada.
7. Vital Statistics, Volume 1; Births and Deaths for 1978, 1979. Statistics Canada.
8. Medical Services, Annual Reviews, 1978 and 1979. Department of National Health and Welfare, Ottawa, Canada.
9. FY 1984 Budget Appropriation, Indian Health Service, "Chart series" (and tables). Office of Program Statistics, Division of Resource Coordination, Indian Health Service, U.S. Department of Health and Human Services.
10. Duval B, Therrien F. Demography, mortality and morbidity of the northern Quebec Inuit. In: Harvald B, Hart Hansen JP, eds. Circumpolar Health 81. Nordic Council Arct Med Res Rep 1982; 33:206-211.
11. Young TK. Mortality pattern of isolated Indians in northwestern Ontario: a ten year review. Public Health Reports 1983; 98:467-475.

Elizabeth Robinson
Department of Community Health
Montreal General Hospital
2100 Guy Street
Montreal, Quebec   H3H 2M8
Canada

Circumpolar Health 84:170-172

LENGTH, WEIGHT, AND HEAD CIRCUMFERENCE IN QUEBEC CREE CHILDREN

MICHAEL E.K. MOFFATT, C. KATO AND G.V. WATTERS

In the course of providing tertiary pediatric care and maternal and child health program consultation to the Cree Regional Health Board in the James Bay area of Quebec, it became apparent that we were seeing a lot of very heavy infants and children referred for investigation of large head size. Data from a study of the effects of methylmercury on the James Bay Cree Indians performed at McGill University (1,2) provided a unique opportunity to develop growth and head circumference norms for this group of Cree children.

METHODS

We re-analyzed the growth and head circumference data on the 232 Cree children in four communities in the James Bay area, representing 90.6% of the eligible children between 12 and 30 months of age at the time of the study in July 1978. Birth measurements were available for 213 of these children (104 boys and 109 girls). The birth weights and lengths and average measurement for children of each month of age between 12 and 30 months, plus and minus two standard deviations, were plotted on standard growth charts of Hamill et al. for U.S. children from the National Center for Health Statistics (3) supplied by Ross Laboratories.

Birth measurements of head circumference were available for only 85 children (39 boys and 46 girls) but this appeared to be a chance sample. To decrease the variance, head circumferences for children were grouped by 3-month intervals and the average plotted at the middle of this interval on standard Nelhaus graphs for Caucasian children.

The curves for this mean were hand drawn in a best fit fashion and for head circumference the upper 97.5th and lower 2.5th percentile lines were also drawn.

RESULTS

From Figures 1 and 2 it can be seen that Cree children are on the average very heavy at birth, and they remain very heavy compared to American children throughout the

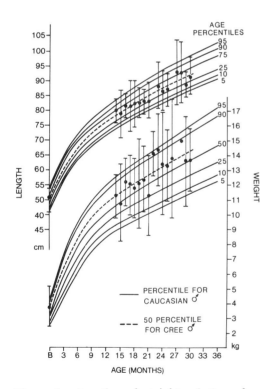

Figure 1. Length and weight of Cree boys (±2 S.D.) superimposed on standard Caucasian growth charts.

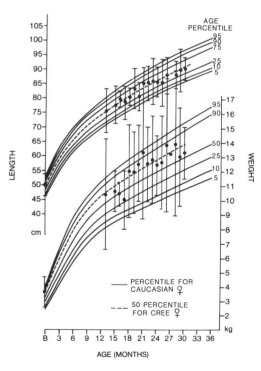

Figure 2. Length and weight of Cree girls (±2 S.D.) superimposed on standard Caucasian growth charts.

first 30 months of life. The mean birth weight of boys was 3,800 g, with a standard deviation of 680, and girls weighed 3,700 g ± 540.

By contrast, the average birth length was 50.2 cm for boys and 49.5 cm for girls. These are exactly the same as American children. The mean lengths for Cree children appear to continue right along the 50th percentile for Caucasian children.

Head circumferences are plotted in Figures 3 and 4. Cree children have large heads at birth (36.2 ± 1.7 cm for boys and 35.7 ± 1.3 cm for girls). This is more than 1 cm greater than the American average for both sexes. Head growth appears to follow along a curve well above the 50th percentile for Caucasian children. The 2.5th percentile is larger and the 97.5th percentile is considerably larger than the Caucasian.

DISCUSSION

There are several clinical implications of this study. The first is that Cree children in this region have large head circumference measurements, and before becoming concerned about hydrocephalus, health care workers should consult these norms, examine the child, and take serial head measurements. Considerable savings of investigative effort can arise through a better understanding of these norms. The social effects of evacuating an infant from the far north for investigation in southern

hospitals are considerable and we favor minimizing such separations. A single measurement of head circumference on Cree children would result in 11.3% of these children having head circumferences greater than the 98th percentile on the Nelhaus chart.

The growth data are equally interesting in that Cree children are heavy but not too long for their age compared with Caucasian standards. The birth weight ±2 S.D. for girls shows that the lower limit for birth weight would be about 2,600 g and not 2,500 g which is usually considered low birth weight. For boys the figure is less certain because the range of birth weights (1,616 to 5,475 g) is much wider than for girls (2,298 to 5,210 g). It is virtually certain that some premature boys are included, but we did not have such ascertainment available. Thus, for boys we found the mean minus 2 S.D. to be 2,440 g. We suspect that if prematures were eliminated, this standard deviation would decrease and the mean would increase slightly, and that boys would also show a low birth weight level higher than the standard 2,500 g. Perhaps such a study could be done prospectively in the James Bay region.

We could not find data on expected growth patterns of Indian tribes in infancy, so we do not know whether these growth patterns are unusual.

Elsewhere in these Proceedings, Postl et al. (5) present growth patterns of

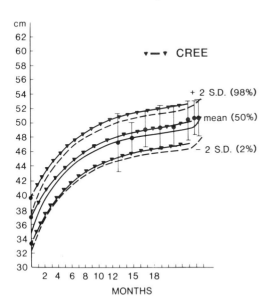

Figure 3. Head circumference of Cree boys (±2 S.D.) superimposed on standard Nelhaus head circumference chart.

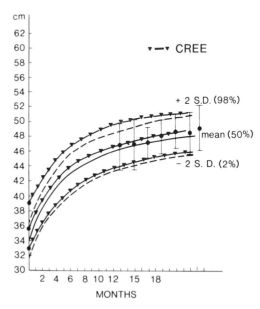

Figure 4. Head circumference of Cree girls (±2 S.D.) superimposed on standard Nelhaus circumference chart.

Keewatin Inuit children over the first seven days of life which show similar length and weight patterns. They also present ponderal indexes which suggest that the extra weight is mainly lean body mass, not fat. They do not present head circumferences.

Partington et al. (6) studied an extended population of Cree Indians in the same general region in the 1960s and found that the mean birth weight of 768 infants was 3,780 g, which was about 450 g heavier than the Canadian average for Indians, suggesting that the Cree may be unusual among Indian groups.

Diabetes is fairly prevalent among the James Bay Cree but no relevant data on gestational diabetes are available for the children in this study. Pettit et al. (7) have shown that there is a higher perinatal mortality in Pima Indian infants who were large for gestational age (>90th percentile Caucasian standards) versus those who were not large. This resulted almost entirely from a five-fold increase in stillbirths rather than an increase in neonatal mortality. The large-for-gestational-age babies were much more common in mothers whose two-hour glucose tolerance curve showed values greater than 160 mg/dl. More recently the same group has presented evidence that long-standing obesity is more common in the offspring of mothers whose glucose tolerance curve was abnormal during pregnancy (8).

The possibility that these growth patterns are due to a metabolic disorder such as diabetes must be further explored. The traditional Cree diet contained very little carbohydrate and thus even if the genes for diabetes were common, the manifestations would have been few. Dietary change in this population occurred several centuries ago, however, with the advent of the fur trade. Flour and sugar became essential staples for Indians then, and there is of course no way to go back and measure infants prior to this period.

Further investigation is clearly needed to determine whether there are secular trends in this growth pattern, and whether a distinct metabolic cause can be found.

REFERENCES

1. The McGill Methylmercury Study: A study of the effects of exposure to methylmercury on the health of individuals living in certain areas of the Province of Quebec. Montreal: McGill University Press, 1980.
2. McKeown-Eyssen GF, Ruedy J, and Neims A. Methylmercury exposure in northern Quebec. II. Neurologic findings in children. Am J Epidemiol 1983; 118: 470-479.
3. Hamill PVV, Drizd TA, Johnson CL et al. Physical growth: National Center for Health Statistics percentiles. Am J Clin Nutr 1979; 32:607-629.
4. Nelhaus G. Head circumference from birth to eighteen years: Practical composite international and interracial graphs. Pediatrics 1968; 41:106-114.
5. Postl BP, Carson J, Spady D et al. Northwest Territories perinatal and infant morbidity and mortality study: Follow up 1982. II. Physical examination. In: Fortuine R, ed. Circumpolar Health 84. Seattle: University of Washington Press, 1985 (this volume).
6. Partington NW and Roberts N. The heights and weights of Indian and Eskimo school children in James Bay and Hudson Bay. Canad Med Assoc J 1969; 100:502-509.
7. Pettit DJ, Knowler WC, Baird HR, and Bennet PH. Gestational diabetes: Infant and maternal complications in relation to third trimester glucose tolerance in Pima Indians. Diabet Care 1980; 3:458-464.
8. Pettit DJ, Baird HR, Kirk AA et al. Excessive obesity in offspring of Pima Indian women with diabetes during pregnancy. N Engl J Med 1983; 308: 242-245.

Michael E. K. Moffatt
Northern Medical Unit
University of Manitoba
61 Emily Street
Winnipeg, Manitoba R3E 1Y9
Canada

Circumpolar Health 84:173-180

DEVELOPMENTAL MILESTONES IN JAMES BAY CREE INDIAN CHILDREN

MICHAEL E.K. MOFFATT and C. KATO

INTRODUCTION

Child development in North American Indians has not been studied systematically. Erikson made a major contribution to psychoanalytic theory through his studies of the Oglala Sioux Indians (1) and Dinges (2) has written about developmental intervention in Navajo children, but to our knowledge nobody has established when it is normal for any group of Indian children to perform certain tasks. Nevertheless, Indian children are regularly assessed for developmental progress by health professionals, using tests like the Denver Developmental Screening Test (DDST) (3) which takes as its norm a Colorado Caucasian population. Children who fail to meet these norms are sometimes subjected to extensive investigations in southern hospitals.

Studies from around the world have given varying results as to the cross-cultural validity of the DDST (4-8). Often it is only on a few specific items that cultures differ, but occasionally important differences are found in whole areas of development.

In 1978 a study was undertaken by the Department of Pharmacology of McGill University to determine the effects of methylmercury exposure on adults and the unborn child (9,10), but no effects on child development were demonstrated. Since a virtually complete birth cohort was examined during this study, we re-analyzed these data for the purpose of establishing norms for the DDST milestones for Cree children.

METHODS

The original study population consisted of all living children 12 to 30 months of age as of July 1, 1978, in four northern Cree communities in the James Bay region of Quebec (Great Whale River, Fort George, Mistasini, Waswanipi). These communities account for two-thirds of the Quebec Cree population.

The Cree inhabit a boreal forest area, and have maintained a fair degree of cultural identity. The traditional economy was based on hunting, trapping, and fishing and there are still many people engaged in these activities. In 1975 they signed an agreement with the Quebec and Canadian governments in which they traded the right to some of their land to the province in return for a cash settlement plus control of social and health programs affecting them and some economic programs, including a guaranteed income for trappers. The economic benefits of these programs were just beginning to be felt at the time of this study. Social disruption in the form of alcoholism and family breakdown were relatively rare. The average educational achievement of the parents was still low by comparison to southern standards, with mothers having completed 6.1 and fathers 5.5 years of schooling.

The total known number of births in the cohort was 269, but 13 children had died prior to the study, leaving a total of 256 eligible subjects. Nine children were living off the reserve and 15 children had incomplete data. Thus the study population was reduced to 232 or 90.6% of eligible subjects.

Field examinations consisted of two separate maternal interviews, the first conducted by a pediatrician assisted by a Cree interpreter, and the second undertaken solely by the Cree interpreter. A complete physical and neurological examination was carried out on each child by one of two pediatricians or two pediatric neurologists. Neurological abnormalities were always corroborated by the pediatric neurologist. Developmental examinations were carried out with the aid of three trained Cree interpreters. Although no formal testing of consistency between raters was performed, the physicians involved underwent training sessions and during the course of the examinations they talked with each other extensively to ensure that they were all doing the same thing. Some of the items were obtained by history through the interpreter. In the opinion of the physicians involved, the interpreters were extremely conscientious.

The cross-sectional data on developmental milestones were analyzed by the probit transformation technique (11) to obtain expected ages and 95% confidence intervals at which the 25th, 50th, 75th, and 90th percentile of the population would have achieved each milestone. Twelve children with abnormal or suspected abnormal neurological examination were eliminated from the probit analysis to make it more comparable with the population on which the original DDST was standardized. Thus the norms are derived from 220 children. These were compared with the North American norms of Frankenburg and Dodds (3) for the DDST. If the 95% confidence interval for our data did not incorporate the published norm, we considered our norm to be different from the North American figure.

Because there is a postulated effect of chronic otitis media on language development

GROSS MOTOR NORMS FOR DENVER AND CREE CHILDREN

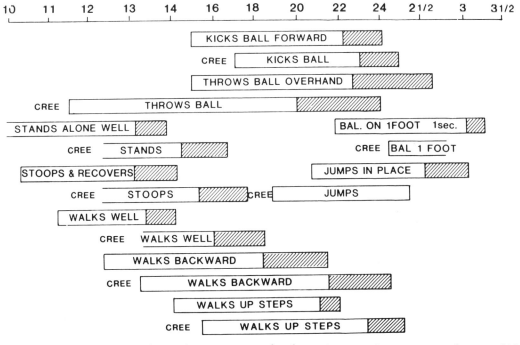

Figure 1.   Graphic comparison of gross motor development norms for Denver and Cree children.

FINE MOTOR – ADAPTIVE

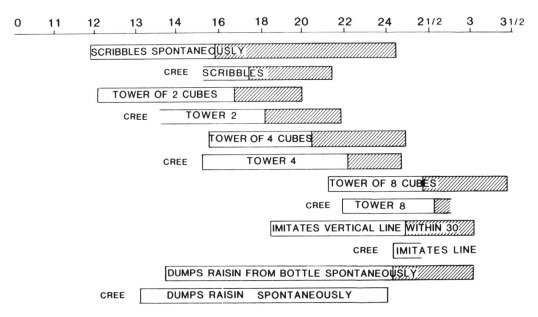

Figure 2.   Graphic comparison of fine motor development norms for Denver and Cree children.

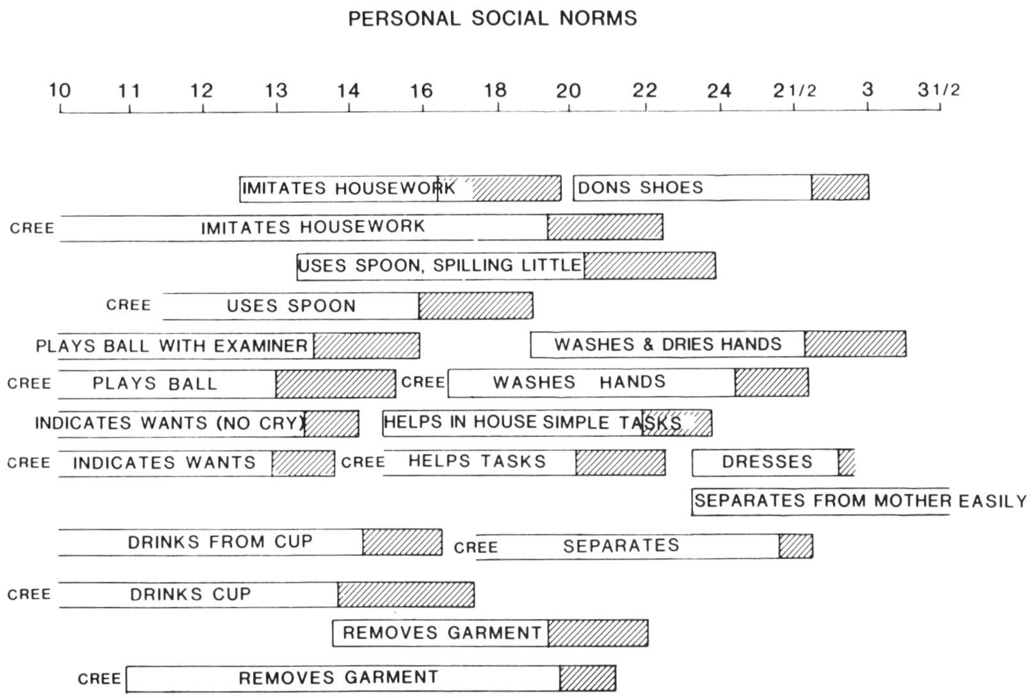

PERSONAL SOCIAL NORMS

10   11   12   13   14   16   18   20   22   24   2 1/2   3   3 1/2

IMITATES HOUSEWORK
CREE   IMITATES HOUSEWORK
DONS SHOES

USES SPOON, SPILLING LITTLE
CREE   USES SPOON

PLAYS BALL WITH EXAMINER
CREE   PLAYS BALL
WASHES & DRIES HANDS
CREE   WASHES HANDS

INDICATES WANTS (NO CRY)
HELPS IN HOUSE SIMPLE TASKS
CREE   INDICATES WANTS   CREE   HELPS TASKS
DRESSES
SEPARATES FROM MOTHER EASILY

DRINKS FROM CUP   CREE   SEPARATES
CREE   DRINKS CUP

REMOVES GARMENT
CREE   REMOVES GARMENT

Figure 3. *Graphic comparison of personal-social development norms for Denver and Cree children.*

LANGUAGE NORMS

10   11   12   13   14   16   18   20   22   24   2 1/2   3   3 1/2

3 WORDS OTHER THAN MAMA DADA
CREE   3 WORDS

COMBINES 2 OF DIFFERENT WORDS
CREE   COMB. 2 WORDS

DADA OR MAMA SPECIFIC   POINTS TO 1 NAMED BODY PART
CREE   DADA MAMA   CREE   BODY PART

FOLLOWS 2 OF 3 DIRECTIONS
CREE   FOLLOW 2/3 DIRECTIONS

USES PLURALS
CREE   USES PLURALS

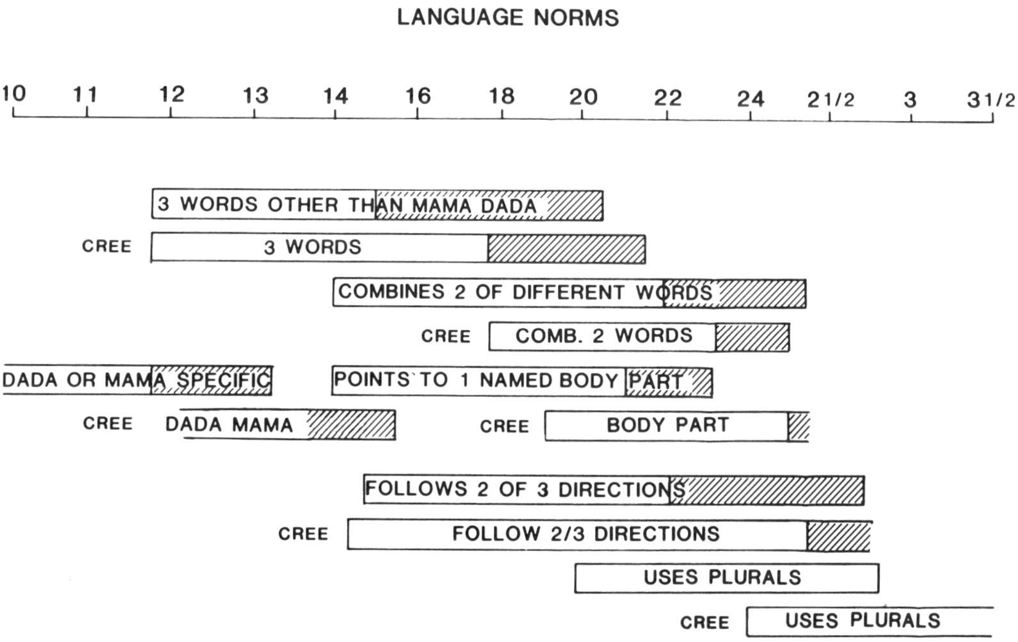

Figure 4. *Graphic comparison of language development norms for Denver and Cree children.*

Table 1. *Milestones in gross motor development by James Bay Cree children. Age of achievement in months, for 25th, 50th, 75th, and 95th percentiles, with associated 95% Confidence Intervals (C.I.).*

Milestone	Percentile 25th Age	C.I.	50th Age	C.I.	75th Age	C.I.	90th Age	C.I.
Stands alone well			12.1	8.0 / 13.7	14.5	12.4 / 15.7	16.6	15.4 / 18.5
Stoops and recovers			12.4	8.8 / 14.1	15.3	13.4 / 16.5	17.8	16.6 / 19.7
Walks well			13.6	11.3 / 14.9	16.1	14.8 / 17.2	18.4	17.3 / 20.2
Walks backwards	13.0	7.0 / 15.7	17.1	13.8 / 19.0	21.2	19.3 / 23.7	24.9	22.7 / 29.5
Walks up steps	15.3	13.0 / 16.7	19.1	17.8 / 20.2	23.0	21.9 / 24.5	26.5	24.9 / 28.9
Kicks ball forwards	17.2	15.7 / 18.3	20.2	19.2 / 21.1	23.2	22.3 / 24.5	25.9	24.7 / 27.8
Throws ball overhand	11.5	7.6 / 13.8	15.8	13.5 / 17.3	20.1	18.8 / 21.6	24.0	22.4 / 26.5

(12,13) we compared the language norms for 37 children with evidence of current or old middle ear disease to the overall norms.

RESULTS

The results are presented for each of the four areas of development in Tables 1 to 4 with the upper and lower 95% confidence levels, and then graphically, analogous to the standard DDST forms (Figures 1 to 4) with the lower bars representing Cree children. Milestones achieved by half of the children before or after the ages 12 and 30 months respectively render the probit transformation analysis too speculative and they are therefore not presented.

Gross Motor

At lower levels, gross motor achievement seems similar to Denver norms, but the 75th percentile is later for stooping and recovering, walking well, walking backwards, and walking up steps. At the 90th percentile, standing alone and kicking are added

to this list and the differences between the lower 95% confidence limit and the Caucasian norms appear to widen.

Fine Motor

There are relatively few milestones in fine motor development completed in this time period. Only building a tower of 2, 4, or 8 cubes appears to be slightly behind at one or more percentiles, but not consistently so. Drawing a line is behind but may reflect lack of exposure to writing materials.

Personal-Social

The majority of the items on personal-social criteria for development are achieved appropriately or early by Cree children. It is only at the 90th percentile achievement level that any milestones appear to develop late: these are in using a cup, imitating housework, and removing a garment. The 25th and 50th percentiles were often reached early. Separation from mother was achieved very early by all the children.

Table 2. Milestones in fine motor development by James Bay Cree children.

Milestone	Percentile 25th Age	C.I.	50th Age	C.I.	75th Age	C.I.	90th Age	C.I.
Scribbles spontaneously					15.5	10.6 17.8	21.3	19.1 24.8
Tower of 2 cubes			13.1	5.2 16.1	18.3	14.9 10.8	23.1	20.6 28.2
Tower of 4 cubes	14.9	12.4 16.5	18.9	17.5 20.1	22.9	21.7 24.4	26.5	24.9 29.0
Tower of 8 cubes	23.1	21.8 24.3	26.7	25.5 28.5	30.4	28.6 33.4		
Imitates vertical line within 30°	25.4	23.1 28.5	29.8	27.1 36.9				
Copies circle	26.8	25.5 28.7	30.3	28.5 33.9				
Dumps raisins spontaneously	13.3	9.3 15.6	18.8	16.8 20.3	24.3	22.7 26.6		

Language

The largest proportion of delayed percentiles (one-half) occurred in the language area. At the 90th percentile only one out of three milestones was delayed and that was the age at which children say three words clearly. Combining two words was late at the 75th percentile, but not at the 90th. The projected values for the 90th percentile for two other receptive language milestones (points to one named body part, and follows two of three directions) were also delayed but fell outside the 30th month limit.

The postulated relationship between otitis media and language delay could not be demonstrated in this small sample.

DISCUSSION

The developmental norms from these data are unique but before being accepted they should be repeated. It is possible that difficulties encountered in asking questions through interpreters have produced some distortion. A further complicating factor is that it was sometimes difficult to get the cooperation of shy Indian children and some items were thus tested by history alone.

On the other hand, the DDST is widely used on Native·populations by public health nurses and the developmental and neurological training of the examiners in this study was greater than that of the nurses who use this test.

Whatever the accuracy of the actual testing, the clinical implication is that other Caucasian health workers would obtain similar results in similar circumstances and, therefore, these norms should be taken into account when interpreting DDST's applied to this population of Cree.

The major strengths of this study are the completeness of the birth cohort (90.6%) and the limited number of highly skilled observers who did the testing. Since all of the study children were examined by a pediatrician, it is unlikely that serious chronic diseases affecting development were missed. The DDST has been standardized on several other populations outside Denver, including children from Cardiff (4), Tokyo (5), Okinawa (6), British Columbia, Canada (7), and the Yucatan Peninsula of Mexico (8).

Minor differences were found between most of these populations and the Denver population. The most striking and interesting differences were presented by Ueda (5),

Table 3.   Milestones in personal-social development by James Bay Cree children.

Milestone	Percentile 25th Age	C.I.	50th Age	C.I.	75th Age	C.I.	90th Age	C.I.
Plays ball		2.7		7.2		11.5		14.4
	10.0		11.9		13.8		15.6	
		12.0		13.4		15.0		17.5
Indicates wants (not cry)		2.0		6.7		11.2		14.3
	9.8		11.8		13.8		15.6	
		11.9		13.3		15.0		17.4
Drinks from cup		3.1		8.8		14.2		17.9
	9.1		12.6		16.1		19.3	
		11.7		14.4		17.5		21.4
Uses spoon		-17.4		-4.2		8.3		16.3
	7.4		11.4		15.4		19.0	
		12.1		14.8		18.1		24.4
Imitates housework		1.4		9.4		16.7		21.5
	8.2		13.4		18.6		23.3	
		11.5		15.6		20.2		26.2
Helps in house, simple tasks		10.5		15.1		19.0		21.7
	13.8		17.1		20.4		23.3	
		15.7		18.5		22.0		26.0
Washes and dries hands		14.3		19.8		24.2		27.7
	16.6		21.1		25.7		29.8	
		18.1		22.4		27.8		33.2
Removes garment		6.4		12.8		18.4		22.3
	10.8		15.3		19.8		23.9	
		13.2		16.9		21.3		26.5
Separates from mother easily				9.9		24.0		
			16.6		27.0			
				19.5		34.7		
Dresses with supervision		21.5		25.1		28.0		
	22.8		26.2		29.6			
		23.8		27.6		32.1		

who found Tokyo children to be earlier for most Personal-Social items, similar in Fine Motor-Adaptive items, generally slower in expressive language at all ages, and slower in Gross Motor prior to the age of 18 months, than their Denver counterparts. This pattern bears some resemblance to our norms for the Cree children, and in view of the Mongolian origin of Canadian Native people, leads to some speculation regarding genetic contribution.

One possible explanation for the differences found in Cree children is that they were economically underprivileged. An example of the way that a developmental milestone can change with socioeconomic development is presented by Harriman and Lukosius (14) who found that there was a 2.5-month advance in the age of walking in Hopi Indian children over the period from 1940 to 1979. The delayed onset of walking (15 months) had been attributed to cultural factors such as the use of a cradle board, but it now appears that nutritional and general health factors were to blame. In 1940 the infant mortality rate in Hopi Indian children was 180 per 1,000 and by 1979 it had dropped close to the American average at 21.1 per 1,000, and the use of the cradle board had no effect on age of walking.

To try to control for social class, we compared our norms with the norms of Denver children from social classes IV and V. Very

Table 4. Milestones in language development by James Bay Cree children.

Milestone	Percentile Age	25th C.I.	50th Age	C.I.	75th Age	C.I.	90th Age	C.I.
Dada or Mama specific							16.2	9.2 20.8
Three words other than Mama or Dada	11.9	5.7 14.6	15.6	12.0 17.5	19.3	17.3 21.4	22.6	20.6 26.4
Combines 2 different words	18.6	15.2 20.5	21.6	19.6 23.6	24.7	22.9 27.8	27.5	25.2 32.3
Points to one named body part	19.5	17.2 21.0	25.0	23.5 27.3	30.6	28.2 35.1		
Follows 2 of 3 directions	14.5	9.8 16.9	21.2	19.6 22.9	27.8	25.6 32.0		
Uses plurals	26.6	25.0 28.9						
Comprehends cold, tired, hungry	22.6	20.8 24.2	28.0	26.1 31.2				

few of the differences disappeared. The developmental pattern found in Cree children does not appear in lower class Denver children. The Cree did not live under such appalling conditions as the Hopi did in 1940. Infant mortality was under 30 per 1,000 and abject poverty was rare. However, we cannot rule out some subtle effects on the finer aspects of development due to socioeconomic conditions.

Finally, it may simply be that cultural differences in child-rearing are responsible for the developmental patterns found in this study. Miller et al. (15) have suggested that this is the explanation for certain differences in results for specific items on the DDST when applied to Southeast Asian children immigrating to the U.S. They found that games like pat-a-cake did not exist in these cultures, and that linguistic differences led to failures in use of plurals and recognition of colors. We do not know enough about Cree culture and the importance placed on gross motor or language development to know whether the pattern found in this study could be simply a function of child-rearing attitudes, and this would be worthy of further investigation.

Whether the developmental pattern we have found is cultural, social, hereditary, or simply due to testing difficulties, requires further research. The study should be replicated and expanded to older children. It should be repeated again when socioeconomic conditions have improved. Meanwhile, health care workers should be cautious in their diagnosis of developmental delay.

The language development pattern is of particular interest and if found in other studies may have educational implications, since the current approach to education is based on verbal skills. McShane (16) reviewed the literature on intelligence testing in Indian school children and found a consistent pattern of low scores on verbal scales. Environment has been blamed for the low scores, but our results suggest that very early language development in Cree children even as determined through an interpreter in their own language may be slower than in Caucasian children, raising the possibility that genetic or cultural factors are important. If this proves to be true, the whole approach of Indian children may need re-thinking, with major input from the Cree themselves.

SUMMARY

The James Bay Cree children studies exhibited a different developmental pattern from Caucasian children, with definitely slower gross motor and probably slower language development, and perhaps earlier personal-social development. Serial follow-up could lead to valuable information about the relationship between social and cultural environment, genetics, and child development.

REFERENCES

1. Erikson EH. Childhood and society. 2nd ed. New York: WW Norton and Co Inc, 1963.
2. Dinges N. Mental health promotion with Navajo families. In: Manson S, ed. New directions in prevention among American Indian and Alaska Native communities. Portland: Oregon Health Sciences University, 1982.
3. Frankenburg WK, Dodds JB. Denver developmental screening test manual. Denver: University of Colorado Medical Center, 1969 ed.
4. Bryant GM, Davies KJ, Newcombe RG. Standardization of the Denver development screening test for Cardiff children. Develop Med Child Neuro 1979; 21:353-364.
5. Ueda R. Standardization of the Denver developmental screening test on Tokyo children. Develop Med Child Neuro 1978; 20:647-656.
6. Ueda R. Child development in Okinawa compared with Tokyo and Denver, and implications for developmental screening. Develop Med Child Neuro 1978; 20:657-663.
7. Barnes KE, Stark A. The Denver developmental screening test: a normative study. Am J Public Health 1975; 65:363-369.
8. Solomons HC. Standardization of the Denver developmental screening test on infants from Yucatan, Mexico. Int J Rehab Research 1982; 5:179-189.
9. The McGill methylmercury study: A study of the effects of exposure to methylmercury on the health of individuals living in certain areas of the Province of Quebec. Montreal: McGill Univ Press, 1980.
10. McKeown-Eyssen GE, Ruedy J. Methylmercury exposure in northern Quebec. II. Neurological findings in children. Am J Epidemiology 1983; 118:470.
11. Collquhoun D. Lectures on biostatistics. Oxford: Clarendon Press, 1974: 345-364.
12. Zinkus PW, Gottlieb MI, Shapiro M. Developmental and psychoeducational sequelae of chronic otitis media. Am J Dis Child 1978; 132:1100-1104.
13. Kaplan GJ et al. Long term effects of otitis media. A 10 year cohort study of Alaska Eskimo children. Pediatrics 1973; 52:577-585.
14. Harriman AE, Lukosius PA. On why Wayne Dennis found Hopi infants retarded in age at onset of walking. Perceptual Motor Skills 1982; 55:86-99.
15. Miller V, Onotira RT, Dernhand AS. Denver developmental screening test: cultural variations in Southeast Asian children. J Pediatr 1984; 104:481-482.
16. McShane D. A review of scores of American Indian children on the Wechsler intelligence scale. White Cloud Journal 1978; 1:3-10.

Michael E. K. Moffatt
Northern Medical Unit
University of Manitoba
61 Emily Street
Winnipeg, Manitoba R3E 1Y9
Canada

CHANGING PATTERN OF CHILDBIRTH IN NORTHERN FINLAND OVER THE PAST THREE DECADES

JUKKA PUOLAKKA, PENTTI A. JARVINEN and A. KAUPPILA

INTRODUCTION

Over the last few decades both maternal and perinatal health in Finland have improved greatly, leading to decreased maternal and perinatal mortality and morbidity (1). At the same time, operative interventions in the course of gestation, delivery by different methods, including artificial interruption of early pregnancy, and reliable family planning using various contraceptive means have become common and popular (2). To obtain a more exact picture of the changes in childbirth practice, we performed a retrospective analysis of parturitions in Oulu University Central Hospital district from 1950 through 1982. Special attention was paid to seasonal and diel variations in deliveries because we live in an area with great seasonal variation in day length: the sun shines for 22 hours a day in June, but only for 2 hours in December.

MATERIAL AND METHODS

Data were recorded from 16,949 deliveries in a single area, the Oulu University Central Hospital district, in northern Finland. All deliveries in the years 1950,

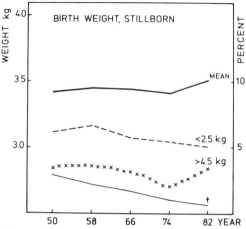

Figure 2. Mean birth weight (solid line) and the percent frequency of stillborns (thin solid line) and newborns weighing 2,500 g or less (dashed line), or 4,500 g or more (dotted line with x-symbols).

1958, 1966, 1974, and 1982 were recorded, the corresponding number of births being 2,786, 3,235, 3,877, 3,246, and 3,885. The data recorded and analyzed by computer included maternal age, parity, and mortality; presentation, weight, and sex of the newborn; stillborns; date and time of delivery; and operative procedures. The significance of the results was tested by Student's t-test and the chi-square test.

RESULTS

Mothers

There were 6 deaths (3 in 1950, 2 in 1966, and 1 in 1974) during the observation years, resulting in a maternal mortality of 2.5 per 10,000 births. Mean maternal age decreased from 28.3 years in 1950 to 25.8 years in 1974 but increased again to 27.5 years in 1982 (Figure 1). At the same time the corresponding figures for mean parity were 2.8, 2.1, and 2.4 (Figure 2). In 1950, 33% of the parturients were primiparas. This percentage increased to 47 (p < 0.01) in 1974 and declined to 38 (p < 0.01) in 1982. At the same time the frequency of grand multiparas (≥ 5 children) decreased from 28% to 6% of the total (p < 0.001).

Newborns

In 1950, 3% of the newborns were stillborn but this percentage declined to only 0.7% in 1982 (p < 0.001) (Figure 3).

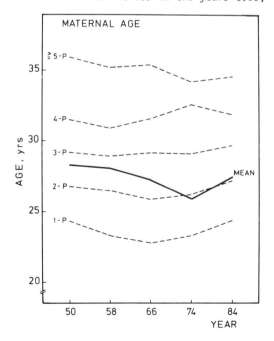

Figure 1. Mean (solid line) and the parity-specific (dotted line) age of the parturients in Oulu district.

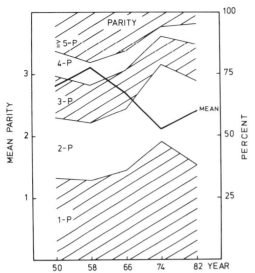

Figure 3. Mean parity and percent distribution of parturients into different parity groups.

The mean birth weight increased from 3,414 g in 1950 to 3,501 g in 1982 (p < 0.01). The frequency of prematurity (birth weight < 2,500 g) decreased from 6.3% to 5.1% (p < 0.001) over the same time. Over the years observed, 51.9% of the newborns were boys and 48.1% girls.

Parturition

The birth rate was about 5% higher from March to August and 5-10% lower from October to February when compared with the mean monthly birth rate (Figure 4). The conception rate was therefore significantly higher (p < 0.01) during the summer than the winter months. This seasonal variation also existed in the period from 1974 to 1982, years of effective family planning.

There was no diel variation of birth rate in the early years of the study period (Figure 5). In 1974 and 1982 the majority of the deliveries took place during the daytime, especially the induced ones.

The frequency of cesarean sections increased greatly in the later years as also did the use of vacuum extraction. Induction of labor peaked in 1974 (33%) but decreased to 8% in 1982. Breech extractions decreased significantly (p < 0.001) and the use of forceps was mimimal all the time (Figure 6).

DISCUSSION

The improvements in maternal and prenatal mortality and morbidity reported here are in accordance with previous reports from Finland (1) and other Scandinavian countries (2). The mean maternal age was fairly constant throughout the study period

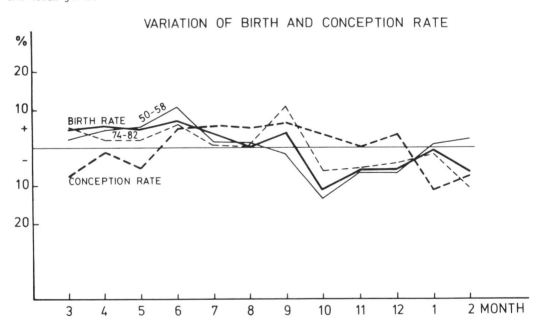

Figure 4. Mean monthly birth (solid line) and conception rate (dashed line) for the whole sample (N=16,949) in the periods 1950-1958 (thin solid line) and 1974-1982 (thin dashed line). The percentage deviations were calculated from the mean monthly birth rate. The length of the months has been accounted for.

but the proportion of primiparas increased and that of multiparas decreased significantly, reflecting the efficacy of family planning. In spite of the increase in the proportion of primiparas, the mean birth weight increased, suggesting improvement in maternal well-being and care over the past three decades. Although the frequency of prematurity decreased, this decline is unsatisfactory if compared with the improvement in the rate of stillborns. A proportion of the improved perinatal results can be attributed to the effective management of pregnancy and delivery. This is counterbalanced by the markedly increased frequency of such operative procedures as artificial rupture of membranes, vacuum extraction, and cesarean section. Nowadays the normal temporal rhythm of deliveries is disturbed and the liberal use of amniotomy and oxytocic agents and frequent interruption of pregnancy by cesarean section have led to an afternoon peak in the birth rate.

Consistent with the findings of other investigators (3,4) we observed a clear seasonal variation in the birth rate, the highest conception rate being in the summer months. A new observation is that, in spite

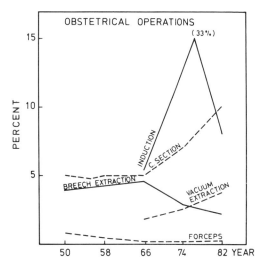

Figure 6. *Percent frequency of different obstetrical intervention in the years from 1950 to 1982. Percentages were calculated from all the annual deliveries.*

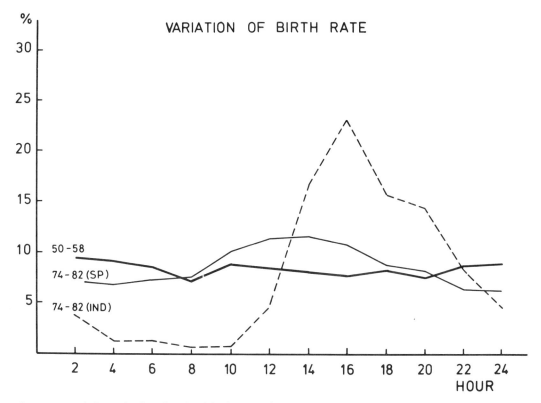

Figure 5. *Diel variation in the birth rate in 1950-1958 (solid line) for the total sample and in 1974-1982 separately for spontaneous delivery (thin line, SP) and for induced delivery (dashed line, IND).*

of the use of seasonal contraceptives, this seasonal variation still prevailed in 1974 and 1982. As has been discussed (4), social factors are perhaps more dominant than biological ones in the regulation of conception and birth seasonality. Our observation may indicate, however, that daylight, acting via pineal gland hormones, affects pituitary-ovarian function so strongly that even in modern communities the day-length related difference in the fertility pattern is not abolished in humans.

REFERENCES

1. Finnish Medical Association: Report of perinatal status in Finland, 1975.
2. Brody S. Obstetrik och gynekologi. Almqvist and Wiksell Förlag AB. Stockholm, 1982.
3. Editorial. Lancet 1974; ii:1235.
4. Leppäluoto J. Seasonal variation of human reproductive functions. Nordic Council Arct Med Res Rep 1983; 36:10-14.

Jukka Puolakka
Department of Obstetrics and Gynecology
University of Oulu
SF-90220 Oulu 22
Finland

SECTION 4. INFECTIOUS DISEASE

Circumpolar Health 84:187-190

COMMUNICABLE DISEASE CONTROL IN THE EARLY HISTORY OF ALASKA I. SMALLPOX

ROBERT FORTUINE

No disease struck more fear into the hearts of men and women of the 18th and 19th centuries than smallpox. In Europe the disease had long been a grim companion, periodically snuffing out the lives or scarring the faces of persons from all walks of life, from beggar children to royalty. Among the more "primitive" peoples of the world, however, smallpox was a terrible angel of death which stalked through households and villages, leaving in its wake few, sometimes mutilated, survivors to tell the tale. There was no defense against such an enemy in their religious beliefs or their healing traditions.

The purpose of this paper is to describe briefly the story of smallpox in 18th and 19th century Alaska, but more particularly to relate the crude but well meant efforts to control the disease undertaken and carried out by officials of the Russian-American Company.

Smallpox probably first appeared in Alaska about 1770, spreading northward from the Stikine River district in southeastern Alaska and causing a high mortality in the Indian villages (1). The disease probably reached Alaska Indians through their regular contact with other Indian tribes of the Northwest coast. Captain Nathaniel Portlock on his trading voyage in 1787 observed several Tlingit with the typical scars of smallpox and speculated, from the ages of the youngest persons affected, that the disease had been introduced into Alaska in 1775 by the Spanish (2), perhaps Perez and Bodega y Quadra who were in Alaska waters that year. The narratives of these voyages, however, make no mention of smallpox either among the crews or among Native peoples, and thus it is more likely once again that the disease spread to the coast through trade channels from the interior. Other 18th century records confirm the presence of the disease as far north as Yakutat Bay (3,4).

As early as 1808, a mere decade after an English rural physician named Edward Jenner had reported his successful experiments in preventing smallpox by the use of a vaccine derived from cowpox, the directors of the Russian-American Company in St. Petersburg sent a supply of the new vaccine to the colonies with instructions for its administration. The officers of the company were told to vaccinate all Russians and as many Natives as possible. Dr. Mordgorst, surgeon on the Imperial Naval Ship *Neva*, was charged with demonstrating the technique and teaching the method to capable employees (5). Among those who learned to vaccinate were the Orthodox missionaries, who seemed to have accepted the responsibility reluctantly (6).

Although the decision to vaccinate was an enlightened one, it no doubt involved a healthy measure of company self-interest, since smallpox was known to cause great devastation and economic loss wherever it struck a population without previous exposure to it. Already in these early years the company had had promising young Creoles (an old term for individuals of mixed Russian and Native parentage), sent to Russia for training, die of the disease while in route to the capital (7).

Despite these good intentions, however, many problems became apparent in the vaccination program. Vaccine was chronically in short supply and what there was of it had often lost its potency on the long sea voyage to Alaska, if indeed it had ever been potent. Methods of administration were not standardized, and poor technique probably contributed to the lack of "take." Few seemed eager to receive the vaccine, least of all the Native peoples who needed it the most.

By 1822, the 200 or so Russians, Creoles, and Aleut hunters at Sitka were finally vaccinated, thanks to the arrival of a large shipment of vaccine from Okhotsk. The following year the chief manager ordered that the employees at all outlying company posts be similarly vaccinated, but vaccine supplies ran out before his task could be completed (8). In October 1828, however, a new shipment of vaccine permitted the feldsher at Kodiak to send his Creole assistant to vaccinate in the outlying villages. By April 1829 over 500 persons in Russian America were vaccinated against smallpox (9). Over the next five or six years, however, new supplies of vaccine were constantly in short supply.

Smallpox broke out in Alaska in the fall of 1835, probably brought overland from the British territories to the east and south. At Tongass, the southern border of the Russian colonies, some 250 died out of a population of 900 (10). The disease appeared at Sitka in November, quickly killing several Aleut hunters there. It raged out of control over the next few months, leaving in its wake 100 dead out of 161 persons who became ill, a case fatality rate of 62% (11). Dr. Edward Blaschke, the chief medical officer at the capital, did his utmost to care for the sick but his ministrations were ineffective. Much more useful was his effort to vaccinate some 200 Russians, Creoles, and Aleuts who had not become sick (12).

Panic was already seizing many of the Tlingit of the surrounding villages as they saw their family members die around them with high fever, utter prostration, and a cruel disfiguring rash. Their own methods of treatment, including the best efforts of their shamans, were totally ineffective. As the disease spread from household to household the survivors abandoned their families, both the sick and the dead, and fled to other villages (13), often carrying with them the virus in the incubation stage. According to the Orthodox missionary Veniaminov, during the months of January and February 1836, some 300 Indians died near the fort, sometimes as many as eight to twelve in a single day (14). By the time the epidemic burned itself out in southeastern Alaska, some 400 Indians but only one European had died (15)--eloquent testimony to the effectiveness of vaccination.

The Tlingit initially refused vaccination, but their own high mortality, the helplessness of their shamans, and the fact that the Russians did not get sick finally persuaded even the skeptics that the Russians possessed a superior technology. Finally, but too late to save many, the Tlingit clamored for vaccination, which was freely given by Dr. Blaschke. This acceptance of Russian ways, incidentally, also marked the beginning of the acceptance by the Tlingit of the teachings of the Orthodox missionaries (16).

At the height of the epidemic in Sitka, Chief Manager Kupreianov recognized that the disease posed a grave threat to the safety and economic stability of the other Russian trading posts. In March 1837 he issued regulations to all captains of company ships requiring them to vaccinate their crew members, air out thoroughly all items taken on board, remain at anchor for two days upon arrival at port, isolate persons with smallpox from the crew, and prohibit crew members from mingling with people on shore (17). Dr. Blaschke was also asked to prepare, for the benefit of all outlying company posts, a set of instructions on how to prevent spread of the disease.

In spite of these precautions, however, smallpox broke out at Kodiak on July 8, 1837, although the news did not get back to Sitka until the end of August. Fearing the worst, Kupreianov dispatched Dr. Volynskii to Kodiak, together with two feldshers, Kalugin and Zykov, who were to vaccinate the Natives in the outlying villages of the island. By the time the team reached Kodiak in October, however, some 265 Koniags had already died. Despite the best efforts of the medical team a total of 736 persons, nearly one-third of the population, had perished before the epidemic died out there in January 1838 (18,19). Factors contributing to this high mortality included the unwillingness of the Koniags to accept vaccination, their continued reliance on their own shamans, the lateness of the vaccination effort, and the doubtful quality of the vaccine itself (20).

Kupreianov sent Dr. Blaschke himself to try to prevent a similar disaster in the Unalaska District. Sailing on the ship *Polyfem*, the doctor arrived at Unalaska May 28, 1838, armed with strict instructions from the chief manager to company officials to see that the Aleuts cooperated. By the end of the summer Blaschke had vaccinated 1,086 Aleuts, of whom only five later succumbed to smallpox. Among the unvaccinated, some 129 died of smallpox when the disease struck in August (21).

Meanwhile, the feldsher Galaktion was instructed to vaccinate the people of the Atka District, but his program was delayed pending the arrival of a new supply of vaccine from Kamchatka. Father Netsvetov, a Creole missionary stationed there, was specifically requested by the chief manager to encourage his flock to accept vaccination (22). It is uncertain whether the Atka Aleuts were ever afflicted during the epidemic or indeed whether they even became vaccinated at all until some years later. A smallpox outbreak is not mentioned in Netsvetov's detailed diary of those years.

The vaccination campaign also extended northward from Kodiak to the Alaska Peninsula, Cook Inlet, Prince William Sound, Bristol Bay, and even the shores of Norton Sound. On the peninsula, a company foreman named Kostylev succeeded in vaccinating some 243 persons, despite resistance, and in his district only 27 persons died of smallpox, all of them unvaccinated (23). In Bristol Bay the vaccination effort was too late, despite the best efforts of Surgeon's Apprentice Fomin who labored there from February 1835 through the following year. Some 522 smallpox deaths were reported from Alexandrov Redoubt (Nushagak) and Kuskokwim Territory (24). The people of Cook Inlet and Prince William Sound resisted all efforts to vaccinate them and consequently mortality there was also very high (25).

The vaccinators also encountered resistance in the Yukon-Kuskokwim valley, with a consequent mortality as high as 36%, according to one account (26). An example of open hostility occurred when a dozen Eskimos from the lower Kuskokwim travelled across to the Yukon and burned the Russian post at Ikogmiut (Russian Mission), apparently in retaliation for what they thought was the deliberate introduction of the disease among them (27). When Lt. Zagoskin travelled through these parts a few years after the epidemic he found many recently abandoned village sites, the survivors of the disease having pulled up stakes and consolidated with the remnants of other villages (28).

At St. Michael Redoubt, the principal Russian post in the North, the employees of the company were vaccinated but the Eskimos of the surrounding district for the most part refused, from suspicion of the Russians' motives. Mortality was predictably high near the fort. A populous Eskimo village on St. Michael Island was reduced to only 19 persons by the time of Zagoskin's visit in 1842. The epidemic also reaped a grim harvest along the southern coast of Norton Sound and in the area around Unalakleet (29). From here it spread to the Athapaskan Indian villages along the Yukon and its tributaries as far upriver as Nulato (30). The epidemic seems to have burned itself out in 1840.

The consequences of this devastating epidemic were far-reaching. The true death toll cannot be known, but it was estimated by contemporary witnesses to have been one-third to one-half of the Native population. Many died of starvation in the years following the outbreak because of the loss of hunter husbands, sons, and brothers. Others died of intercurrent disease, such as tuberculosis, because of their weakened state. The survivors lost faith in their religion, their culture, and their future.

In the aftermath of this terrible destruction of life, the Russian-American Company mounted a regular vaccination program to prevent a recurrence. During the administration of Chief Manager Etolin (1840-45) some 1,200 vaccinations were performed at Sitka alone (31). Vaccinations were also carried out regularly at Kodiak, where the population now enthusiastically received them, and at all the other principal outposts of the company as far away as St. Michael. By 1845 Dr. Romanowsky felt that the colonies were "with certainty" protected from the threat of smallpox (32). In truth, there could have been few persons remaining who had not either been vaccinated or had not recovered from the disease itself. As the adult population became solidly immunized, the emphasis on vaccination properly shifted to the children (33).

During the later years of the Russian-American Company the task of keeping the vaccinations current fell to the feldshers, their assistants, and in some cases to priests and store managers at the smaller posts. Such individuals performed the job grudgingly, sometimes keeping poor records or grumbling to their superiors that vaccination responsibilities interfered with their regular work (34,35). In 1859 Chief Manager Furuhjelm took a doctor with him to vaccinate on his initial inspection tour of the colonies, presumably because the program of regular immunization was beginning to falter (36).

Smallpox appeared again in southeastern Alaska in 1862, apparently spreading northward once more from the British possessions to the south. Sitka was spared because of the relatively high immunity of its people, but the disease exacted a heavy toll among the British Columbia Indians (37).

After the sale of Alaska to the United States in 1867, the policy of regular vaccinations was allowed to lapse. There is no indication that the Army, the Navy, or the civil government ever undertook any effort to vaccinate the population against a disease that had already demonstrated its appalling capacity for destruction.

Smallpox did return, almost inevitably, but did not gain a foothold again in Alaska until June of 1900, during the peak of the Nome Gold Rush. Curiously, the epidemic was quickly brought under control by means of a strict policy of ships' quarantine, without the use of vaccination for susceptibles (38).

Smallpox was probably the single most destructive force in the 19th century Alaskan history. In a five-year period, the disease demonstrated its awesome power by sharply reducing the entire Native population living in contact with the Russians and probably extending far beyond into the little-known interior. The impact of this disaster on the Native peoples and their cultures will never be fully known, but certainly life and beliefs were never the same in the wake of the epidemic.

Perhaps the only positive aspect of this great human tragedy was the effort to prevent, or at least slow down, the inexorable sweep of the epidemic by the use of vaccination--the same method which in our own day has succeeded in eradicating the scourge of smallpox from the world. The officials of the Russian-American Company who conceived, organized, and carried out this program of vaccinating the population over a period of nearly six decades and despite resistance and overwhelming logistical problems deserve recognition as public health pioneers.

REFERENCES

1. Khlebnikov KT. Colonial Russian America. Kyrill T. Khlebnikov's reports 1817-1832. Dmytryshyn B, Crownhart-Vaughan EAP, trans. Portland: Oregon Historical Society, 1976:29.
2. Portlock N. A voyage round the world: but more particularly to the north-west coast of America: performed in 1785, 1786, 1787, and 1788, in the King George and Queen Charlotte. Captains Portlock and Dixon. 1789. Reprint. Amsterdam: N. Israel/New York: Da Capo Press, 1968:271.
3. Fleurieu CPC. A voyage round the world performed during the years 1790, 1791, and 1792, by Etienne Marchand. 2 vol. 1801. Reprint. Amsterdam: N Israel/New York: Da Capo, 1969: 2: 271.

4. Bancroft HH. History of Alaska 1730-1885. 1886. Reprint. New York: Antiquarian Press Ltd, 1959:350.
5. Tikhmenov PA. A history of the Russian-American Company 1861-63. Pierce RA, Donnelly AS, trans and eds. Seattle and London: Univ. Washington Press, 1978:161-2.
6. Documents relative to the history of Alaska. Alaska History Research Project 1936-38. College: Univ Alaska, 1936-38. 15 vol. 4:169.
7. Ibid:142.
8. Sarafian WL. Russian American Company employee policies and practices 1799-1867. PhD Dissertation. Los Angeles: Univ California, 1971:297.
9. Sarafian WL. Smallpox strikes the Aleuts. Alaska Journal 1977; 7:46-49.
10. Bancroft, op cit:560.
11. Sarafian op cit, 1971:199.
12. Ibid.
13. Belcher E, Simpkinson FG. H.M.S. Sulphur on the northwest and California coasts, 1837 and 1839. Pierce RA, Winslow JA, eds. Kingston, Ont: Limestone Press, 1977:22.
14. Veniaminov I. The condition of the Orthodox Church in Russian America. Nichols R, Croskey R, trans and eds. Pacific Northwest Quarterly 1972; 63(2):41-54.
15. Tikhmenov, op cit:198.
16. Veniaminov, op cit:47-48.
17. Sarafian 1977, op cit:48.
18. Ibid.
19. Veniaminov, op cit:49.
20. Sarafian 1977, op cit:48.
21. Sarafian 1971, op cit:202.
22. Netsvetov I. The journals of Iakov Netsvetov: The Atkha years. 1828-1844. Black L, trans. Kingston, Ont: Limestone Press, 1980:163-164, 176.
23. Tikhmenov, op cit:199.
24. VanStone JW. Ingalik contact ecology: An ethnohistory of the lower and middle Yukon, 1790-1835. Fieldiana: Anthropology 1979; 71:58-59.
25. Bancroft, op cit:562 f.n.
26. Oswalt WH, VanStone JW. The ethnoarcheology of Crow Village, Alaska. Smithsonian Institution, Bureau of American Ethnology. Bull 199. Washington: Government Printing Office, 1967:80-81.
27. Oswalt WH. Kolmakovskiy Redoubt. The ethnoarcheology of a Russian fort in Alaska. Los Angeles: Institute of Archeology, Univ California, 1980:12.
28. Zagoskin LA. Lieutenant Zagoskin's travels in Russian America, 1842-44. The first ethnographic and geographic investigations in the Yukon and Kuskokwim valleys of Alaska. Michael HN, ed. Arctic Institute of North America. Toronto: Univ Toronto Press, 1967:204, 281.
29. Ibid:100, 92.
30. Ibid:147.
31. Tikhmenov, op cit:371.
32. Romanowsky A. Five years of medical observations in the colonies of the Russian American Company. Part I. Alaska Med 1962; 4:33-37.
33. Frankenhauser A. Five years of medical observations in the colonies of the Russian American Company. Part II. Alaska Med 1962; 4:62-64.
34. Golovnin PN. The end of Russian America. Captain P.N. Golovnin's last report 1862. Dmytryshyn B, Crownhart-Vaughan EAP, trans. Portland: Oregon Historical Society, 1979:63.
35. Documents relative to the history of Alaska, (see ref. 6) 2:57.
36. Tikhmenov, op cit:371.
37. Arctander JW. The apostle of Alaska: The story of William Duncan of Metlakatla. Fleming H Revell Co, 1909:155-6, 38.
38. White JT. Report of the Medical Officer of the U.S. Steamer Nunivak, Yukon River, Alaska. In: Cantwell JC. Report of the operations of the U.S. Revenue Steamer Nunivak on the Yukon River Station Alaska, 1899-1901. Washington: Government Printing Office, 1902:257-8.

Robert Fortuine
1615 Stanton Avenue
Anchorage, Alaska 99508
U.S.A.

Circumpolar Health 84: 191-194

COMMUNICABLE DISEASE CONTROL IN THE EARLY HISTORY OF ALASKA II. SYPHILIS

ROBERT FORTUINE

During the 18th and early 19th centuries syphilis became a serious plague in Alaska not only among the Alaska Native peoples but also among the Europeans who lived in or visited the territory. The disease was chronic and conspicuous, often manifested by indolent skin ulcers and crippling lesions of the extremities, or in chronic untreated cases by heart disease and insanity. Syphilis was also not infrequently transmitted *in utero*, leaving in the infant tragic stigmata such as blindness, crippling bone lesions, and facial deformity.

The disease was almost certainly introduced into Alaska from outside, although at different times and on multiple occasions. It was probably first brought to the Aleutian islands by Russian fur traders in the mid-18th century, for by the time of Captain Cook's third voyage in 1778, venereal disease, presumably syphilis, was well established in the Aleut population of Unalaska (1,2). Only Russian ships had been to this area before those of Cook. The Orthodox missionary Father Veniaminov felt certain that syphilis was the "gift of the Russians." The disease, he said, spread widely among the Aleuts, reaching a peak about 1798, at which time whole families were affected. Thereafter it declined rapidly for reasons that remain obscure (3).

Syphilis was already present on Kodiak Island in the mid-1780s and indeed was the only communicable disease observed there by the trader Shelikhov (4). It was again probably introduced by the Russian fur hunters, who had recently expanded their operations to Kodiak. The disease spread rapidly through the island, and by the early 1800s was among the commonest afflictions of the Native people there (5). Although it continued to be a problem, syphilis apparently declined somewhat in prevalence over the next few decades until about 1840, when a flare-up occurred.

The disease did not become established in southeastern Alaska until the early 1800s (6), probably during the first years of Russian fur trading there, and soon was very common in the capital at New Archangel, or Sitka. In 1818 the Russian official Golovnin expressed his view that the Russian American Company employees acquired it from the Tlingit Indians, who, he believed, had become infected by the crews of foreign ships, especially from New England, that were illegally trading in the archipelago (7). The sailors in turn had probably become infected in the Pacific islands, where the disease was then raging out of control (8). Although the Yankee traders no

doubt contributed their share to the spread of the disease, the Russian settlement itself was also a significant source of infection, since the class of persons employed by the company at this time was not known for its standard of morality. Indeed, Zagoskin in 1844 remarked that since the chief manager in those earlier years, Alexander Baranov, was a bachelor, he was "obliged to permit his subordinates free reign with Indian and Aleut women" (9).

By the 1840s syphilis had spread to Prince William Sound (10) and to the company posts in Cook Inlet (11,12), Bristol Bay, and even Norton Sound (13). The Yukon-Kuskokwim area seems to have been spared, perhaps because the vast area was difficult to reach except on foot or in small boats.

As early as 1831 Baron von Wrangell became convinced that the decline of the Native population at Kodiak due to disease was one of the main reasons for the company's lack of profits there. He accordingly sent Dr. Gregorii Meier from Sitka to oversee the removal of sick Natives (particularly those with venereal disease) from their villages to the hospital at Kodiak. Wrangell considered venereal disease to be widespread at this time on the island and that there would be "disastrous consequences" if the situation was not promptly brought under control (13). About a decade later a doctor was sent to the company post at Nuchek, in Prince William Sound, to round up cases of syphilis among the Chugaches and send them to Kodiak for treatment (14).

By the 1840s, syphilis was alarmingly prevalent in and around the principal posts of the Russian American Company in New Archangel and Kodiak. Not only were many of the Russian employees infected but also the mixed-blood Creoles and Natives of the surrounding countryside. Attempts to control the disease were fruitless since it was continually being reintroduced by infected Native women, and by the crewmen of visiting, usually foreign, ships. The seriousness of this situation moved the medical department of the company to undertake an organized program of control. Our principal source of information on this subject is Dr. Romanowsky, a Russian staff physician based at Sitka in the early 1840s (15).

In the capital, beginning in 1822, the company had permitted about 700 Tlingits to settle near the northwestern wall of the redoubt, principally in order to be able to keep a closer watch on them. These Indians had daily interactions with the Russians and Creoles at the fort, trading in foodstuffs and other commodities. These regular commercial relations almost inevitably led to a more personal type of relationship and before long a number of Russians were consorting with some of the Tlingit women, especially a group who lived year round in the woods near the fort. Virtually all of these women engaging in what the doctor called "clandestine debauchery" ultimately became infected with syphilis and were thus a vital link in the chain of infection at the fort (16). The women for their part treated the disease with indifference, considering it a necessary evil in their line of work (17).

The authorities tried various unsuccessful means of coping with the problem but finally hit on the idea of capture and enforced treatment of the women. The chief manager at Sitka issued the necessary orders in 1842, apparently after consultation with the Tlingit elders. These latter had a special stake in the matter, since at least some of the infected women were their slaves and household consorts. Over the next few years many Indian women were captured by the Russian soldiers and brought to the fort for examination. In 1845, for example, some 70 women were rounded up, of whom 33 were found to be syphilitic and confined in a special section of the hospital until they were rendered non-infectious. The treatment method used, incidentally, involved the ingestion, external application, or inhalation of mercury in some form (18). After the full course of treatment the women were discharged and allowed to return to their homes (19).

These measures, although helpful, had definite limitations. The Tlingit were a proud and independent people who resisted the imposition of outside authority. Tlingit women, whether slave or free, avoided treatment and hid from the soldiers whenever possible. Moreover, the leaders themselves came to resent the enforced treatment of their women and often insisted on their return to the village before therapy was completed. They believed that the disease in any event was a manifestation of sorcery and should be treated by their own shamans. Another factor limiting success of the program was that the Indians were engaged in considerable trade with neighboring tribes, thus ensuring that the disease was being recycled. Infected slaves were one item of commerce.

In spite of all these limitations, however, Romanowsky noted that after several years the program enjoyed some measure of success, as the Tlingit began to see the more effective means of treatment proffered by the Russians and the value of keeping on good terms with them for purposes of trade and employment at the fort.

Meanwhile, the situation with respect to syphilis was also a source of concern at the company's second major post at Kodiak.

The chief manager temporarily assigned Dr. Romanowsky there in the early 1840s to deal with the mounting problem. According to his report, the doctor examined all the people of Kodiak Island and sent the infected ones to the hospital at Kodiak for enforced treatment. These measures (only partially successful at Sitka) were fully effective at Kodiak because there was less opportunity for the disease to be re-introduced from outside, as Kodiak at this time was off limits to ships other than those of the Russian American Company. All ships clearing for Kodiak from the capital or other company posts were required to have their crew certified free from syphilis both before departure and again before landing (20).

A few years later another medical officer at the capital, Dr. Frankenhauser, complained that syphilis could not be eradicated at Sitka under the system of enforced treatment because the policy could not be effectively carried out. Among the Russians only the men were infected, yet even if they were all treated the disease continued to be propagated by the women of the forest, who were often successfully evading treatment, or by the influx of new cases from other villages being visited by ships carrying on illicit trade in the Russian territories. Despite the setbacks, however, he acknowledged that the program was producing some results, the number of syphilitic men at the fort falling from 62 in 1842 to only 24 in 1843 (21).

These measures must have lapsed somewhat over the next decade and a half, however, for when Chief Manager Furuhjelm arrived in the colonies in 1859, syphilis had again gotten out of hand at the capital. As a first step toward control he ordered the destruction of all the huts near the fort which were being used for illicit relations, then had a special building constructed near Lake Lebiazhe and posted a sentry on top. Infected women were once again sought out, rounded up, and brought to the hospital for enforced treatment. The women of course resented their confinement and usually managed to escape to the village after a few days, where they were difficult to locate again. The chief manager then solemnly proclaimed that any woman who ran away from the infirmary before her treatment was finished would, if caught, have half her head shaved, a punishment which the Tlingit found most humiliating. Once they learned that Furuhjelm meant business in this regard the women began to cooperate, the more so when they began to appreciate that the mercury treatments were indeed effective (22).

The continual problem at Sitka was of course not solely the responsibility of the women, for many of the soldiers, workmen, and probably the officers as well were infected. Despite the best efforts of the priests to discourage sexual liaisons with the Indian women, such relationships were widespread. Those with enough money purchased uninfected Indian slaves as mistresses, but the rank and file still depended on casual unions with the women of the forest and thus often became infected themselves. Some even seemed to welcome infection so that they could escape the daily round of hard work and lie at ease in the hospital. The chief manager effectively dealt with this attitude by docking the pay of a worker while under treatment for syphilis.

Finally, by a combination of enforced treatment of the Indian women and a stricter enforcement of company rules among the Russians, syphilis began to decline once more toward the end of the Russian administration (23).

The change of government from that of Imperial Russia to that of the United States in 1867 led not only to lost ground in control efforts but to many opportunities for fresh introduction of the disease, as hundreds of tough, battle-weary Civil War veterans were assigned to army garrisons in Sitka, Kodiak, Unalaska, and other posts.

In Sitka, the Army assistant inspector general blamed the renewed spread of syphilis on the Indian women, piously noting that "no one ... could believe that they were corrupted by the troops" (24). The Army's senior medical officer, nevertheless, felt that it was a serious mistake to station troops among the Indians, since they "mutually debauch[ed] each other" (25). Many records of this period describe the licentiousness, immorality, and drunkenness of the soldiers who were assigned to Alaska to keep the peace (26-28). In effect, the Russians blamed the American soldiers for the resurgence of the disease, the soldiers blamed the women, visitors blamed the previous Russian administration, and the missionaries blamed everyone. When the Army left Alaska in 1877, the Navy took its place and bore its own share of responsibility for the problem. The situation improved under civil rule, beginning in 1884, but by then a new element of lawlessness represented by miners and prospectors contributed to the persistence and spread of syphilis (29). By the late 1880s "hereditary diseases" (a polite name for syphilis at this time) were "frightfully prevalent", according to a medical survey commissioned by the governor (30).

In the Aleutians and on Kodiak Island syphilis was "almost non-existent" by the end of the Russian administration (31). Within 20 years, however, Dr. Robert White of the U.S. Revenue Marine Service found a "marked prevalence" of venereal diseases in all forms in the Aleutians, due, as he thought, to the large numbers of Caucasians fishing in the region (32). A similar situation prevailed in certain Kodiak villages (33).

Although of less importance for this paper, it might be noted here that syphilis also spread widely in northern Alaska during the latter third of the 19th century, in large measure because of the influx of American ships which overwintered or established shore stations for processing whale carcasses. Somewhat later, syphilis was introduced to communities of the interior by the countless prospectors and gold-seekers who overran northwestern Alaska in the last few years of the century.

Thus, syphilis had become by the beginning of the 20th century a chronic disease of considerable importance to many of the people of Alaska. Though rarely fatal by itself, it caused crippling, large unsightly skin ulcers, and other forms of disability. Congenital syphilis was rampant as well, leading to cruel deformities and disabilities, such as blindness, among the children.

This grim disease was introduced repeatedly into the Native population by people of many nationalities, following almost inevitably the intimate liaisons that occur in the wake of overwhelming cultural invasions. Once established in the Native population, the disease became endemic throughout whole communities, often spreading further afield by trade or warfare.

Very little was known about the control of this noxious plague in the 18th and 19th centuries because modern methods of sexually transmitted disease control, such as the identification, isolation, treatment, and follow-up of cases, plus contact investigation and treatment, were yet to be developed. Prevention of diseases by planned community action was then a novel concept, not to reach fruition for a long time.

In this setting it is therefore all the more remarkable that officials of the Russian American Company in the first half of the 19th century recognized syphilis as a health problem, gauged its impact, identified its possible causes, and took community action consistent with contemporary scientific knowledge to combat the problem. These efforts, moreover, were effective in controlling if not eradicating the disease in the population. That the measures taken were a bit draconian should not divert us from the fact that they worked reasonably well as long as they were in force, and they were no different in principle from measures used in our time for the control of tuberculosis and other hazards to the public health.

REFERENCES

1. Cook J. The journals of Captain James Cook on his voyages of discovery. 3 vol. Beaglehole JC, ed. Cambridge: The Hakluyt Society, 1967. The voyage of the Resolution and Discovery 1776-1780. 3(1):468.
2. Ibid, 1144.
3. In: Hrdlicka A. The Aleutian and Commander Islands and their inhabitants. Philadelphia: Wistar Institute of Anatomy and Biology, 1945:172.
4. Shelikhov GI. A voyage to America 1783-1786. Pierce RA, trans. Kingston, Ont: Limestone Press, 1981:55.
5. Lisianski U. A voyage round the world in the years 1803, 4, 5, and 6; performed by order of his Imperial Majesty Alexander the First, Emperor of Russia, in the ship Neva. London: John Booth, Longman, Hurst, Rees, Orme and Brown, 1814:201.
6. Tikhmenov PA. A history of the Russian American Company (1861-63). Pierce RA, Donnelly AS, trans and eds. Seattle and London: Univ Washington Press, 1978:83.
7. In: Bancroft HH. History of Alaska 1730-1885. 1886. Reprint. New York: Antiquarian Press, Ltd, 1959:712 f.n.
8. Romanowsky A. Five years of medical observations in the colonies of the Russian-American Company. Part I. Alaska Med 1962; 4:33-37.
9. Zagoskin LA. Lieutenant Zagoskin's travels in Russian America, 1842-1844. Michael HN, ed. Arctic Institute of North America. Toronto: Univ Toronto Press, 1967:68.
10. Romanowsky, op. cit.
11. Tikhmenov, op cit:83.
12. Zagoskin, op cit:110.
13. Sarafian WL. Russian-American Company employee policies and practices 1700-1867. PhD dissertation. Los Angeles: Univ California.
14. Romanowsky, op cit.
15. Ibid.
16. Ibid.
17. Golovnin PN. The end of Russian America. Captain P.N. Golovnin's last report 1862. Dmytryshyn B, Crownhart-Vaughan EAP, trans. Portland: Oregon Historical Society, 1979:64.
18. Romanowksy, op cit.
19. Romanowsky, op cit.
20. Ibid.
21. Frankenhauser [A]. Five years of medical observations in the colonies of the Russian-American Company. Part II. Alaska Med 1962; 4:62-64.
22. Golovnin, op cit:64.
23. Ibid.
24. U.S. Army Alaska. Building Alaska with the U.S. Army 1967-1962. Pamphlet No. 35505. Anchorage, 1962:20.
25. Colyer V. Report of the Hon. Vincent Colyer, United States Special Indian Commissioner. In: Report of the Secretary of the Interior. Washington: Government Printing Office, 1869:1023-4.
26. Bancroft, op cit:606-607.
27. Morris W.G. Report upon the Customs District, public service and resources of Alaska Territory. Washington: Government Printing Office, 1879:62.
28. Teichmann E. A journey to Alaska in the year 1868 being a diary of the late Emil Teichmann. Teichmann O, ed. New York: Argosy-Antiquarian Ltd, 1963: 187.
29. Morris, op cit:62.
30. U.S. Department of the Interior. Report of the Governor of Alaska for the fiscal year 1889. Washington: Government Printing Office, 1889:21.
31. Golovnin, op cit:63.
32. White R. Notes on the physical condition of the inhabitants of Alaska. In: Bailey GW. Report on Alaska and its people. Washington: Government Printing Office, 1880:39-40.
33. Shalamov T. Travel journal of Priest Tikhon Shalamov. In: Documents relative to the history of Alaska. Alaska History Research Project. College, 1936-38. 15 volumes. 2:87.

Robert Fortuine
1615 Stanton Avenue
Anchorage, Alaska 99508
U.S.A.

Circumpolar Health 84:195-198

PERSISTENT VIRUS INFECTIONS IN THE ARCTIC

PETER SKINHØJ

Three years ago in Copenhagen, Professor C.E. Albrecht outlined some of the successful campaigns against infectious diseases in the circumpolar area as well as expected forthcoming achievements in this field (1). I will focus here on some infectious disease problems which may still be with us beyond the year 2000, the year of Health for All.

Our improvements during the past have been due to four main principles: better standards of living (hygiene, nutrition), immunization, chemotherapy, and quarantine.

Some diseases are highly susceptible to several of these measures, e.g. tuberculosis, but nevertheless this disease remains a considerable problem in such circumpolar areas as Greenland (2). The reason for this is that tuberculosis is a chronic infection which may become reactivated and transmissible years after the primary infection.

Chronicity is a principal strategy for microbial survival in sparsely populated areas with small communities. Table 1 depicts the main mechanisms for perpetuation of microorganisms. Basically, either the isolation barrier or the individual immune system is insufficient.

Dealing with isolation first, I find it is indeed an effective barrier to many agents. Black et al. in a study of isolated jungle Indians obtained a clear serological distinction between those few microorganisms which had reached and survived in such populations and those which could not (3). However, the highly communicable diseases such as measles, mumps, or rubella are hard to keep out for long periods and when they are introduced into largely susceptible populations, disastrous outbreaks may take place. Under conditions of crowded living

and poor hygiene, even less contagious agents may lead to such outbreaks as was recently observed with hepatitis A in Greenland (4). Non-human reservoirs are essential for the maintenance of many infectious diseases in the tropics but are less important in the north, notable exceptions being trichinosis, tularemia, rabies, and tetanus.

Maintenance of infections, because of deficiency within the immune defenses, involves some of the more serious present and future health problems.

A high frequency of re-infections may obviously maintain an agent even within a small population. The principal example in Greenland is gonorrhoea, which continues to be a health problem in spite of its susceptibility to ordinary penicillin (2). An example among the chronic infections is tuberculosis, mentioned above. In what follows, I will concentrate on viral infections.

Much interest has been shown in hepatitis B, which tends to cause chronic infection if the infection occurs early in life or in an immunocompromised host.

It is well documented that HBV is present in all circumpolar populations, although considerable differences exist from one village to another regarding the prevalence rate of HBsAg (0-25%) as well as HBeAg positivity (5-7) (Table 2).

An important point in the understanding of hepatitis B infection is that the presence of HBsAg is not a static phenomenon: 1-2% of carriers turn negative each year and most will become negative for HBeAg well before this event. The duration of the carrier state may be under genetic control and seems to vary from location to location. Most important is the HBeAg status of women in childbearing age; if such a woman is still HBeAg positive following prior infection, vertical infection to the newborn occurs, resulting in chronic infection in the neonate. Otherwise, the virus is

Table 1. *Maintenance of microorganisms in isolated small populations.*

General problems	Mechanisms	Examples
Isolation insufficiency	Importation	Measles, hepatitis A
	Non-human reservoir	Rabies, bunyaviruses
Immune insufficiency	Reinfection	Gonorrhoea
	Chronic infection	Tuberculosis, hepatitis B

Table 2. *Hepatitis B infection in Eskimo populations.*

Area		No. studied	HBsAg prevalence rate	HBeAg positive fraction
Alaska	1974	3,053	6.4%	69%
Canada	1979	671	4.2%	0
Greenland	1965	1,450	11.4%	24%

dependent on horizontal transmission among children or adults. Relevant data on this point are essential for the planning of vaccination campaigns (Table 3).

A second problem in the evaluation of the hepatitis B problem is the presence of cohort phenomena. In a Canadian study the prevalence of HBsAg and antibodies increased by age after 20 years of age (5). This increase may indicate that infection takes place among adults, but may also indicate that early childhood infections stopped 20 years ago. Similar data were obtained in Greenland (8). When the results are compared to those from sera obtained 10 to 15 years ago showing a high number of HBsAg positive children, we must conclude that a cohort effect is indeed present and that this infection without specific measurements is in a significant retreat. Such data are also important before vaccination is initiated.

The third point on the management of hepatitis B concerns the clinical morbidity and mortality caused by this infection. Beside clinical hepatitis, which may increase in incidence as childhood infections and immunity decrease, severe cases of vasculitis or polyarteritis may occur (9). Most HBsAg carriers are, however, healthy and according to a small number of biopsy-studied cases, only low grade inflammatory lesions are found in the liver.

Sudden exacerbation of clinical manifestations in such carriers has recently been found to be due to superinfection with the delta-agent, a small incomplete virus consisting of an RNA fragment (10). This agent can only infect HBsAG positive individuals; it apparently requires HBsAG for its existence. Transmitted parenterally, it is mainly found in drug addicts or Italians. In a study of Greenlanders we were able to identify one case with antibody to the delta-agent among 105 individuals studied.

A chronic sequela of HBV infection is cirrhosis. Strangely enough, we have been unable to detect any increased mortality from cirrhosis in Greenland in spite of the high HBsAg prevalence rate (11). More important, however, is the carcinogenic effect of HBV. Patients with persistent infection carry a risk of primary hepatocellular carcinoma(PHC) of up to 400 times that of non-carriers (12).

In contrast to these data, however, we were unable to find any increased rate of PHC in Greenland compared to Denmark where HBV is a negligible problem (11). To try to verify such unexpected results, we have recently extended our observation period by a further 6 years, but over a total of 22 years have identified only 7 cases of PHC (8). Compared to expected rates for Taiwan or even Alaska an unexplained number of cases are missing in Greenland. In Alaska, however, the rate of PHC also varies, since a few villages account for a high proportion of all cases (13). Thus, it must be stressed that with respect to carcinogenicity as well the pattern of HBV infection is extremely variable even within the populations living in the circumpolar areas. Therefore, we can at present make no overall judgment on the need for large-scale vaccination. In Greenland I would not consider it appropriate.

Leaving HBV infection, I will now turn to the herpes virus group. They have a greater capacity to induce chronic infection, typically latent, with clinically overt reactivations, for example, zoster and herpes labialis, or inapparent viral excretion, as cytomegaloviruria in pregnancy or intermittent Ebstein-Barr virus (EBV) in saliva. Due to these characteristics they have no trouble maintaining themselves even in small circumpolar settlements.

In collaboration with Dr. Ebbesen's group in Arhus, we have studied age-specific infection rates by these agents in Greenland and compared them with similar rates in Danish children (8).

Table 3. *HBeAg in HBsAg carriers in Greenland.*

Area	Age group	No. studies	HBeAg No. (%)	Anti-HBe No. (%)
West coast	10-19	9	1 (11)	7 (78)
	20+	18	0	17 (94)
East coast	10-19	15	12 (80)	3 (20)
	20+	20	2 (10)	14 (70)
Total		62	15 (24)	41 (66)

Table 4. *Primary hepatocellular carcinoma (PHC) and hepatitis B infection in Greenland.*

Incidence/Population	Number
Male Eskimo population	20,000
Adult male HBsAg carriers (11.5%)	1,500
PHC observed 1960-81	7
PHC expected I. (Taiwan: 4/1,000 HBsAG carrier/year)	132
PHC expected II. (Alaska: 11.2/100,000 population/year)	49

For herpes simplex (SV) and cytomegalovirus (CMV), identical patterns are seen. Acquisition of antibody occurs in more than 75% within the first 5 to 6 years of age. These viruses are obviously more efficiently circulated in Greenland than in Denmark.

EBV appears even more adapted to this Greenlandic community, 75% being infected by one year of age and all by 3 years--leaving practically no susceptibles for adult infection with its clinical manifestation of mononucleosis. On the other hand, in temperate areas with a high standard of living, 75% are already infected before puberty.

Similar figures for Varicella-zoster virus (VZV) infection were not available, but according to other studies zoster eruptions will be regular sources of virus for maintenance of chicken pox. A fairly constant number of cases in Greenland each year confirms that a stable endemicity exists (2).

The clinical problems with these persistent viruses are generally moderate in this part of the world. The stable relation with the host population prevents potentially serious primary infections in the adults.

The more important point, as in the case of hepatitis B, is the relationship of these viruses to malignancies. Others have dealt with this subject at greater length, but here I would like to point out the high rates of EBV-associated cancers; namely, nasopharyngeal and salivary gland carcinoma, which are present in Greenland. The differences in these cancer rates compared to those from Denmark are, however, larger than the difference, in crude infection rates of EBV between Greenland and Denmark, can account for (8).

The relationship of HSV infection to cervical carcinoma is controversial, but in comparing the incidence rate of cancer to the infection rate of HSV, a two-fold higher rate of cervical carcinoma in Greenland than in Denmark is epidemiologically in accordance with this theory. Kaposi's sarcoma may be associated with CMV infection. No case had been found in Greenland in recent years, and the present epidemic of acquired immune deficiency syndrome (AIDS) has not spread to Greenland.

In conclusion, I would like to emphasize that much has been achieved in the control of infectious diseases in the circumpolar area. These achievements have been possible mainly through intelligent use by the local health care workers of often limited resources. The infectious disease problems that are still with us are nevertheless complex, as in the case of persistent viruses. A number of studies in the fields of epidemiology and molecular biology are still needed before these disorders can be properly dealt with.

REFERENCES

1. Albrecht CE. The eradication of infectious diseases in the Arctic. In: Harvald B, Hart Hansen JP, eds. Circumpolar Health 81. Nordic Council for Arct Med Res Rep 1982; 33:381-384.

2. The state of health in Greenland. Annual Report from the Chief Medical Officer in Greenland for the years 1979-1982.

3. Black FL, Hierholzer WJ, Pinheiro FP, Evans AS, Woodall JP, Opton EM, Emmons JE, West BS, Edsall G, Downs WG, Wallace GD. Evidence for persistence of infectious agents in isolated human populations. Amer J Epidemiol 1974; 100:230-250.

4. Skinhøj P, Mikkelsen F, Blaine Hollinger F. Hepatitis A in Greenland: Importance of specific antibody testing in epidemiologic surveillance. Amer J Epidemiol 1977; 105:140-147.

5. Minuk GY, Nicolle LE, Postl B, Waggoner JG, Hoofnagle JH. Hepatitis A and B virus infection in an isolated Canadian Inuit settlement. In: Harvald B, Hart Hansen JP, eds. Circumpolar Health 81. Nordic Council for Arct Med Res Rep 1982; 33:407-409.

6. Schreeder MT, Bender TR, McMahon BJ, Moser MR, Murphy BL, Sheller MJ, Heyward WL, Hall DB, Maynard JE. Prevalence of hepatitis B in selected Alaskan Eskimo villages. Amer J Epidemiol 1983; 118:543-549.

7. Skinhøj P. Hepatitis and hepatitis B-antigen in Greenland. II: Occurrence and interrelation of hepatitis B associated surface, core, and "e" antigen-antibody systems in a highly endemic area. Amer J Epidemiol 1977; 105:99-106.

8. Melbye M, Skinhøj P, Nielsen NH, Vestergaard BF, Ebbesen P, Hart Hansen JP, Biggar RJ. Virally associated cancers in Greenland: Frequent hepatitis B virus infection but low primary hepatocellular carcinoma incidence. In press.

9. McMahon BJ, Bender TR, Templin DW, Finley JC, Clement D. Clinical and epidemiological aspects of hepatitis B vasculitis in Alaskan Eskimos. In: Harvald B, Hart Hansen JP, eds. Circumpolar Health 81. Nordic Council for Arct Med Res Rep 1982; 33:398-400.

10. Redeker AG. Delta agent and hepatitis B. Ann Int Med 1983; 98:542-543.

11. Skinhøj P, Hart Hansen JP, Højgaard Nielsen N, Mikkelsen F. Occurrence of cirrhosis and primary liver cancer in an Eskimo population hyperendemically infected with hepatitis B virus. Amer J Epidemiol 1978; 108:121-125.

12. Beasely RP. Hepatitis B virus as the etiologic agent in hepatocellular carcinoma-epidemiologic considerations. Hepatology 1982; 2:215-265.

13. Heyward WL, Lanier AP, Bender TR, Hardison HH, Dohan PH, McMahon BJ, Francis DP. Primary hepatocellular carcinoma in Alaskan Natives, 1969-1979. Int J Cancer 1981; 28:47-50.

Peter Skinhøj
Medical Department A
Rigshospitalet
Copenhagen
Denmark

Circumpolar Health 84:199-202

HEPATITIS B IN THE BAFFIN REGION OF NORTHERN CANADA

R.P.B. LARKE, G.J. FROESE, R.D.O. DEVINE and V.P. LEE

Previous seroepidemiologic studies in Alaska and Greenland, as well as preliminary evidence from northern Canada, indicated that the prevalence of hepatitis B virus (HBV) infection among Inuit (Eskimo) populations is appreciably higher than among the inhabitants of southern Canada or the continental United States (1-4). Prevalence rates of hepatitis B differ markedly from one northern community to another, even those in close proximity (1).

Hepatitis B vaccine was licensed for use in Canada in November 1982; its safety and efficacy have been well documented. We are conducting a seroepidemiologic survey throughout the Northwest Territories (N.W.T.) to establish a data base for the development of a hepatitis B vaccination strategy adjustable to the pattern of infection in each community. This paper presents the initial results from the eastern arctic region of Canada.

MATERIALS

For purposes of administration of Federal health services, the Baffin Zone is composed of nine communities (Arctic Bay, Nanisivik, Pond Inlet, Clyde River, Broughton Island, Pangnirtung, Frobisher Bay, Lake Harbour and Cape Dorset) on Baffin Island (area 507,454 sq. km), as well as Hall Beach and Igloolik on the Melville Peninsula, Resolute Bay on Cornwallis Island and Grise Fiord on Ellesmere Island. The population of the Baffin Zone is estimated to be 8,062 (June 1982 statistics), of which approximately 84% are Inuit and the remainder predominantly White. All of the communities were included in the survey except Nanisivik, a lead/zinc mining site with about 275 inhabitants, less than half of them Inuit.

An information package was sent in advance to the field visit of the mayor/settlement chairman of each community. Upon arrival of the team, meetings were usually held with council or local health committee to explain the hepatitis B control program and to arrange clinics to obtain sera from those interested in participating. Assurances were provided concerning medical confidentiality of the results, which were returned to the senior nurse in each village.

Blood samples were collected by venepuncture, the sera transferred to sterile glass vials and frozen for transport to Edmonton. Specimens were tested for hepatitis B surface antigen (HBsAg) and antibody to hepatitis B surface antigen (anti-HBs) by radioimmunoassay; sera positive for HBsAg were further tested for hepatitis B e antigen (HBeAg) and its antibody, anti-HBe, using a radioimmunoassay. All serologic tests employed commercial reagents purchased from Abbott Laboratories, North Chicago, Illinois.

RESULTS

During the spring and fall of 1983 we collected 3,271 serum samples; over 90% were from Inuit and 49.6% were from females. The age range of participants was 6 months to 85 years, with a mean age of 21.5 years and median age of 15.6 years. The age distribution of 2,795 of the participants is compared to the age distribution of the population of Baffin Zone in Table 1. No particular effort was made to involve infants and children up through 4 years of age, largely due to technical difficulties in blood sampling; hence, this age group is underrepresented in he serologic survey. The majority of school-aged children were included in each community. Most participants were reputedly healthy at the time of sampling and only a few volunteered a previous history of liver disease.

Table 1. Age distribution of persons screened for hepatitis B virus markers compared to age distribution of total population,* Baffin Zone, N.W.T.

	Age range (years)			
	0-4	5-14	15-64	≥65
Approximate age distribution Baffin Zone, 1980* (N=5,173)	16%	30%	52%	2%
Hepatitis B serologic sample Baffin Zone, 1983* (N=2,795)	5%	44%	50%	2%

* Excludes Nanisivik (not surveyed), Frobisher Bay (predominantly schools surveyed) and Grise Fiord (1980 population analysis not available).

Table 2. Age distribution of Hepatitis B virus (HBV) markers in 3,271 persons, Baffin Zone, N.W.T., 1983.

HBV serologic marker	Age range (years)							Total
	0-10 N=951	11-20 N=1,122	21-30 N=423	31-40 N=334	41-50 N=220	51-60 N=121	>61 N=100	N=3,271
HBsAg	12	22	16	37	36	21	23	167
% positive	1.3	2.0	3.8	11.1	16.4	17.4	23.0	5.1
Anti-HBs only	97	272	179	165	139	88	71	1,011
% positive	10.2	24.2	42.3	49.4	63.2	72.7	71.0	30.9
Total HBV markers	109	294	195	202	175	109	94	1,178
% positive	11.5	26.2	46.1	60.5	79.6	90.1	94.0	36.0

Table 2 displays the age-specific prevalence rates of HBV markers; rates for HBsAg and anti-HBs increased with age through the sixth decade and HBV markers were detected in 94% of the persons 61 years of age or older. Of 167 persons positive for HBsAg, 67 (40%) were also positive simultaneously for anti-HBs (Table 3). In other tables, persons with both HBsAg and anti-HBs were considered positive for HBsAg only for statistical purposes. The male/female ratio of persons positive for HBsAg was 1.4 and for anti-HBs was 0.9. HBeAg was detected in 14 (8%) of 166 HBsAg-positive persons tested, anti-HBe was present in 129 (78%), one had both markers, and 23 (14%) were negative for HBeAg and anti-HBe. In striking contrast to the mean (39.6 years) and median age (40.4 years) of the total group positive for HBsAg, the mean age of the 14 persons who also had detectable HBeAg was 16.4 years and their median age was 13.8 years.

Table 4 lists the 12 communities surveyed, designated A through L, in ascending order of the percentage of persons positive for HBV markers; the table also indicates the proportion of the total population of each community who were screened. There was wide variation from place to place in the percentage of participants found to be positive for HBsAg, ranging form 0.4% to 11.7%. In many of the communities there were few, if any, persons with HBsAg in the first three decades of life.

DISCUSSION

This serologic survey in the Baffin Zone confirms previous reports of a higher prevalence of HBV markers among Inuit in N.W.T. relative to inhabitants of southern Canada (3,4). Our results are similar to those from Alaska, where the overall prevalence rate of HBsAg-positive persons was

Table 3. Age distribution of persons with both hepatitis B surface antigen (HBsAg) and antibody (anti-HBs) in 167 sera positive for HBsAg, Baffin Zone, N.W.T., 1983.

HBV serologic markers	Age range (years)							Total
	0-10	11-20	21-30	31-40	41-50	51-60	>61	
HBsAg only	9	15	9	25	20	8	14	100
HBsAg + anti-HBs	3	7	7	12	16	13	9	67
Total with HBsAg	12	22	16	37	36	21	23	167
Proportion of total HBsAg-positive sera with both markers	25%	32%	44%	32%	44%	62%	39%	40%

Table 4. Percentages of persons sampled in each community and percentages positive for hepatitis B virus (HBV) Markers, Baffin Zone, N.W.T., 1983 (N=3,271).

Community	% of total popu-lation sampled	% of sera positive for HBsAg	% of sera positive for anti-HBs	% of sera positive for HBV markers
A	35.9	1.6	14.8	16.4
B	72.5	5.1	17.0	22.1
C	44.9	1.6	21.7	23.2
D	16.5	3.9	22.6	26.4
E	51.9	0.8	25.9	26.7
F	65.7	3.5	23.2	26.8
G	63.8	0.4	27.0	27.4
H	66.9	5.3	29.4	34.7
I	61.2	7.4	38.2	45.6
J	45.7	6.5	42.2	48.7
K	54.0	10.7	39.3	50.0
L	57.5	11.7	51.7	63.4
Total	43.0	5.1	30.9	36.0

6.4% among 3,053 Central Yupik Eskimos surveyed in 1973-1975 (1). However, in the report by Schreeder et al. (1), the basis for selecting the 12 villages in their study included hospital admissions of village residents with acute clinical HBV infection and results of a previous serologic survey of military personnel indicating high village prevalence of HBsAg. Our extensive 1983 survey of the Baffin Zone excluded only one small, predominantly White mining settlement and involved 55% of the inhabitants of the other 11 communities with a population of less than 1,000 people.

The prevalence of HBeAg was much higher, 69.1%, in the Alaskan study compared to our rate of only 8% among 166 HBsAg-positive sera assayed. All but one of the 14 HBeAg-positive individuals in Baffin Zone were 20 years of age or less and lived in one of three communities; this contrasts with mean and median ages of about 40 years for the entire group of 167 HBsAg-positive persons. In Alaska, the proportion of the study population with HBsAg was significantly higher in those under the age of 13 years (1).

The high HBsAg and HBeAg seropositivity observed in Alaskan Eskimo children suggested that children were both more recently infected with HBV and were more involved in HBV transmission in their villages (1). Hyland and Shanley (5) have commented on the relationship between carriage of HBeAg and HBsAg with respect to different prevalences of HBV infection in two neighboring Gambian villages. They speculated that factors other than age distribution, such as genetic variations in viral antigenicity and host response and regional and international differences in social and cultural patterns may influence the HBsAg and HBeAg carriage rates (5). We presently have no adequate explanation for the considerable variation in the prevalence of HBV infections among the 12 Baffin Zone communities nor the apparent paucity of HBsAg-positive persons 20 years of age or less noted in several settlements.

An unexpected observation in our serologic survey was that 40% of the 167 sera found positive for HBsAg also had detectable anti-HBs; this occurred in each of the 10-year age groupings. The simultaneous presence of both HBsAg and anti-HBs in the serum of chronic HBV carriers has been detected by radioimmunoassay and electron microscopy in South African populations (6,7) and may occur in a small percentage of asymptomatic HBsAg-positive Canadian blood donors. The possible clinical significance of higher rates of the two HBV markers being detectable simultaneously in sera of Inuit from the Baffin Zone has not yet been determined. A recent report by Hadler et al. (8) presents some disconcerting data regarding the nonspecificity of results in which anti-HBs tests fall into the low range of positivity (2.1 to 9.9 sample ratio units) by radioimmunoassay. The contribution of non-specific test results to our overall rates of anti-HBs positivity and to the apparent presence of both HBsAg and anti-HBs in the same serum sample will have to be examined. Hadler et al. (8) have emphasized the importance of their findings when serologic tests are used for epidemiologic studies of HBV infection or to determine susceptibility before using hepatitis B vaccine.

McMahon et al. (9) reported delayed development of anti-HBs among young Alaska Eskimos after symptomatic infection with HBV. We have not had the opportunity for such a prospective study in the eastern Arctic. The immune response to HBV infection may be different in Inuit compared to White population groups and may contribute to the present endemicity of hepatitis B among Eskimo groups. Such differences in immune responsiveness may also account for the relatively high incidence of primary hepatocellular carcinoma and necrotizing vasculitis as complications of chronic HBV infections in Alaska Natives.

ACKNOWLEDGMENT

We thank the Donner Canadian Foundation for a generous grant in support of this project. Mr. V.P. Lee held a Studentship from the Alberta Heritage Foundation for Medical Research.

REFERENCES

1. Schreeder MT, Bender TR, McMahon BJ, et al. Prevalence of hepatitis B in selected Alaskan Eskimo villages. Am J Epidemiol 1983; 118:543-549.
2. Skinhøj P. Hepatitis and hepatitis B-antigen in Greenland. II: Occurrence and interrelation of hepatitis B associated surface, core, and "e" antigen-antibody systems in a highly endemic area. Am J Epidemiol 1977; 105:99-106.
3. Larke RPB, Eaton RDP, Schaefer O. Epidemiology of hepatitis B in the Canadian Arctic. In: Harvald B, Hart Hansen JP, eds. Circumpolar Health 81. Nordic Council for Arct Med Res Rep 1982; 33:401-406.
4. Minuk GY, Nicolle LE, Postl B, Waggoner JG, Hoofnagle JH. Hepatitis virus infection in an isolated Canadian Inuit (Eskimo) population. J Med Virol 1982; 10:255-264.
5. Hyland CA, Shanley BC. Relationship between carriage of HBeAg and HBsAg. Lancet 1983; 2:1140-1141.
6. Stannard LM, Moodie J, Keen GA, Kipps A. Electron microscope study of the distribution of the Australia antigen in individual sera of 50 serologically positive blood donors and two patients with serum hepatitis. J Clin Pathol 1973; 26:209-216.
7. Wiggelinkhuizen J, Sinclair-Smith C, Stannard LM, Smuts H. Hepatitis B virus associated membranous glomerulonephritis. Arch Dis Childr 1983; 58:488-496.
8. Hadler SC, Murphy BL, Schable CA, Heyward WL, Francis DP, Kane MA. Epidemiological analysis of the significance of low-positive test results for antibody to hepatitis B surface and core antigens. J Clin Microbiol 1984; 19:521-525.
9. McMahon BJ, Bender TR, Berquist KR, Schreeder MT, Harpster AP. Delayed development of antibody to hepatitis B surface antigen after symptomatic infection with hepatitis B virus. J Clin Microbiol 1981; 14:130-134.
10. McMahon BJ, Bender TR, Templin DW, et al. Vasculitis in Eskimos living in an area hyperendemic for hepatitis B. JAMA 1980; 244:2180-2182.
11. Heyward WL, Lanier AP, Bender TR, et al. Primary hepatocellular carcinoma in Alaskan Natives, 1969-1979. Int J Cancer 1981; 28:47-50.

R.P.B Larke
Provincial Laboratory of Public Health
University of Alberta
Edmonton, Alberta T6G 2J2
Canada

Circumpolar Health 84:203-205

HEPATITIS B VIRAL MARKERS IN TWO EPIDEMIOLOGICALLY DISTINCT CANADIAN INUIT (ESKIMO) SETTLEMENTS

G.Y. MINUK, B. POSTL, N. LING, J.G. WAGGONER, C. POKRANT and J.H. HOOFNAGLE

INTRODUCTION

Hepatitis B viral (HBV) infections are endemic in the Inuit (Eskimo) populations of the world. Hepatitis B surface antigen (HBsAg) positive carrier rates have been reported as high as 20 to 25% in some studies (1,2). We recently reported the results of a large sero-epidemiologic survey of HBV infection in an isolated Canadian Inuit settlement, Baker Lake, where the HBsAg carrier rate was 4% and serologic evidence of previous HBV infection was 27% (3). One of the striking features of that study was an unusual correlation between the prevalence of HBV markers and age, such that only 6% of those under the age of 20 were sero-positive, in contrast to 93% of those over the age of 60. Moreover, serologic evidence of recent hepatitis B viral infection, including hepatitis B e antigen (HBeAg), DNA polymerase, HBV-DNA and liver enzyme abnormalities were absent in all 31 HBsAG carriers identified. These two findings (the unusual age-specific prevalence rate and the lack of serologic evidence for recent viral infection) led us to believe that HBV infection in this particular Inuit community had, for unknown reasons, become uncommon over the course of the past 20 to 30 years.

Because the community studied had only recently been established (some 30 years previously), and because socioeconomic conditions in the settlement were better, for the most part, than in other communities in the area, we set out to determine if demographic and/or socioeconomic differences might explain the apparent decrease in the incidence of hepatitis B infection in this particular community. We therefore carried out a similar serological survey on an older, less prosperous community in the area where population growth has been static and living conditions are poor.

MATERIALS AND METHODS

Chesterfield Inlet, a coastal community on the western shore of Hudson Bay, is the oldest settlement in the Keewatin District of Canada's Northwest Territories. (Figure 1). The population is approximately 220 individuals. Its inhabitants are, for the most part, dependent on government-sponsored welfare programs for assistance. Socioeconomic conditions in the community are relatively poor.

A total of 172 of the 220 residents (75%) agreed to take part in the study. Distribution of the population by age, sex,

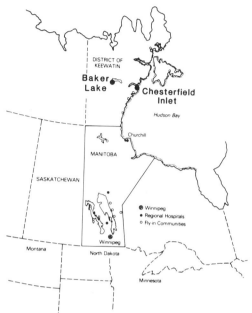

Figure 1. Location of communities surveyed in the N.W.T.

and race is shown in Table 1, with the study population from Baker Lake, N.W.T., provided for comparison. In both communities approximately 95% of the study population were Inuit. Males made up a larger portion of

Table 1. Composition of the two study populations compared by race, sex, and age.

	Baker Lake (1980)	Chesterfield Inlet (1982)
Population	850	220
Study Population:	720 (85%)	172 (75%)
Inuit	671 (93%)	164 (95%)
White	49 (7%)	8 (5%)
Male	364 (51%)	63 (37%)
Female	356 (49%)	107 (63%)
Age (2 months - 78 years)		
< 20	406 (56%)	98 (57%)
20 - 40	190 (26%)	42 (24%)
> 40	213 (18%)	33 (19%)

the study population from Baker Lake (p < 0.05 chi-square analysis). The majority of individuals from both communities were under the age of 20. Approximately one-fourth were between the ages of 20 and 40, and one-fifth over the age of 40.

Informed consent was obtained through a nursing station interpreter from all adults, and from parents of guardians of children involved in the study.

Five milliliters of blood were drawn from all study participants, and the serum frozen until serologic testing was performed approximately one week later. All 1972 sera were screened for antibody to hepatitis A virus (anti-HAV), hepatitis B surface antigen (HBsAg), antibody to hepatitis B surface antigen (anti-HBs) and antibody to hepatitis B core antigen (anti-HBc) by commercial solid phase radioimmunoassays (HAVAB, AUSRIA II, AUSAB and CORAB, respectively: Abbott Laboratories, North Chicago, Ill.). Serum samples positive for HBsAg were then tested for IgM anti-HBc (4), hepatitis B e antigen (HBeAg) and antibody to hepatitis B e antigen (anti-HBe) by immunodiffusion and radioimmunoassay (5), and DNA polymerase using ^{3}H-thymidine according to the method of Kaplan (6). Antibody to hepatitis B virus-associated delta agent was tested by radioimmunoassay (courtesy of Dr. J. Gerin) (7).

RESULTS

The results of anti-HAV testing in Chesterfield Inlet and Baker Lake are shown in Figure 2. Of those from Chesterfield Inlet, 76% had serologic evidence of exposure to this virus, as compared to 71% in Baker Lake. The differences observed in the 20-29 year age group between the two communities were not statistically significant by chi-square analysis (p > 0.05).

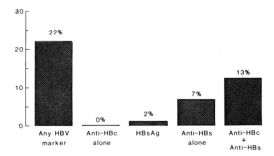

Figure 3. Components of HBV-positive test results for the Chesterfield Inlet population.

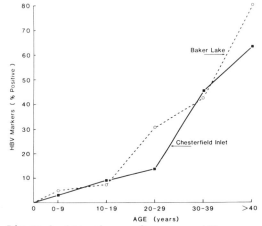

Figure 4. Comparison of age-specific prevalence of HBV markers in Chesterfield Inlet and Baker Lake populations.

Testing for the presence of any HBV marker revealed that 22% of the inhabitants of Chesterfield Inlet had serologic evidence of HBV infection (Figure 3). This figure consists of 2.3% who were positive for HBsAg, 7% positive for anti-HBs alone and 13% positive for both anti-HBc and anti-HBs. The four HBsAg positive carriers included a father, aged 50, and three sons, aged 12, 14, and 15. The mother and four daughters were anti-HBs and anti-HBc positive. Each of the carriers was negative for HBeAg, DNA polymerase, HBV-DNA, IgM anti-HBc and anti-delta.

The results of the age-specific prevalence rates for HBV markers were shown in Figure 4, with the results from the Baker Lake study included for comparison. As in Baker Lake, a marked correlation was found between the prevalence of HBV markers and age. Thus a relatively low prevalence of HBV markers was obtained in the under 20 age group (7 of 172, or 4%), while among individuals over the age of 60, 10 of 16 (67%) had serologic evidence of infection.

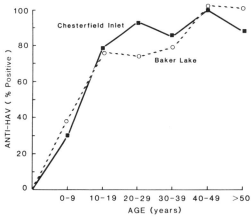

Figure 2. Results of anti-HAV testing in Baker Lake and Chesterfield Inlet.

DISCUSSION

The results of this study indicate that HBV infection is relatively uncommon in the children of these two Canadian Inuit communities. The results also indicate that the majority of the HBsAg positive carriers identified appear to have acquired their infection some time in the distant past, as all serologic markers for recent HBV infection (HBeAg, HBV DNA, DNA polymerase and live enzyme tests) were consistently negative. Together, these results suggest that HBV infection has become relatively uncommon in the Canadian Inuit during the past 20 to 30 years, and that demographic and socioeconomic changes in the area do not appear to have played a major role in bringing about that decline. Alternative explanations must therefore be considered.

In areas of the world where HBV is endemic, continuous viral transmission requires the presence of a "critical mass" of chronic HBsAg-positive carriers. Any changes resulting in the loss of this "critical mass" of carriers would ultimately result in a significant decrease in the prevalence of HBV infection within the community. The possibility exists that government-sponsored programs for the control of other infectious diseases in the area may have indirectly influenced the number of HBsAg positive carriers present in these communities. One such program involved the evacuation of Native individuals with active pulmonary tuberculosis to TB sanatoriums in southern Canada (8). This measure resulted in the prolonged absence (2 to 3 years) of a large number of fertile women who in endemic areas act as the primary source of HBV transmission (via "vertical" or maternal-infant transmission) (9). A second consideration was the introduction of widespread BCG vaccination programs for all Native newborn Inuit children. BCG vaccinations have previously been reported to have a beneficial effect on eradicating the HBsAg carrier state of children (10). It is conceivable, therefore, that neonatal vaccination with BCG may have resulted in fewer HBsAg-positive carrier children and hence less "horizontal" transmission within the community. Further supporting this possibility is recent evidence presented by McGlynn and colleagues at an international symposium on viral hepatitis in San Francisco, indicating that the presence of cell-mediated immunity to *Mycobacterium tuberculosis* (as manifested by a positive Mantoux skin test) was associated with a lower HBsAg and HBeAg carrier rate in 2,100 Indochinese refugees than in those refugees who were Mantoux-negative.

The temporal association between the government-sponsored evacuation and BCG programs with the decrease in the prevalence of HBV infection in these Canadian Inuit settlements underscores the need for further consideration of the potential effect that the control of other infectious agents may have had on the prevalence of HBV in the Canadian North.

REFERENCES

1. Skinhøj P. Hepatitis and hepatitis B antigen in Greenland. II. Occurrence and interrelation of hepatitis B associated surface, core and "e" antigen-antibody systems in a highly endemic area. Amer J Epidemiol 1977; 105:99-106.
2. Barrett DH, Burks JM, McMahon B, Elliot S, Berquist KR, Bender TR, Maynard JE. Epidemiol 1977; 105:118-122.
3. Minuk GY, Nicolle LE, Postl B, Waggoner JG, Hoofnagle JH. Hepatitis virus infection in an isolated Canadian Inuit (Eskimo) population. J Med Vir 1982; 10:255-264.
4. Lemon SM, Gates NL, Simms et al. IgM antibody to hepatitis B core antigen as a diagnostic parameter of acute infection with hepatitis B virus. J Infect Dis 1981; 193:803-809.
5. Mushahwar IK, Overby LR, Froesner G, Deinhardt F, Ling CM. Prevalence of hepatitis B e antigen and its antibody as detected by radioimmunoassays. J Med Vir 1978; 2:77-87.
6. Kaplan PM, Greenman RL, Gerin JL, Purcell RH, Robinson WL. DNA polymerase associated with human hepatitis B antigen. J Vir 1973; 995-1005.
7. Rizzetto M, Shih JWK, Gerin JL. The hepatitis B virus associated antigen: isolation from liver, development of solid phase radioimmunoassays for antigen and anti-δ and partial characterization of δ antigen. J Immunol 1980; 125:318-324.
8. Schaefer O. Ethnology, demography and medicine in the arctic. In: Harvald B, Hart Hansen JP, eds. Circumpolar Health 81. Nordic Council for Arct Med Res Rep 1982; 33:187-193.
9. Steven CE, Beasley RP, Tsui T et al. Vertical transmission of hepatitis B antigen in Taiwan. N Engl J Med 1975; 292:771-774.
10. Brzosko WJ, Debski R, Derecka K. Immunostimulation for chronic active hepatitis. Lancet 1978; 2:211.

G. Y. Minuk
Department of Medicine
University of Calgary
3330 Hospital Drive N.W.
Calgary, Alberta T2N 4N1
Canada

Circumpolar Health 84:206-208

INCREASED PREVALENCE OF HEPATITIS B SURFACE ANTIGEN IN PREGNANT ALASKA ESKIMOS

DAVID T. ESTROFF, JACQUELINE A. GREENMAN, WILLIAM L. HEYWARD, BRIAN J. MCMAHON, H. HUNTLEY HARDISON and THOMAS R. BENDER

INTRODUCTION

In 1973, serologic testing for hepatitis B surface antigen (HBsAg) and antibody (anti-HBs) among Yupik Eskimos in two villages of southwestern Alaska revealed a high prevalence of infection with hepatitis B virus (HBV) (1). Children less than 10 years of age had the highest prevalence of HBsAg. These findings led to expanded serological surveys which revealed that HBV infection was hyperendemic in many villages of southwestern Alaska (2). In some villages HBsAg was detected in up to 23% of the residents and up to 50% of the residents were positive for anti-HBs.

Since parenteral mechanisms of transmission were not evident in this population, other mechanisms of infection were investigated. One investigation revealed the presence of HBsAg in saliva and exudates of impetiginous skin lesions, and HBsAg was detected on many environmental surfaces in schools and households (3).

Since other studies in Asian populations hyperendemic for HBV infection have suggested that perinatal transmission of HBV is common, a study was undertaken in 1978-1979 to determine if perinatal transmission of HBV was occurring in the Alaska Native population. In 1982, routine serologic screening for HBsAg in all pregnant women was begun as part of the hepatitis B control program now underway in Alaska. Results of this more recent screening are compared to the earlier study in 1978.

MATERIALS AND METHODS

In the first study, all women seen at the prenatal clinic at the Public Health Service Alaska Native Hospital at Bethel (now Yukon-Kuskokwim Delta Regional Hospital) between October 2, 1978 and August 30, 1979, were tested for serologic markers of HBV infection at their first visit, at 32 and 36 weeks gestation, and at 2 days postpartum. HBsAg-positive mothers were retested at 6 to 16 months after delivery, and their offspring were tested at 2 to 19 month intervals and were followed until 7 to 23 months of age.

Routine serologic screening of all pregnant women in the third trimester was begun in April 1982, and all infants born to HBsAg-positive mothers (since 1983) have received both hepatitis B immune globulin (HBIG) and hepatitis B vaccine (Heptavas--TM). HBsAg results on all women who delivered from January 1, 1983 through December 31, 1983 were analyzed.

All women tested were residents of the villages of the Yukon-Kuskokwim Delta region, an area of 120,000 square kilometers with a Native population in 1980 of approximately 13,760 (4). Medical care is delivered by the hospital in Bethel, and in the villages by community health aides, itinerant public health nurses, and visiting physicians from Bethel.

Serum specimens were tested for HBsAg and anti-HBs by radioimmunoassay (RIA) or enzyme-linked immunosorbent assay (ELISA) (AUSRIA-II, AUSAB, and EIA, Abbott Laboratories, Chicago, Illinois). When appropriate, sera were tested for anti-HBc by RIA (CORAB, Abbott Laboratories) and HBeAg and anti-HBe by RIA or EIA. All testing was performed at the Hepatitis Laboratories Division, Center for Infectious Diseases, Centers for Disease Control, (CDC), Phoenix, Arizona, or the Arctic Investigations Laboratory, CDC, Anchorage, Alaska.

RESULTS

In the first study (1978-1979), 7 of 267 prenatal women tested, (2.6%) were positive for HBsAg at the time of delivery and 3 of the 7 were sisters (Table 1). Of those 7, 5 were positive for anti-HBe and 2 were negative for both markers (Table 2). Two (28.5%) of the infants born to these 7 HBsAg-positive mothers developed serologic evidence of infection between 7 and 11 months of age. One infant born to a mother negative for both e markers was HBsAg-positive at 7 months of age, but converted to anti-HBs at 20 months of age. The other infant, born to a mother who was anti-HBe positive, was positive for anti-HBc only at 11 months and positive for both anti-HBs and anti-HBc at 27 months of age.

In 1983, after the start of a routine prenatal screening program, 554 prenatal women were tested and 25 (4.5%) were positive for HBsAg prior to delivery (Table 1). The mothers who were positive for HBsAg were younger than those who were negative. ($z=-1.94$, $p=0.05$). Six (24%) of these HBsAg-positive women were positive for HBeAg, 18 (72%) had anti-HBe, and one was negative for both e markers (Table 2).

DISCUSSION

Transmission of HBV infection from HBsAg-positive mothers to their newborn infants has been extensively studied. Previous studies have shown that up to 90%

Table 1. Age distribution of mothers and HBsAg prevalence.

Age	Total Births 1978-9	1983	No. HBsAg Pos. 1978-9	1983	Prevalence (%) 1978-9	1983
<15		0	0	0		0
15-19		72	3	5		6.9
20-24		207	2	14		6.8
25-29		155	1	2		1.3
30-34		78	1	3		3.8
35-39		35	0	1		2.9
>40		7	0	0		0
TOTALS	267	554	7	25	2.6%	4.5%

of infants born to HBeAg-positive mothers were infected with HBV, but less than 20% of those born to anti-HBe-positive mothers developed HBV infection (5-7). Infants infected by HBeAg-positive mothers during the perinatal period and in infancy are likely to become chronic carriers of HBsAg and thus be a continuing source of infection in the household and community (1,2,12). These carriers are also at increased risk of the complications of HBV infection such as chronic liver disease, primary hepato-cellular carcinoma, vasculitis, and glomeru-lonephritis (9,10,13). All of these compli-cations of HBV infection have been found in infants and children in southwestern Alaska. Symptomatic hepatitis is rare in infancy, but can be fulminant and fatal if it occurs (6).

The results of the initial study showed evidence of HBV infection before 1 year of age in 2 of 7 (28.6%) infants born to HBsAg positive mothers. In these cases, it is not possible to determine whether transmission occurred at the time of delivery or subse-quently in a horizontal fashion. Previous epidemiologic studies in this population have suggested that perinatal transmission is not a major factor in the clustering of HBV seropositivity among household members (1,2). The precise route of horizontal transmission in these households remains unclear and several mechanisms have been proposed. Premastication of food, a common practice in this area, has been suggested as one possible route of postnatal transmission (12), as well as close person-to-person contact with HBsAg-positive family members.

The prenatal screening program now in effect in the Yukon-Kuskokwim Delta region showed that 4.5% of the women who delivered in 1983 were HBsAg-positive. This is similar to the 6.4% prevalence of HBsAg among the general population and is 12.5-fold higher than the rate (0.36%) found among 3,067 prenatal women in Denver, Colorado in 1974 (8). Over 75% of the HBsAg-positive mothers were in the 15 to 24 year age group, which accounted for only 50% of the total deliveries. The observed increase in prevalence of HBsAg among prenatal females between 1978 and 1983 was not significant and could be attributed to seasonal variation, chance, or the generally increasing incidence of infection. Another explanation for this finding might be that the children who were previously shown to have high rates of HBsAg developed the chronic carrier state and have now advanced into the childbearing age.

In conclusion, HBsAg is relatively common among Eskimo women of childbearing

Table 2. HBeAg and Anti-HBe in HBsAg-positive prenatal females in the Yukon-Kuskokwim Delta Service Unit.

Year	No.HBsAg+	No.HBeAg+(%)	No.Anti-HBe+(%)	No.Neg for HBeAg/Anti-HBe(%)
1978-79	7	0 (0%)	5 (71.4%)	2 (28.6%)
1983	25	6 (24%)	18 (72%)	1 (4%)

age. The prevalence of HBeAg is much lower than in populations where perinatal infection is the predominant mode of transmission, and this may account for the relatively low incidence of perinatal transmission in the Alaska Native population.

An effective HBV control program must include the use of HBIG and hepatitis B vaccine in infants born to all HBsAg-positive mothers, as well as vaccination of high risk seronegative individuals, especially young children (11). Such a program is currently being implemented in Alaska Natives.

REFERENCES

1. Barrett DH, Burks JM, McMahon B, et al. Epidemiology of hepatitis B in two Alaskan communities. Amer J Epidemiol 1977; 105:118-122.
2. Schreeder MT, Bender TR, McMahon BJ, et al. Prevalence of hepatitis B in selected Alaskan Eskimo villages. Amer J Epidemiol 1983; 118:543-549.
3. Petersen NJ, Barrett DH, Bond WW, et al. Hepatitis B surface antigen in saliva, impetiginous lesions, and the environment in two remote Alaskan villages. Appl Envir Micro 1976; 32:572-574.
4. 1980 Census of Population Vol I. General social and economic characteristics Alaska PC 80-1-C-3 Washington: US Govt Print Off 1983; 3:175-180.
5. Stevens CE, Beasley RP, Tsui J, Lee WC. Vertical transmission of hepatitis B antigen in Taiwan. New Eng J Med 1975; 292:771-774.
6. Isenberg, JN. The infant and hepatitis B virus infection. Adv Pediat 1977; 24:455-463.
7. Dupuy JM, Giraud P, Dupuy C, et al. Hepatitis B in children. II. Study of children born to chronic HBsAg carrier mothers. J Pediat 1978; 92:200-204.
8. Kohler PF, Dubois RS, Merrill DA, Bowes WA. Prevention of chronic neonatal hepatitis B virus infection with antibody to the hepatitis B surface antigen. New Eng J Med 1974; 291:1378-1380.
9. McMahon BJ, Bender TR, Templin DW, Finley JC, Clement D. Clinical and epidemiological aspects of hepatitis B vasculitis in Alaskan eskimos. In: Harvald B, Hart Hansen JP, eds. Circumpolar Health 81. Nordic Council Arct Med Res Rep 1982; 33:398-400.
10. Heyward WL, Lanier AP, Bender TR, Hardison HH, et al. Primary hepatocellular carcinoma in Alaskan natives 1969-1979. Int J Cancer 1981; 28:47-50.
11. Maupas P, Chiron JP, Barin F, Coursagnet P, et al. Efficacy of hepatitis B vaccine in prevention of early HBsAg carrier state in children. Lancet 1981; 1:289-292.
12. Beasley RP, Hwang LY. Postnatal infectivity of hepatitis B surface antigen-carrier mothers. J Infect Dis 1983; 147:185-190.
13. Maupas P, Werner B, Larouze B, et al. Antibody to hepatitis B core antigen in patients with primary hepatic carcinoma. Lancet 1975; 2:9.

David T. Estroff
Mt. Edgecumbe Alaska Native Hospital
Box 4577
Mt. Edgecumbe, Alaska 99835
U.S.A.

Circumpolar Health 84:209-212

BUNYAVIRUSES THROUGHOUT THE WESTERN CANADIAN ARCTIC

DONALD M. McLEAN

Isolation of two bunyaviruses, snowshoe hare (SSH) virus within the California serogroup of arboviruses, and Northway (NOR) virus within the Bunyamwera serogroup, from mosquitoes collected in east-central Alaska near Northway (63°N, 142°W) during the summer of 1970 (1) revealed for the first time the existence of a natural focus of bunyavirus infection in subarctic North America. Following isolation of 12 strains of SSH virus from *Aedes* sp. mosquitoes collected in the boreal forest of the Yukon Territory, Canada, near Whitehorse (61°N, 135°W), about 500 km east of Northway, during 1971 by our own team (2), we undertook extensive epidemiological investigations throughout the western Canadian Arctic during 12 successive summers from 1972 through 1983 (3).

METHODS AND RESULTS

Bunyavirus Infections in Adult Mosquitoes

Throughout 12 summers from 1972 through 1983, a total of 58 bunyavirus strains, including 54 SSH and 4 NOR strains, were isolated from 136,854 mosquitoes of 7 species (Table 1) (3). Overall mosquito infection rates ranged from 0.024% for *A. hexodontus* to 0.120% for *Culiseta inornata*. Although 32 SSH isolates were achieved from 86,400 *A. communis* during 8 of 12 years, thus clearly demonstrating the importance of this species as a natural vector, the overall mosquito infection rate of 0.037% was only marginally above that for *A. hexodontus*, which was the lowest rate for any species. Most SSH isolations were achieved from *A. communis* and *A. nigripes* which were collected from early June onwards throughout summer. *C. inornata*, which yielded 5 SSH isolates, was found only during spring from mid-May to early June, and *A. hexodontus*, which yielded another 5 SSH isolates, emerged only during full summer in late June. Isolations of NOR virus were restricted to *A. hexodontus* and *C. inornata*.

The 58 bunyavirus isolates were made at a total of 12 different localities. [Ed. note: Tabular data reductions showing locations and foci are available from the author.] Mosquito infection rates per week ranged from 1:61 (1.63%) *A. nigripes* at Marsh Lake to 1:1,029 (0.097%) *A. communis* at the same location and 1:3,003 (0.033%) *A. communis* at Inuvik. At Marsh Lake, SSH virus was isolated from adult mosquitoes during 6 of 10 years on one or more occasions each week between week no. 22 and no. 31, except week no. 30. In 2 additional years, SSH virus was isolated from larvae in week no. 17 or no. 18. A single NOR isolation was achieved from *C. inornata* during 1978. Along the Dempster Highway from km 26 to 342, but mainly between km 68 and 197 (66°N, 138°W), SSH virus was isolated during 7 of 10 years on one or more occasions each week between week no. 24 and no. 31, except no. 26 and no. 27. At Inuvik (69°N, 135°W), both SSH and NOR viruses were isolated from *A. hexodontus* in 1976 and SSH virus from *A. communis* in 1978. In the southern Mackenzie District, N.W.T., between latitudes 60 and 62°N, SSH virus was isolated near Fort Smith during week no. 28 and at Fort Simpson during weeks no. 28 and 29.

Mosquito infection rates were highest (0.082%) at a boreal forest location, Marsh Lake, some 30 km east of Whitehorse (61°N, 135°W) in the southern Yukon (3). At other southern Yukon locations between latitudes 60 and 63°N, the infection rate of 0.052% was somewhat lower, but it was comparable with the 0.049% rate at boreal forest locations in the northern Yukon, principally along the Dempster Highway to 67°N. In the boreal forest of the southern Mackenzie District, N.W.T. between Fort Smith and Fort Simpson, the mosquito infection rate was 0.030%, but this rate was reduced to 0.009% in open woodland extending northwards from 62°N to Inuvik at 69°N.

Bunyavirus Infections in Mosquito Larvae

Larval *Aedes* sp. mosquitoes were collected at Marsh Lake during the spring of each of 5 years, before the emergence of *Aedes* adults, and larval mosquitoes were collected elsewhere in the Yukon less regularly. Isolations of SSH virus were achieved from 4 of 453 pools during 3 of 5 years. These included 1 of 8 larval pools collected near Kusawa Lake (61°N, 136°W) in 1974 (4), 2 of 12 larval pools at Marsh Lake in 1975 and 1 of 5 larval pools at the same site in 1983 (3). Isolation of SSH virus both from larval and adult mosquitoes at these two locations illustrates the importance of transovarial transfer as a mechanism of overwintering of this serotype at these natural foci.

Vector Competence of Yukon Mosquitoes

Replication of SSH isolates representative for each of three years 1980 (80-Y-123), 1981 (81-Y-121) and 1982 (82-Y-46) was demonstrated in salivary glands and thoraces of *A. communis* mosquitoes after intra-thoracic injection with 1 to 0.01 PFU virus and incubation at 13°C for 14 to 28 days. [Ed. note: Tabular data are available from the author.] Isolates from 1980 and 1982 multiplied in salivary glands and thoraces of *A. hexodontus* after intrathoracic injection of 0.1 or higher doses of virus. Isolate 82-Y-46 also multiplied in salivary glands and thoraces of *C. inornata* after intrathoracic injection of 1 PFU or more virus. The minimum infectivity dose of 1.0 to 0.01 PFU of the above 3 isolates of SSH virus for *A. communis* and other arctic vector species is consistent with previous results (5).

Results summarized in Table 2 show that *A. communis* transmitted the 74-Y-234 topotype after feeding on 1.0 to 0.01 mouse LD_{50} virus and after intrathoracic injection of 0.1 to 0.01 mouse LD_{50}. *C.*

inornata also transmitted after injection of 0.1 mouse LD_{50} 74-Y-234 and 30 mouse LD_{50} 71-Y-23 topotypes.

Northway virus multiplication was also detected in *A. communis* and *C. inornata* after feeding of 30 PFU of the 76-Y-330 topotype. Transmission by *A. communis* was achieved after injection of 300 PFU of the 76-Y-330 and 78-Y-284 topotypes, both of which replicated in *A. communis* and *C. inornata* after injection of 3.0 PFU (Table 2).

Indirect immunofluorescent staining was applied to head-squash preparations of 83 mosquitoes injected with SSH strains from 1980, 1981, and 1982. SSH antigen was

Table 1. Bunyavirus isolations from Yukon and N.W.T. mosquitoes 1972-1983.

Year	Mosquito species							Total
	Culiseta inornata	*Aedes communis*	*Aedes hexodontus*	*Aedes punctor*	*Aedes nigripes*	*Aedes canadensis*	*Aedes cinereus*	
1972	0/18	6/9048[S]				0/1251		6/10317
1973	1/1648[S]	1/2932[S]				1/519[S]	1/1179[S]	4/6278
1974[1]	0/112	3/5676[S]	0/3133			1/970[S]		4/9891
1975	0/40	0/7990	0/2080			0/103	0/268	0/10481
1976[2]	0/477	2/12716[S]	5/5096 (4S 1N)	2/2808[S]	2/2650			9/23747
1977[2]	0/146	0/8677	0/7884	0/638	0/421			0/17766
1978[2]	7/3726 (4S 3N)	9/13311[S]	0/1961		0/1307			16/20305
1979	0/3	0/7915	0/1079					0/8997
1980[2]	0/217	7/5772[S]	0/1443					7/7432
1981	0/20	3/7017[S]	0/1063		3/2088[S]			6/10188
1982[2]	0/79	1/3099[S]	1/1227[S]		3/2583[S]			5/6988
1983	0/175	0/2247	0/524		1/1520[S]			1/4466
Total	8/6661 (5S 3N)	32/86400 (32S)	6/25490 (5S 1N)	2/3446 (2S)	7/10567 (7S)	2/2843 (2S)	1/1447 (1S)	58/136854 (54S 4N)
Rate[3]	0.120	0.037	0.024	0.058	0.066	0.070	0.069	0.042

S   Snowshoe hare virus
N   Northway virus
1. One larval SSH isolate during 1974, two during 1975 and one during 1983.
2. Collected both in Yukon Territory and Northwest Territories.

3. Rate: $\dfrac{\text{number of virus isolations}}{\text{number of mosquitoes tested}} \times 100$

visualized by immunofluorescence in 50 mosquitoes. Infectious virus was detected in 48 salivary glands which contained 1.0 to 2.8 log PFU per gland and in 63 thoraces which contained 1.0 to 3.6 log PFU per thorax. This paralleled earlier findings that SSH virus antigen was detected frequently by immunofluorescence in salivary glands of infected mosquitoes (5).

Antigenic Analysis

Employing single injection (6) rabbit antisera to two SSH topotypes, 74-Y-234 and 76-Y-316 (from 53 *A. hexodontus* collected at Fort Smith N.W.T. on 23 July 1976), no significant differences of plaque reduction neutralization antibody titer were observed in tests with both sera against 37 of 39 isolates, and merely fivefold differences were shown with the remaining 2 isolates. Rabbit antisera prepared against the Alaska 1970 NOR prototype and the Yukon 78-Y-245 topotype revealed fivefold or smaller titer differences between each of the 4 Canadian isolates and the Alaskan prototype. Thus virtual antigenic homogeneity was observed among all SSH isolates and all NOR strains respectively.

DISCUSSION

Isolation of SSH virus from adult mosquitoes at one or more Yukon locations during 8 of 10 sampling years, and from *Aedes* sp. larvae during 3 sampling years, in one of which no virus was isolated from adult mosquitoes, demonstrates clearly the endemic prevalence of SSH virus throughout the boreal forest of the Yukon Territory. Virus recovery from larvae at Marsh Lake on two springtime occasions separated by 8 years, during which SSH virus was isolated from adult mosquitoes in 4 intervening years, clearly points towards transovarial transfer as an important mechanism of virus in midwestern USA (7), Keystone virus along the Atlantic Seaboard (8), and California encephalitis virus in California (9).

Abundance of SSH virus isolation from *A. communis* mosquitoes, together with its ability to transmit virus following incubation at 4°C and 13°C in the laboratory after oral feeding or intrathoracic injection (10) illustrates clearly the dominance of *A. communis* as the natural vector species throughout summer. Field collections of *A. communis* in the Northwest Territories and in the Canadian Provinces of Alberta and Manitoba (12) have also yielded SSH virus (11). In the Yukon Territory *A. nigripes*

Table 2. *Minimum infectivity doses of SSH and NOR **viruses** for Yukon mosquitoes after incubation at 13°C following virus feeding or **intrathoracic** injection.*

Serotype	Topotype	Passage route	Route	Aedes communis	Aedes cinereus	Aedes hexodontus	Culiseta inornata	Virus assay
					Minimum dose[1]			
SSH	71-Y-23	3 mouse	INJ		3.0 TR[2]	300	0.3 TR[4]	LD_{50}
	74-Y-234	zero	FED	1.0 TR[2]				
			INJ	0.1 TR[2]				
		1 mouse	FED	0.01 TR[2]			100	
			INJ	0.01 TR[2]			0.1 TR[2]	
	75-L-10	1 mouse	FED	300		30	300	
			INJ	0.1		0.1	1.0	
	78-Y-133	1 mouse	INJ	3.0			3.0	PFU
	80-Y-123	1 mouse	INJ	0.01		0.1		
	81-Y-121	1 mouse	INJ	0.1				
	82-Y-46	1 mouse	INJ	0.01		0.1	1.0	
NOR	76-Y-330	3 mouse	FED	30			30	PFU
			INJ	3.0	3.0 TR[3]		3.0	
	78-Y-284	1 mouse	INJ	3.0 TR[3]			3.0	
	78-Y-289	zero	INJ	3.0				

1. Minimum virus dose which induced virus multiplication in salivary glands.
2. Transmission (TR) was also demonstrated after administration of this dose.
3. Transmission (TR) was demonstrated after injection of 300 PFU virus.
4. Transmission (TR) was demonstrated after injection of 30 mouse LD_{50} and incubation at 27°C.

appears to serve as a subsidiary vector species throughout summer. Repeated SSH isolations from *C. inornata*, which is the first species to emerge in spring, together with its transmission in the laboratory after incubation at 0-4°C and 13°C (10) and its persistence in mosquitoes as long as 329 days (5), demonstrate its role as a spring-time vector. Collections of *C. inornata* in Alberta, Saskatchewan and Manitoba (11) have also yielded SSH virus. *Aedes hexodontus*, which emerges during midsummer, has yielded SSH virus repeatedly in the Yukon Territory and the Mackenzie District N.W.T. and during summer 1973 in the Keewatin District N.W.T. (11). Present and previous (5) observations reveal susceptibility to infection of salivary glands following oral feeding or intrathoracic injection of virus. Thus *A. hexodontus* appears to be a vector species during late summertime.

Between 1963 and 1983, bunyaviruses, especially SSH virus, have been isolated from adult mosquitoes in all regions of Canada (11) and from sentinel rabbits in central and western Canada also. Serological evidence of SSH infection has been demonstrated to date in 11 non-fatal cases of aseptic meningitis or encephalitis in central and eastern Canada (11,12). Although no clinically manifested SSH infections were documented in the Yukon or the Northwest Territories between 1972 and 1983, possibly due to the sparse population and lack of serological surveillance, subclinical infections with California serogroup virus have been detected in east-central Alaska (1) and in western and central Canada (11). In each of these regions, SSH antibodies have been detected in snowshoe hares (*Lepus americanus*), and also in the arctic ground squirrel (*Citellus undulatus*) in the Yukon, and SSH virus was isolated from a wild-caught *L. Americanus* in Alberta (11).

This twelve-year study has demonstrated that SSH virus is maintained in nature throughout boreal forest and open woodland portions of the western Canadian Arctic involving snowshoe hares and arctic ground squirrels as summertime vertebrate reservoirs, 4 principal mosquito species as arthropod vectors during part or all of the arctic summer season, and with transovarial transfer as an important overwintering mechanism. Human infections may be acquired tangentially to this natural cycle of SSH infection.

REFERENCES

1. Ritter DG, Feltz ET. On the natural occurrence of California encephalitis virus and other arboviruses in Alaska. Can J Microbiol 1974; 20:1359-1366.

2. McLean DM, Goddard EJ, Graham EA, Hardy GJ, Purvin-Good KW. California encephalitis virus isolations from Yukon mosquitoes, 1971. Amer J Epidemiol 1972; 94:347-355.

3. McLean DM, Lester SA. Isolations of snowshoe hare virus from Yukon mosquitoes, 1983. Mosq News 1984; 44. (In press).

4. McLean DM, Bergman SKA, Gould AP, Grass PN, Miller MA, Spratt EE. California encephalitis virus prevalence throughout the Yukon Territory, 1971-74. Amer J. Trop Med Hyg 1975; 24:676-684.

5. McLean DM, Grass PN, Judd BD, Stolz KJ. Bunyavirus development in arctic and *Aedes aegypti* mosquitoes as revealed by glucose oxidase staining and immunofluorescence. Arch Virol 1979; 62:313-322.

6. McLean DM. Immunological investigation of human virus disease. In: Nairin RC, series ed. Practical methods in clinical immunology, Vol 5. Edinburgh: Churchill Livingstone, 1982.

7. Watts DM, Thompson WH, Yuill TM, DeFoliart GR, Hanson RP. Overwintering of La Crosse virus in *Aedes triseriatus*. Amer J Trop Med Hyg 1974; 23:694-700.

8. LeDuc JW, Suyemoto W, Eldridge BF, Russell PK, Barr AR. Ecology of California encephalitis viruses on the DelMarVa Peninsula. II. Demonstration of transovarial transmission. Amer J Trop Med Hyg 1975; 24:124-126.

9. Turell MJ, LeDuc JW. The role of mosquitoes in the natural history of California serogroup viruses. In: Calisher CH, Thompson WH, eds. California serogroup viruses. New York: Alan R Liss Inc., 1983:43-55.

10. McLean DM. Yukon isolates of snowshoe hare virus, 1972-1982. In: Calisher CH, Thompson WH, eds. California serogroup viruses. New York: Alan R Liss Inc., 1983:247-256.

11. National Research Council of Canada. Biting flies in Canada: Health effects and economic consequences. NRCC Publ No 19248, 1982.

12. Artsob H. Distribution of California serogroup viruses and virus infections in Canada. In: Calisher CH, Thompson WH, eds. California serogroup viruses. New York: Alan R Liss Inc., 1983:277-290.

Donald M. McLean
Medical Microbiology
University of British Columbia
301-6174 University Boulevard
Vancouver, British Columbia   V6T 1W5
Canada

VIRUS ISOLATIONS FROM SEWAGE IN FINLAND

KAISA LAPINLEIMU, M. STENVIK and LEENA SOININEN

INTRODUCTION

More than 100 different virus types are known to be excreted into sewage in human feces:

-- enteroviruses, including polio-, coxsackie-, echo- and several recently discovered enteroviruses numbered in order of discovery, e.g. enterovirus 72, which is hepatitis A, a well-known virus type, transmitted via water;

-- adenoviruses;

-- reoviruses, including rotaviruses, which are the most important etiological agents of diarrhea in infants;

-- parvoviruses, including Norwalk agent, which also causes gastro-intestinal infections;

-- oncogenic viruses, e.g. papova viruses, which are resistant and presumably present in sewage.

The conventional virological laboratories working with cell cultures are nowadays mostly able to detect entero-, adeno- and reoviruses. The epidemiologically important types like rotavirus, Norwalk agent and hepatitis A virus do not grow in conventional cell cultures. Studies on these types are limited to specially equipped laboratories. The results of tests made at a public health laboratory therefore present only a fraction of the total virus content.

Viruses multiply only in living cells, but in a natural environment they may survive and remain infective for long periods. Factors affecting the survival of enteric viruses include temperature, exposure to sunlight, pH, and the presence of organic matter. Viruses readily adsorb to particles, especially at low pH levels, and this prolongs their survival. The colder the environment the longer viruses survive. If frozen, enteroviruses may survive for months, even for years. Their survival time in permafrost areas is unknown.

MATERIALS AND METHODS

Studies on viruses in sewage were carried out during two periods in Finland. The first study was started in 1960 during a polio type 1 epidemic and stopped at the end of 1961, when the epidemic was over (1). A total of 156 samples from influents to three sewage treatment plants were studied. The aim was to compare virus isolations from sewage with viruses isolated simultaneously from patients.

The second study was begun in 1971 as part of an intensive search for polio-viruses. The elimination of poliomyelitis solely by the use of inactivated poliovirus vaccine raised a suspicion that latent polioviruses were circulating in this country. At a sewage plant in Helsinki a sample of influent was taken once a week and investigated immediately. All together 399 samples were studied by the end of 1980.

In the north of Finland a study of viruses in the sewage influent and effluent has been carried out since 1979. The aim was to compare viruses found there with those found in Helsinki. Both influent and effluent (about 1 liter of each) were collected once a month in our northernmost community, Inari-Utsjoki, with 8,200 inhabitants, about 1,000 km north of Helsinki. Some 49 samples from both the influent and the effluent were investigated.

In all these studies the main features of the methods used were similar: concentration of sewage, inoculation into cell cultures, incubation at +36°C and identification with conventional antisera.

The methods of concentration, however, has been changed. In the first study sewage was concentrated about tenfold by dialyzing it against 59% gum arabic, while during 1971-1980 it was concentrated with alginate membranes. In 1975, a shortage of suitable alginate membranes in Finland interrupted the study until 1976. Since then sewage has been concentrated about 100-fold by a two-phase system according to Albertson (2).

The concentrated samples throughout the studies have been treated with chloroform to eliminate bacteria. The pretreated samples were inoculated into different cell cultures, in the first study into three and then into five bottles with different cell monolayers: primary human amnion cells, human fibroblasts, Vero, GMK and HeLa cells. The cultures were then incubated at +36°C until a cytopathogenic effect (CPE) was noted. If no CPE occurred, one subculture was made from each cell culture.

When CPE was noted, the virus was titrated and identified with conventional antisera. Only the virus with the highest titer from each cell culture was identified, because the main purpose of our study was to look for polioviruses, which are known to grow rapidly and to high titers. Obviously there were many types of viruses in each sample, but we had no facilities for neutralizing the known types in order to look for others. The use of different cell cultures made it possible to show the presence of several virus types even in the first inoculation.

RESULTS AND DISCUSSION

The results of the first study were published two decades ago (1). During the polio epidemic we isolated polio type 1 viruses both from sewage and from patients' stool samples. The conclusion drawn from that study was: "Sewage samples representing a large number of stool specimens could serve as a good source of material to determine the enteric viral flora of the population." But, a confusing discrepancy was found between the abundance of echo 11 strains in sewage and only a few in stools of patients. Our explanation at that time was that echo 11 was circulating latent in the country.

The results of the second study in Helsinki during 1971-1980 are shown in Table 1. There were 357 virus isolations from 399 sewage samples. Not a single strain of polioviruses was found. Most of the isolations, 230 strains, were coxsackie B viruses. Of 108 echo isolations 80% were echo 11 or echo 6 strains. There were only four isolations of adeno- and four of reoviruses.

The dominant virus types isolated from patients did not always correspond to the viruses detected in sewage. The virus types isolated most frequently from patients (echo 18 in 1972, echo 22 throughout the study and echo 30 in 1980) were not found among the viruses isolated from sewage.

The discrepancy between the viruses in sewage and those obtained from patients may be explained by our isolation methods. The coexistence of many virus types in sewage is generally accepted (3). When such a mixture of viruses is inoculated into cell cultures, the most rapidly adsorbing viruses gain the ascendancy. The etiological agents of epidemics, even if present in abundance, are not necessarily the first to multiply in cell cultures. Polio, coxsackie B, echo 11 and echo 6 may have been the most rapidly growing virus types in our studies. Obviously they had occupied the cells and so prevented viruses of other types from growing.

In any case, the results of our second study do not support the conclusion drawn from our first study that the virus isolations from sewage reflect the etiological agents of epidemics in the community. There may be a correlation, if the etiological agent is a rapidly growing virus type. The laborious work of isolating viruses from sewage by the present methods seems to be pointless epidemiologically.

The results of the study at Inari are shown in Table 2. The virus types isolated were similar to those found in Helsinki. Again the isolations mostly belonged to coxsackie B, echo 11 and echo 6 types. In 1981 we found echo 6 viruses causing aseptic meningitis in Finland. At the same time echo 11, which since 1979 had been the only echo type isolated from sewage in Inari, was replaced by echo 6 strains. Otherwise there was no correspondence between the isolations from sewage and the findings in patients.

Table 1. Virus isolations from sewage in Helsinki, 1971-1980.

Virus types	Year:	1971	1972	1973	1974	1976	1977	1978	1979	1980	Sub-total	Total
Polio		0	0	0	0	0	0	0	0	0		0
Coxsackie A9										1	1	
	B1	6	10				1		1		18	
	B2	1	5	2	1	1	5	2	4	19	40	
	B3	3		1	8	1	2	14	11	6	46	
	B4		6	1	6	5	14	3	13	5	53	
	B5	3	5	25	11		14	7	3	5	73	
												231
Echo	6			1		2	3	15	12	2	35	
	11			1		1	1	2	15	31	51	
Other types				1		2	2	7	8	2	22	
												108
Adeno	1, 2			1						3		4
Reo	2, 3							4				4
Untyped, non polio		2	2		3		3					10
No. samples studied		15	52	52	52	15	52	52	52	52		357

Table 2. Virus isolations from sewage in Inari.

Time of collection	Influent			Effluent		
1979: October	E11*	CB3**		E6,11		
December	E11					A2***
1980: January	E11					A1
February	E11					
March		Not Done			Not Done	
April	E11	CB5	A5		CB5	A1
May		CB5				A1
June	E11	CB5		E11	CB5	
July		CB5		E11	CB5	
August		Not Done			Not Done	
September	E11			E11	CB5	
October	E11	CB4		E11	CB4	
November		CB2,5			CB5	
December	E11	CB2	A2	E11		A2
1981: January	E11	CB2				
February	E11	CB5				
March		CB2,5	A2			
April	E11	CB4		E11		
May						
June						
July	E6	CB2				
August	E6	CB2		E6		
September	E6	CB2		E6	CB2	A1
October	E6			E6		
November	E6	CB2		E6	CB2	
December	E6		A2	E6		
1982: January						
February	E6					
March			A2			
April			A1			A1
May			A2			A2
June			REO2			REO3
July		CB4	A2		CB2,4	
August	E6		REO2			REO2
September	E3	CB2			CB2	
October		CB2			CB2	
November		CB2			CB1,2	
December	E22	CB1		E22	CB2	
1983: January		CB2			CB5	
February	E22	CB1				
March		CB1	A2	E22	CB1	A2,5
April		Not Done			Not Done	
May						A1
June			A2			A2
July	E6	CB1	A2	E6	CB1	
August	E6			E3,6		
September	E11			E11		
October	E11			E11		A1
November	E6,11	CB1		E6		
December	E11	CB2		E11		

* = Echo 11; ** = Coxsackie B3; *** = Adeno 2

The Inari study was also directed to the treatment of sewage. Without going into details of the purification procedures, we may accept that sedimentation, and especially biological treatment with activated sludge, removes about 90% of viruses, but many nevertheless survive the present treatment processes (4). Inari sewage is treated by the biological process supplemented by ferro-sulfate coagulation. Table 2 also shows the viruses isolated from effluents. Unfortunately, we had no quantitative method in our routine work, but the slower detection of viruses from effluents than from influents indicated a reduction in the quantity of viruses. Viruses were isolated from effluents in 72%, but from influents in 92% of samples.

The strains isolated from effluents and from influents tested at the same time sometimes belonged to different virus types. The reason may be a difference in sensitivity to treatment or a difference in growth rate. The seasonal role of enteroviruses in the fall is seen better in the effluents than in the influents.

In a small study carried out in the fall of 1981 after isolation of echo 6 strains, a pailful of influent and one of effluent were put out of doors. Both pails were sampled monthly for 5 months (as long as the sewage lasted). Echo 6 viruses were found in every sample from the influent but not any from the effluent, likewise indicating a reduction in the viruses in the effluent.

There is a great need for a simple viral marker to supplant the laborious, time-consuming and expensive work of isolation and identification of viruses. Unfortunately, a negative *E. coli* test affords no certainty of the absence of viruses, which are more resistant to treatment than bacteria (4).

The aim of this paper is to draw attention to the presence of pathogenic viruses in sewage. Especially in the north, where viruses in a frozen condition may survive for years, maybe longer than we imagine, the importance of adequate treatment of waste waters should be known not only to medical officers, but also to technical experts and to politicians who decide about measures affecting public health.

SUMMARY

Viruses in sewage in Finland were studied in 1960-1961 during a polio type 1 epidemic, weekly during 1971-1980 as a routine in Helsinki, and in 1979-1980 once a month in our most northern community of Inari- Utsjoki.

The isolations of polio type 1 viruses in sewage during the epidemic in 1960 led us to conclude that viruses isolated from sewage are a good indicator of viruses causing diseases in the community. In the other studies, however, the virus types isolated from sewage did not correspond to those isolated from patients at the same time. Our hypothesis is that the virus types most frequently isolated by our methods (coxsackie B viruses, echo 11 and echo 6), are those that grow most rapidly in cell cultures, thus preventing the multiplication of slower viruses. In consequence, virus isolations from sewage have practical value only in special studies, and not epidemiologically.

The virus types of the north were similar to those isolated in Helsinki.

REFERENCES

1. Lapinleimu K, Penttinen K. Virus isolations from sewage in Finland in 1960-61. Arch Ges Virusf 1963; 12:72-75.
2. Albertson P. Two-phase separation of viruses. In: Maramorosch K, Koprowski H, eds. Methods of virology. New York: Academic press, 1967:303-321.
3. Feachem R, Garelick H, Slade J. Enteroviruses in the environment. World Health Forum 1982; 3:170-180.
4. Human viruses in water, wastewater and soil. WHO Tech Rep Ser 1979; 639:1-49.

Kaisa Lapinleimu
National Public Health Institute
Mannerheim intre 166
Helsinki
Finland

TUBERCULOSIS IN THE JAMES BAY CREE INDIAN POPULATION 1980-1983

LISE RENAUD and CHARLES DUMONT

INTRODUCTION

Historically, health care for the Cree Indians has been under the jurisdiction of the Canadian Department of Health and Welfare. The exception was the Ste-Thérèse de l'Enfant-Jésus Hospital in Fort George, now known as Chisasibi, which was administered by the Quebec provincial government. The Anglican and Catholic missions also offered parallel health services to the Cree. In 1978, the James Bay Agreement transferred the administration of all health services to the Cree Health Council, under the jurisdiction of the Department of Social Affairs of the Quebec provincial government. The Department of Community Health of the Montreal General Hospital (DSC-MGH) and the Cree Board of Health and Social Services are beginning cooperatively to develop and evaluate health programs for the Cree Indian population.

The anti-tuberculosis campaign has slowly gained momentum. A provincial tuberculosis screening program has been in effect in all the coastal villages since 1978, while the inland villages were added to the tuberculosis screening program in 1980.

The regional hospital is in Chisasibi, and each community has its own clinic (Figure 1).

This paper describes the epidemiology of tuberculosis in the northern Quebec Cree Indian population between 1980 and 1983, and examines the efficiency of mass chést x-rays in screening for cases of active tuberculosis. A complete and detailed document is available from the senior author's institution (DSC-MGH). The full document examines the epidemiology of tuberculosis: mortality, morbidity, and infection among the Cree. It describes the coverage of the Cree population by the prevention program, and examines the diagnostic efficiency of large scale, mass chest x-rays as a screening tool.

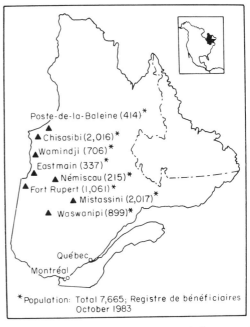

Poste-de-la-Baleine (414)*
Chisasibi (2,016)*
Wamindji (706)*
Eastmain (337)*
Némiscau (215)*
Fort Rupert (1,061)*
Mistassini (2,017)*
Waswanipi (899)*
Québec
Montréal

*Population: Total 7,665; Registre de bénéficiaires October 1983

Figure 1. Cree Indian communities and populations of James Bay, Quebec.

METHODS

The data sources included:

-- the mandatory tuberculosis declaration form, Ministry of Social Affairs (M.A.S.)

-- the chest x-ray reports, Community Health Department, Hôtel-Dieu de Lévis

-- the medical records from the community clinics

-- the permanent tuberculosis register in each clinic.

It should be noted that the data for active and reactivated cases may be subject

Table 1. Evolution of tuberculosis: Quebec and Native populations, 1973-1981. New and reactivated cases per 100,000.

	1973-77	1974-78	1975-79	1976-80	1977-81
Quebec population	17.0	15.3	14.5	13.6	12.8
Native population	147.6	105.9	98.8	88.9	86.5

Source: ref. 3.

Table 2. Incidence of new active and reactivated cases of tuberculosis among the James Bay Cree Indians, 1980-1983.

Year	New active cases	Reactivated cases	Total cases	Annual incidence rate (per 100,000)
1980	7	2	9	120.1
1981	4	1	5	66.7
1982	15	3	18	240.1
1983	3	3	6	80.1
Average for the 4 years	7.3	2.2	9.5	126.8

to an "under-reporting" bias, which is difficult to determine. However, the continued presence of active tuberculosis in the Cree population indicates that some active cases are never identified, and, therefore, never declared.

RESULTS AND DISCUSSION

In general, tuberculosis is declining in the Quebec population. It continues to be a major problem within the Native population, however, although there is a tendency towards a decline here as well (Table 1). The Native population, which represents 0.8% of the total Quebec population, accounts for 5.1% of all active tuberculosis cases recorded in 1981 in Quebec. The incidence of active and reactivated cases among the Cree Indians of James Bay during the 1980-83 period is shown in Table 2. In 1982, the recorded incidence of active tuberculosis cases was much higher than in the preceding or following years. This increased incidence coincides with the onset

of a systematic and uniform screening process. We assume that many active or reactivated cases of tuberculosis which had not been previously identified, due to the absence of any systematic screening, was identified in 1982. Identification and treatment of tuberculosis patients in 1982 would, in turn, reduce the pool of persons able to transmit the tubercle bacillus, thus reducing the number of tuberculosis patients in 1983.

The annual incidence rate of active tuberculosis cases provides us with an overall picture of the problem. This rate among Cree Indians is 126.8/100,000, which is 10 times greater than that found in the total Quebec population, and almost twice that of the general Native population of Quebec (Table 3).

The incidence of tuberculosis varies among the different Native communities. The frequency of tuberculosis found in the Cree population is 30% higher than that of other Quebec Indians, but one-third that observed in the Inuit population (Table 4).

Table 3. New and reactivated tuberculosis cases for certain populations.

	Year	Average annual rate (per 100,000)
Province of Quebec	1977-81	12.8*
Native population	1977-81	86.5*
Cree Indians	1980-83	126.8

*Source: ref. 3.

Table 4. New and reactivated tuberculosis cases for American Indian communities, Cree and Inuit, Quebec, 1981.

Communities	Annual incidence rate (per 100,000)
American Indian, excluding Crees*	51.4
Quebec Crees	66.7
Inuit*	202.4

*Source: ref. 3.

Reactivated Cases

A reactivated case may be defined as one in a person who has had active tuberculosis in the past and who has currently a new episode of the disease.

The proportion of reactivated cases of tuberculosis found in Cree Indians is 23% (Table 5), a percentage similar to that of the Inuit population, and comparable to that of the general Quebec population, excluding Native peoples and immigrants.

Many years tend to elapse between two episodes of tuberculosis (Table 6). Among the 9 reactivated cases, at least half occurred 20 years after the first episode, and one untreated case after 7 years. The results are similar to those obtained by Grzybowski et al. (1) for the Inuit of the Northwest Territories. The risk of reactivation among the Inuit is small during the first years following the original episode. This risk slowly increases, attaining a maximum level 10 years after the original episode. This situation differs from the non-Native population, where the risk of reactivation is highest in the years closest to the original attack of tuberculosis.

Distribution by Age and Sex

The distribution of tuberculosis differs among the Crees from that in the general Quebec population. The new and reactivated cases are equally distributed among males and females of the Cree population (Table 7). Approximately 40% of the active cases are found in those less than 14 years of age. In the general Quebec population the number of active cases under the age of 34 is the same for males and females. After the age of 35, the prevalence of tuberculosis is almost twice as high in males as in females. Only 4% of the active tuberculosis cases are found in the general Quebec population under 14 years of age, or

Table 6. Number of years between the two episodes of tuberculosis among the James Bay Cree Indians, 1980-1983.

Years between episodes	Number of reactivated cases
7	1 (untreated)
20	1
25	2
28	1
31	1
Unknown	3
Total	9

one-tenth the proportion of this age group in the Cree population.

The age distribution of tuberculosis among the Quebec Crees is similar to that among the Ontario Crees and Ojibwas. Young states between 1975 and 1979, a third of the active tuberculosis cases in Ontario Crees and Ojibwas were under 25 years of age. Grzybowski et al. (1) made a similar observation among the Inuit of the Northwest Territories where more cases of active tuberculosis were found in those under 25 years of age than any other age groups.

Distribution by Village

The distribution of new and reactivated cases of tuberculosis is not uniform over the James Bay area. Inland communities (Mistassini and Waswanipi) report 4 times more active tuberculosis cases than coastal villages. This difference may be explained by the fact that many Crees from the inland communities live in camps year round and have less access to the screening program. These camps are possibly the source of undetected and untreated cases of tuberculosis.

Table 5. Distribution of new active and reactivated cases of tuberculosis by community, 1981.

	New active cases	Reactivated cases	Total
Inuit*	8 (80%)	2 (20%)	10 (100%)
Cree Indians (average 1980-83)	7.3 (77%)	2.2 (23%)	9.5 (100%)
Quebec population (excluding Native and immigrants)	442 (85.6%)	74 (14.4%)	56 (100%)

*Source: ref. 3

Table 7. Distribution of new and reactivated tuberculosis cases for Cree Indians of James Bay and population of Quebec.

Age Group	Cree Indians 1980-83				Quebec* 1981			
	M	F	Total	%	M	F	Total	%
0-4	4	2	6	15.8	7	6	13	2.0
5-14	3	5	8	21.1	6	7	13	2.0
15-34	7	7	14	36.8	61	65	131	19.4
35-54	4	1	5	13.1	132	51	183	28.1
55+	2	3	5	13.2	192	124	316	48.5
Total	20	18	38	100.0	398	253	651	100.0

*Source: Ministère des Affaires sociales, Rapport annuel de tuberculose, 1981.

Value of Mass Chest X-Rays in Screening

Over 3 years, only 3.2% of the chest x-rays were abnormal and required follow-up (Table 8). Among these, only one case of active tuberculosis was identified by x-ray, and this case was also identified by a test in one of our tuberculosis clinics. The diagnostic value of mass chest x-rays were therefore judged negligible, and they were abandoned in 1984. Other methods will have to be used to screen for tuberculosis. It has been shown that 75% of the active cases of tuberculosis among the Cree Indians were identified after consultation for symptoms and a subsequent investigation of contacts (Table 9).

This finding suggests that better health education would be useful for the population. More information should also be

Table 9. Distribution of new tuberculosis cases based on initial investigation procedures, Cree Indians of James Bay, 1981-1983.

Initial investigation procedures	Number of cases	%
Contact history	11	37.9
Consultations due to symptoms	11	37.9
Routine PPD	6	20.7
Routine x-rays	1	3.5
Total	29	100.0

Table 8. Results of mass x-ray screening for tuberculosis in Cree Indians, James Bay, 1981-1983.

Year	Total number of mass x-rays	Number of cases identified at screening	Number of cases confirmed tuber- culosis positive*
1981	3,196	114 (3.6%)	0
1982	2,320	72 (3.1%)	1
1983	2,731	81 (2.9%)	0

*   The cases identified at the x-ray screening were tested tuberculosis positive by one of the following methods: sputum culture, urine analysis, PPD 5TU, presence or absence of clinical symptoms.

made available to the health professionals, so that they can be familiar with, and watchful for the diversity of the clinical symptoms of tuberculosis.

REFERENCES

1. Grzybowski S et al. Tuberculosis in Eskimos, Tubercle 1976; 57:S1-S55.

2. Young T Kue. Epidemiology of tuberculosis in remote native communities, Can Fam Phys 1982; 28:67-74.

3. MAS Annual Report on Tuberculosis-- 1981. Province of Quebec, Infections Diseases Division, June 1982:23.

Lise Renaud
Department of Community Health
Montreal General Hospital
1597 Pine Avenue West
Montreal, Quebec H3G 1B3
Canada

Circumpolar Health 84:222-225

REACTIVATION OF TUBERCULOSIS IN MANITOBA, 1976 TO 1981

IAN L. JOHNSON, M. THOMSON, J. MANFREDA and E.S. HERSHFIELD

INTRODUCTION

The rates of reported cases of tuberculosis in Canada decreased between 1965 and 1980. A similar decrease occurred in the province of Manitoba (1), although variability in the trend was greater (Figure 1). The proportion of reactivations in Manitoba has remained relatively stable at 8 to 14% of all cases of tuberculosis (2). Because reactivation is an important source of tuberculous infection in a community, this study was initiated to describe the characteristics of reactivators and to identify groups at relatively high risk of reactivation.

MATERIALS AND METHODS

The Canadian Tuberculosis Standards (3) define reactivation as "the repeat isolation of the tubercle bacillus on culture or the presence of clinical symptoms and chest x-ray changes compatible with disease activity following a period of inactivity." A period of inactivity is considered to be a minimum of 6 continuous months in which there are no signs of tuberculous activity in a patient who is receiving or has received anti-tuberculous therapy (3).

All cases listed as tuberculosis reactivation by the Central Tuberculosis Registry (C.T.R.) of the Manitoba Lung Association from the years 1976 to 1981 were included in this study. The C.T.R. is the official registry for Manitoba and contains all cases of tuberculosis diagnosed in the province, since registration is required by provincial law. An agreement between the provincial and federal governments to provide treatment through the provincial system ensures that it has complete records for registered Indians in the province.

Validation of the cases was performed by reviewing available hospital and registry records. The diagnosis was confirmed on the basis of positive bacteriological or radiological reports but in the absence of these, the diagnosis of the physician at the time was assumed to be correct. The period of inactivity was verified through reviews of hospital and outpatient records.

Data on age, sex, ethnic origin, bacillary status, and extent of disease at the initial and recurrent episodes were extracted primarily from the registry's records. Analysis of the effects of drug therapy and compliance on the potential for reactivation could not be performed because of incomplete data.

A Treaty Indian is defined as a person, who is registered pursuant to the Indian Act

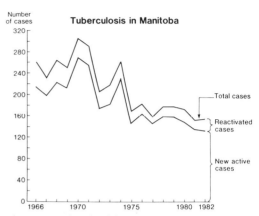

Figure 1. The incidence of tuberculosis in Manitoba 1966-1982.

as an Indian or is entitled to be registered as an Indian. A Métis is a person of mixed ancestry. "Other ethnic group" includes primarily Caucasians. Bacillary status was considered positive if bacilli were identified by smear or culture. The extent of disease was assessed on the basis of radiological findings. The disease was minimal if there was parenchymal involvement without cavitation. Moderate and advanced disease were characterized by more extensive parenchymal involvement plus cavitation. In pleural disease, parenchymal involvement was absent or minor, while in extrapulmonary disease, the site of the disease process was outside the lungs.

To identify the risk factors for reactivation, two controls for each case of reactivation were selected at random from the same registry. A control was defined as a patient who had active tuberculosis in the same year as the case but had no known evidence of reactivation since then. Cases were matched with the controls for sex, all but 3 cases were matched for age within 5 years. Due to the poor quality of the records prior to 1947, controls could not be selected for 13 of the cases of reactivation who had their initial episode prior to 1947.

RESULTS

There were 113 cases listed as reactivated tuberculosis from 1976 to 1981 but after review only 72 (64%) satisfied the definition for reactivation (Table 1). Of the 41 cases deleted, in 5 cases charts were unavailable, 6 cases had no documented evidence of an initial episode of disease, and 2 cases provided insufficient evidence

Table 1. *Validity of the diagnosis of reactivation.*

	No.	Percent
Total cases listed as reactivations	113	100%
Disqualifications	**No.**	**Percent**
Charts unavailable	5	4%
No proof of the initial episode of TB	6	5%
No period of inactivity	26	23%
Non-tuberculous mycobacterial disease	2	2%
No proof of the second episode of TB	2	2%
Valid cases of reactivations	72	64%

Table 2. *Relationship between the initial episode and reactivation.*

Extent of disease at initial episode	Disease at Reactivation		
	Pulmonary	Extra-pulmonary	Total
Pleurisy	5	0	5 (7%)
Minimal	16	4	20 (28%)
Moderate	18	1	19 (26%)
Advanced	12	1	13 (18%)
Extrapulmonary	6	9	15 (21%)
Total	57	15	72 (100%)

118 controls. Case-control comparisons were made on ethnic origin, bacillary status at the initial episode, and extent of disease of the initial episode (Table 3). The association between ethnic origin and reactivation was significant. Treaty and Non-treaty Indians and Métis made up 64% of the reactivators, and only 35% of the controls. Bacillary status at the initial episode was not found to be associated with the risk of reactivation. A greater propor-

Table 3. *Risk factors for reactivation.*

	Cases N=59*		Controls N=118*	
Ethnic origin				
Treaty Indian	25	42%	28	24%
Non-Treaty/ Métis	13	22%	13	11%
Other	21	36%	74	63%
				p=0.001
Bacillary status first episode				
Positive	26	46%	61	53%
Negative	31	54%	55	47%
				p=0.50
Extent of disease first episode				
Moderate/ advanced	22	37%	29	25%
Other	36	63%	86	75%
				p=0.10

* Because of missing information, a case or control was excluded from the analysis, and as a result, not all columns sum to N, or to 100%.

of a second episode of tuberculosis. In 2 cases other non-tuberculosis mycobacteria were cultured (both *M. avium intracellulare*). The largest number of deletions from the list (26) were removed for lack of a documented 6-month period of inactivity.

Of the 72 verified cases of reactivation, the greatest number (21) had their initial episode of disease in the 1950s, and the next largest number (17) in the 1940s. Of the reactivations 57 (79%) were pulmonary while 15 (21%) had extrapulmonary disease. There were 42 (58%) male patients and 30 (42%) female. The average age at the initial episode was 32 years with a range from 2 to 73 years and at the second episode 53 years with a range from 21 to 83. The period of inactivity ranged from 1 to 61 years with an average of 21 years. Ethnically, 28 (39%) of the reactivators were Treaty Indians, 14 (19%) were non-Treaty Indians or Métis, and 30 (42%) were persons of other ethnic origins.

At the initial episode, 39% (54%) of the cases were non-bacillary. The extent of pulmonary disease shown in Table 2 reveals that 20 (28%) had minimal disease, 19 (26%) moderate, 13 (18%) had advanced disease. Pleurisy occurred in 5 (7%) and 15 (21%) had the disease outside the lungs. Of the 15 cases who initially had extrapulmonary disease, 9 reactivated with extrapulmonary disease, and 6 reactivated with pulmonary disease. Similarly, 6 cases out of 51 with initial pulmonary disease reactivated in extrapulmonary sites while the majority (45) reactivated with pulmonary disease.

The 59 cases of reactivation with sufficient documentation were matched with

Table 4. Relationship between the extent of the initial episode and reactivation by ethnic group.

	Extent of disease	Cases	Con- trols	Odds ratio
Treaty Indian	Moderate/ advanced	13	6	
	Minimal/ extra	12	22	4.0
Non-Treaty Indian and Métis	Moderate/ advanced	3	3	
	Minimal/ extra	10	10	1.0
Other ethnic groups	Moderate/ advanced	6	20	
	Minimal/ extra	14	54	1.2
Total	Moderate/ advanced	22	29	
	Minimal/ extra	36	86	1.8

tion of reactivators had moderate and advanced disease at the initial episode than did controls (37% vs. 25%). Although this difference is marginally significant statistically at p = 0.1, when the relationship between the extent of initial disease and reactivation was examined by ethnic groups (Table 4), a significant association was found in Treaty Indians with an odds ratio of 4.

DISCUSSION

Previous studies (4,5) on the accuracy of tuberculosis reporting have concentrated mainly on avoiding duplication and not on the accuracy of the diagnosis. Zaki et al. (6) used procedures similar to ours. They reported disqualifying cases for failing to meet their specific criteria for reactivation, but did not specify the number. Our disqualification of 41 (36%) of the original 113 reactivation cases is significant. The major failure to meet the case definition was in obtaining a 6-month period of inactivity. We believe that most of the 26 patients in this disqualified group began on therapy, were subsequently lost to follow-up, and were listed as reactivations when their therapy was reinstituted.

Since more than half the cases of reactivation in the late 1970s occurred in individuals initially treated prior to 1960, patients who had tuberculosis a long time

ago must be considered as important potential sources of infection for the community. By contrast, the individual's risk of reactivation is maximal soon after therapy and decreases with time (7,8).

The high proportion (39%) of reactivations among Treaty Indians indicates the importance of this group to the overall frequency of reactivations. By the case-control analysis, Treaty Indian status was associated with a significantly increased risk of reactivation, especially if the initial disease was extensive, i.e. with cavitation. The reasons for this increased risk require further study. Poor or incomplete therapy, poor access to health care, and aspects of living conditions in Native communities may be implicated. The unique positive correlation between extent of initial disease and risk of reactivation in Treaty Indians may be attributable to some of the same factors.

Control of tuberculosis in Manitoba should focus on preventing reactivation, especially among Indians because cases of reactivated tuberculosis might be sources of outbreaks of disease in Native communities. Effective preventive techniques are not easy to select. The value of routine screening with chest x-rays is questionable (9), sputum surveys are likely to be unacceptable to the population, and prophylactic treatment with isoniazid is impossible. On the other hand, it seems clear that vigorous treatment, close supervision, and post-treatment monitoring of the initial episode (especially when it occurs with cavitation) should be insisted upon. The only practical way to achieve early detection through clinical suspicion may be to educate physicians and health care professionals on risk factors.

REFERENCES

1. Tuberculosis Statistics: Morbidity and Mortality, 1982, Statistics Canada.
2. Manitoba Lung Association, Annual Report, 1980:10.
3. Classification and reporting of tuberculosis in Canada, 1969, Canadian Tuberculosis and Respiratory Disease Association.
4. Horowitz O, Rossen A, Wilbek E. Control of the efficacy of the Danish notification system for pulmonary tuberculosis. Acta Tuber Scand 1960; 38:119-125.
5. Davies PDO, Citron K, Raynes RH. Ambiguities and inaccuracies in the notification system for tuberculosis in England and Wales. Community Medicine 1981; 3:108-118.

6. Zaki H, Lyon HA, Tizes R, Ali H. Tuberculosis patients: reactivation. NY State J Med 1977, Aug:1441-1446.

7. Horowitz O. Public health aspects of relapsing tuberculosis. Am Rev Resp Dis 1969; 99:183-193.

8. Campbell AH. Relapse in pulmonary tuberculosis. Med J Australia 1967; 2:448-450.

9. Tomon K. Tuberculosis, casefinding and chemotherapy. Geneva: WHO, 1979.

E.S. Hershfield
Department of Medicine
Respiratory Hospital
810 Sherbrook Street
Winnipeg, Manitoba R3A 1R8
Canada

Circumpolar Health 84:226-228

LOWER RESPIRATORY TRACT INFECTIONS AMONG CANADIAN INUIT CHILDREN

JAMES B. CARSON, B.D. POSTL, D. SPADY and OTTO SCHAEFER

In the era of declining importance of pulmonary tuberculosis, Inuit infants and children continue to sustain a high incidence of lower respiratory tract infections (LRTI) (1-3). LRTI and bronchiolitis in childhood are suspected antecedents of chronic respiratory impairment (4,5). Chronic respiratory impairment has been shown to be increasing among Inuit pediatric patients in comparison with other racial groups (6).

With this in mind, and as part of a larger follow-up study on health of children in the Canadian Northwest Territories, we retrospectively surveyed at age 8 years Inuit children who had been subjects of the Perinatal and Infant Morbidity and Mortality Survey (PIMM) of 1973-74 (1).

The original PIMM study involved a one year follow-up of all infants born to residents of the Canadian Northwest Territories for a calendar year. The present study involved locating and examining surviving Native children in their home settlements and was conducted in 1982. Subjects for this report are the Inuit children of the eastern Arctic--namely the Keewatin and Baffin districts of the Northwest Territories.

There were 314 live births from this geographic area during the original study, but 25 had died by age 8, most in infancy, and over one-quarter from LRTI. We located 260 or 90% of survivors for follow-up.

Of the 260, we examined 234. Spirometry was obtained for 219 children with a McKessan wedge spirometer. Spirometry was not performed on children with acute upper or lower respiratory tract infections. Also, spirometry was not done on children with neurologic or neuromuscular abnormalities. A further small number of children were too shy to be tested. Chest radiographs were not obtained.

Medical records were reviewed for all subjects at nursing stations and at referral hospitals. Hospitalizations for lower respiratory tract infections were reviewed in detail. The diagnosis of bronchiolitis was confirmed on clinical grounds with the documentation of cough, fever, tachypnea, and wheeze occurring prior to age 2 (5).

Of the 260 Inuit children (Figure 1), 81 (31%) had been hospitalized one or more times for a confirmed LRTI, and of those, 46 children were hospitalized at least once for bronchiolitis. A further 109 children (42%) had one or more LRTI treated on an outpatient basis, but had not been hospitalized. The remaining 70 children (27%) had no documented LRTI.

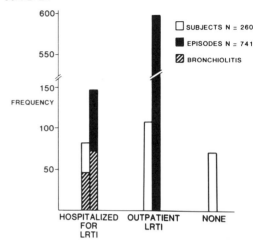

Figure 1. Lower respiratory tract infections (LRTIs) in Inuit children from birth to 8 years.

There were 741 episodes of LRTI. This includes 147 hospitalizations of which 71, almost half, were considered to be bronchiolitis. The remaining 594 episodes occurred among outpatients. There were 3 cases of pulmonary tuberculosis.

The incidence of LRTI per 100 children per year is shown for three age groups (Figure 2). Among infants, there were 41 hospitalizations per 100 children per year and 110 out-patient episodes per 100 per year. Rates for the second year were 9 and 42 respectively, and declined to 1 and 11 thereafter. The incidence of hospitalization for bronchiolitis was 24 per 100 per year in infancy.

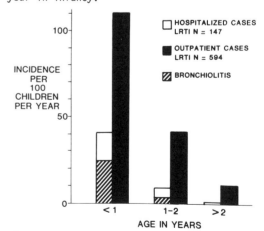

Figure 2. Age-related incidence of lower respiratory tract infections in 260 Inuit children.

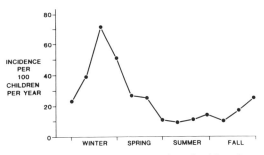

Figure 3. *Seasonality of hospitalizations for bronchiolitis in 260 Inuit children.*

Hospitalization for bronchiolitis in infancy by month is shown (Figure 3). A peak incidence of 71 per 100 children per year was noted during winter months.

Breast-feeding was associated with a significant reduction in hospitalization for 244 Inuit on whom feeding information was available (Figure 4). Of those hospitalized for LRTI, 67% were never breast-fed; 15% were breast-fed less than three months and 18% were breast-fed three or more months. Among those never hospitalized, 38% were never breast-fed, 19% were breast-fed less than three months and 43% were breast-fed three or more months.

Birth-weight, sex, adoption, number of siblings, maternal smoking, and current weight and height were not associated with the incidence of hospitalization for LRTI.

Spirometry for 119 of the Inuit boys at age 8 is shown (Figure 5). Forced expiratory volume in 1 second (FEV_1), and forced vital capacity (FVC) are plotted for hospitalized and never hospitalized subjects. FEV_1 was 1.68 liters for hospitalized boys and 1.77 liters for those never hospitalized

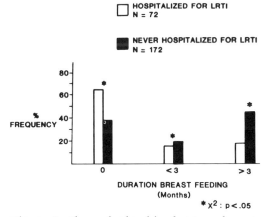

Figure 4. *The relationship between breast-feeding and hospitalization for lower respiratory tract infections in 244 Inuit children from birth to 8 years.*

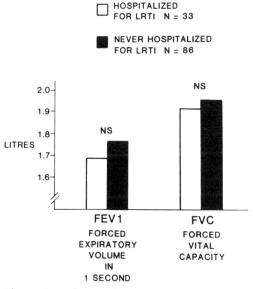

Figure 5. *Spirometric performance of 119 Inuit boys, age 8, with different histories of lower respiratory tract infections. (NS = statistically not significantly different.)*

for LRTI. FVC's were 1.92 liters and 2.01 liters respectively. Analysis of co-variance controlling for height revealed no significant difference between groups.

Similar spirometry data are shown (Figure 6) for 100 Inuit girls at age 8. FEV_1 was 1.63 liters for hospitalized girls and was 1.64 liters for those never hospitalized for LRTI. FVC's were 1.78 liters and 1.85 liters respectively. Again, controlling for height, no significant difference was noted between hospitalized and non-hospitalized subjects. Comparing FEV_1 and FVC for children hospitalized with bronchiolitis with children never hospitalized for LRTI similarly revealed no significant difference for Inuit boys or girls.

A group of 19 children, 7% of the total, was identified as having frequent or recurrent LRTI, defined as five or more episodes post-infancy. Twelve of these children were boys and seven were girls, with 14 being hospitalized at least once for a LRTI. Only one of these children was identified as having a chronic respiratory impairment, namely bronchiectasis.

Spirometry is available for 15 of these 19 children including 10 boys and 5 girls. FEV_1 and FVC are shown for these 15 children and are expressed as percent of predicted for sex and height (Figure 7). Predicted values are based on prediction equations generated for each sex from the spirometer data of the 219 tested children. The method described by Hsu (7) was used to develop the

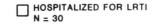

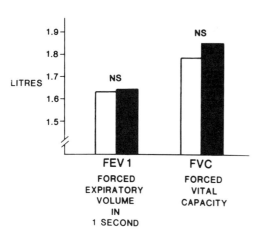

Figure 6. Spirometric performance of 100 Inuit girls, age 8, with different histories of lower respiratory tract infections. (NS = statistically not significantly different.)

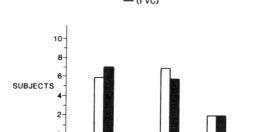

Figure 7. Spirometric performance at age 8 for 15 Inuit children with histories of frequent post-infancy lower respiratory tract infections. Observed performances are compared to those predicted for normal children, corrected for sex and body size.

prediction equations. FEV_1 was reduced in 6 cases and FVC was reduced in 7 cases to values of less than 80% of predicted, defining a sub-group with significant respiratory impairment.

In summary, these Inuit children by age 8 have had a very high incidence of LRTI, especially in infancy. Bronchiolitis, based on clinical criteria, accounted for almost half of all hospitalizations for LRTI. Frequent or recurrent LRTI, defined as five or more episodes post-infancy, was observed for 19 children or 7% of all subjects. One-third of this group (7 children), had significant reduction of FEV_1, FVC or both, defining a small sub-group with respiratory impairment.

REFERENCES

1. Spady DW, Covill FC, Hobar CW, et al. Between two worlds: The report of the Northwest Territories perinatal and infant mortality and morbidity study. Occasional publication 16, Boreal Institute for Northern Studies. University of Alberta, 1982.

2. Morrell RE, Marks MI, Champlin R, Spence L. An outbreak of severe pneumonia due to respiratory syncytial virus in isolated arctic populations. Amer J Epidemiol 1975; 101:231-237.

3. Lembke EC. Bronchiolitis epidemic: Repulse Bay, 1978. U Man Med J 1981; 51:24.

4. Burrows B, Knudson RJ, Lebowitz MD. The relationship of childhood respiratory illness to adult obstructive airway disease. Amer Rev Resp Dis 1977: 115:751-760.

5. Wohl MEB, Chernick V. Bronchiolitis. Amer Rev Resp Dis 1978; 118:759-781.

6. Fleshman JK, Wilson JF, Cohen JJ. Bronchiectasis in Alaska Native children. Arch Environ Health 1968; 17:517-523.

7. Hsu KHK, Jenkins DE, Hsi BP, Bourhofer E, Thompson V, Tanakawa N, Hsick GSJ. Ventilatory functions of normal children and young adults--Mexican-American, white and black. I. Spirometry. J Ped 1979; 95:14-23.

James B. Carson
Northern Medical Unit
Division of Community and Northern Medicine
University of Manitoba
61 Emily Street
Winnipeg, Manitoba R3E 1Y9
Canada

Circumpolar Health 84:229-234

PERTUSSIS: A STUDY OF INCIDENCE AND MORTALITY IN A YUKON-KUSKOKWIM DELTA EPIDEMIC

BELINDA IRELAND, LISA KNUTSON, WALLACE ALWARD and DAVID B. HALL

INTRODUCTION

Pertussis ("whooping cough") is a disease of decreasing importance in developed countries and is rarely discussed at any length in medical schools today. Yet, because of the controversy regarding pertussis vaccination, it is important that we re-examine the morbidity and mortality patterns of this childhood disease. The 1961-1962 Alaska Eskimo cohort provides an excellent opportunity for us to examine an epidemic in an unimmunized infant population.

Between October 1960 and December 1962, 643 live births from 27 Eskimo villages in the Yukon-Kuskokwim Delta area of southwestern Alaska were identified and entered into a study of perinatal morbidity and mortality (1). This cohort was followed beginning in the third trimester of the mother's pregnancy, with quarterly visits by a research nurse during the first two years of life and intermittently thereafter. Information was gathered on pregnancy and delivery, growth, nutritional practices and illnesses. Health-related data such as hemoglobin levels and records of immunization were also collected.

This cohort has been maintained as a study group. Data have been collected on psychological development, physical growth, illness, vision, teenage alcohol and tobacco use, nutrition, and a host of other personal characteristics of research interest. Preliminary examination of this data set revealed exceptional village to village variation in almost all measures. It also revealed patterns of epidemic spread for measles, respiratory disease, and a pertussis syndrome.

Our purpose in this report is threefold. We want to describe the spatial and temporal pattern of the epidemic of disease characterized by a pertussis syndrome, explore factors related to symptomatic illness, and explore factors related to mortality involving this infection. In the process we will attempt to document epidemiologic evidence that this clinically diagnosed pertussis syndrome was caused by *Bordetella pertussis*. The examination of factors associated with symptomatic illness is a cohort study. The examination of factors associated with mortality after infection is a matched case-control study.

Pertussis is an acute respiratory disease with a reported communicability rate of 85% in unimmunized children (2). It exists worldwide, occurs as epidemics, and infects humans as its only host. Spread by droplets, it is most communicable during the early catarrhal stage and before development of the paroxysmal cough. The incubation period usually lasts from one to two weeks but can last up to three weeks. While susceptibility is general, 80% of those infected are less than five years of age (2), and 64% of the deaths are in infants under one year of age (3). Both morbidity and mortality are greater in females than males. No apparent protection is offered infants of immune mothers. One attack of pertussis confers prolonged but not lifelong immunity.

Clinical diagnosis is easier to establish in the older child who follows the characteristic pattern. The catarrhal stage, lasting two weeks, begins with nonspecific symptoms of nasal discharge and mild cough. The paroxysmal stage follows in which the distinct "whoop" develops as a result of the deep, forced inspiration to rapidly replace air lost during the coughing episode. During this stage, vomiting often follows and the child becomes exhausted. The very young infant will not have the paroxysmal cough and may die with the disease undiagnosed during a period of apnea. Fever is absent throughout the disease and develops only if complications are present (4).

Prevention by active immunization is effective in most individuals. At present, controversy exists regarding the risk/benefit of pertussis immunization due to the relatively high incidence of neurologic complications following vaccination.

In Alaska, pertussis remained a serious health problem even after the development of the vaccine. The remoteness of much of the state's population prevented its widespread use. Once the disease was contracted, lack of available health care often prevented its diagnosis and treatment. Pertussis was an important cause of morbidity and mortality, ranking fifth in incidence among communicable diseases in Alaska in 1950 (5).

MATERIALS AND METHODS

As a part of this and other studies, the original records kept on each cohort member were reviewed, and a history of severe infectious disease was abstracted for each person. Episodes of infectious disease were identified and recorded with date of onset, duration, signs, symptoms, and diagnoses. Possible diagnoses included rubella, rubeola, chickenpox, bronchiolitis, and pneumonia as well as pertussis. The original diagnoses were reviewed for consistency and surety.

For this study persons were considered to have had pertussis when their respiratory symptoms included the characteristic cough and/or coughing until vomiting, or when they had been admitted to the hospital with a diagnosis of pertussis.

The pattern of illness from pertussis, as defined symptomatically, was examined to define the epidemic which passed through this region. The path of the epidemic was determined using graphical techniques (6) supplemented with anecdotal information. Villages were divided into those with documented pertussis cases and those with none.

For the cohort study of factors related to illness, cohort members with pertussis were compared with other cohort members alive at the time of the epidemic. We explored possible predisposing factors for illness, including age, sex, birthweight, illness history preceding the pertussis and diphtheria-pertussis-tetanus (DPT) immunization status. Analysis was restricted to those villages with at least one documented episode of pertussis in a cohort member, and, whenever necessary, analyses were adjusted for village as a confounding factor. Analytic techniques included Mantel-Haenszel statistics, the Wilcoxon rank sum test for blocked data (7) and logistic regressions as appropriate.

Feeding practices were also evaluated in the cohort study to distinguish between breast-feeding and bottle-feeding. In examining the relationship to symptomatic pertussis infection two observations were considered: the first observation which was usually during the first three months of life and the last observation immediately preceding the epidemic. Information was available for 178 cohort members from villages involved in the epidemic. For 73 cohort members there is only one analysis, since they were visited only once before the pertussis epidemic in their villages. Analysis was performed using Mantel-Haenszel tests to adjust for village.

For the case-control study of mortality related to pertussis, deaths in the cohort during this period were reviewed for cause of death and possible connection to pertussis. Those deaths with such a connection were classified into "probable" or "possible" pertussis-related deaths. The "probable" group included those with a diagnosis of pertussis in their fatal illness episode, though the final cause of death was often bronchopneumonia. The "possible" group included individuals who died as a result of non-specific respiratory illness during the period when other cohort members in that village were diagnosed as having pertussis. When infants are less than six months old,

the cough which characterizes pertussis is often not observed (8). Each pertussis-related death was matched to a control subject with a non-fatal episode of pertussis. The control was the cohort member from the same village as the case subject with a date of onset of illness from pertussis closest to that of the case subject. When no such person existed, the control subject was selected from the cohort members in the nearest village with pertussis episodes who met the definition for control subjects. This case-control study examined possible predisposing factors for mortality such as age at illness, sex, birthweight, breast-feeding and preceding illness. Statistical techniques such as McNemar's test and the Wilcoxon signed rank test were used to account for the matched nature of the data.

RESULTS

Episodes of a pertussis syndrome were identified in 15 of the 27 cohort villages. There had been 475 births by May 1962, when the last pertussis episode in this epidemic occurred. Of these, 221 lived in the villages which were involved in the epidemic. The crude incidence was 168 per 1,000 infants, while the incidence in villages documented to have been exposed was 362 per 1,000 infants. All members of the study cohort were less than 18 months of age at the time of the epidemic. Median age at diagnosis for those ill was 7 months.

All of these diagnoses were made between August 1961 and May 1962 (Figure 1, a-f). For three months in 1961, the infection was seen in a cluster of three villages at the mouth of the Yukon River (Figure 1b). During the last two months of 1961, the infection spread down the coast, with a major outbreak in the village of Hooper Bay to the south of the first villages (Figure 1c). In January of 1962, coastal incidence had subsided, and sporadic cases were reported at the mouth of the Kuskokwim River and in several small villages near Bethel, the transportation and commercial hub for Yukon-Kuskokwim Delta (Figure 1d). The epidemic spread rapidly in this area, and in February and March of 1962, all eight villages near Bethel experienced a high incidence of disease (Figure 1e). The departure of the epidemic was as dramatic as its arrival, with no cases in the Kuskokwim River villages during the remainder of 1962 (Figure 1f). The spread of pertussis to Mekoryuk, a particularly isolated village on Nunivak Island, was documented anecdotally in the terminal illness records of one child who died in March 1962. The record states: "2 Bethel children (with cough) in village for 2-3 weeks early in February. Whooping cough reported 03/04/62, 9 cases."

Using as the population at risk all cohort members in the pertussis villages

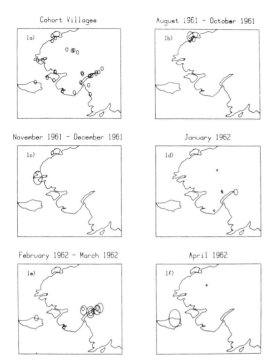

Cohort Villages

August 1961 - October 1961

November 1961 - December 1961

January 1962

February 1962 - March 1962

April 1962

Figure 1. The course of a pertussis epidemic in the Yukon-Kuskokwim Delta region of Alaska, 1961-1962.

alive at any time during the epidemic in each village, morbidity was slightly higher in females at 37.3% (44/118) than in males at 35.0% (36/103), although the difference is not statistically significant. The proportion ill in cohort villages varied from 0.17 (2/12) in Kipnuk to 1.00 (2/2) in Oscarville (Table 1). The median age of

those who became ill was 7 months and of those without documented pertussis it was 6 months (Wilcoxon rank sum z = -0.772, p = 0.4402). Other factors, including birth weight, respiratory illness preceding the epidemic, and immunization status, also showed no association with morbidity.

The level of immunization was very low in this population; of the cohort members in the pertussis villages alive on December 31 1961, (midway through the epidemic) 21.5% had received at least one injection and only 6.7% (14/209) had received two or more injections.

At their first visit, while less than 3 months of age, 66 infants were exclusively breast-feeding (37%), 32 were exclusively bottle-feeding (18%) and 80 were both breast- and bottle-feeding (45%). Before the epidemic these percentages had shifted to 16%, 44% and 40%, respectively, for the 105 individuals who had subsequent visits (Table 2). Pertussis was most prevalent in the group that was feeding from both sources at first visit, diagnosed for 54% of such infants. Prevalence in first visit breast-feeding infants was 35% and in bottle-feeding infants was 28%. The difference between those who were both breast- and bottle-feeding when first observed and those who were exclusively feeding either way was statistically significant (Mantel-Haenszel chi-square = 7.55, p = 0.006). This relationship had disappeared before the epidemic, and there was not association between feeding habits at the last visit before the epidemic and symptomatic pertussis infection. For the 105 cohort members with more than one observation on feeding habits the first visit indicated increased risk for children both breast- and bottle-feeding (Mantel-Haenszel chi-square = 4.37, p =

Table 1. Pertussis in 1960-1962 cohort members from 15 affected villages in Alaska.

Village	Date of last case	Pertussis cases (N)	Persons at risk (N)	Proportion ill
Sheldon's Point	08/61	1	5	0.20
Alakanuk	10/61	4	17	0.24
Emmonak	12/61	8	23	0.35
Hooper Bay	12/61	8	23	0.35
Akiachuk	03/62	4	19	0.21
Akiak	03/62	4	10	0.40
Kipnuk	03/62	2	12	0.17
Pilot Station	03/62	3	14	0.21
Kasigluk	03/62	4	16	0.25
Napakiak	03/62	7	13	0.54
Napaskiak	03/62	4	19	0.37
Nunapitchuk	03/62	7	19	0.37
Oscarville	03/62	2	2	1.00
Kwethluk	03/62	9	19	0.47
Mekoryuk	05/62	13	20	0.65

0.04), while the last visit indicated no relationship (Mantel-Haenszel chi-square = 0.01, p = 0.92).

The review of mortality indicated 10 deaths possibly associated with pertussis. Seven (6 female, 1 male) were classified as probable pertussis deaths, while the other three (1 female, 2 male) were all infants under 2 months of age who died of respiratory infections. All were in pertussis villages during the epidemic and for one of the "possible" cases there is documentation of siblings with pertussis. Combining both categories, this gives a case-fatality rate of 8 per 100 in males and 16 per 100 in females (chi-square 0.462, df=1, p = 0.5). The case-control study of fatal versus non-fatal cases did not indicate significant differences in birthweight (Wilcoxon signed rank p = 0.469), sex (McNemar's test p = 0.5), breast-feeding (McNemar's test p = 0.5) or previous lower respiratory infection (McNemar's test p = 0.5). The age at which a child contracted pertussis appeared to be associated with mortality (Wilcoxon signed rank p = 0.084, 2-sided). The median age at diagnosis for children who died was 3.5 months, as opposed to 6.5 for the controls.

DISCUSSION

The rate of documented symptomatic infection in affected villages and the nature of the case ascertainment supports the contention that many cases of infection were not identified as pertussis. Our primary objective was to demonstrate that, despite this problem, we could document the epidemic as it spread across the Yukon-Kuskokwim Delta. Similar methods will be applied to epidemics of measles and respiratory infections.

The characteristics of the epidemic which passed through the Yukon-Kuskokwim Delta during the fall and winter of 1961-1962 are consistent with those caused by *Bordetella pertussis*. Recorded clinical symptoms included whooping cough, often continuing until vomiting occurred. *B. pertussis* is known to have been present in the Yukon-Kuskokwim region during the spring of 1962 (9). In addition, morbidity and mortality from this illness followed the pattern known for pertussis. The proportion of females with recorded illness episodes exceeded that of the males; this is consistent with pertussis and in contrast to other respiratory infections (10). The same relationship is present in the deaths associated with this epidemic with a female case-fatality rate twice that for the males, another pattern unique to pertussis (3). These deaths were concentrated among the younger cases; all infants who died were under 10 months of age at the onset of their illness. Approximately 70% of pertussis deaths occur in those under one year of age at illness and the majority under six months (8). The deaths themselves also indicate *B. pertussis* rather than *B. parapertussis*, which often resembles mild pertussis, seldom with complications (3).

The one piece of evidence that the infection might not be due to *B. pertussis* is the high incidence at Mekoryuk, despite vaccination records of three or four doses before symptomatic illness.

Important in the study of any disease is the search for risk factors predisposing one to the disease. Pertussis is widely recognized as a disease of childhood with incidence highest in those under seven years of age. A sex predilection also exists with females at higher risk than males. Other

Table 2. *Feeding habits in cohort members from villages involved in the pertussis epidemic.*

	One visit			Two or more visits			Total*		
	Breast-fed	Bottle-fed	Both	Breast-fed	Bottle-fed	Both	Breast-fed	Bottle-fed	Both
(First visit)									
No pertussis	18	16	10	25	21	13	43	37	23
Pertussis	7	19	3	16	24	6	23	43	9
Total	15	35	13	41	45	19	66	80	32
(Last visit)									
No pertussis				11	24	24	29	40	34
Pertussis				6	18	22	13	37	25
Total				17	42	46	42	77	59

*Mantel-Haenszel tests controlling for village. Both vs. (Breast-fed + Bottle-fed).
First visit chi-square = 7.55, p = 0.006.
Last visit chi-square = 0.85, p = 0.355.

than these, no risk factors have been documented.

Our analysis of risk factors revealed only one statistically significant outcome. Our unanticipated finding was that being fed by both breast and bottle during the first three months of life was associated with pertussis infection. This relationship was stronger than that between feeding habits at the time of the epidemic and symptomatic illness. We do not consider this finding remarkable. Many analyses were performed on these data, and the result may be just a chance association. While infant feeding practices may be a factor in disease susceptibility, it is equally plausible that they are the consequence of a factor which increases risk. Feeding habits are affected by many factors including the health of the mother, the health of the infant, access to the mother, and attitudes in the mother's social group. Any of these could affect exposure or susceptibility to infection. The existence of many plausible alternatives with differing implications for the epidemiology of pertussis make speculation unattractive.

The high attack rate for this population (36.2%) reflects the very young age (less than 18 months) and unimmunized status (78.5% having no DPT immunization) of this population. Crowded living conditions and increased contacts could play an important role in increased exposure to the disease in the very young infant compared to the infant in the nuclear family of an industrial society. The Eskimo population lives a subsistence lifestyle with much importance placed on extended families. Large families with closely spaced children are common.

Published reports to date give varying mortality rates for this disease. Most values reported, however, are given as deaths per total population and thus understate the importance of the disease in the very young. It is important to look at this disease in terms of case fatality rates in infants since 75% of the deaths from pertussis occur in infants less than 1 year of age (4). Our population exhibits a high case fatality rate of 8/100 in males and 16/100 in females. The mortality pattern in our population follows that known for the disease. Mortality is greatest in females and in the very young (median age among infants who died is 3.5 months, among controls it is 6.5 months).

While vaccine efficacy is not precisely established for pertussis, it is generally accepted as effective in the "majority of individuals" (2) and Koplan et al. estimate it to be effective in 70% of vaccinees (based on studies of intrafamilial secondary cases) (11). Results from several studies indi .te that when cases do occur in immunize children, severity of the disease is substantially lessened (12). With the extremely low vaccination rate in our population (only 21.5% receiving at least one injection) it is impossible to examine efficacy of the vaccine in this infant group.

The epidemic, presumed to be *B. pertussis*, was of short duration and followed a simple, documentable pattern as it moved from village to village. Risk of symptomatic infection was associated with feeding habits. Disease-related mortality was associated with age of the child at infection. The ability to detect these relationships, despite small numbers and lack of precision in the data, is encouraging for future research using this cohort data base. This study of pertussis will be a model for studies of other epidemics which spread through this cohort, particularly measles and lower respiratory infections. Finally, the morbidity and mortality associated with the epidemic serve as a timely reminder of the public health importance of an effective pertussis vaccination program.

REFERENCES

1. Maynard JE, Hammes LM. A study of growth, morbidity and mortality among Eskimo infants of western Alaska. Bull Wld Hlth Org 1970; 42:613-622.
2. Harrison TR. Principles of internal medicine. New York: McGraw Hill, 1977:852-854.
3. Bradford WL. The *Bordetella* group. In: Dubos RJ, Hirsch JG, eds. Bacterial and mycotic infections of man. Philadelphia: JB Lippincott, 1965:742-751.
4. Beeson PB, McDermot W. Textbook of medicine. Philadelphia: WB Saunders, 1971:553-556.
5. Field GE. Alaskan work to control communicable diseases. Alaska's Health 1951; 9:1-46.
6. Cliff AD, Haggett P, Ord JK, Versey GR. Spatial diffusion: An historical geography of epidemics in an island community. Cambridge: Cambridge University Press, 1981.
7. Lehmann EL. Nonparametrics: Statistical methods based on ranks. San Francisco: Holden-Day, Inc., 1975.
8. Morse SI. Whooping cough. In: Hoeprich PD, ed. Infectious diseases. Philadelphia: Harper and Row, 1977: 277-280.
9. Nelson JD, Hempstead B, Tanaka R, Pauls FP. Fluorescent antibody diagnosis of infections. JAMA 1964; 188:1121-1124.
10. Miller DL, Ross EM. The authors reply. Am J Epidemiol 1984; 119:137-139.
11. Koplan JP, Schoenbaum SC, Weinstein MC, Fraser DW. Pertussis vaccine--An analysis of benefits, risks and costs. N Engl J Med 1979; 17:906-911.

12. Miller DL, Alderslade R, Ross EM.
    Whooping cough and whooping cough
    vaccine: The risks and benefits
    debate. Epidemiologic Rev 1982;
    4:1-23.

Belinda Ireland
Arctic Investigations Laboratory
Centers for Disease Control
225 Eagle Street
Anchorage, Alaska 99501
U.S.A.

THE EPIDEMIOLOGY OF NASOPHARYNGEAL CARRIAGE OF NEISSERIA MENINGITIDIS IN AN ISOLATED NORTHERN COMMUNITY

L.E. NICOLLE, B.D. POSTL, G.K.M. HARDING, W. ALBRITTON and A.R. RONALD

Sporadic outbreaks of group B meningococcal disease have been reported from isolated northern communities in Canada and Alaska over the past several decades. In the winter of 1980, following one such epidemic, we assessed the efficacy of community-wide prophylaxis for meningococcal disease in one northern community. In that study, the *Neisseria meningitidis* carrier rate in the community was studied to assess efficacy prior to and following chemo-prophylaxis. Prior to prophylaxis, we observed a relatively high proportion of carriers of N. meningitidis amongst Inuit members of the community (1,2).

To assess whether this observed high carriage reflected the prior epidemic year, or was usual for that community at that time of year, a survey of *N. meningitidis* carriage was repeated in the community in April of 1981. No meningococcal disease had been identified in the community in the intervening year.

MATERIALS AND METHODS

These studies were undertaken in the community of Baker Lake, Northwest Territories. This community has a population of approximately 1,000 individuals, 90% of whom are Inuit and permanent residents, with the remainder Caucasians, a high proportion of whom are resident in the community for only one or two years. The hamlet council agreed to the participation of the community in the study. The survey had been advertized in the community through announcements at the school, broadcasts over the radio station, and poster displays in the post office. All children attending school were given a printed consent form to be signed by their parents.

A study team of three individuals, together with necessary equipment and supplies, travelled to Baker Lake from Winnipeg, Manitoba. On the first morning, nasopharyngeal swabs were obtained at the school from all children whose parents had consented to their participation. Naso-pharyngeal swabs were obtained from adults when they presented to the Nursing Station during the two days of the study. Nasopharyngeal swabs were obtained using a calcium alginate swab and plated directly onto a split plate containing one-half Thayer-Martin medium and one-half chocolate agar. These plates were incubated for 24 hours at 37°C in a carbon dioxide-enriched environment in Baker Lake, then packed and transported by commercial carrier to Winnipeg for further isolation and identification.

Neisseria meningitidis were identified as oxidase positive gram negative diplococci which utilized glucose and maltose but not lactose or sucrose. Serogrouping was performed using a standard slide agglutination test, and susceptibility testing was performed by an agar dilution technique on Mueller Hinton agar.

RESULTS

In April 1981, nasopharyngeal swabs were obtained from 508 Inuit (67% of the total population) and 71 Caucasians (esti-mated 76% of the population). This compared with 709 (94%) Inuit in 1980 and 71 (82%) Caucasians. The proportion of the Inuit population participating declined signifi-cantly in 1981 ($p < 0.001$, chi-square analy-sis).

The prevalence of nasopharyngeal carriage of *N. meningitidis* in April 1981 was 105 (21%) of 508 Inuit and 10 (14%) of 71 Caucasians. This compared with carriage of 33% and 5.6%, respectively, in February 1980. Nasopharyngeal carriage was signifi-cantly lower ($p < 0.001$) in Inuit in the second year compared with the first. While there was a significantly increased carrier rate in Inuit compared with Caucasian in 1980, this trend was not significant.

Because 82% of all resident Caucasians were surveyed in 1980, the assumption was made, for 1981, that any Caucasians surveyed in 1981, who were not included in the 1980 survey, were resident in the community for one year or less. Of Caucasians who had been resident in the community for over 1 year, only 1 (4.2%) of 24 was a carrier while for those resident less than 1 year, 9 (19%) of 47 were carriers of *N. meningitidis* ($p < 0.05$, Fischer's Exact Test).

There was a trend to increased carriage among Inuit males compared with females for both 1980 and 1981, with 35% and 21% of males and 28% and 16% of females carriers in the respective years. These differences were not significant in either year, howev-er. The proportion of Caucasian females who were carriers was 8% for both years, but the proportion of Caucasian males who were carriers increased significantly ($p < 0.05$) from 2.5% in 1980 to 21% in 1981. The male Caucasian carriers in 1981 were virtually all resident in the community for under one year.

The age specific prevalence of naso-pharyngeal carriage of *N. meningitidis* for the Inuit population for 1980 and 1981 is shown in Figure 1. The two years are consistent in showing peak rates of carriage at the age of two years and again in late adolescence. In 1980 elderly individuals in the community also had a very high carrier rate, whereas in 1981 the carrier rate in this age group was relatively lower than other ages of peak carriage.

The distribution of *N. meningitidis* isolates by serogroup is shown in Table 1. There were no significant differences between the two years, with serogroup B the predominant serogroup in both years, and group W135 second in frequency.

While 7.8% of all isolates of *N. meningitidis* in 1980 were resistant to sulfonamides, all isolates identified in 1981 were susceptible with the minimum inhibitory capacity (MIC) greater than 10 micrograms/ml. The distribution of susceptibilities to both minocycline and rifampin, which were used as prophylactic agents in 1980, were similar for the two years, with the MIC 50 for rifampin, 0.03 µg/ml (range 0.007 to 0.5 µg/ml) for both years, and the MIC 50 for minocycline, 0.25 µg/ml (range 0.01 to 1 µg/ml).

DISCUSSION

For two consecutive years we observed a fairly high rate of carriage of *N. meningitidis* in this Inuit community. While the rate was higher in the first year compared with the second, suggesting yearly fluctuations in *N. meningitidis* carriage in the community, it is possible that the lower rate observed in the second year is actually an artifact. In the second year the survey was obtained in April during warmer weather and longer hours of sunlight, compared with February. The cold weather and short days would facilitate crowding and, hence, transmission of *N. meningitidis* may well be decreased in April compared with February.

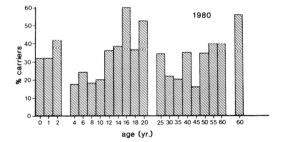

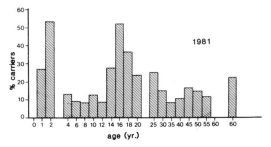

Figure 1. Age specific prevalence of nasopharyngeal carriage of N. meningitidis among the Inuit population for two consecutive years in one northern community.

Supporting the suggestion that we may be seeing a seasonal variation between the two years rather than a true yearly variation is our observation in April 1980, at the second survey following prophylaxis (2), that the *N. meningitidis* carrier rate for members of the community who had not received prophylaxis was 22%, similar to the April rate in 1981. However, the two April surveys cannot be considered comparable because of the likely effect of prophylaxis on the carrier rate in individuals not receiving prophylaxis in the community.

Community participation in the second nasopharyngeal survey was, for the Inuit inhabitants, not as complete as that in the first year. It is unlikely that the decreased participation artifactually altered the nasopharyngeal carriage rates, but this possibility cannot be excluded. The reasons for the poor participation in the second year are probably multifactorial. These include, as discussed above, the fact that the survey was in April in 1981, with better weather, and more community members may have been "out on the land." In addition, it had been over a year since a case of meningitis had occurred in the community and there was less interest in the problem of meningitis. Finally, the survey in 1981 was performed for 2 days, while the initial survey in 1980 was obtained over 3 days.

There are two other reports in the literature of community nasopharyngeal

Table 1. Distribution of serogroups of N. meningitidis isolated from nasopharyngeal carriers in an isolated northern community for two consecutive years.

| Serogroup | No. of isolates (%) | |
	1980	1981
B	99 (64)	62 (55)
C	6 (3.9)	4 (3.5)
Y	8 (5.2)	3 (2.6)
W135	22 (14)	32 (28)
29E	9 (5.8)	5 (4.4)
Autoagglutinable	6 (3.9)	7 (6.2)
Non-typable	5 (3.2)	

carriage of *N. meningitidis* in remote northern communities. One of these, by Reed et al. (3), reports the meningococcal carriage, of serogroup B only, in an Alaskan Eskimo village at the time of an outbreak of group B meningitis, followed by three subsequent surveys obtained over the ensuing two months. The initial carrier rate of group B was 20%, which fell to 13% over the subsequent two months of observation. The carrier rates for group B alone in our surveys were 13.5% (1980) and 10% (1981), which are comparable to carrier rates observed in the Alaska study at surveys temporally removed from the epidemic. Reed et al. observed no sex differences, and the age specific prevalence was highest in the age group 15 to 19 years and in individuals over 40 years of age. This is consistent with our observation of highest carriers for group B among older adolescents.

A report by Holten et al. (4) examined nasopharyngeal carriage of *N. meningitidis* in the population of an island off the coast of Norway following a case of group B meningitis in that community. They found a carrier rate in over 1,000 individuals sampled of 39% for all serogroups at the time of sampling, and also observed maximal carriage in two year olds and in the 15 to 19 year old group. Our findings of a fairly high overall carriage rate, as well as specific age variations in carriage, appear to be consistent with this report from Norway.

The carrier rate of *N. meningitidis* in a community in southern North America has been found to range from 4 to 11% (5). In certain settings, such as institutions, carriage rates may be much higher. Thus, our findings and those in other reports suggest the carrier rate for *N. meningitidis* is higher in northern communities. Factors which promote the transmission of *N. meningitidis* from person to person and increase the carriage rate include the susceptibility of individual members of the population as well as crowding that facilitates the spread of the organism. As discussed above, conditions during the winter months in northern communities may well facilitate the spread of *N. meningitidis* through crowding. Crowding may explain the relatively high carrier rates observed by ourselves and others. If so, modifications in living conditions that decrease crowding seem to be one method to prevent recurrences of epidemic serogroup B meningococcal disease in such communities.

REFERENCES

1. Nicolle LE, Postl B, Albritton WA, Harding GKM, Hildes J, Ronald A. Meningitis in an isolated northern Canadian community: Nasopharyngeal carriage of *N. meningitidis* and *H. influenzae*. In: Harvald B, Hart-Hansen JP, eds. Circumpolar Health 81. Nordic Council Arctic Med Res Rep 1982; 33:429-432.
2. Nicolle LE, Postl B, Kotelewetz E, Remillard F, Bourgeault AM, Albritton W, Harding GKM, Ronald A. Chemotherapy for *Neisseria meningitidis* in an isolated arctic community. J Inf Dis 1982; 145:103-109.
3. Reed D, Brody J, Huntley B, Overfield T. An epidemic in an Eskimo village due to group-B meningococcus. J Amer Med Assoc 1966; 196:383-387.
4. Holten E, Bratlid P, Bovre K. Carriage of *Neisseria meningitidis* in a semi-isolated Arctic community. Scand J Infect Dis 1978; 10:36-40.
5. Greenfield S, Sheehe P, Feldman HA. Meningococcal carriage in a population of 'normal' families. J Inf Dis 1971; 123:67-73.

L. E. Nicolle
Office of Infection Control
Calgary General Hospital
844 Centre Avenue East
Calgary, Alberta T2E 0A1
Canada

Circumpolar Health 84:238-240

THE EVOLUTION OF CHRONIC OTITIS MEDIA IN THE INUIT OF THE EASTERN CANADIAN ARCTIC AND ITS MANAGERIAL IMPLICATIONS

JAMES D. BAXTER

In Canada there is no consensus among physicians regarding the treatment of so-called chronic otitis media in the Inuit. The type of ear disease that is usually seen in an Inuk is confined to the middle ear; attic involvement with cholesteatoma is unusual and complications seldom occur. Medical and surgical methods of treatment have been applied and have been reported (1-4).

In the Eastern Canadian Arctic (Baffin Zone) reconstructive middle ear surgery in Inuit children has not been recommended during the past decade because of what has been observed in the region and elsewhere. Since the early 1970s the Department of Otolaryngology, McGill University, through the McGill-Baffin Zone Project, has provided service to the region and conducted two population surveys.

The initial survey (1972-73) was carried out to determine the extent and ramifications of the chronic otitis media problem across the region (5). This survey revealed that chronic otitis media was widespread (9% of ears examined) affecting up to 20% of the population in certain settlements, with most found among the children. A great deal of scarring of the tympanum was observed (21% of ears examined) in ears of children and adults that were essentially disease free and in hearing were functionally adequate. One-third of Cape Dorset Inuit who were identified in 1968 (6) as having discharging ears were found, 4 years later, to have scarred, intact tympanic membranes and hearing within normal limits. Finally, sensorineural hearing loss secondary to noise exposure was found in up to 85% of the adult males examined.

Following this survey a predicament arose. We were intrigued by the observations at Cape Dorset and by the amount of tympanic scarring seen across the Baffin Zone. We wondered what had been achieved by surgery and turned to the Central and Western Canadian Arctic for answers, since reconstructive middle ear surgery on Inuit had been performed there since the mid-1960s. Conflicting reports were received from these regions. Surgical success up to 94% was reported by the surgeons (7). The nursing stations, however, reported that the majority of the post-surgical ears discharged from time to time and required treatment.

In December 1973 it was agreed at a meeting convened by Canada National Health and Welfare that an independent review should be made of these surgical cases. Subsequently, in the spring of 1975 an inter-university otolaryngology group visited the Inuvik and Fort Smith Zones in the Western Canadian Arctic and examined the Inuit there who had had reconstructive middle ear surgery (8).

It was found in a series of 240 operations performed in 186 ears that the operative success rate judged on the basis of an intact tympanum was only 39%. The total number of ears judged to have had successful tympanoplasty type I after one or more operations was 50% of the ears surgically treated. When judged on the basis of hearing, 53.4% of them had inadequate hearing post-operatively.

In the ears judged to be successful tympanoplasty type I, there was documented evidence that 10% of the successful results could be attributed to spontaneous healing after surgery. In approximately 20% of these ears, there was clinical evidence of complications, many of which could be related to the surgery. There was no statistical evidence that the age of the patient at surgery had any bearing upon the success or lack of success of the operation. At the time of the initial surgery, 81% of the patients were 15 years of age or younger.

Following this surgical review it was agreed that in the Eastern Canadian Arctic a medical method of treatment would be applied across the region and that we would observe the results. A hearing aid program was expanded, directed predominantly at the children of school age in certain settlements.

During 1979-80 we surveyed the region to assess again the otolaryngological status of the Inuit and to determine what evolved in the ear disease during the interval since our 1972-73 survey (9). (The response of the Inuit to each survey was interesting. During the 1972-73 survey 74.8% of the Inuit in the Baffin Zone were examined while only 32.1% were examined during the 1979-80 survey. The reasons for this decreased response is that in the last decade the attitude of the Inuit has changed dramatically. In the early 1970s they would come by families to be examined. Today they do not respond unless it is in their interest. It is still possible to examine most of the school children as they are a relatively accessible group in their classrooms. The majority of adults who responded did so because they were seeking assistance for problems.)

This survey revealed that chronic otitis media and hearing loss was still widespread (12.7% of ears examined); again, a great deal of scarring of the tympanic membranes was observed (29.4% of ears examined) in ears which were essentially disease-free and in which hearing was functionally adequate. The majority of the adult males tested were found to have a high-frequency sensorineural hearing loss which was secondary to noise (snowmobiles and firearms). Many of the pre-teenage and teenage males tested in the schools were found to have a significant sensorineural hearing loss. A significant number of children in the school population had an unrecognized hearing loss which was impeding their educational progress. Hearing aids had generally been well accepted but lack of counselling and ongoing maintenance had almost nullified their use.

Longitudinal observations on the so-called chronic otitis media (1972-73 and 1979-80) were revealing. Since the first phase of the 1972-73 Baffin Zone Survey the examination records have been left in the nursing stations. Of the 1,989 Inuit examined during the 1979-80 surveys, 962 or 48.4% had 1972-73 examination records available in their charts. The records of the initial examination and the latest examinations were recorded on special forms which were brought south for analysis.

Since what evolves in chronic otitis media, especially during the second decade or teen years, was of particular interest to us, these 962 Inuit were divided into two groups for analysis and discussion:

Group I - those born prior to 1960 (20 years of age or older in 1980)

Group II - those born after 1960 (under 20 years of age in 1980).

Group I included 258 Inuit (516 ears). In 1972-73 30 ears (5.8%) were observed with chronic otitis media or chronic suppurative otitis media vs. 26 ears (5.1%) in 1979-80.

A longitudinal study of these ears with chronic otitis media/chronic suppurative otitis media (COM/CSOM) revealed that of the 30 ears having this condition in 1972-73, 10

ears healed (33.3%) and 6 ears acquired the condition in the interval, resulting in 26 ears with COM/CSOM in 1979-80 (Table 1).

In Group II there were 704 Inuit (1,408 ears). In 1972-73, 197 of these ears had COM/CSOM. In 1979-80 it was observed in these 197 ears that 140 or 71% had persistent COM/CSOM and 57 or 29% had healed their disease. In 1979-80, 230 ears had COM/CSOM which necessitated 90 ears acquiring COM/CSOM during the eight year interval between surveys (230-140 = 90) (Table 2).

These observations confirm that COM/CSOM is not rigidly entrenched in an Inuk in the Baffin Zone. During an 8-year period, approximately one-third of the Inuit suffering with the condition healed spontaneously (33.3% in those over 20 years of age and 29% in those under 20 years of age), while others acquired the condition.

From a managerial point of view the situation could be compared to the members of the cast of a very successful Broadway play in which certain actors retired during the course of the production. During the eight years that our production, COM/CSOM, has been running in the Baffin Zone, approximately one-third of our actors retired (underwent spontaneous healing) while others (both children and adults) filled the vacancies in the cast (acquiring COM/CSOM).

The problem is, how can one identify at any given time which actors will stay for the duration of the play and which actors will retire prematurely? It is impossible to identify who will join the cast to fill the vacancies from the general population.

What has been observed in the Baffin Zone during the past decade supports the view that reconstructive middle ear surgery in the Inuit should be deferred in childhood and be applied only in later life to those ears that have not healed as a result of medical treatment or the natural course of the disease. It must be recognized that many children with ear disease have hearing deficiencies and appropriate measures must be taken in the schools to remedy the problem.

Table 1. *Evolution of chronic otitis media (COM) in 516 ears of persons born prior to 1960 (Group I) between 1972-73 and 1979-80.*

Sample size in Group I:	516
Cases of COM in 1972-73:	30
Cases of COM healed:	10 (33%)
Newly acquired cases:	6
Net cases in 1979-80:	26

Table 2. *Evolution of chronic otitis media (COM) in 1,408 ears of persons born after 1960 (Group II) between 1972-73 and 1979-80.*

Sample size in Group II:	1,408
Cases of COM in 1972-73:	197
Cases of COM healed:	57 (29%)
Newly acquired cases:	90
Net cases in 1979-80:	230

REFERENCES

1. Baxter JD, Katsarkas A, Ling D, Carson R. The Nakasuk Project--the conservative treatment of chronic otitis media in Inuit elementary school children. J Otolaryngol 1979; 8:201.
2. Lupin AJ. Ear disease in western Canadian natives--a changing entity and the results of tympanoplasty. In: Shephard RP, Itoh S, eds. Proceedings of the Third International Symposium on Circumpolar Health. Toronto: Univ Toronto Press, 1976:389-397.
3. Brodovsky D, Woolf C, Medd LM, Hildes JA. Chronic otitis media in the Keewatin District. In: Shephard RO, Itoh S, eds. Proceedings of the Third International Symposium on Circumpolar Health. Toronto: Univ Toronto Press, 1976:398-402.
4. McCullough D. Tympanoplasty results in the Canadian Arctic 1970-1980. In: Harvald B, Hart-Hansen JP, eds. Circumpolar Health 81. Nordic Council for Arctic Med Res Rep 1982; 33:364-365.
5. Baxter JD, Ling D. Ear disease and hearing loss among the Eskimo population of the Baffin Zone. Can J Otolaryngol 1974; 3:110-122.
6. Ling D, McCoy RH, Levinson ED. The incidence of middle ear disease and its educational implications among Baffin Island Eskimo children. Can J Public Health 1969; 60:385-390.
7. Mallen R. Report to National Health and Welfare, Canada. Unpublished data, 1973.
8. Baxter JD. Chronic otitis media and hearing loss in the Eskimo population of Canada. Laryngoscope 1977; 87:1528-1542.
9. Baxter JD. Observations on the evolution of chronic otitis media in the Inuit of the Baffin Zone, Northwest Territories. J Otolaryngol 1982; 11:161.

James D. Baxter
Chairman, Department of Otolaryngology
McGill University
Montreal, Quebec H3A 1A1
Canada

Circumpolar Health 84:241-244

FOLLOW-UP OF TYMPANOPLASTIES IN THREE N.W.T. COMMUNITIES 1975-1980

PAMELA H. ORR and D.W. McCULLOUGH

The Northern Medical Unit of the University of Manitoba in Winnipeg provides ear, nose, and throat services to the Keewatin District of the Northwest Territories, including the Inuit communities of Rankin Inlet, Whale Cove, and Chesterfield Inlet. These hamlets, situated on the west coast of Hudson's Bay (Figure 1), comprise a total population of approximately 1,450, of whom 75% are Inuit and 24% are Caucasian.

Over the last decade consultant otolaryngologists have visited each settlement once per year, accompanied by a clinical audiologist. Visits are also made by general practitioners from the Churchill Health Center every four to six weeks. Surgical trips to Churchill are scheduled several times per year by three otolaryngologists. This study reports the results of tympanoplasties performed on Keewatin patients from these settlements at the Churchill Health Center from 1975 to 1980. Outcomes measured include graft healing, audiologic improvement and the results of postoperative tympanometry.

MATERIALS AND METHODS

All Inuit patients from Rankin Inlet, Whale Cove, and Chesterfield Inlet who underwent tympanoplasty between January 1975 and January 1980 were included in the study. Patients were identified through a review of nursing station and Churchill Health Center medical records and surgical lists. Two patients who had moved from the Keewatin were excluded from the study, since both the patients and their medical records were unavailable. Of the remaining 54 patients, 52 had undergone surgery in Churchill. Two subjects underwent surgery in Winnipeg as a matter of convenience and were included in the study. Several patients had repeat or bilateral tympanoplasties. Measurement of outcome was therefore based on total number of tympanoplasties (or "cases") rather than the number of patients operated on.

The nursing station and hospital medical records of all patients were examined retrospectively for data regarding age of onset of middle ear disease, treatment, pre- and postoperative diagnosis, evidence of graft success or failure as observed by either the visiting physician or local nurse-practitioner, and audiogram records. All patients were examined in clinic by the senior author and underwent audiometry and tympanometry.

Criteria for those referred for tympanoplasty included tympanic membrane perforation that was dry and present for greater than two years in patients aged four

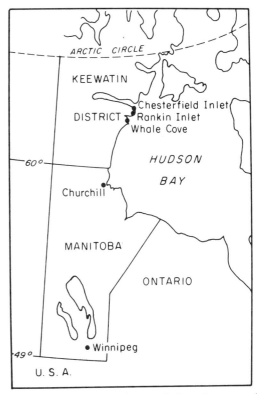

Figure 1. Rankin Inlet, Whale Cove, and Chesterfield Inlet, N.W.T., Canada.

years or greater. All patients were screened both at the nursing station and in Churchill prior to surgery to ensure that their middle ears were dry.

Patients underwent either a Stage 1 or House Plaster tympanoplasty, performed by one of three consulting otolaryngologists. The majority were discharged on the first postoperative day and returned to their settlement on day three or four. All patients received pre- and postoperative antibiotics (erythromycin or amoxicillin) for seven days. They were seen by the nurse-practitioner at seven days for suture removal, and thereafter by the visiting general practitioner and otolaryngologist. All patients were seen by a physician at least twice during the first six months after surgery and thereafter an average of once every six months for the following three years. The criteria for successful tympanoplasty were complete anatomical closure and healing of the graft as determined otoscopically.

Postoperative audiograms were obtained by the author (P.H.O.) and a visiting

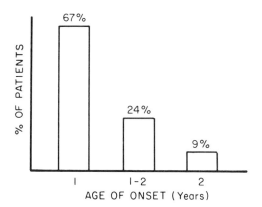

Figure 2. *Age of onset of acute otitis media.*

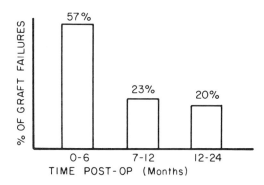

Figure 3. *Timing of graft failure.*

audiologist using a Maico MA-20 portable audiometer. Improvement in hearing was difficult to ascertain as in many cases preoperative audiograms had not been obtained. For those cases in which both pre- and postoperative audiograms were available, however, the classification used by Kaplan et al. in their study of Alaskan Eskimo children (1) was followed: 0 to -25 db in the affected ear (averaged over 500, 1,000 and 2,000 Hz) was considered hearing within normal limits, and -26 db or greater was considered indicative of significant hearing loss. The Alaska study joins a growing body of evidence linking mild to moderate levels of hearing loss in this range with a significant reduction in verbal skills in children with a history of otitis media (2-6). For the purposes of this study, those patients who postoperative hearing in the affected ear improved to less than 26 db were considered successful.

As in other studies, patients have been classified according to the hearing in the affected ear, following evidence that even unilateral hearing loss may have detrimental effects on the development of language skills (7). Such effects are especially important in the case of Inuit children, who are already grappling with linguistic, cultural, and socioeconomic impediments to learning.

Postoperative tympanograms were also obtained by the author using a portable American Electromedics tympanometer. Unfortunately, no preoperative tympanograms were available for comparison. Type A curves were recorded as normal and type A(d), A(s), B, or C curves as abnormal.

RESULTS AND DISCUSSION

A total of 71 tympanoplasties were performed on 54 patients. Seven of these were repeat tympanoplasties and 11 patients underwent bilateral surgery. Patients ranged in age from 4 to 38, with an average age at the time of surgery of 12 years. The ratio of male to female subjects was 1.3:1.

The preoperative diagnosis of chronic suppurative otitis media was made in all cases. The disease was primarily bilateral in 76% of cases and unilateral in 24%. Median age of onset of otitis media was 9 months, with 67% of subjects experiencing their first episode of acute otitis within the first 12 months of life (Figure 2). These results confirm previous studies which have noted the early onset of middle ear disease in Inuit children and its tendency to occur bilaterally (1, 8-10).

Of the 71 tympanoplasties performed, 41 (58%) grafts were intact at least two years after surgery. This indicates a success rate slightly lower than that found by Lupin in northern Alberta and the western Arctic (11) and by McCullough for the Keewatin District as a whole (12), but higher than that noted by Baxter in the western and central Arctic (13). Of the 64 first-time tympanoplasties, 36 (56%) were successful, and 28 (44%) were unsuccessful. Of the 7 repeat tympanoplasties 5 (71%) were successful and 2 (29%) failed. No significant difference was found between success rates in those undergoing initial versus repeat surgery. Similarly, there was no significant association between age of the patient and success rate.

Subsequently, 7 of the 30 (23%) graft failures went on to re-heal when observed over a period of three to seven years. This corresponds to previous reports of spontaneous healing of approximately 2% of tympanic membrane perforations per year (14).

Figure 3 indicates the time lapse between surgery and diagnosis of graft breakdown. Of the 30 unsuccessful results 80% were noted within the first year of surgery, and a total of 57% occurred within the first six months. Variable intervals between follow-up examinations do not allow more accurate assessment of the time of graft failure within the first six months.

Nevertheless, the records reveal frequent nursing notes indicating otorrhea obscuring the tympanic membrane soon after patients returned to the settlement. We suspect that many of the graft breakdowns occur within the first few weeks or even days following surgery. The adverse effects of pressure changes during early air transportation back to the settlements have been proposed as a factor in early tympanoplasty failure, and further study of this variable may be of interest.

Both pre- and postsurgical audiograms were available in only 32 of the 71 tympanoplasties performed. Of the remaining 39 cases, 33 had recorded postsurgical audiograms only, 3 had pre- but no postoperative evaluation and 3 had neither pre- nor postoperative audiograms. The latter cases occurred when the patients were out of the settlement for extended periods at the time of the audiology clinics.

The average preoperative hearing level was 38 db and the postoperative level was 29 db. Of the 32 cases in which both pre- and postoperative assessments were made, only 14 (44%) showed significant improvement in their hearing as previously defined. Only one patient showed significant deterioration of hearing. Surprisingly, although the numbers involved are small, there was no significant difference in hearing improvement between those patients who displayed graft healing and those who did not. These results correspond to Baxter's findings in Labrador and the western and central Arctic in which only 45% of patients post-tympanoplasty were judged to have adequate hearing as defined by an average conductive hearing level of less than 30 db (15).

Tympanometry was performed in 64 of the 71 cases between two and seven years post-tympanoplasty. Seven patients were away from the settlement at school or "on the land" and thus unavailable for testing. Ten patients (16%), all of whom had demonstrated graft healing, displayed normal type A tympanograms, while 54 (84%) had abnormal curves. The 10 patients with normal tympanograms represent 24% of the 41 cases of graft healing. As expected, all patients with tympanoplasty breakdown displayed abnormal tympanograms. Sample size was too small to assess any association between improved hearing and normal tympanogram.

The results of this study and others (15) confirm the discrepancy in success rates, as judged by either graft healing or hearing improvement, between tympanoplasties performed on Inuit versus southern Caucasian people. The reasons for the discrepancy are unknown. Factors for further study include the effects of early transportation by air postoperatively and the degree of compliance with antibiotic regimes and postoperative care in this population. The role of such factors as housing, general nutrition, bottle versus breast-feeding and genetics in the development of chronic otitis media have been discussed by numerous authors, (16-20). The particular clinical features of the disease in Inuit as opposed to Caucasian children--including the early age of onset, more protracted course with fewer sequelae and decreased responsiveness to medical or surgical treatment--have led some researchers to postulate a fundamentally different disease process in the two groups (21).

REFERENCES

1. Kaplan GJ, Fleshman JK, Bender TR, Baum C, Clark PS. Long-term effects of otitis media: A ten-year cohort study of Alaskan Eskimo children. Pediatrics 1973; 52:577.
2. Zinkus PW, Gottlieb MI, Shapiro M. Developmental and psychoeducational sequelae of chronic otitis media. Am J Dis Child 1978; 132:1100.
3. Ling D. Rehabilitation of cases with deafness secondary to otitis media. In: Glorig A, Gerwin KS, eds. Otitis media. Proceedings of the National Conference, Callier Hearing and Speech Center, Dallas, Texas. Springfield: Charles C Thomas, 1972:249.
4. Hamilton P, Owrid HL. Comparisons of hearing impairment and sociocultural disadvantage in relation to verbal retardation. Br J Audio. 1974; 8:27.
5. Downs MP. Minimal auditory deprivation syndrome. Audiology: An Audio J Cont Educ 1979; 4: No 4.
6. Rapin I. Conductive hearing loss: Effects on children's language and scholastic skills. A review of the literature. Ann Otol Rhinol Laryngol 1979; 88:3.
7. Peckham CS, Sheridan M, Butler NR. School attainment of seven-year-old children with hearing difficulties. Develop Med Child Neurol 1972; 14:592.
8. Reed D, Struve S, Maynard JE. Otitis media and hearing deficiency among Eskimo children: A cohort study. Amer J Public Health 1967; 57:1657.
9. Maynard JE. Otitis media in Alaskan Eskimo children: An epidemiologic review with observations on control. Alaska Med 1969; 11:93.
10. Baxter JD, Ling D. Ear disease and hearing loss among the Eskimo population of the Baffin Zone. Can J Otolaryngol 1974; 3:110.
11. Lupin AJ. Ear disease in western Canadian natives--a changing entity--and the results of tympanoplasty. In: Shephard R, Itoh S., eds. Proceedings of the Third International Symposium on Circumpolar Health. Toronto: Univ Toronto Press, 1976:389-397.

12. McCullough DW. Tympanoplasty results in the Canadian Arctic 1970-1980. In: Harvald B, Hart Hansen JP, eds. Circumpolar Health 81. Nordic Council for Arct Med Res Rep, 1982; 33:364-365.

13. Baxter JD. Chronic otitis media and hearing loss in the Eskimo population of Canada. Laryngoscope 1977; 87:1528.

14. Brodovsky D, Woolf C, Medd LM, Hildes JA. Chronic otitis media in the Keewatin district. In: Shephard R, Itoh S, eds. Proceedings of the Third International Symposium on Circumpolar Health. Toronto: Univ Toronto Press, 1976; 398-402.

15. Baxter JD. The evolving attitude in Canada toward the management of chronic otitis media in the Inuit population. J Otolaryngol 1981; 10:81.

16. Ling D, Katsarkas A, Baxter JD. Ear disease and hearing loss among Eskimo elementary school children. Can J Public Health 1974; 65:37.

17. Hayman CR, Kester FE. Eye, ear, nose and throat infection in natives of Alaska: Summary and analysis based on report of the survey conducted in 1956. Northwest Med (Seattle) 1957; 56:423.

18. Hildes JA, Schaefer O. Health of Igloolik Eskimos and changes with urbanization. J Hum Evol 1973; 2:241.

19. Schaefer O. Otitis media and bottle feeding. An epidemiological study of infant feeding habits and incidence of recurrent and chronic middle ear disease in Canadian Eskimos. Can J Public Health 1971; 62:478.

20. Ratnesar P. Chronic ear disease along the coasts of Labrador and northern Newfoundland. J Otolaryngol 1976; 5:122.

Pamela H. Orr
Northern Medical Unit
University of Manitoba
61 Emily Street
Winnipeg, Manitoba R3E 1X9
Canada

Circumpolar Health 84:245-247

THE CURRENT STATUS OF ALVEOLAR HYDATID DISEASE IN NORTHERN REGIONS

ROBERT L. RAUSCH and JOSEPH F. WILSON

The genus *Echinococcus*, in the family Taeniidae, includes four species of very small tapeworms that occur as adults in carnivores. The life cycles of these cestodes are completed by means of the natural predator-prey relationship that exists between the respective final and intermediate hosts, but when eggs of the adult parasites expelled by the final host are ingested incidentally by man, the resulting larval stages of three of the known species cause distinctive forms of hydatid disease.

Two of these cestodes have extensive geographic ranges in arctic and subarctic regions, where infections in man have been diagnosed predominantly among indigenous populations. In northern regions, cystic hydatid disease, caused by the larval stage of the northern form of *Echinococcus granulosus* Batsch, 1786, typically takes a benign course, and surgical intervention or other treatment is rarely necessary. In contrast, alveolar hydatid disease, caused by the larval stage of *Echinococcus multilocularis* Leuckart, 1863, is a serious health problem in northern Eurasia and northern North America.

In the circumpolar zone of tundra, *Echinococcus multilocularis* occurs commonly in the arctic fox, but the red fox also serves as final host. The larval stage of the parasite develops in small rodents of the family Arvicolidae, which make up a high proportion of the diet of foxes. In and around settlements, dogs may capture and eat rodents harboring the larval stage of this cestode. In settlements where such rodents take up a commensal existence, and where dogs are numerous, hyperendemic foci may exist. We consider that dogs are the usual source of infection for the human population. When dogs are numerous, their feces grossly contaminate inhabited areas. In Iakutia, Martynenko et al. (1) found a significant correlation between prevalence of alveolar hydatid disease and the use of potentially contaminated lakes for water supply. Whether wild foxes are a significant source of human infection has not been clearly established. Most human infections are evidently acquired early in life, but alveolar hydatid disease usually does not become clinically apparent before middle age.

Echinococcus multilocularis has an holarctic distribution in the northern hemisphere. In the Arctic and Subarctic, it occurs from Latvia east to the Bering Sea, and from western Alaska at least to Hudson's Bay. It is present on islands in the Bering Sea, and in the Canadian Arctic Archipelago.

The cestode has not been recorded in Greenland, to which arctic foxes periodically migrate from eastern Canada (2). Its range is extensive in the Soviet Union, where the distribution of cases of alveolar hydatid disease has been defined by Lukashenko (3). A single case has been reported in northern India (4), and more than 100 cases have been diagnosed recently on the mainland of China (5). Numerous cases have been found in northern Japan (Hokkaido), where the cestode is extending its range. Robbana et al. (6) reported a singe case also from northern Tunisia, in Africa. In North America, *Echinococcus multilocularis* was first recorded beyond the limits of the zone of tundra in 1964, when Leiby and Olsen (7) found infected animals in North Dakota. Since that time, it has been reported in seven additional states, and in the three adjacent provinces of Canada. The establishment of the cestode in that region appears to be attributable to the dispersal of eggs by arctic foxes that periodically migrate southward from the tundra west of Hudson Bay (8). Continuing spread of *Echinococcus multilocularis* in the United States is predictable, since suitable mammalian hosts are widely present.

With reference to human disease in the Arctic and Subarctic, the highest rates have been recorded in the Iakut Autonomous Republic, northeastern Siberia. According to Martynenko et al. (1), 604 primary cases of alveolar hydatid disease were diagnosed in the principal hospitals in Iakutia during the period 1971 to 1980. Nemirovskaia et al. (9) stated that rates of infection in hunters, trappers, and herders in the same region ranged as high as 50 to 70 cases per 1,000.

The pathogenesis of the larval stage of *Echinococcus multilocularis* in man is attributable to a high degree of incompatibility between the parasite and the host. The larval cestode remains in the early, proliferative phase of development, gradually infiltrating adjacent hepatic tissue. Very large hepatic lesions may develop over a period of years, and encroachment on major hepatic vessels is not unusual. Metastasis to the lungs or brain may occur in patients with advanced hepatic disease.

In Alaska, alveolar hydatid disease is a serious health problem among Eskimos living on St. Lawrence Island and along the western coast of the mainland. Only 37 cases have been diagnosed in Alaska, with about one new case per year. Nonetheless, this disease causes far more morbidity and mortality than does, for example, a disease such as rabies, which receives much greater public attention. During the past four years, patients with alveolar hydatid disease have required 361 days of hospitalization, at a cost of about $157,750 per year, at one hospital alone.

The diagnosis of alveolar hydatid disease is usually made when patients present with an abdominal mass, or a positive serological titer. Serological surveys have been increasingly important, and diagnoses of 9 cases have been made primarily by this means. In an additional 10 cases, serological findings were important in conjunction with other tests in establishing the clinical diagnosis.

In alveolar hydatid disease, the preclinical period may be prolonged, perhaps as much as 10 to 25 years. Detection of early cases while the lesion is small and more amenable to surgical resection has been emphasized in our work. A program for identifying patients at risk of having early-stage lesions by means of serological surveys has been conducted by us for a number of years. Thus far in this effort, we have failed to identify patients at an early stage of infection. We are continuing this work, with the hope that more refined diagnostic techniques, such as more sophisticated CT-scans, will give better results.

Surgical resection of the lesion remains the treatment of choice, but only 19% of our cases have been resectable for cure. These seven patients are all living, with an average survival time post-surgery of 19 years (range: 10 to 31 years). One has evidence of recurring disease. In the management of nonresectable lesions, we have been engaged in a clinical trial of mebendazole therapy since 1974. Results in these patients are still being assessed. On the one hand, it appears that the drug has had a beneficial effect, since it has prolonged survival time, given symptomatic improvement, and shown a possible arrest of metastasis. On the other hand, the parasite tissue in the lesions seems usually to remain viable, probably because of difficulties in obtaining sufficiently high serum levels of the drug.

Traditionally, it has been shown that hydatid disease, in the broad sense, can be controlled by appropriate measures to disrupt the life cycle of the cestode. But prevention of alveolar hydatid disease and the control of the etiologic agent are much more difficult than, for example, the control of cystic hydatid disease. This has been evident in central Europe, where a disjunct, endemic focus of *Echinococcus multilocularis*, recognized since the middle of the last century, has persisted. Alveolar hydatid disease is a natural-focal disease that is perpetuated among wild mammalian populations. Consequently, disruption of the cycle of *Echinococcus*

multilocularis is not feasible. In Alaska, prevention of infection in man would seem to depend on public education and improved sanitation. Whereas numbers of sled dogs have been markedly reduced in many villages during recent years, the potential benefit of that reduction seems to have been offset by the growing popularity of maintaining dogs as pets.

Measures for the prevention and treatment of alveolar hydatid disease require further definition. Of high priority is the need to establish better methods in the medical management of nonresectable lesions. Through cooperation with the Department of Chemistry, University of Alaska (Anchorage), we have assessed serum levels of mebendazole under different modes of administration and dosage. Results to date indicate that serum levels are usually quite low, probably below the effective therapeutic level. Available information suggests that albendazole may give improved therapeutic levels, and we plan to include this drug in chemotherapeutic trials as soon as it becomes available for use. Broader based serological surveys of populations in the endemic regions are being conducted this year (1984) in conjunction with the Alaska state hepatitis studies. The need for more effective screening tests for laboratory use is recognized.

The establishment of better diagnostic methods, the implementation of effective programs of control of the cestode in dogs, and improved chemotherapy of alveolar hydatid disease present some difficult but promising challenges for future investigations. Any success in these efforts in Alaska can be expected to have important implications in other regions of the Arctic and Subarctic, as well as in endemic regions at lower latitudes.

REFERENCES

1. Martynenko VB, Maiorova LA, Zorihina VI, Suvorina VI. Epidemiologiia al'veokokkoza v taezhnoi zone Iakutii. Med Parazit 1983; 61:38-40.
2. Rausch RL, Fay FH, Williamson FSL. Helminths of the arctic fox, *Alopex lagopus* (L.), in Greenland. Can J Zool 1983; 61:1847-1851.
3. Lukashenko NP. Al'veokokkoz (al'veoli-arnyi ekhinokokkoz). Moskva: Meditsina, 1975. (See map, Figure 49).
4. Aikat BK, Bhusnurmath SR, Cadersa M, Chhuttani PN, Mitra AK. *Echinococcus multilocularis* infection in India: first case report proved at autopsy. Trans Roy Soc Trop Med Hyg 1978; 72:619-621.
5. Jiang C. Liver alveolar echinococcosis in the Northwest. Report of 15 patients and a collective analysis of 90 cases. Chinese Med J 1981; 91:777-778.

6. Robbana M, Ben Rachid MS, Zitouna MM, Heldt N, Hafsia M. Première observation d'échinococcose alvéolaire autochtone en Tunisie. Arch Anat Cytol Pathol 1981; 29:311-312.

7. Leiby PD, Olsen OW. The cestode *Echinococcus multilocularis* in North Dakota. Science 1964; 145:1066.

8. Rausch RL. Life cycles and geographic distribution of *Echinococcus* species (Cestoda: Taeniidae). In: Thompson RCA, ed. The biology of *Echinococcus* and hydatid disease. London: Allen and Unwin, 1984 (in press).

9. Nemirovskaia AK, Nekipelov VIa, Iakovleva TA, Iasinskii AA. Problema ekhinokokkoza i al'veokokkoze v RSFSR. Med Parazit 1980; 49:17-21.

Robert L. Rausch
Division of Animal Medicine SB-42
University of Washington
Seattle, Washington 98195
U.S.A.

SECTION 5. NON-INFECTIOUS AND CHRONIC DISEASE

Circumpolar Health 84:249-253

CHRONIC DISEASE SURVEY OF A LABRADOR COMMUNITY

ALISON C. EDWARDS, JOHN R. MARTIN, GORDON J. JOHNSON and JANE GREEN

INTRODUCTION

A survey of ophthalmic conditions in Nain, latitude 56°33'N on the coast of Labrador, was conducted in October 1977 (1). At the same time, data were collected on chronic diseases as noted in the patient's medical records or as known by the nursing station staff.

METHODS

Analyses of the data were performed using a VAX 11/780 computer and the Statistical Package for Social Sciences program (SPSS-X).

The population at Nain is essentially Inuit. There have been a number of Caucasian settlers of English origin living in the area for several generations. When the family history suggested that more than one great-grandparent was Caucasian in the case of an apparent Inuit patient (or Inuit in the case of a Caucasian patient), the patient was classified as "mixed." A number of Caucasians from outside Labrador who were in the community as teachers, nurses, social workers, or technicians were referred to as the "floating population." Four people of North American Indian or mixed Indian-Caucasian ancestry had come in from other parts of Labrador. For the following results the Indian, Indian/mixed, and "floating population" have been omitted due to the small percentage involved.

RESULTS

Data were obtained for 673 people. A recent locally conducted census listed 773 people resident in the community. Of these,

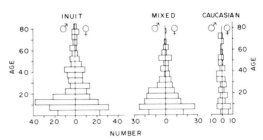

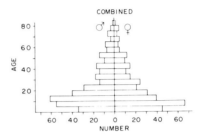

Figure 1. Population structure of Inuit, mixed, and Caucasian sub-groups, 1977.

28 Inuit were away seal hunting, leaving 745 people in the settlement. No information was collected for those people not seen in the ophthalmology study. The study population therefore represents 87% of the total registered population.

Table 1 shows the breakdown of ethnic groups in the study population. The population structures of the 3 main ethnic groups, Inuit, mixed, and Caucasian settlers, are shown in Figure 1. It can be seen that the Caucasian population does not have the characteristic "Christmas tree" shape, probably due to the decreasing number of "pure" Caucasian marriages and offspring. In recent years there has been a trend toward smaller families as well as a significant reduction in the infant mortality rate (2). This may explain the smaller base to the "Christmas tree" for both Inuit and mixed groups.

The diseases were categorized according to the International Classification of Diseases (3). Table 2 shows that the 3 ethnic groups show a similar prevalence for many of the grouped classifications, exceptions being infectious/parasitic, mental, CNS, eye, ear, and respiratory system. This table includes multiple diagnoses; i.e., a patient can have 2 or more problems from the same classification group and all would be counted. The differences between the races for infectious/parasitic and respiratory

Table 1. Number and percentage of population divided into ethnic groups.

Ethnic groups	Number	Percentage
Inuit	329	49
Mixed	237	35
Caucasian settlers	80	12
Indian or Indian/mixed	4	1
"Floating population"	23	3
Number in survey	673	100
Number in recent census (locally conducted, 1977)	773	

Table 2.   Diagnoses expressed as percentage of individuals in ethnic groups, singly and combined.

Diagnoses	Inuit	Mixed	Caucasian	Combined
Infectious/parasitic	34	19	13	26
Neoplasms	2	3	1	2
Endocrine/metabolic	2	3	1	33
Mental	9	6	4	7
CNS	6	5	1	5
Eye	9	6	14	9
Ear	18	10	3	13
Circulatory system	9	9	8	9
Respiratory system	25	19	4	20
Digestive system	9	6	8	8
Genito-urinary system	5	6	9	6
Pregnancy/birth	2	1	0	1
Skin/subcutaneous	2	3	1	2
Musculo-skeletal/connective	4	4	1	3
Congenital	4	5	0	4
Perinatal period	2	1	0	2
Ill-defined conditions	4	1	3	3
Injury/poisoning	9	3	5	6
External causes	7	3	5	5
Total diagnoses	535	270	63	868
Number in survey	329	237	80	646

diseases may be a reflection of lowered socioeconomic status with its associated poor conditions of sanitation, overcrowding, and nutrition, especially in the case of the Inuit and mixed ethnic groups.

Certain diseases were chosen to demonstrate the distribution of "problem diseases" and to pinpoint the ethnic variability in those group diagnoses as seen in Table 2. Sixteen conditions are shown in Table 3, divided into the number of cases in each ethnic group. This table does not include multiple diagnoses but rather shows the actual number of patients with each complaint. For example, if a patient has 2 or more diagnoses of middle ear disease, he is counted only once. It can be seen that certain diseases are much more prevalent in the Inuit and mixed groups (i.e. pulmonary tuberculosis, alcohol dependence, middle ear disease, pneumonia, and bronchitis) while eye disorders and hypertension are more prevalent in the Caucasians, but not to a large extent.

Pulmonary tuberculosis, pneumonia, and bronchitis are most likely increased in the

Table 3. Number and percentage of individuals with certain diseases.

Diagnoses	Inuit	Mixed	Caucasian
Pulmonary tuberculosis	68 (21)	20 (8)	2 (3)
Middle ear disease	52 (16)	19 (8)	2 (3)
Pneumonia	38 (12)	22 (9)	0
Bronchitis	24 (7)	11 (5)	1 (1)
Eye disorders	23 (7)	12 (5)	10 (13)
Hypertension	9 (3)	9 (4)	4 (5)
Meningitis	10 (3)	6 (3)	0
Alcohol dependence	11 (3)	2 (1)	0
Developmental delay	5 (2)	2 (1)	0
Diabetes mellitus	2 (1)	2 (1)	1 (1)
Benign neoplasms	2 (1)	1 (1.4)	1 (1)
Malignant neoplasms	3 (1)	1 (0.4)	0
Unspecified neoplasms	0	5 (2)	0
Depressive	4 (1)	2 (1)	1 (1)
Viral hepatitis	4 (1)	1 (.4)	0
Self-inflicted poisonings	3 (1)	2 (1)	0
Number in survey	329	237	80

Inuit, and to a lesser extent in the mixed groups, because of lowered socioeconomic status. Little ear disease was present in the Inuit prior to 1950 (4,5). The increase since then is said to be associated with

-- a high incidence of bottle-feeding (6),
-- significantly shorter, straighter, and wider eustachian tubes in the Inuit children when compared to Caucasians (6), and
-- the increase in crowding with the associated high temperature and low humidity in southern-type homes (4).

Ratnesar in a survey of chronic ear disease on the coasts of Labrador and northern Newfoundland found the variation in the different ethnic groups to be related to the aeration of the middle ear cleft with its associated incidence of cholesteatoma (7).

Alcohol dependence may be higher in the non-Caucasians because of their cultural breakdown and depressed socioeconomic circumstances with its associated feelings of worthlessness and frustration (8).

Breast cancer is said to be rare in Inuit women, a result of the traditional practice of breast-feeding each child until the next is born, an average of three and one-half years later (4,9). The noted decline in the number of breast-fed infants may be a reason why 2 cases of breast cancer were found in the Inuit in Nain.

Note was made from the patients' records whether tuberculosis was "active," "prophylaxis," or "contact." One hundred and seven patients (16.6% of the total Inuit, mixed, and Caucasian population) had at some time had active tuberculosis, 11 (1.7%) had been given prophylaxis treatment, and 37 (5.7%) had been in contact with tuberculosis.

Table 4. Diagnoses expressed as percentage of individuals in each age group: Inuit, mixed, and Caucasian combined.

Diagnoses	0	1-4	5-9	Age in years 10-19	20-29	30-39	40+
Infectious/parasitic	0	2	9	18	40	64	42
Neoplasms	0	0	0	1	1	5	6
Endocrine/metabolic	0	2	1	2	0	2	9
Mental	0	5	4	6	8	17	10
CNS	0	8	11	4	3	2	2
Eye	0	3	2	4	8	7	26
Ear	0	18	22	18	8	3	3
Circulatory system	7	0	0	1	7	14	33
Respiratory system	14	46	39	9	7	3	21
Digestive system	7	0	2	1	1	14	29
Genito-urinary system	0	0	1	1	14	5	18
Pregnancy/birth	0	0	0	0	7	0	2
Skin/subcutaneous	0	6	0	0	5	0	5
Musculo-skeletal/connective	0	0	2	1	0	9	10
Perinatal period	14	8	1	1	0	0	0
Ill-defined conditions	0	6	2	3	0	0	4
Injury/poisoning	0	0	1	3	9	9	17
External causes	0	2	3	4	7	14	6
Total diagnoses	6	75	125	135	114	98	315
Number in survey	14	65	121	171	88	58	129

In Table 4 it can be seen that various age ranges show a predominance for certain diagnoses. The 30 to 39 range shows peak percentages for infectious, mental, and accidents by external causes (e.g. firearms, fights, fire, water immersion, etc.), the 40+ range for neoplasms, eye disease, circulatory, digestive and genito-urinary systems, and injury/poisoning, the 1 to 9 range for CNS and the respiratory system, and the under 20s for ear disease. This table includes multiple diagnoses as described for Table 2 above.

The number and percent of patients currently using medications is shown in Table 5. Medications were grouped according to ailment, and the number of patients using any one or more of a grouped drug have been tabulated. Patients using medication for more than one group were included in all the relevant groups. Cardiovascular drugs were the most commonly used medication (3.7% of the patients, age range 33 to 81, mean 61 years), followed closely by antimicrobials (3.3%, age range 6 to 76), including 14 patients (2.2%, age range 6 to 53) who were

Table 5. *Number and percentage of patients currently using medication: Inuit, mixed, and Caucasian combined.*

Medication	Number	Percentage
Cardiovascular	24	3.7
Anti-microbials	21	3.3
Psychotropic and CNS	12	1.9
Anti-glaucoma	7	1.1
Anti-inflammatory	5	0.8
Gastro-intestinal	3	0.5
Hypoglycemic	1	0.2
Number with at least one medication	58	9.0
Number in survey	646	

currently taking antituberculosis drugs, of whom 13 were taking only these medications. Psychotropic/CNS drugs were used by 12 patients (1.9%), four of them being children (age range 1 to 7, mean 3.5) who were prescribed phenobarbital. There was one case of dietary supplement in an 81-year-old Inuit.

CONCLUSION

A high prevalence of infectious/parasitic, respiratory, and chronic ear diseases was noted in the Inuit, and to a lesser extent in the people of mixed blood, possibly a reflection of their lowered socioeconomic circumstances.

REFERENCES

1. Johnson GJ, Paterson GD, Green JS, Perkins ES. Ocular conditions in a Labrador community. In: Harvald B, Hart Hansen JP, eds. Circumpolar Health 81. Nordic Council for Arct Med Res Rep 1982; 33:352-359.
2. Williams, JH. Personal communication, 1984.
3. International Classification of Diseases, 9th Revision, Clinical Modification (ICD.9.CM), 1978.
4. Martin JD. Health care in northern Canada--an historical perspective. In: Harvald B, Hart Hansen JP, eds. Circumpolar Health 81. Nordic Council for Arct Med Res Rep 1982; 33:180-187.
5. Baxter JD. Ear disease among the Eskimo population of the Baffin Zone. In: Shephard RP, Itoh S, eds. Proceedings of the Third International Symposium on Circumpolar Health. Toronto: University of Toronto Press, 1976:384-389.
6. Timmermans FJW, Gerson S. Chronic granulomatous otitis media in bottlefed Inuit children. Canad M Assoc J 1980; 22:545-547.
7. Ratnesar P. Chronic ear disease along the coasts of Labrador and northern Newfoundland. J Otolaryng 1976; 5:122-130.
8. Schaefer O, Metayer M. Eskimo personality and society--yesterday and today. In: Shephard RP, Itoh S, eds. Proceedings of the Third International Symposium on Circumpolar Health. Toronto: University of Toronto Press, 1976:469-479.
9. Thomas GW, Williams JH. Cancer in native populations in Labrador. In: Shephard RP, Itoh S, eds. Proceedings of the Third International Symposium on Circumpolar Health. Toronto: University of Toronto Press, 1976:283-289.

Alison C. Edwards
Program of Northern Medicine and Health
Memorial University of Newfoundland
Health Sciences Center
St. John's, Newfoundland A1B 3V6
Canada

Circumpolar Health 84:254-255

CURRENT TRENDS IN CANCER INCIDENCE IN GREENLAND

N. HØJGAARD NIELSEN and JENS PETER HART HANSEN

Greenland has the largest population group of Eskimo origin in the world (1983: 42,700). The general pattern of malignant diseases among Greenlanders shows great similarities to the pattern in the Eskimo populations of Alaska and northern Canada. The cancer incidence since 1955 up to 1975 has been presented at the 2 most recent international symposia on circumpolar health (1).

Analysis of the 574 cancers diagnosed among indigenous Greenlanders during the 9-year period from 1975 through 1983 revealed almost the same characteristic pattern as found for the previous 10 years, 1965 to 1974. Table 1 gives the total number of newly diagnosed cancers among males and females in the 2 periods. The observed numbers of cancers are compared to expected numbers calculated by assuming the cancer incidence in Greenland to be the same as in Denmark at any given time. Expected numbers for 1975 to 1983 are based on the latest published incidence rates from Denmark covering the period 1973 to 1977. The ratios of observed numbers divided by expected numbers represent the relative risk.

Total cancer incidence was significantly lower than in Denmark for males but not for females. Compared to the Danish population the risks were significantly higher for the following sites: nasopharynx, salivary glands and esophagus in both males and females, and cervix uteri and lung in females (Table 2). Significantly lower risks were found for male bladder cancer and male rectal cancer, prostate cancer, cancer of the testes, cancer of the endometrium, and breast cancer. Malignant diseases of the combined lymphatic and hematopoietic tissues were fewer than expected compared to Denmark mainly due to a very low incidence of Hodgkin's disease.

The overall risks for the remaining cancer types did not significantly deviate from the risks in Denmark. This applies particularly to cancer of the liver, gall bladder, thyroid, and kidney, which have been reported to occur among Eskimos in North America with frequencies differing from those in the U.S. population in general (2).

Infection with hepatitis-B virus is endemic in Natives in Alaska, Canada, and Greenland. This has been followed by a high incidence of primary liver cancer in Alaska and Canada but strangely enough not in Greenland.

Adjusted rates (world population) for the 2 periods 1970 to 1974 and 1975 to 1983 revealed increased rates (per 100,000) for lung cancer in both sexes in the latter period, most pronounced for women (21.4) where incidence exceeds that in Denmark for 1979 (15.9). Increasing rates were also found for cervical cancer (64.2), now almost four times the incidence among women in Denmark (16.8). Rates for breast cancer decreased slightly from 31.5 in 1970-1974 to 27.1 in 1975-1983. Variation in the rates for the remaining cancer types listed was not statistically significant.

A changing picture of neoplastic diseases has recently been reported from the western and central Canadian Arctic (3). However, despite an increasing "westernization" of the Greenlandic society with changes of life and lifestyle, habits of diet and environment, most of the traditional pattern of malignant disorders is so far unchanged according to the most recent data.

Table 1. *Greenland 1965-1983. Observed (O) number of cancers, all sites, and observed-to-expected (O/E) ratio by time and sex, in Greenland cancer patients 1965-1983.*

Period	Males		Females	
	O	O/E	O	O/E
1965-1974	188	0.8*	298	1.1
1975-1983	233	0.8*	341	1.0

* = p < 0.01

Table 2. Observed (O) number of cancers among indigenous Greenlanders and observed-to-expected (O/E) ratios. Expected numbers are based on incidence in Denmark 1965-74 and 1973-77.

Site	Period	Males		Females	
		O	O/E	O	O/E
Nasopharynx	1965-74	14	22.6**	9	25.0**
	1975-83	13	17.1**	13	29.0**
Salivary glands	1965-74	5	6.2**	12	10.5**
	1975-83	4	6.2**	7	13.7**
Esophagus	1965-74	15	5.7**	9	7.3**
	1975-83	20	5.7**	13	8.3**
Cervix uteri	1965-74			70	1.9**
	1975-83			100	3.1
Lung	1965-74	34	0.8	15	1.4
	1975-83	57	1.1	27	1.7
Urinary bladder	1965-74	6	0.4**	3	0.5
	1975-83	9	0.4**	6	0.8
Rectum	1965-74	10	0.7	5	0.5
	1975-83	6	0.4**	11	0.8
Prostate	1965-74	1	0.1**		
	1975-83	2	0.1		
Testis	1965-74	3	0.3*		
	1975-83	5	0.4*		
Endometrium	1965-74			6	0.4*
	1975-83			8	0.5*
Breast	1965-74			32	0.5**
	1975-83			38	0.5**
Lymphatic and hematopoietic system	1965-74	7	0.3**	9	0.6
	1975-83	11	0.5**	9	0.5*

* $p < 0.05$ ** $p < 0.01$

REFERENCES

1. Nielsen NH, Hart Hansen JP. Cancer incidence in Greenlanders. In: Harvald B, Hart Hansen JP, eds. Circumpolar Health 81. Nordic Council Arct Med Res Rep 1982; 33:265-267.
2. Lanier AP, Bender TR, Blot WJ, Fraumeni JF and Hurlburt WB. Cancer incidence in Alaska Natives. Int J Cancer 1976; 18:409-412.
3. Hildes JA, Schaefer O. The changing picture of neoplastic disease in the western and central Canadian Arctic (1950-1980). Can Med Assoc J 1984; 130:25-32.

Jens Peter Hart Hansen
Gentofte Hospital
DK-2900 Hellerup
Denmark

Circumpolar Health 84:256-260

CANCER INCIDENCE IN NORTHERN FINLAND: A REGISTRY AND AUTOPSY STUDY

FREJ STENBÄCK

Reports of cancer incidence in the Nordic countries are regarded as being among the most reliable owing to long clinical experience, extensive reporting systems, and the high standard of medical facilities. As part of a series of ongoing studies about morbidity in northern regions, we have focused our attention on cancer incidence and its relationship to environmental, occupational, etiological, and other conditions. Certain differences among the Nordic countries and between different parts of these countries have been reported (1,2). However, few studies have explained the underlying figures, their reliability, and accuracy.

Studies of cancer incidence in the north are few. In general, the occurrence of cancer in northern areas in other parts of the world, such as Greenland, Alaska, or Labrador, is of the same magnitude but has a distinctly different pattern from that of the European countries or North America (3,4). Some types of tumors such as nasopharyngeal tumors, hepatocellular carcinomas, and esophageal carcinomas are relatively common, while others, such as mammary tumors, are less frequent.

Cancer incidence data are based on information from clinicians, hospitals,

Table 1. The mean population of the twelve counties of Finland in 1979, by sex.

Country	Males	Females
	Thousands	
Uedenmaan	522.9	592.6
Turun ja Porin	337.5	363.9
Ahvenanmaa	11.2	11.4
Hämeen	315.7	346.2
Kymen	168.4	177.0
Mikkelin	102.5	106.8
Pohjois-Karjalan	87.8	88.9
Kuopion	123.1	128.6
Keski-Suomen	119.1	123.0
Vaasan	209.6	219.5
Oulun	207.4	206.4
Lapin	98.6	96.6
Total for Finland	2,303.8	2,460.9

pathology laboratories, and death certificates. The latter are the sources of much medical and epidemiological information, although it has long been recognized that certified causes of death vary greatly in

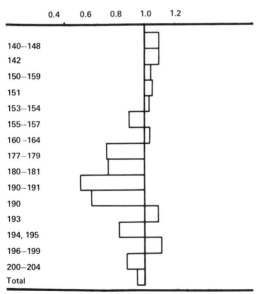

Figure 1. Ratio of incidence of tumors in males in the province of Oulu compared to all of Finland using WHO code numbers (see Material section).

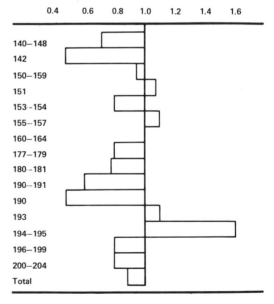

Figure 2. Incidence of tumors in females in the province of Oulu compared to all of Finland using WHO code numbers.

accuracy (5,6). Some diseases are diagnosed earlier than others and in consequence cause-specific mortality statistics could be misleading.

This study attempts to determine how cancer incidence in northern Finland differs from that in the rest of the country and to examine the effect of latitude. Autopsy diagnoses and clinical diagnoses made prior to autopsy are also compared in relation to the effect on the incidence of different types of tumors.

MATERIAL

The tumor incidence data were based on the Finnish Cancer Society Annual Report (7), a compilation of the data on cancer cases diagnosed in 1980. Hospitals, pathological laboratories, and practicing physicians are requested to report to the registry all cases of cancer which come to their attention, both new cases and those registered previously. The listing of all deaths was checked against the registry. The diagnosis was based on histological confirmation in 88% of the cases, and in 1.6% of the cases was based on death certificate alone. A latitude gradient is also reported based on data from Teppo et al. (2).

The clinical and autopsy data derive from a series of 400 consecutive cancer patients in northern Finland. In the autopsy study, diagnoses made by the clinician prior to autopsy were compared with diagnoses of cancer made by the attending pathologist. A complete autopsy was performed on all patients included in this study. All parenchymatous organs were studied and all tumors verified histologically. Uncertain or borderline cases were reviewed; this group comprised very few patients, and the cases were assigned proper designations. The autopsy designations were based on actual autopsy findings, additional information being obtained from clinical studies. The diagnosis code numbers are based on the WHO code (International Classification of Diseases ICD Code 7th Revision, 1955). The estimates are based on the incidence for the whole country being 1.0 and the averages for the two northern countries, Oulu and Lapland, in fractions thereof.

RESULTS

Table 1 shows the population involved in this study (12% of the total population of Finland) as well as the sex distribution. The location of the area, northern Finland, encompasses approximately half of the total area of Finland on either side of the Arctic Circle.

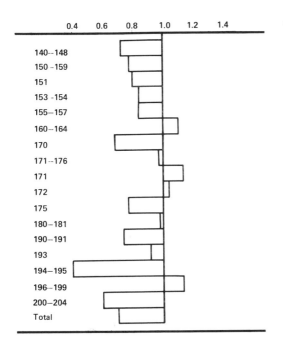

Figure 3. Incidence of tumors in males in the province of Lapland compared to all of Finland using WHO code numbers.

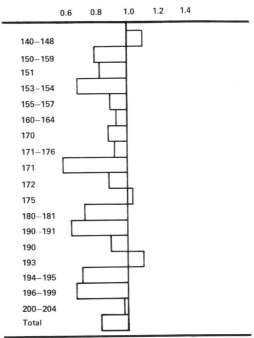

Figure 4. Incidence of tumors in females in the province of Lapland compared to all of Finland using WHO code numbers.

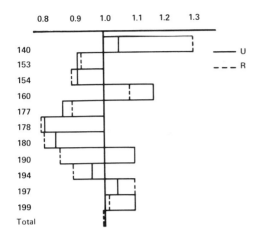

Figure 5. *Latitude gradient of cancer in males. Ratio of tumor incidence in northern areas compared to all of Finland using WHO code numbers. U = urban, R = rural.*

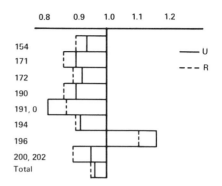

Figure 6. *Latitude gradient of cancer in females. Ratio of tumor incidence in northern areas compared to all of Finland using WHO code numbers. U = urban, R = rural.*

In comparing cancer incidence in Oulu province with that for the entire country for males (Figure 1) and for females (Figure 2), several differences are found. In males, pancreas, stomach, and thyroid tumors were more common in the north, while most other tumors were less common. Female cancer incidence data from Oulu province (Figure 2) showed a lower incidence for many tumor forms, in particular tumors of the

reproductive tract and breasts. In the province of Lapland a similar pattern was observed, with comparatively low tumor incidence in both males (Figure 3) and females (Figure 4). Tumors of particular interest, salivary gland tumors, esophageal tumors, or hepatocellular carcinomas, were very few or nonexistent.

A negative latitude gradient for the whole country of Finland was observed for total tumor incidence in males (Figure 5). A positive latitude/incidence relationship was to be seen only for tumors of the lip and pharynx, nose and sinuses, and soft

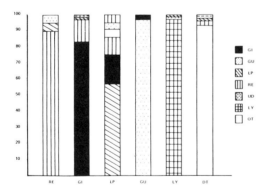

Figure 7. *Clinical confirmation rate of tumors detected at autopsy. RE = respiratory, GI = gastrointestinal, LP = lymphomas, leukemias, GU = genitourinary, LY = lymphoma, OT and DT = other, UD = undefined tumors. Vertical = clinical diagnoses, horizontal = autopsy diagnoses.*

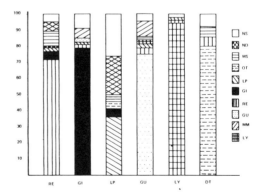

Figure 8. *Clinical detection rate of tumors diagnosed at autopsy. Abbreviations same as in Figure 7. Also, NS = not suspected, ND = not detected, MS = malignancy suspected, and MM = miscellaneous malignancies suspected prior to autopsy. Vertical = clinical diagnoses, horizontal = autopsy diagnoses.*

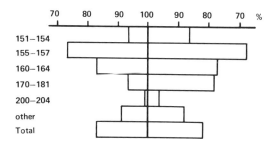

Figure 9. Detection and confirmation rate of clinical diagnoses at autopsy in percent. Left = tumors not detected clinically only at autopsy, right = tumors diagnosed clinically but not confirmed at autopsy.

tissues. A negative latitude gradient was more common, being particularly distinct for colo-rectal and genital tumors. The overall incidence of tumors in females was also inversely related to latitude (Figure 6), most significantly for gynecological, rectal, and endocrine tumors. Of particular interest was the indistinct latitude relationship for skin tumors, as UV-radiation is significantly less in the north of Finland.

In the second part of the study we compared antemortem and postmortem diagnoses of the same patients. As shown in Figure 7, clinical diagnoses prior to autopsy were frequently not verified at autopsy, though this did depend upon the organ concerned. Thus, lymphomas were rarely disputed while pulmonary, pancreatic, and liver tumors were less frequently agreed upon. A similar pattern was seen with regard to the clinical detection of tumors found at autopsy. The average failure of antemortem diagnosis was 82% (Figure 8). This related particularly to liver and pancreatic tumors and less frequently to gastrointestinal and genito-urinary neoplasms. A number of tumors were frequently not assigned any specific site or number of sites, the final decision being made at autopsy.

The detection rate and confirmation is compared in Figure 9. Under-diagnosis (lack of clinically observed cancer) leads to an under-reporting of cancer incidence. This applies to tumors of the liver and pancreas as they have a low detection rate. Over-reporting (clinical diagnosis of cancer not confirmed at autopsy) would lead to erroneously high cancer incidence rates had autopsies not been performed. In Figure 9 this is reflected as a low confirmation rate, i.e., for respiratory tumors.

DISCUSSION

The population included in this study, 307,000 males and 303,000 females, is almost entirely Caucasian, the Native Lapp population being less than 1%. The size of the area, virtually one-half of the country, indicates the sparse population and a lack of contact between people. This and the location explain the low industrial output and a low level of pollution. The location around the Arctic Circle is farther north than any other population of comparable size.

The tumor incidence in the northern part of Finland, as shown in Figures 1 and 4, was slightly lower than in the rest of the country, with some exceptions. This is in agreement with the findings of a higher tumor incidence in industrialized parts of the world (8). The north of Finland is generally less industrialized, the country's major factories and plants being in the southernmost part of the country.

In males, stomach cancer incidence was slightly higher, while that of rectal cancer was slightly lower. Similar findings have been reported for Labrador (9) and Greenland Eskimos (4). Cancer of the lung, the most important fatal neoplasm in males, has increased distinctly during the last decades in northern Finland. Lung cancer was previously reported as less common there (7), as well as in many other northern areas (1,10). A positive latitude gradient correlation, shown in Figure 6, was obtained for cancer of the lip and cancer of the nose and sinuses. The incidence of lip cancer was higher in northern Finland (Figure 5), as shown previously (2,11), seen also in northern Canada (12). This is in accordance with findings on the association between risk of lip cancer and socioeconomic status: northern Finland is less developed than southern Finland.

The tumor incidence in females was also lower than average in both provinces in the present study. As shown in Figures 2, 4, and 6, a negative latitude gradient correlation was obtained and applied to almost all types of tumors. The incidence of tumors of the genital system had a lower incidence in the north except for cervical tumors; this has been shown in other studies on northern populations (4, 13). Cancers of the cervix have a distinct association with extraneous causes, sexual behavior, and the number of sexual partners. The low incidence in the province of Oulu is possibly associated with an aggressive prevention program (14) now being conducted in the province of Lapland.

Certain types of cancers, such as nasopharyngeal carcinoma (NPC) or salivary gland carcinoma, are common in Alaska and Greenland (3,4), but tumors of this kind were not found in the current study. A high incidence of esophageal tumors has been reported in some parts of the north (4). These tumors, possibly caused by the presence of nitrosamines, were not found in our study. Skin tumor incidence is the one most expected to have a distinct negative latitude gradient correlation, since this tumor is most clearly associated with latitude and sunlight. In southern countries, Caucasians show a many-fold increase in skin cancer, basal cell carcinomas, squamous cell carcinomas, and melanomas (15). In the present study, the correlation is not strong, the difference in men in particular being rather small.

In determining the significance of registry data, the source of information has to be taken into account. As we have shown before (16), and seen also in other studies (6,17), information regarding tumors is frequently disputable. As shown in Figures 7 and 8, both confirmation and detection accuracy is variable and can be a source of considerable misinterpretation. Published incidence rates may vary as certain tumor types are suggested based on less evidence than others. The reporting of cases which were clinically suspected but not confirmed at autopsy, combined with the reporting of cases clinically not suspected but observed at autopsy, may result in fairly accurate total figures. A low clinical detection rate may cause a misleading low incidence rate, and a low confirmation rate at autopsy the opposite.

The need for studies of population in the northern parts of the world is indicated owing to the specific environmental, geographic, genetic, and cultural background of these people. Such studies may offer valuable conclusions applicable to many other countries. As shown here, additional studies are needed to explain the existing differences. Also, caution has to be exercised in drawing conclusions from epidemiological data, and extra care is called for when collecting information from the many sources necessary to provide meaningful, comparable data.

REFERENCES

1. Ringertz N. Cancer incidence in Finland, Iceland, Norway and Sweden. Acta Path Microbiol Scand Sect A 1971; suppl 224:1-37.
2. Teppo L, Pukkala E, Hakama M, Hakulinen T, Herva A, Saxen E. Way of life and cancer incidence in Finland. Scand J Soc Med Suppl 1980; 19:1-84.
3. Lanier AP, Bender TR, Blot WJ, Fraumeni JF, Hurlburt WB. Cancer incidence in Alaska Natives. Int J Cancer 1976; 18:409-412.
4. Nielsen NH, Hansen JPH. Cancer incidence in Greenlanders. In: Harvald B, Hart Hansen JP, eds. Circumpolar

Health 81. Nordic Council Arct Med Res Rep 1982; 33:265-267.
5. Bauer FW, Robbins SL. An autopsy study of cancer patients: I. Accuracy of the clinical diagnoses (1955 to 1965) Boston City Hospital. JAMA 1972; 221:1471-1475.
6. Steer A, Land CE, Moriyama IM, Yamamoto T, Asano M, Sanefuji H. Accuracy of diagnosis of cancer among autopsy cases. JNIH-ABCC population for Hiroshima and Nagasaki. Gann 1976; 67:625-632.
7. Finnish Cancer Society. Cancer incidence in Finland 1980. Helsinki, 1983:1-38.
8. Doll R, Peto R. The causes of cancer: Quantitative estimates of avoidable risks of cancer in the United States. J Nat Cancer Inst 1981; 66:1192-1228.
9. Thomas GW, Williams JH. Cancer in native populations in Labrador. In: Shephard RJ, Itoh S, eds. Proceedings of the Third International Symposium on Circumpolar Health. Toronto: University of Toronto Press, 1976:283-289.
10. Schaefer O, Hildes JA, Medd LM, Cameron DG. The changing pattern of neoplastic disease in Canadian Eskimos. In: Shephard RJ, Itoh S, eds. Proceedings of the Third International Symposium on Circumpolar Health. Toronto: University of Toronto Press, 1976:277-283.
11. Lindqvist C. Risk factors in lip cancer. A questionnaire study. Amer J Epidemiol 1979; 169:521-528.
12. Spitzer WO, Hill GB, Chambers LW, Murphy HB. Clinical epidemiology of the lip in Newfoundland. Ann Roy Coll Phys Surg Canada 1974:44.
13. Larsson L-G, Sandström A. Epidemiology of breast and gynecologic cancers in northern Sweden. Nordic Council Arct Med Res Rep 1983; 36:42-48.
14. Stenbäck F, Karttunen T, Vuopala S, Kauppila A. Cervical cancer and its precursors in northern Finland, effect of mass screening. Nordic Council Arct Med Res Rep 1983; 36:35-41.
15. Stenbäck F. Life history and histopathology of ultraviolet light induced skin tumors. NIH Mon 1978; 50:57-70.
16. Stenbäck F, Päivärinta H. Relation between clinical and autopsy diagnoses, especially as regards cancer. Scand J Soc Med 1980; 8:67-72.
17. Berge T, Lundberg S. Cancer in Malmö 1958-1969. An autopsy study. Acta Pathol Microbiol Scand Suppl 1977; suppl 206:1-234.

Frej Stenbäck
Nordic Council for Arctic Medical Research
Aapistie 3
90220 Oulu 22
Finland

Circumpolar Health 84:261-265

ENVIRONMENTAL FACTORS, DIETARY BEHAVIORS, AND NASOPHARYNGEAL CARCINOMA: ANTHROPOLOGICAL APPROACH

ANNIE HUBERT, JOËLLE ROBERT-LAMBLIN and MARGARIDA HERMANN

INTRODUCTION

The collaboration between social sciences and biomedical sciences has long been a desired goal, but in practice scientists keep to their own territory and are still rather suspicious of the other's approach. We would like to show the value of an anthropological approach preceding the setting up of classic epidemiological studies.

The aim of analytical epidemiology is the characterization of the causes of disease on a population level. One of the aims of anthropology is to give an account of culture and behavior (socio-cultural patterns) of homogenous groups, either large or small. The anthropologist's approach is different and at the same time complements that of the epidemiologist.

Anthropologists try to understand a group through the analysis of details of the life and customs of a given cultural unit. Analytical epidemiology compares, within a single group, 2 series of individuals differentiated by the presence or the absence of a particular pathology. This comparison between cases and controls, realized by means of a questionnaire applied by an interviewer, must be based on hypotheses needing verification.

It is for the formulation of such hypotheses that the anthropological approach can, before the start of any epidemiological study, bring a determinative contribution.

The purpose of this study was to search for one or several possible environmental factors related to the etiology of nasopharyngeal cancer (NPC). This tumor represents the most frequent cancer in man in certain areas of Southeast Asia, particularly among the Cantonese, who have an incidence of 30 per 100,000. It is also frequent in North Africa (9 per 100,000) and in the Arctic (among the Eskimo, 25 per 100,000). For the Cantonese and Eskimo, the peak incidence is between 45 and 55 years of age. In North Africa, a first peak appears between ages 10 and 24, followed by a second peak between 55 and 60.

Three factors seem to be related to this tumor: a) a presumed genetic factor, linked to the HLA system (1), b) a herpes virus, the Epstein-Barr virus (EBV), closely associated with NPC without any geographical restriction (2), and c) an environmental factor. This latter could be associated with specific dietary behavior.

In their study on risk factors and cancer, Doll and Peto (3) showed that food and diet (any substance willingly ingested by humans) were dominant risk factors for the development of a majority of cancers in industrial countries as well as in developing countries. Moreover, classic case-control epidemiological studies carried out in Hong Kong and Singapore did not point to any definite risk factor among patients (4-7) other than a "traditional way of life," more common in the patients' families compared to controls.

Facing the very complex sphere of environmental and dietary factors, we thought it might be more fruitful to tackle the problem from an anthropological angle, by developing a comparative study among the 3 high-risk groups for NPC, to determine common factors (or effects) which could represent an oncogenic risk. Thus, we could elaborate new hypotheses for further research in the field as well as in the laboratory.

It was then necessary to elaborate a method through which one could collect ethnographic data among families (with and without NPC) in various populations so as to carry out a comparative study. The data should not only cover diet, but also habitat, genealogies, and a history of diseases in the family, which could also point to other factors bearing on etiology of the disease under study.

METHODS

In Greenland, as in the 2 other high risk areas, the following methodology was applied in the choice of families with cases of NPC. Certain criteria must be observed: it is best to have living cases, and if that is not possible, it is desirable to have cases in which the patient died recently. It is also important that the patient and his family should be able to give an account of the patient's childhood and youth. If the parents are not available, one must find brothers, sisters, or any other relative or close friend who spent his childhood in the same household as the patient, and is able to give an account of diet and life at that period. The various households visited should of course be willing to cooperate with the researcher.

Sample Selection

Twenty families per sample were a maximum for the first survey. Since this was an ethnographic type of study, not an epidemiological survey, and given the time necessary for minute observations of the daily way of life and the lengthy conversa-

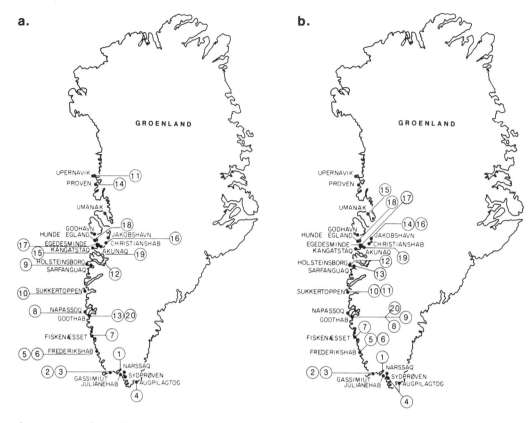

Figure 1.   Each patient's place of birth (a) and each patient's place of residence in 1982 or at death (b).

tions carried out with the members of the household, this number 20 already represents a high figure for a field stay of about 2 months.

Since there is no particular concentration of NPC in any area of Greenland, we chose the most recent cases from the list of 40 patients proposed by Dr. Hart Hansen in order to gather the most reliable information. Further, we decided to cover the widest possible geographical area; from Julianehåb/Qaqortoq (60°30'N) to Umanak (70°30'N), in order to point out local differences.

The 20 cases included 11 men and 9 women. Eight were living patients (3 men, 5 women); the remainder (8 men, 4 women) were deceased. Only one case could be considered as "adolescent" (22 years old at death).

Geographical Distribution

In the sample, cases were distributed as follows: Narssaq (2), Julianehåb/Qaqortoq (2), Frederikshåb/Paamiut (2), Godthåb/Nuuk (4), Sukkertoppen/Maniitsoq (2), Holsteinborg/Sisimiut (2), Egedesminde/Aasiaat (3), Jakobshavn/Ilulissat (2), and Umanak (1) (Figure 1).

Field Work

Anthropological research on food, diet, and habitat requires the observation *in situ* of the various households under consideration. In no case should these inquiries be carried out in hospital or in the work place. What is needed is a knowledge of how people live and behave at home, in their own surroundings. The observations of the facts and acts are as important as the questions asked.

A thorough knowledge of the ethnography of the group under study is necessary as a starting point, requiring teamwork with a specialist of the ethnic group concerned (in the case of Greenland, J. Robert-Lamblin and M. Hermann). In comparative studies of this type, it is also essential that the same researcher (in this case, A. Hubert) be present on each field survey, so that the same methods could be uniformly applied.

The local hospital contacted the families with NPC cases who had accepted our coming into field inquiries and we personally visited each household. No medical or administrative personnel accompanied us, so that people would feel free in their answers. The visit to the household included interviews (following a uniform inquiry pattern, not presented as a questionnaire but rather as an informal conversation) and observations. These include the following subjects:

1. Genealogy of the family with a history of diseases in its members, pointing out, if appropriate, possible genetic transmissions or factors.

2. The history of the disease, as it is perceived by patient and family, is important not only to define cultural perception of the disease, relevant in any efficient treatment on a personal level or for public health, but also because it can point out interesting facts. For example, in all the histories collected among high-risk groups for NPC, clear differences have appeared in the description of symptoms among North Africans on the one hand, and Cantonese and Greenlanders on the other. These differences might just be on a cultural level, but they could equally point to some real differences between these groups on the pathological level.

3. A life history of the patient and family to note all changes, movements, professions, transformations of the material surroundings, etc. This type of data is useful to follow the evolution of a disease on an epidemiological level throughout transformations in the group's lifestyle.

4. Data on habitat, past and present, to include:
a) Description of the village, neighborhood, or housing complex; useful for knowing how the various households share a given space, and which can be the geographical points of transmission of pathogens; and
b) Description of the house, such as building material, division of space, air, light, number of inhabitants, presence of animals, etc., relevant to horizontal transmission of viruses and diseases. A description of furnishings, bedding, etc., gives details on possible modes of transmission (sleeping several in the same bed, babies with parents, with brothers and sisters, etc.).

5. Observations on conditions of hygiene, relating again to possibilities of horizontal transmission. They also include body techniques, gestures and physical behavior of the household, notions of hygiene, washing, changing, washing children, etc. Gestures of affection must also be noted, such as kissing on the mouth of babies or premasticating food (in our particular case for early EBV transmission).

6. Diet and foods, to include:
a) Description of the cooking area, implements, fuel (presence of smoke or toxic substances), a list of usual foods throughout the year, to determine seasonal factors and constant factors, and a study of techniques of food transformation such as food preserving and cooking. This type of data is relevant to search for dietary oncogenic factors, or other factors affecting the group's health.
b) Conversations with members of the family, completing visual observations: table manners (hand washing, common plates, eating with fingers, etc.), special diets, types of meals, changes in diet during life span, weaning, diet in childhood, etc. A dietary history of the family concentrating on the patient's childhood is thus obtained. The importance of the latter on risk for diseases with a long period of latency is well known.
c) All data on food and diet obtained among the various households are then completed by the study of any existing document on the subject, for each area under study and a basic document is established completing the files on each household.

7. Traditional therapies, if any, such as herb teas, etc.

Conversations were carried out in the local language. In Greenland, they were recorded, translated by M. Hermann, and written out.

RESULTS

Environment and Lifestyle

Three-quarters (15 out of 20) of the families came from small villages. Ten had moved to a town, 5 of them before the patient was 20; 5 of them much later in life. Eighteen of the 20 came from hunting and/or fishing families and had a traditional lifestyle in their youth. The fathers of two were wage earners but could obtain traditional food by exchange. Half of the patients were hunters or fishermen themselves, and ten others became wage earners in adult life. In the past all the families (10 out of 20) had eaten the following traditional foods: meat (fresh and dried) of sea mammals, reindeer (for the middle of the west coast), and sheep (for a small area in the south), sea mammals being a constant factor. They had also eaten dried fish and sea mammal fat (raw, boiled, and in oil) and seasonal foods: berries (*Empetrum nigrum* and *Vaccinium uliginosum*), angelica, birds, Arctic char ('*Salvelinus alpinus*), and capelin (*Mallotus villosus*). Members of 2 families ate sizeable amounts of imported foods in their childhood, and all others had access, in various degrees, to bread, sugar, tea, and coffee. Eleven out of 20 had a strong taste for putrefied foods (highly fermented sea mammal meat and fish). Slightly fermented food was eaten by all families in the way cod fish is sometimes prepared prior to boiling. Eight of the 20 had important food changes in their adult life, generally when they moved to town and entered a wage-earning activity, whereas 12 out of 20 had only very minor changes in diet since they continued hunting and fishing together with wage-earning activities, or had hunters and fishermen in the family to supply food. Fifteen out of 20 were born and raised in traditional housing, with the remaining five living in more modern type housing, but without electricity, running water, or toilets, at least during their youth. All of them now live in modern apartment buildings or individual houses.

One of our aims was to establish a profile of NPC patients in Greenland, a region which is undergoing very rapid evolution, with urbanization, modernization, increased medical assistance, and schooling.

It appears that the great majority of the patients came from small villages where they spent their childhood and adolescence. They had a traditional way of life; that is, they depended mostly on local resources prepared according to ancestral techniques and lived in old style housing, fairly similar to ancient Greenlandic habitations. Today they all have a completely different lifestyle, more Westernized, living in modern housing, with access to imported products available at the local shops.

If traditional lifestyle and food habits in the first years of life are important or decisive factors in NPC etiology, it appears that the younger generations, who considerably changed their way of life and eating habits as compared to their parents, should show a drastic drop in the curve of incidence. For example, promiscuity in sleeping conditions, spitting, the way of eating and drinking in communal containers, which were practices common to a great majority of the patients interviewed, certainly played a role in the early transmission of EBV. These cultural practices are now rapidly disappearing among the young generations.

Concerning food habits, for all patients interviewed we must emphasize:

- The extreme importance of protein foods: meat (sea mammals, reindeer, birds) and fish.
- The very heavy consumption of sea mammal fat (polyunsaturated fatty acids) and reindeer fat.
- The very small amount of plant food, most of it seasonal.
- The great importance of dried foods: meat and fish.
- The importance of foodstuffs which are eaten raw.
- A frequent preference among the people interviewed (mostly older generation) for strong tasting, dried, and putrefied foods and fats.

Fermentation has been a way of processing food to give it a variety of tastes, particularly for arctic people who traditionally had no sapidity agent (not even salt except sea water). This liking for strong tastes is disappearing with the young, who now at the local store find enough different food stuffs to satisfy a variety of tastes. They favor, much more than their parents, imported foods and Danish cooking techniques.

Family Aggregation

The genealogical data have revealed some multiple cases of NPC in families and some cases of salivary gland carcinoma in families with an NPC patient, both tumors being related to EBV. Cases 2, 3, and 5 had one other case of NPC in their family (cases 2 and 3 being related), whereas cases 5, 8, 18, and 19 had a case of salivary gland carcinoma in their family.

The various cases mentioned were medically diagnosed. Families interviewed mentioned other cases where symptoms were close to NPC but could not be traced back for medical diagnosis. It would be advisable to make such genealogical inquiries among all new NPC patients, to help determine whether a genetic factor is present or not (HLA typing of multiple case families). In searching for a possible genetic factor, one must keep in mind that the mixed parentage with Caucasians goes back several centuries for Western Greenland. Part of the local population remained in isolation nevertheless, since the Caucasian genitors were for the most part whalers. Greenland's opening to the outside world after World War II led to a rapid increase of blood admixture. At the same time, the Caucasian population residing in Greenland is regularly increasing (Table 1). It seems logical to presume that the younger generation will present a genotype different from that of their forefathers.

Table 1. Numbers of Greenlanders and Caucasians living in Greenland, 1945 to 1980.

Year	Greenlanders	Caucasians
1945	20,939	473
1950	22,581	1,061
1960	30,378	2,762
1970	38,912	7,620
1980	41,459	9,184

Any future study on NPC in Greenland will have to take into consideration these changing biological (genetic) and cultural (lifestyle) factors. It is now essential to follow the trend for NPC incidence in Greenland. If it drops, it would be circumstantial evidence of the importance of an environmental factor involving traditional lifestyle and diet. This factor should in any case be more important than a genetic one, since most of the NPC patients we saw had some Caucasian blood.

CONCLUSIONS

The preliminary comparative study, carried out with the same methods, among Cantonese, North Africans (Tunisia), and Greenlanders, leads to the following remarks:

Some common points have been found: 1) A traditional lifestyle during childhood (traditional housing with lack of light and air), promiscuity due to crowded living conditions, and lack of hygiene. 2) A regular consumption of dried foods since infancy (dried fish and meat for all 3 groups and dried vegetables for Cantonese and Tunisians). 3) A fairly regular consumption of fermented food (meat or fish for all 3 groups, vegetables for Cantonese and Tunisians).

These traditional preserving techniques, common to all 3 high-risk groups, involve drying and fermentation, leading to growth of various types of fungi. It seems to us that a close examination of these methods of traditional food preservation should be made in order to study the presence of possible mycotoxins or other oncogenic or EBV reactivating factors.

For Greenland, the study showed a much higher number of family aggregation for NPC and salivary gland carcinoma (7 out of 20).

ACKNOWLEDGMENTS

This study was carried out thanks to international cooperation between Dr. Jørgen Bøggild of Greenland, Dr. J. P. Hart Hansen of Denmark, and Prof. Guy de Thé of France. Further, it could not have been carried out without the kind collaboration of local medical officers and Greenlandic health personnel.

REFERENCES

1. Simons MJ, et al. Immuno-genetic aspects of nasopharyngeal carcinoma (I). Differences in HLA antigen profiles between patients and comparison groups. Int J Cancer 1974; 13:122-134.

2. de Thé G. Epidemiology of Epstein-Barr virus and associated diseases. In: Roizman B, ed. The herpes viruses. Vol. I. A. New York: Plenum Press, 1982:25-100.

3. Doll R, Peto R. The causes of cancer: quantitative estimates of avoidable risks of cancer in the United States today. J Nat Cancer Inst 1981; 6:1191-1308.

4. Shanmugaratnam K, et al. Etiological factors in nasopharyngeal carcinoma: A hospital-based, retrospective case-control questionnaire study. In: de Thé G, Ito Y, eds. Nasopharyngeal carcinoma: Etiology and control. IARC Sci Publ Lyon, 1978; 20:199-212.

5. Geser A, et al. Environmental factors in the etiology of nasopharyngeal carcinoma: Report on a case-control study in Hong Kong. In: de Thé G, Ito Y, eds. Nasopharyngeal carcinoma: Etiology and control. IARC Sci Publ Lyon, 1978; 20:213-229.

6. Anderson E N Jr, et al. A study of the environmental backgrounds of young Chinese nasopharyngeal carcinoma patients. In: de Thé G, Ito Y, eds. Nasopharyngeal carcinoma: Etiology and control. IARC Sci Publ Lyon, 1978; 20:231-239.

7. Henderson BE, et al. Risk factors associated with nasopharyngeal carcinoma. NEJM 1976; 295:1101-1106.

Annie Hubert
Laboratoire d'Epidémiologie
  et Immunovirologie des
  Tumeurs
Faculté de Médecine Alexis Carrel
Rue G. Paradin
69372 Lyon Cedex 2
France

Circumpolar Health 84:266-267

DIETARY SELENIUM INTAKE IN GREENLAND RELATED TO MERCURY EXPOSURE

JENS C. HANSEN

It has been known for several years that population groups in arctic areas are to a higher extent than others exposed to mercury through the diet. High blood mercury concentrations have been found in Alaska (1) and in Canada (2,3).

To evaluate the mercury exposure in Greenland, a survey was started in 1979 and is still going on. Selenium, as shown in animal experiments, is a powerful antagonist to toxic effects of methyl mercury; this element was included in the program from 1982.

MATERIALS AND METHODS

At present a total of 608 persons, corresponding to 1.2% of the total population, has been investigated. Blood samples and in most cases also hair samples have been collected from 7 different districts, giving a good geographical distribution. Also, 24 samples of typical Eskimo food items have been collected.

All samples have been analyzed by atomic absorption spectroscopy. The analytical method has been carefully controlled and is described elsewhere (4-6).

RESULTS AND DISCUSSION

Blood mercury as well as blood selenium concentrations were found to be closely related to the amount eaten per day of meat from marine mammals (4-6). This is illustrated for mercury in Figure 1, where the arithmetic means of blood mercury concentrations found in various geographical regions are plotted against the amount of meat available per person per day, taken from official hunting statistics. This is done based on the assumption that the amount eaten reflects the amount available. For comparison, figures from Denmark are included.

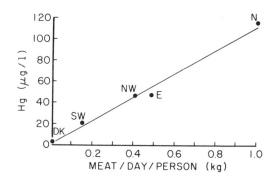

Figure 1. *Relationship between available meat from marine mammals per person per day in Greenland and Denmark. N: North Greenland, E: East Greenland, NW: Northwest Greenland, SW: Southwest Greenland, DK: Denmark.*

The same tendency is observed for selenium where only data from 2 districts are obtained, namely Angmagssalik on the east coast with an overall arithmetic mean of 164±83 µg/l (N=119) and Thule in the north with a mean of 1,609±1,116 µg/l (N=86).

The very high mercury concentrations found in Thule with a mean of 117 µg/l and highest recorded concentration of 267 µg/l does not necessarily indicate a higher mercury concentration in animals in the north, but more likely reflects the varying conditions of life and consequently of eating habits.

The results of analysis of the 22 samples of meat from various typical Eskimo prey animals are shown in Table 1.

Terrestrial animal meat (reindeer and sheep) is without importance with regard to

Table 1. *Selenium and mercury concentrations in Greenlandic food items.*

	No.	Hg x̄ mg/kg	Hg range	Se x̄ mg/kg	Se range
Seal and whale	8	0.35	0.09-0.87	0.39	0.20-0.85
Fish	7	0.12	0.04-0.25	0.43	0.20-0.90
Reindeer and lamb	4	0.04	0.01-0.07	0.11	0.05-0.20
Auk	2	0.22	0.18-0.27	0.73	0.40-1.05

both mercury and selenium. This kind of meat plays only a minor role in the diet of the hunting district, but is commonly used in the developed areas of the southwest coast of Greenland. Also, seabirds play only a quantitatively modest role in the total diet.

In the hunting districts the main source of dietary mercury is marine mammals. With a mean concentration of 0.35 mg per kg the WHO (7) provisional tolerable weekly intake of 0.2 mg per person per week as methyl mercury will be reached with a daily intake of only 80 g of meat. Generally an Eskimo will eat several hundred grams of meat daily and consequently the WHO limit will regularly be exceeded among sealers in Greenland.

With regard to selenium concentrations no differences were found between the concentration in marine mammals and in fish with mean values at 0.39 and 0.43 mg per kg, respectively. The nutritional requirement of 50 to 200 µg per day is thus easily obtained.

On a molar basis selenium is found in surplus to mercury in food and in human blood samples. Selenium has a role as an antagonist to neuro-toxic effects of methyl mercury (8). The mechanism of this effect is not known in detail, but is probably due to formation of the less toxic bis-methyl-mercuric selenide (9). The alleviation of mercury toxicity by selenium has so far only been described in laboratory animals. In all probability, however, dietary selenium can be regarded as a protective agent against adverse effects of natural methyl mercury exposure in humans as well.

CONCLUSION

The typical Eskimo diet with a very high intake of meat from marine mammals will, in spite of the moderate mercury concentrations in meat, provide an excess intake compared to the WHO recommendations.

The diet is rich in selenium also. Selenium is found in higher concentrations than mercury in food as well as in blood. This may be a protective factor against hazards from mercury ingestion. Careful epidemiological investigations are, however, needed to prove this.

REFERENCES

1. Galster WA. Environmental Health Perspectives. 1976; 15:135-140.
2. Bernstein AD. Int Symp Proc: Recent Advances in the Assessment of the Health Effects of Environmental Pollution. Paris June 1974. CEC Luxembourg, 1975; 1:105-117.
3. Charlebois C. Ambio 1978; 7:204-210.
4. Hansen JC. Meddr Grønland, Man and Soc 1981; 3:1-36.
5. Hansen JC, Wulf HC, Kromann N, Albøge K. Sci Total Environ 1983; 26:233-243.
6. Hansen JC, Kromann N, Wulf HC, Albøge K. Sci Total Environ 1984; 38:33-40.
7. WHO Tech Rep Ser 1972; 505.
8. Task Group on Metal Interactions: Environmental Health Perspectives 1978; 25:3-41.
9. Masakawa T, Kito H, Haynshi M, Iwata H. Biochem Pharmacol 1982; 31:75-78.

Jens C. Hansen
Institute of Hygiene
University of Aarhus
DK 8000 Århus C
Denmark

Circumpolar Health 84:268-275

COMPARISONS OF TOTAL SERUM CHOLESTEROL AND TRIGLYCERIDES BETWEEN TOWN AND FARM DWELLING ICELANDIC YOUTHS

ANTHONY B. WAY, JÓHANN AXELSSON, GUDRUN PÉTURSDÓTTIR and NIKULAS SIGFÚSSON

INTRODUCTION

A comparative study of cardiovascular risk factors in young Icelanders was conducted in 1979. This study had 3 purposes: 1) to acquire data for comparison with future data from Canadian youths of pure Icelandic descent (1), 2) to test for differences among town, farm, and city dwelling youths in Iceland, and 3) to provide data for comparison with other populations.

The study was conducted in rural eastern Iceland. We studied 211 comparable boys and girls aged 7 to 20 who lived either on farms or in a small town. Data were collected on hematological, morphological, physiological (2), behavioral, and genealogical characteristics and on general health status. This paper presents the findings on serum cholesterol and triglycerides (triacylglycerols).

A consistent epidemiological observation is that many characteristics are associated with cardiovascular diseases. The recognition that degenerative cardio-vascular disease is the result of a chronic process has aroused interest in the appearance of cardiovascular risk factors in children (3,4). Our preliminary reports (5,6) suggest that Icelandic youths have levels of cardiovascular risk factors that are similar to those of adults, including high serum cholesterol.

MATERIALS AND METHODS

Fljótsdalshérad is a farming district with a total population of about 2,700, including the town of Egilsstadir (population ca. 1,200). Our sample was drawn from about 1,000 youths who were probably genetically comparable because their parents and grandparents had lived in Fljótsdalshérad. We measured 224 individuals aged 7 to 20. In the analysis, the sample was reduced to 211 because of some missing values. Subjects were recruited so that each two-year subgroup provided 8 boys and girls from both farms and town (Table 1). Our unpublished analyses suggest that both the town and farm youths are similar in body morphology except

Table 1. Sample size, cholesterol, triglycerides, and age by sex and residence.

	Town		Farm	
	Boys	Girls	Boys	Girls
Number	55	48	54	54
Cholesterol, mg/dl*				
Mean	197.4	205.3	203.9	213.2
95% Confidence limit	8.27	9.61	8.28	10.03
Maximum	260	275	303	315
Minimum	106	137	145	151
Triglycerides, mg/dl				
Mean	49.2	53.9	58.7	56.9
95% Confidence limit	6.54	6.12	6.97	4.01
Maximum	131	134	148	106
Minimum	22	24	23	27
Age, yrs				
Mean	12.22	13.29	12.72	12.63
95% Confidence limit	0.966	1.048	1.007	0.900
Maximum	20.6	20.6	19.7	19.4
Minimum	7.2	7.0	6.8	6.8

* 38.7 mg/dl cholesterol = 1 mmol/l

possibly that the farm youths are slightly fatter.

Blood samples were obtained by venipuncture in the morning, after an overnight fast. The cooled serum was frozen within 18 hours to $-22°C$ while awaiting analysis. Total cholesterol was determined colorimetrically using a ferric chloride and acid technique (7). Triglycerides (triaglycerols) were determined fluorometrically using a saponification and oxidation technique (8). Quality control was maintained through the WHO (9).

Comparisons were made between the town and farm dwellers by using multiple regression analyses to adjust for possible effects due to other factors such as sex, age, size, and fitness. Stepwise analyses were used to determine which variables other than residence were important, and whether complex interactions needed to be considered. The categorical variables of sex and residence were coded as $+1$ for males and town, and -1 for females and farm. This is equivalent to an analysis of covariance and to a t-test. Interaction variables between 2 or more main effect variables were created by multiplying them together. Since the coefficient of each variable in a multiple regression can be interpreted as its effect when all other independent variables are equal to zero, the restricted meaning of the lower order coefficients of the interactions was enhanced by adjusting all the independent variables to have means of zero (by subtracting the means). The interactions were standardized by multiplying the standardized main effect variables and then subtracting the mean of that product (algebraically equivalent to subtracting the mean of the product and adding the product of the means). Incidentally, such standardization makes the intercept equal to the mean of the dependent variable (Appendices 1 and 2).

RESULTS

Cholesterol

The mean total serum cholesterol for 211 youths was 205 mg/dl (Appendix 1). The difference between town and farm youths was checked both before and after testing for the effects of sex, age, body morphology, and exercise capacity.

The simple difference in mean cholesterol between town and farm youths is marginally nonsignificant (Appendix 1). However, adjusting by multiple regression for the most important variable, height (Figure 1), reveals that the town youths have cholesterol levels 11 mg/dl lower than the farm youths: $2 \times -5.4 = -10.8$. Thus at the mean height of 153 cm, the farm youths have a cholesterol of 210 mg/dl: 204.9 -

5.4 x -1.033, and the town of 200 mg/dl: 204.9 - 5.4 x 0.967. Residence and height, however, only account for 14% of the variation in cholesterol.

No significant difference in cholesterol appeared in our subjects when also compared by sex or any of its interactions (such as sex-residence, sex-weight, etc.). These findings refute our preliminary report (6) of a sex-age interaction with serum cholesterol. Age is also not significantly correlated with cholesterol when adjusting for height (see below).

Height correlates with cholesterol. Detailed analyses suggest that, in a stepwise multiple regression, height is merely a slightly better indicator of growth and development than any other variable tried, including chronological age. Cholesterol declines by 0.7 mg/dl per centimeter of increasing height for both town and farm dwellers. When adjustment is made for this relationship, other variables such as body size, obesity, physical fitness, age, and their interactions did not further account for the variation in serum cholesterol.

Triglycerides (Triacylglycerols)

The mean serum triglycerides for 211 youths was 55 mg/dl (Appendix 2). The difference between town and farm dwelling youngsters was checked both before and after testing for the effect of sex, age, body morphology, exercise capacity, and serum cholesterol. Adjustment for cholesterol was considered because of the concern that triglycerides may only be an apparent risk factor due to its correlation with cholesterol.

No significant difference in mean serum triglycerides was found when our subjects were compared simply by residence or by residence when adjusting for other important main effect variables (Appendix 2, Figures 2 and 3). However, a difference may exist between the town and farm youths if interactions are considered. Triglycerides are found to decrease more rapidly (Appendix 2, Figure 4) with maximum oxygen consumption in farm dwelling than in town dwelling youngsters: $(-.016 + .0044 \times residence) \times$ maximum oxygen consumption. Furthermore, the difference in triglycerides between the sexes is more marked, and in the opposite direction, in the farm youths than in the town youths, the farm boys being higher than the farm girls: $(1.51 - 2.96 \times residence) \times$ sex. Residence, the other 8 main effect variables, and 11 of their interactions account for 40% of the variation in triglycerides.

When adjustment is made for differences due to the main effects of age, body morphology, and exercise capacity, we found no

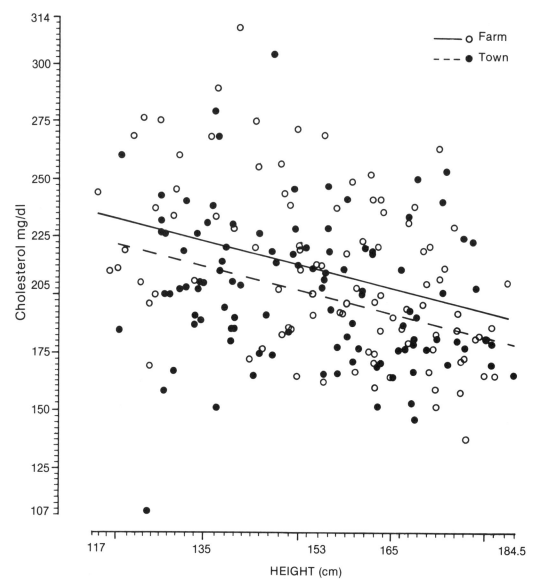

Figure 1. Plot of data points for total serum cholesterol (mg/dl) and height (cm), by residence (location). The predicted values demonstrate the regression lines of the second equation in Appendix 1. Height is the difference from the mean of 152.7 cm.

significant difference between the sexes. There is, however, a sex-residence interaction as described above, as well as sex interactions with height and sum of skin folds (subcutaneous fat). We previously reported (6) a difference between the sexes in mean serum triglycerides. This is now seen to apply to the farm dwelling youths only. Similarly, when the main effects of the other measures of growth and development are considered, age is not an important correlate of triglycerides. Thus our reported interaction between sex and age (6) is now found to be better explained by differences between the sexes in the association of triglycerides with height and with body fat. However, when interactions are considered, age is important as an interaction with cholesterol (each increasing the other's effect).

The variation in triglycerides is significantly and independently associated

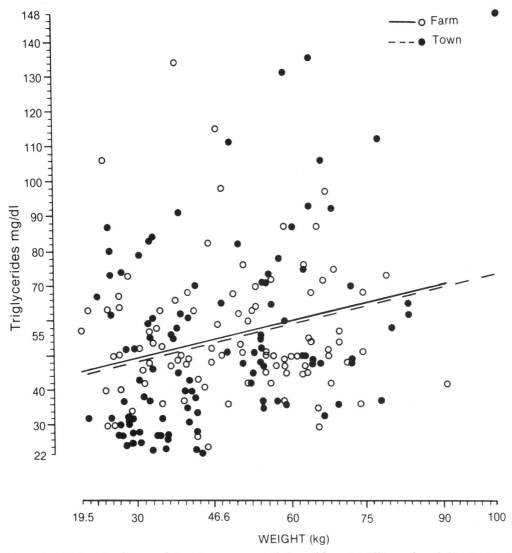

Figure 2. *Plot of data points for serum triglycerides (mg/dl) and weight (kg), by residence (location). The predicted values demonstrate the regression lines of the second equation in Appendix 2. Weight is the difference from the mean of 46.6 kg.*

with many measurements of body morphology, physiology, and serum cholesterol, including their interactions. However, body weight (adjusted for the other variables) is the most consistently important variable for the prediction of triglycerides. As suspected, there is a significant correlation of triglycerides with total serum cholesterol.

DISCUSSION

Total serum cholesterol levels are high in adult Icelanders. They are 254 mg/dl in men of the capital city of Reykjavik (9) and 220 mg/dl in men and women of the rural

district of Fljótsdalshérad (5). Our rural Fljótsdalshérad youths have a similarly high cholesterol of 200 to 299 mg/dl (95% confidence limit). This is considerably higher than the mean of 186 mg/dl found in urban Reykjavik youths (unpublished data). Thus there is a rural-urban gradient in mean serum cholesterol with values of 210 mg/dl for farm, 200 mg/dl for town, and 186 mg/dl for city dwelling Icelandic youngsters. Preliminary analysis of our nutritional data is consistent with these differences. Sixty-four of these rural Fljótsdalshérad youths have a higher intake of cholesterol

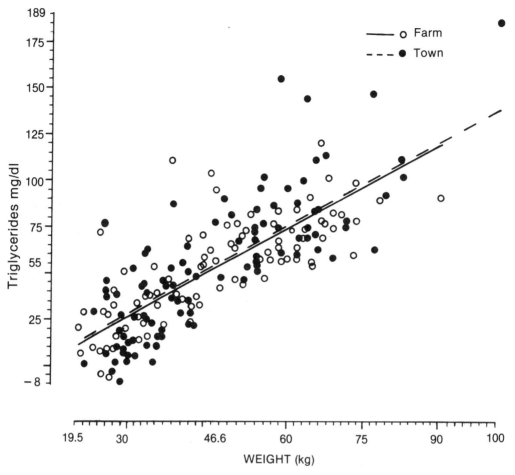

Figure 3. Plot of data points (residuals) for serum triglycerides (mg/dl) and weight (kg), by residence (location), adjusted for the other main effects. The predicted values demonstrate the regression lines of the third equation in Appendix 2. Weight is the difference from the mean of 46.6 kg.

(24%), fat (7%), and saturated to unsaturated fatty acids ratio (6%) than 179 urban Reykjavik youths (unpublished results).

This level of total serum cholesterol in rural Icelandic youngsters is among the highest reported (H. K. Åkerblom, unpublished, presented at this symposium). It is substantially higher than those reported in U.S. youths: 176 mg/dl (3), and 161 to 164 mg/dl (4). Furthermore, these higher levels are not accounted for by differences in height (Appendix 1).

The serum triglyceride level of 52 to 58 mg/dl (95% confidence limit) found in our rural youths is low compared to those of Icelandic adults. Rural Fljótsdalshérad men and women have a mean of 91 mg/dl (5), and urban Reykjavik men have a mean of 96 mg/dl (9). However, the mean for our rural youths is similar to the low mean of 58 mg/dl we find in urban Reykjavik youths (unpublished data).

In contrast with cholesterol, the serum triglycerides of our rural Icelandic youngsters are substantially higher than those reported from the U.S.: 67 to 78 mg/dl (3). Again, this difference is not due to the differences in the other independent variables (Appendix 2).

CONCLUSIONS

Currently proposals are under consideration to induce people, including youths, to modify their dietary customs for disease prevention. The value of dietary change, however, especially for youths, is debated. Our study demonstrates that moderate differences in lifestyle may be associated with differences in cardiovascular risk factors. These occur not only between nations, but

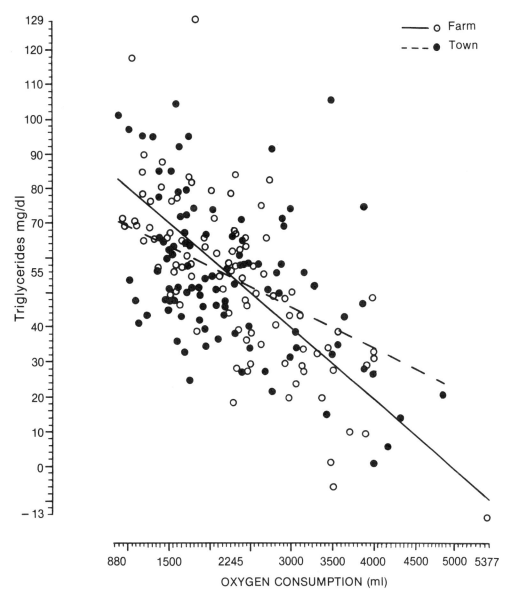

Figure 4. Plot of data points (residuals) for serum triglycerides (mg/dl) and maximum oxygen consumption (ml), by residence (location), adjusted for the other main effects and interactions. The predicted values demonstrate the regression lines of the fourth equation in Appendix 2. Maximum oxygen consumption is the difference from the mean of 2,245 ml.

also within one culture. The general genetic homogeneity of Iceland and the common district parentage of our rural youths argue against a genetic explanation of our results. The differences are quite clear for cholesterol but are more complex for triglycerides.

Our study suggests that health benefits might be obtained by lifestyle modifications

as simple as the differences that exist among a city, a rural town, and farms in Iceland. This may be an important observation since recommendations to the general public will be effective only if they are acceptable to the population. Of course, the relevant lifestyle differences remain to be identified, but our data suggest that diet may be among the important factors.

Appendix 1.   Total serum cholesterol versus residence, regression equations.

Intercept (Mean) = 204.9 mg/dl, 95% CL = 4.5, N = 211
Main Effect Variables
RSQ = .02, 95% CL of the Intercept = 4.5, DF = 209
R = 04.4, p = 0.52
RSQ = .14, 95% CL of the Intercept = 4.2, DF = 208
H = -.69, p < .0001

CL = confidence limit; N = sample size; DF = degrees of freedom; RSQ = correlation coefficient squared; p = probability; $\bar{x}$ = mean; R = Residence, town = +1, farm = -1, $\bar{x}$ = 0.033; H = Height; $\bar{x}$ = 152.67 cm. Independent variables considered and rejected: Weight, Maximum Oxygen Consumption, Bone Width (see Appendix 2), Skin Folds (see Appendix 2), Sex, Age, and up to four-way interactions. E.g. Cholesterol mg/dl = 204.9 - 5.4 x (Residence - .033 - .69 x (Height - 152.67).

Appendix 2.   Serum triglycerides (triacylglycerols) versus residence, regression equations.

Intercept (Mean) = 54.7 mg/dl, 95% CL = 3.0, N = 211
Main Effect Variables: 2-Way Interactions
RSQ = .001, 95% CL of Intercept = 3.0, DF = 209
R = -.80 p = .6
RSQ = .07, 95% CL of Intercept = 2.9, DF = 208
R = -.41 p = .8
W = .36 p < .0001
RSQ = .20, 95% CL of Intercept = 2.7, DF = 204
R = .75 p = .6
W = 1.58 p < .0001
O = -.011 p = .0008
H = -.53 p = .04
C = .18 p < .0001
F = -.53 p = .04
RSQ = .40, 95% CL of Intercept = 2.4, DF = 190
R = -.17 p = .9   :RO =   .0044 p = .01   HC = -.026   p = .009
W = 1.82 p < .0001 :RS = -2.96 p = .04   BC = .011   p = .0005
H = -.83 p = .02   :   AC = .078   p = .02
O = -.016 p < .0001 :   WC = .015   p = .057
F = -.95 p = .001 :   OC = -.00026 p = .009
A = 1.94 p = .047 :   HS = .33   p = .002
C = .16 p = .0002 :   BF = .021   p = .009
S = 1.51 p = .5   :   WH = -.016   p = .050
B = -.043 p = .7   :   FS = -.48   p = .02

See Appendix 1 for other abbreviations and values. W = Weight, $\bar{x}$ = 46.61 kg; O = Maximum Oxygen Consumption, $\bar{x}$ = 2245.0 ml/min; F = Sum of skin folds (triceps and subscapular), $\bar{x}$ = 20.00 mm; A = Age, $\bar{x}$ = 12.70 yr; C = Cholesterol, $\bar{x}$ = 204.9 mg/dl; S = Sex, male = +1, female = -1, $\bar{x}$ = -0.24; B = Sum of bone widths (radio-ulnar heads, femoral condyles), $\bar{x}$ = 284.7 mm; RO $\bar{x}$ = 25.7; RS $\bar{x}$ = .033; HC $\bar{x}$ = 31089.17; BC $\bar{x}$ = 58059.7; AC $\bar{x}$ = 2567.101; WC $\bar{x}$ = 9371.68; OC $\bar{x}$ = 452401.6; HS $\bar{x}$ = -1.19; BF $\bar{x}$ = 5728.77; WH $\bar{x}$ = 7369.09; FS $\bar{x}$ = -3.66. All other two, three, and four way interactions considered and rejected.

REFERENCES

1. Axelsson J, Pálsson JOP, Pétursdóttir G, Sigfússon N, Way AB. Comparative studies of Icelandic people living in Canada and Iceland. In: Harvald B, Hart Hansen JP, eds. Circumpolar Health 81. Nordic Council for Arct Med Res Rep 1982; 33:201-205.

2. Axelsson J, Oskarsson JG, Pétursdóttir G, Way AB, Sigfússon N, Karlsson M. Rural-urban differences in lung size and function in Iceland. In: Fortuine R, ed. Circumpolar Health 84. Seattle: University of Washington Press, 1985. (this volume)

3. Abraham S, Johnson CL, Carroll MD. Total serum cholesterol levels of children, 4-17 years, United States, 1971-1974. Vital and Health Statistics: Series 11, Data from the National Health Survey; No. 207, 1978.

4. Berenson GS. Cardiovascular risk factors in children: The early natural history of atherosclerosis and essential hypertension. New York: Oxford University Press, 1980.

5. Axelsson J, Sigfússon N, Way AB, Pétursdóttir G. Serum lipids in 21 to 60 year old people from eastern Iceland. In: Harvald B, Hart Hansen JP, eds. Circumpolar Health 81. Nordic Council for Arct Med Res Rep 1982; 33:304-307.

6. Pétursdóttir G, Way AB, Sigfússon N, Axelsson J. Serum lipids in children and adolescents from eastern Iceland. In: Harvald B, Hart Hansen JP, eds. Circumpolar Health 81. Nordic Council for Arct Med Res Rep 1982; 33:295-299.

7. Block WD, Jarrett KJ, Levine JB. An improved automated determination of serum total cholesterol with single color reagent. Clin Chem 1966; 10:681-689.

8. Kessler G, Lederer H. Fluorometry measurements of triglycerides. Automation in analytical chemistry, Technicon Symposia. New York: Medical Inc., 1965.

9. Bjornsson OJ, Davidsson D, Olafsson O, Sigfússon N, Thorsteinsson Th. Survey of serum lipid levels in Icelandic men aged 34-61 years. An epidemiological and statistical evaluation. Acta Med Scand (suppl) 1977; 616:1-150.

Anthony B. Way
Department of Preventive Medicine
  and Community Health
School of Medicine
Texas Tech University
Lubbock, Texas 79413
U.S.A.

Circumpolar Health 84:276-281

PREVALENCE OF DIABETES MELLITUS AMONG THE CREE-OJIBWA OF NORTHWESTERN ONTARIO

T. KUE YOUNG and L. LYNN MCINTYRE

INTRODUCTION

The pattern of health and 'sickness among Native peoples in Canada has undergone significant changes as a result of rapid lifestyle alterations, especially since World War II (1,2). Whereas infectious diseases have declined in importance as causes of mortality and morbidity, the burden of chronic conditions in the community has increased substantially. Among practitioners familiar with Native health care, it is widely perceived that chronic diseases such as diabetes are being recognized more frequently.

A considerable literature has accumulated on diabetes among American Indians, as the extensive reviews and bibliographies by Kelly West have indicated (3,4). With over 100 citations in the literature, covering some 80 tribes in the New World, West concluded that diabetes was extremely uncommon in all tribes prior to 1940, but that an "epidemic" began among many tribes in the postwar years. Certain tribes, however, continued to be spared.

While several studies among the Inuit in Canada have been reported by Schaefer (5,6), published data on the prevalence of diabetes among Canadian Indians are scarce. This paper reports on the epidemiological features of diabetes mellitus among the Cree-Ojibwa in northwestern Ontario.

MATERIALS AND METHODS

The Sioux Lookout Zone is an administrative area of the Medical Services Branch which serves approximately 10,000 Algonkian-speaking Cree and Ojibwa Indians living in 25 communities scattered in the eastern subarctic boreal forest of northwestern Ontario. The health care system and epidemiologic pattern of this area have been previously described (7,8).

All Indians who had contact with the Sioux Lookout Zone health service and were given a diagnosis of diabetes mellitus (ICD-code 250) were included in a case registry. Cases were ascertained from:
(1) discharges from the Sioux Lookout Zone Hospital, the secondary care facility for all the communities in the Zone, available from HMRI (Hospital Medical Records Institute) computerized summaries from 1975 onward;
(2) ambulatory care visits to outpost nurses, community health auxiliaries, and physicians in the communities, available from encounter logs coded and stored in computer tapes from 1978 onward;
(3) nursing station chronic disease card indices maintained by outpost nurses for regular follow-up of patients in the communities;
(4) drug dispensing records of diabetic medications from the Sioux Lookout Zone Hospital pharmacy.

All cases living in the Zone on January 1, 1983 were collected from these sources and their clinical histories abstracted from their medical files. The biochemical criteria for diagnosis were those recommended by the National Diabetes Data Group (NDDG) (9). No attempt was made to classify cases further into insulin-dependent (IDDM)

Table 1. Age-sex distribution of diabetic cases and age group specific prevalence rates.

Age group	Number of cases			Percent	Prevalence rate per 1,000 population
	Male	Female	Total		
0 - 14	0	2	2	1.1	0.6
15 - 24	1	4	5	2.6	2.8
25 - 44	20	52	72	37.7	43.6
45 - 64	20	61	81	42.4	98.8
65 and over	8	23	31	16.2	86.1
Total	49	142	191	100.0	23.3

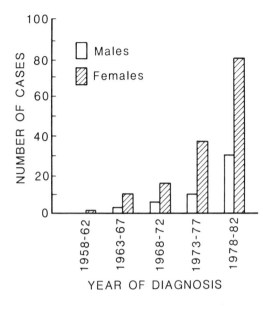

Figure 1. Year of diagnosis of Indian diabetic cases: Sioux Lookout Zone 1958-1982.

or non-insulin dependent (NIDDM) diabetes, although data on therapy status were collected. Gestational diabetes, "secondary" diabetes, and patients with only impaired glucose tolerance were excluded. A total of 191 cases were available for analysis.

Data were coded, keypunched, and entered into the University of Manitoba Health Sciences Computing Facility. The software package Statistical Package for the Social Sciences (SPSS) was used. Stratified analysis was performed on certain variables using the method described by Mantel and Haenszel (10) and Miettinen (11).

RESULTS

An overall prevalence rate of 2.3% was found for this population. The age-sex distribution of cases and age group specific prevalence rates are given in Table 1. The male:female ratio was 1:2.9. Of the 191 cases ascertained, only two were diagnosed when they were under 15 years of age (2 girls aged 8 and 12 at the time of diagnosis). The prevalence rate varied between communities in the zone. However, such rates were not stable due to the small number of cases and small population (varying from 50 to 2,000 people in each community).

Over half of the cases were diagnosed within the past 5 years (Figure 1). The age distribution of cases in more recent years did not differ significantly from that of earlier years.

Data on height and weight recorded at the time of diagnosis were available for 188 (98%) and 142 (74%) cases, respectively. The values of BMI (body mass index; wt in kg/height in square cm) ranged from 18 to 52 among those aged 15 and over. Using the NDDG's criteria of 27 and over for obesity in males and 25 and over for females, 59% of

Table 2. Clinical features of diabetic cases at time of diagnosis.

	Male		Female		Total	
	No.	%	No.	%	No.	%
Fasting plasma glucose						
< 200 mg/dl	16	36.4	68	50.4	84	46.9
200-300 mg/dl	20	45.5	50	37.0	70	39.1
> 300 mg/dl	8	18.2	17	12.6	25	14.0
2-hour PC plasma glucose						
< 200 mg/dl	5	11.9	25	21.0	30	18.6
200-300 mg/dl	13	31.0	46	38.7	59	26.6
> 300 mg/dl	24	57.1	48	40.3	72	44.7
Blood pressure						
≥ 140/90	18	36.7	51	36.2	69	36.3
Glycosuria	41	93.2	105	79.0	146	82.5
Ketonuria	10	22.7	15	11.3	25	14.1

males and 84% of females can be considered "obese."

Using Canadian national standards from the Nutrition Canada Survey of the early 1970s (12), the distribution of cases by quartiles of weight-for-age and weight-for-height-for-age was determined. About 27% of male diabetics had weight at diagnosis below the 50th percentile of national standards compared to only 11% for females.

Forty-four percent of cases were diagnosed because of the presence of "classical" symptoms while in the remainder diabetes was discovered while the patients were being investigated for other conditions. No systematic community-wide screening had been attempted in the zone. Age group and sex had no significant effect on the method of diagnosis. Other clinical laboratory features present at time of diagnoses are summarized on Table 2.

One or more diabetes complications were present in 57 patients at the time of the survey, an overall prevalence rate of 30% (37% in males and 27% in females). Only 5 individuals had 3 or more complications each. The frequencies of the different types of complications (non-mutually exclusive categories) are given in Table 3.

The role of various risk factors associated with complications was investigated by stratified analysis of a series of 2 X 2 tables, controlling for age and sex (Table 4).

When diagnosed initially, over half of the cases were treated with oral hypoglycemic agents, 9% with insulin, while 37% were nominally managed by diet alone. Among oral agents, chlorpropamide was used most frequently. Tolbutamide was popular during the earlier years but had not been used since 1978.

Overall 17% of the cases had been prescribed insulin at some time during the course of illness. Such cases were more likely to have been glycosuric and ketonuric at the time of diagnosis. Insulin use, however, was not associated with weight status or duration of disease. There had also been considerable change in therapy status among insulin users:
--of 16 initially discharged on insulin at the time of diagnosis, the drug was discontinued subsequently in half of the cases;
--of 25 current users of insulin, about 70% had been switched over from other forms of treatment.
With the exception of the 2 young girls whose diabetes was diagnosed when they were under the age of 15, few of the insulin users can be considered as IDDM cases. Ketoacidosis was recorded in only 4 patients.

DISCUSSION

The prevalence reported in this remote Indian population is low on a world-wide scale (13,14). Among North American Indians, the prevalence of diabetes in Cree-Ojibwa of northwestern Ontario was higher than that of Athapaskan Indians in Alaska (15), but far below that of the Pimas (16) and many U.S. tribes (3). Within Canada there have been few published data on Indians. During the 1930s a physician working in Aklavik, N.W.T., remarked on the near absence of diabetes among the Athapaskans (17). More recently, an unpublished study based on nursing station and health center chronic disease registers estimated the prevalence of diabetes among Indians in Saskatchewan to be 1.4% (3.4% among the 20+ age group and 0.05% among the under 20) (18).

The Canada Health Survey provided estimates of diabetes prevalence among Canadians nationally. The prevalence rate of diabetes was 1.5% in the 15 to 64 age group and 6.7% among the over 65 group with an overall male to female ratio of 1:1.5.

Table 3. Proportion of diabetic cases with one or more complications.

	Type	Male (%)	Female (%)	Total (%)
Macrovascular:	Coronary heart disease	22.4	15.5	17.3
	Cerebrovascular disease	12.2	5.6	7.3
	Peripheral vascular disease	4.1	0	1.1
Microvascular:	Retinopathy	2.0	3.5	3.1
	Nephropathy	6.1	4.2	4.7
Neurological:	Peripheral neuropathy	12.2	4.2	6.3
Metabolic:	Ketoacidosis	4.1	1.4	2.1

The highest prevalence was also reported among the lowest income group (19).

One should be cautious in comparing prevalence rates of different populations based on different methods of estimation: self reports (as in the Canada Health Survey), registers of physician-diagnosed cases, or mass screening. The biochemical criteria used also varied widely, but with the publication and increased acceptance of the NDDG's criteria there should be improved uniformity in reporting.

This study is based on known diagnosed cases in a remote population with a single source of medical care. The method of case selection has a high specificity; the application of NDDG criteria to cases labelled by various health professionals as "diabetic" probably eliminated most "false positive" cases. Without population screening using standardized glucose tolerance tests, however, many cases in the communities which had not come to medical attention may have been missed. It has been suggested that for every known diabetic there are at least 1 or 2 undetected cases (13,14).

In a glucose tolerance study of Dogrib Indians in the Northwest Territories where clinical diabetes was reportedly unknown, 13% and 7% of male and female subjects surveyed satisfied the NDDG criteria for diabetes (20).

It is now recognized that IDDM and NIDDM are at least two or even more distinct clinical syndromes. To classify individual cases in this study accurately would probably require an expert panel of diabetologists and further laboratory tests. Although 17% of cases had received some insulin, their clinical features suggested that most of these were likely to have been NIDDM, and the use of insulin probably reflects individual clinician preference. The rarity of ketoacidosis among diabetics with marked hypoglycemia has been recognized in many American Indian tribes (4).

It is hazardous to infer incidence trends from a prevalence study, as the effects of out-migration and mortality among diabetics have not been determined. However, with over 50% of the cases diagnosed within the last 5 years of a 25 year period,

Table 4. Risk factors associated with presence of diabetic complications after adjustment for age and sex. (Percentages do not add up to 100%, as categories are not mutually exclusive.)

Risk factor	No. of cases	Complications		Mantel-Haenszel χ^2	Adjusted odds ratio (95% confidence level)
		No.	Rate (%)		
Duration of illness					
≥ 5 years	82	24	41	4.5*	2.11 (1.06-4.2)
< 5 years	107	23	22		
Blood pressure					
≥ 140/90	69	29	42	4.1*	2.04 (1.02-4.1)
< 140/90	119	28	24		
Weight status					
≥ 75%tile	121	35	29	1.05	1.51 (0.69-3.3)
< 75%tile	65	20	31		
Fasting plasma glucose					
≥ 300 mg/dl	25	9	36	0.12	1.17 (0.48-2.84)
< 300 mg/dl	152	44	29		
Symptoms					
present	79	19	24	2.95	0.54 (0.26-1.09)
absent	103	38	37		

* $p < 0.05$.

a dramatic increase in incidence has likely occurred in this population. Part of the increase can be attributed to increased accessibility to and availability of medical care, and improved health record storage and retrieval. Accelerated environmental, lifestyle, and dietary changes, which have been invoked to explain the dramatic increase of diabetes in other aboriginal populations in Oceania and the New World (21,3) may have played a role in northwestern Ontario as well.

Obesity is well established as one of the most important risk factors for the development of diabetes (13,14,22). In Canada, the Nutrition Canada Survey from the early 1970s indicated that Indian men had lower mean weight-for-age than Canadians up to age 40 to 49 but showed substantial gain beyond age 50. Among women, Indians were heavier at all age groups (12). A similar pattern of obesity was observed in the distribution of risk groups based on the ponderal index (23).

The WHO multinational study of vascular complications of diabetes showed variable prevalences in different populations (24, 25). Direct comparison with the present study is invalid since it involved only record review without special standardized examination. There was probably more underreporting of microangiopathic and neurologic complications than macrovascular diseases. In this study, duration of illness and hypertension were identified as risk factors for diabetic complications, which have been combined and dichotomized for the purpose of analysis. The sample size was not large enough to detect significant relative risks associated with the other factors. In a multivariate analysis of a cross-sectional survey of Oklahoma Indian diabetics, West et al. found that duration of diabetes and plasma glucose level at the time of examination were significant risk factors for retinopathy and proteinuria (26). It should be noted that a cross-sectional design is least suited for etiologic inferences.

This study provided "benchmark" epidemiological data in a population of Canadian Indians. Further surveys involving Indians in different regions in both urban and rural environments as well as longitudinal observational studies should help elucidate the influence of rapid social changes on the pattern of chronic diseases. Reliable and adequate data are essential for appropriate planning and delivery of health services to Native peoples in anticipation of such an increased need.

REFERENCES

1. Schaefer O. Western diseases: Their emergence and prevention. Cambridge: Harvard University Press, 1981:113-128.

2. Young TK. Changing pattern of health and sickness among the Cree-Ojibwa of northwestern Ontario. Med Anthropol 1969; 3:191-223.

3. West KM. Diabetes in American Indians and other Native populations of the New World. Diabetes 1974; 23:841-855.

4. West KM. Diabetes in American Indians. Advan Metab Disord 1978; 9:29-48.

5. Schaefer O. Glycosuria and diabetes mellitus in Canadian Eskimos. Can Med Assoc J 1968; 99:201-206.

6. Schaefer O. Glucose tolerance testing in Canadian Eskimos: A preliminary report and a hypothesis. Can Med Assoc J 1968; 99:252-262.

7. Young TK. Primary health care for isolated Indians in northwestern Ontario. Public Health Reports 1981; 96:391-397.

8. Young TK. Mortality pattern of isolated Indians in a remote Indian population in northwestern Ontario: A ten year review. Public Health Rep 1983; 98:467-475.

9. National Diabetes Data Group. Classification and diagnosis of diabetes mellitus and other categories of glucose intolerance. Diabetes 1979; 28:1039-1057.

10. Mantel N, Haenszel W. Statistical aspects of the analysis of data from retrospective studies of disease. J Nat Cancer Inst 1959; 22:719-748.

11. Miettinen OS. Estimability and estimation in case referent studies. Am J Epidemiol 1976; 103:226-235.

12. Health and Welfare Canada. Nutrition Canada Anthropometry Report: Height, weight, and body dimensions. Ottawa, 1980.

13. Zimmet P. Type 2 (non-insulin-dependent) diabetes--an epidemiological overview. Diabetologia 1982; 22:399-411.

14. West KM. Epidemiology of diabetes and its vascular complications. New York: Elsevier, 1978.

15. Mouratoff GJ, Carroll NU, Scott EM. Diabetes mellitus in Athabaskan Indians in Alaska. Diabetes 1969; 18:29-32.

16. Bennet PH, Rushforth NB, Miller M, LeCompte PM. Epidemiological studies of diabetes in the Pima Indians. Rec Prog Horm Res 1976; 32:333-376.

17. Urquhart JA. The most northerly practice in Canada. Can Med Assoc J 1935; 33:193-196.

18. Gillis D. A diabetes profile in Saskatchewan region. Regina, Saskatchewan: Medical Services Branch, Health and Welfare Canada, 1980.

19. Health and Welfare Canada and Statistics Canada. The health of Canadians: Report of the Canada health survey. Ottawa, 1981.

20. Szathmary EJE, Holt N. Hyperglycemia in Dogrib Indians of the Northwest Territories, Canada: Association with age and a centripetal distribution of body fat. Hum Biol 1983; 55:493-515.
21. Zimmet P. Epidemiology of diabetes and its macrovascular manifestations in Pacific populations: The medical effects of social progress. Diabetes Care 1979; 2:144-153.
22. World Health Organization Expert Committee on Diabetes Mellitus. Second Report. Tech Rep Ser 646. Geneva: WHO, 1980.
23. Health and Welfare Canada. Nutrition Canada Indian Survey. Ottawa, 1975.
24. Keen H, Jarrett RJ. The WHO multinational study of vascular disease in diabetes: 2. Macrovascular disease prevalence. Diabetes Care 1979; 2:187-195.
25. Jarrett RJ, Keen H. The WHO multinational study of vascular disease in diabetes: 3. Microvascular disease. Diabetes Care 1979; 2:196-201.
26. West KM, Erdreich LJ, Stober JA. A detailed study of risk factors for retinopathy and nephropathy in diabetes. Diabetes 1980; 29:501-508.

T. Kue Young
Northern Medical Unit
Faculty of Medicine
University of Manitoba
750 Bannatyne Ave.
Winnipeg, Manitoba   R3E 0W3
CANADA

Circumpolar Health 84:282-284

THE PREVALENCE OF PERIPHERAL ARTICULAR SYMPTOMS AND SIGNS IN TWO ADJACENT IRON ORE MINES IN LABRADOR

JOHN R. MARTIN and ALISON C. EDWARDS

INTRODUCTION AND METHODS

Musculoskeletal complaints of a non-specific nature are frequent in the working population but progressive systemic sclerosis (PSS) is the only inflammatory arthropathy that has been reported to occur in a higher incidence in miners (1,2). In an epidemiologic survey of the current workforce of two open ore mining operations (Companies X and Y) in Labrador West, questionnaires were administered to each participant in the survey: one is for peripheral articular complaints present or past, and the other is the questionnaire used by Olsen (3) to ascertain the prevalence of Raynaud's phenomenon. Any participant with one or more positive responses to the articular questionnaire, or admitting to having had Raynaud's phenomenon was referred to a physician for examination of the peripheral articular system and for diagnosis.

RESULTS

The distribution of the different articular systems and signs is recorded in Table 1 and was similar at both companies. The most striking point was the high percentage of those admitting to painful joints (33%), more than double those admitting to swollen joints or morning stiffness. The latter two are present in almost the same proportion of 10% and 14% respectively.

With respect to signs, the proportion of the tested population with each of the articular signs was low, the highest being deformed joints (2%).

Positive respondents were separated into those with increasing number of symptoms and the proportion of those with one or more articular signs in each category calculated (Table 2). It is apparent that with each additional symptom, the percentage of the tested population with positive responses decreased by at least one half. Furthermore, with each additional symptom the percentage of those with one or more signs doubled.

The examining physician's diagnoses in those employees with one or more articular signs are tabulated in Table 3. Injuries were responsible for 45% of those with one articular sign (post-traumatic arthritis, traumatic amputation, and meniscal tears), 28% of those with 2 signs (post-traumatic arthritis and meniscal tears) and 33% of those with 3 symptoms (post-traumatic arthritis). The percentage of rheumatoid arthritis (RA) increased with each additional sign to a total of 11 cases, of which four had "definite" RA (4), a prevalence of 0.16%. There were two miners with PSS, both in the one articular sign category, a prevalence of 0.08%.

The number of employees with Raynaud's phenomenon and the proportion with articular signs are listed in Table 4. There were 328 employees (13% of respondents) with this

Table 1. Number and percentage of employees with articular symptoms and signs at companies X and Y.

	Company X	Company Y	Companies X and Y combined
Total tested population	1,946 (100)	499 (100)	2,445 (100)
Symptoms:			
At least 1 symptom	739 (38)	209 (42)	948 (39)
Painful joints	633 (33)	183 (37)	816 (33)
Swollen joints	189 (10)	50 (10)	239 (10)
Morning stiffness	265 (14)	78 (16)	343 (14)
Signs:			
At least 1 sign	72 (4)	27 (5)	99 (4)
Deformed joints	38 (2)	9 (2)	47 (2)
Swollen joints	15 (1)	5 (1)	20 (1)
Tender joints	18 (1)	12 (2)	30 (1)
Limited movement	22 (1)	11 (2)	33 (1)

Table 2. *Number and percentage of employees at companies X and Y with zero to three symptoms and the percentage with one or more articular signs. Total tested population = 2,445.*

	Number of symptoms			
	0	1	2	3
Number (a)	1,497	589	268	91
Percentage of tested population	61	24	11	4
Number in (a) with one or more signs	35	26	21	17
Percentage of (a)	2	4	8	19

symptom, of whom 24 had one or more articular signs. Included in this number were five with post-traumatic arthritis, four with RA, two with PSS, and two with an undefined diffuse connective tissue disease.

CONCLUSIONS

One-third of the current workforce at 2 mining operations admitted to having painful joints at one time or another; however, swollen joints and morning stiffness were admitted to by a much smaller percentage. Articular signs were present in only a small proportion of those with symptoms. There were 11 cases diagnosed as RA (four defi-

nite), a prevalence of 0.16, within the range of 0.12 to 3.0% for definite RA noted by others (5). Included in the arthritis NYD was one case of psoriatic arthritis and two of diffuse connective tissue disease. There were 2 cases of PSS, less than the prevalence of 0.21% found by Erasmus (1). The prevalence of Raynaud's phenomenon in 13% of the workforce was less than the 22% noted by Olsen and his colleagues in a population of Scandinavian physiotherapists (3).

In conclusion, the prevalence of peripheral articular symptoms and signs as well as Raynaud's phenomenon in the current workforce showed no unusual trends, apart

Table 3. *Number and percentage of musculo-skeletal diagnoses on employees with one, two, three, and four signs.*

Diagnosis	Number of signs			
	1 N = 73 (100)	2 N = 22 (100)	3 N = 3 (100)	4 N = 1 (100)
Post-traumatic arthritis	25 (34)	5 (23)	1 (33)	
Traumatic amputation	5 (7)			
Ankylosing spondylitis	1 (1)			
Arthritis NYD	2 (3)	3 (14)	1 (33)	
Rheumatoid arthritis (RA)	6 (8)	3 (14)	1 (33)	1 (100)
Psoriatic arthritis		1 (5)		
Osteoarthritis (generalized)	4 (5)	1 (5)		
Osteoarthritis (localized)	3 (4)	1 (5)		
Polyarthralgia NYD	1 (1)			
Bursitis/tendonitis/tenosynovitis	4 (5)	3 (14)		
Meniscal tear	3 (4)	1 (5)		
Scleroderma (PSS)	2 (3)			
Osteochorditis	1 (1)			
Gout		1 (5)		
Connective tissue disease (NYD)		2 (9)		
Congenital anomaly	10 (14)			
Developmental anomaly	2 (3)			
Miscellaneous/unclassified	4 (5)	1 (5)		

Table 4.   Number and percentage of Raynaud's phenomenon and the percentage with one or more articular signs.

	Company X	Company Y	Companies X and Y combined
Total tested population	1,946	499	
Number (a)	242	86	328
Percentage of tested population	12	17	13
Number in (a) with one or more signs	12	12	24
Percentage of (a)	5	14	7

from a possible increase in the number of cases of PSS.

REFERENCES

1.   Erasmus LD.   Scleroderma in gold-miners on the Witwatersrand with particular reference to pulmonary manifestations. S Afr J Lab Clin Med 1957; 3:209-230.
2.   Rodnan GP, Benedek TG, Medsger TA Jr, Cammarata RJ.   The association of progressive systemic sclerosis (sclero-derma) with coal miners' pneumoconiosis and other forms of silicosis.   Ann Intern Med 1967; 66:323-334.
3.   Olsen N, Neilsen SL.   Prevalence of primary Raynaud Phenomenon in young females.   Scan J Clin Lab Invest 1978; 38:761-764.
4.   Ropes MW, Bennet GA, Cobb S, Jacox RA. Revision of diagnostic criteria for rheumatoid arthritis.   Bull Rheum Dis 1958; 9:175-176.
5.   Masi AT, Medsger TA Jr.   In: McCarthy DJ.   Arthritis and allied conditions, textbook of rheumatology, 9th edition. Philadelphia, Lea and Febiger 1979: 11-35.

John R. Martin
Faculty of Medicine
Memorial University of Newfoundland
Room 3307A
Health Sciences Centre
St. John's, Newfoundland   A1B 3V6
Canada

Circumpolar Health 84:285-287

THE SEASONAL OCCURRENCE OF PEPTIC ULCER DISEASE AMONG THE INUIT OF NORTHERN LABRADOR

G. WILLIAM N. FITZGERALD and JOEL R.L. EHRENKRANZ

Hippocrates wrote,

Whoever wishes to pursue properly the science of medicine must proceed thus: First, he ought to consider what effects each season of the year can produce; for the seasons are not alike, but differ widely both in themselves and at their changes. For with the season men's diseases, like their digestive organs, suffer change.

In temperate climates peptic ulcer disease is reported to occur more frequently in the spring and fall (1). The present study was undertaken to determine if this phenomenon is evident or indeed exaggerated among the Inuit of northern Labrador, an area subject to extreme seasonal variation in ambient lighting conditions.

METHODS

A review was undertaken of admissions to the Charles S. Curtis Memorial Hospital, St. Anthony, Newfoundland, from April 1974 to March 1984. During this 10-year period 15 Inuit patients from Nain, Labrador (population 938, 1981 census; lat. 57°N) occasioned 23 admissions to the hospital for the management of peptic ulcer disease. The diagnosis of gastric or duodenal ulcer was confirmed by gastroscopy in all cases; however, these figures exclude admissions solely for repeat gastroscopy done to ensure healing in cases of gastric ulcer.

RESULTS

This group of 15 patients includes 10 males and 5 females ranging in age from 24 to 65 years. Ten patients required only one admission, three patients required two admissions, one required three admissions, and one other required four admissions.

Twenty-one admissions, a surprisingly large number, were occasioned by gastric ulcer disease occurring in 13 patients. Only two patients suffered from duodenal ulcer disease and each of these was admitted only once. Eleven patients required a total of seventeen admissions for the non-operative management of their disease. Two of these subsequently returned and required surgery. A total of six patients, all suffering from gastric ulcer disease, came to surgery for either intractable pain or bleeding.

In order to detect any seasonal variation in the incidence of peptic ulcer disease, admissions were grouped by the month of the year in which they occurred. No admission occurred in either February or July. One admission occurred in each of the months of January, June, November, and December. Two patients were admitted during March, May, and August; three in October; and five in April and September. These results are depicted graphically in Figure 1, which demonstrates a remarkable and significant clustering of admissions in the spring and fall of the year (chi squared value 7.45, p < 0.01).

DISCUSSION

The preponderance of gastric ulcer disease is striking. It may be that difficulties in the interpretation of symptomatology, the natural reluctance of the Inuit to complain, and the unavailability of diagnostic facilities conspire to select only the severest disease for referral. Referral in the spring and fall, however, is mitigated again by break-up and freeze-up.

The seasonal rhythm of biological phenomena has long been observed among northern peoples. In 1891, the surgeon F.A. Cook, accompanying Peary on his first North Greenland Expedition, wrote:

These people [Greenland Inuit] live in a region of constant night for four months, followed by a period of part day and part night, then four months of constant day. This endless night has a peculiar effect on the secretions and upon the passions. During the whole of this long Arctic night the secretions are diminished and the passions suppressed, resulting in great muscular debility. Our own party suffered in the same way. This peculiar condition is due to the prolonged absence of the sun, and I should judge from this that the presence of the sun is essential to animal as it is to vegetable life. The passions of these people are periodical, and their courtship is usually carried on soon after the return of the sun. In fact, at this time they almost tremble from the intensities of their passions and for several weeks most of their time is taken up in gratifying them. Naturally enough, then, the children are usually born at the beginning of the Arctic night, or about nine months from this time. (2)

The Moravian church has been ministering to the Inuit of Northern Labrador since

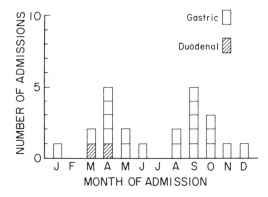

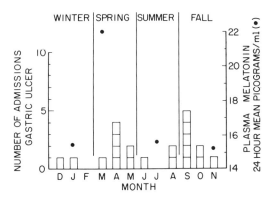

Figure 1.   *Admissions of Inuit patients from Nain, Labrador to the Charles S. Curtis Memorial Hospital, St. Anthony for peptic ulcer disease from April 1974 to March 1984, by month of admission.*

Figure 2.   *The number of admissions for gastric ulcer disease by month compared with the 24-hour mean concentration of plasma melatonin in each season.*

the 1760s. A review of Moravian records documenting more than 3,700 Inuit births in the communities of Hebron and Okak over more than 160 years from 1778 to 1940 has revealed a remarkable and consistent seasonal variation in birth rate (3). This annual cycle demonstrates a peak in March, a 50% fall during June, July, and August, a slight rise in the autumn, and a 30% decrease in December and January. Further work is underway to elucidate the physiological factors which may contribute to this phenomenon. The light-dark cycle is known to regulate the onset of reproduction in a number of plant and animal species. In hamsters, birds, and some species of sheep this phenomenon appears to be mediated through the pineal gland (4). Cook, in his observations of 1891, alluded to the possible role of light in determining the breeding pattern of the Inuit. The secretion of the pineal hormone, melatonin, is influenced by ambient lighting conditions. Melatonin is known to alter gonadal function and may therefore influence reproductive patterns.

A study of plasma melatonin levels among adult male Inuit residents of Nain for 24-hour periods in each of the 4 seasons of the year has demonstrated seasonal variation of both the circadian profile and the 24-hour mean levels of plasma melatonin (5). Mean 24-hour levels of plasma melatonin were greater in March (21.96 picograms/ml) than at any other time of the year. The corresponding values in the other months studied are as follows: January 15.57, July 15.73, and November 15.40 picograms/ml. The greatest fluctuation in circadian profile

was seen in the winter and the least in the summer.

Iguchi and colleagues from Japan recently published data documenting grossly elevated serum melatonin levels during the hours of darkness in patients suffering from gastric ulcer disease (6). These levels were comparable to those seen in other patients with cirrhosis of the liver, in whom the clearance of melatonin was prolonged. When our values for the seasonal 24-hour mean concentration of plasma melatonin in the Labrador Inuit are compared with the seasonal incidence of gastric ulcer disease in the same population, a striking similarity is observed, with a springtime peak occurring in each (Figure 2).

CONCLUSIONS

In summary, we have documented a seasonal variation in the incidence of peptic ulcer disease among the Labrador Inuit. Further, study of the biological rhythm of the same population has disclosed wide seasonal fluctuations in both the circadian rhythm and the 24-hour mean plasma melatonin concentration of the pineal hormone, melatonin. Others have demonstrated a grossly exaggerated circadian profile for serum melatonin in patients suffering from gastric ulcer disease. We postulate that the seasonal occurrence of gastric ulcer disease may be due, in part, to the seasonal variation in plasma melatonin levels. This preliminary study forms the basis for continuing clinical investigation of the neuroendocrine mechanisms influencing gastric physiology.

ACKNOWLEDGMENTS

We are indebted to Evelyn Walker and Zilda Hillier and their respective staff, Charles S. Curtis Memorial Hospital, for assistance with records research, to Alison Edwards and Dr. David Bryant, Memorial University of Newfoundland, for the statistical analysis, to Thomas Budgell and Anthony Cronhelm for technical assistance, and to Hazel Noel for the preparation of the manuscript.

REFERENCES

1. Welsh JD, Wolf S. Geographic and environmental aspect of peptic ulcer. Am J Med 1960; 31:754-760.
2. Cook FA. Medical observations among the Esquimaux. Trans NY Obstet Soc 1893-1894; 3:282.
3. Ehrenkranz JRL. Seasonal breeding in humans: birth records of the Labrador Eskimo. Fertility and Sterility 1983; 40:485-489.
4. Lincoln GA, Short RV. Seasonal breeding: Nature's contraceptive. Recent Prog Horm Res 1980; 36:1.
5. Ehrenkranz JRL. Seasonal alteration of the 24 hour plasma melatonin profile in man. In press.
6. Iguchi H, Kato K, Ibayashi H. Melatonin serum levels and metabolic clearance rate in patients with liver cirrhosis. J Clin Endocrinol Metab 1982; 54:1025-1027.

G. William N. Fitzgerald
Charles S. Curtis Memorial Hospital
St. Anthony, Newfoundland AOK 4SO
Canada

Circumpolar Health 84:288-290

LOW INCIDENCE OF URINARY CALCULI IN GREENLAND ESKIMOS AS EXPLAINED BY A LOW CALCIUM/MAGNESIUM RATIO

BJARNE BO JEPPESEN and BENT HARVALD

In Greenland Eskimos the average serum calcium has been reported to be lower than that in Danes, whereas the average serum magnesium is higher (1,2). The low serum calcium is probably due to a relatively low calcium intake in the Arctic, where dairy products make up a minor dietary contribution. Thus, a surprisingly low 24-hour urinary calcium output has been found in Canadian Eskimos (3). Similarly, the high serum magnesium may be due to a high magnesium content in a diet rich in fish and meat of sea mammals. Furthermore, the absorption of magnesium may be enhanced by the low calcium content of the diet, as the absorption of calcium and magnesium are competitive.

A low serum calcium and high serum magnesium will bring about a low urinary calcium/magnesium ratio. Theoretically this low ratio involves a lowered risk of urinary stone formation. It should therefore be of interest to examine the occurrence of urinary calculi in Eskimos.

MATERIAL AND METHODS

Serum calcium and serum magnesium were determined in Greenlanders and Danes living in Greenland, and for comparison, in selected groups of Greenlanders and Danes living in Denmark. The Greenlanders living in Denmark were all adolescents in boarding schools, whereas the Danish "controls" were chosen among the outpatients of the ear, nose, and throat department of a Danish county hospital. The calcium and magnesium analyses were by titration fluorometry and atom absorption photometry respectively. The serum values of both calcium and magnesium were corrected to a serum albumin concentration of 45 grams per liter according to the equations:

$$\text{ser-Ca}_{corr} = \text{ser-Ca}_{obs} + 0.0163(45 - \text{ser-alb}_{obs})$$

$$\text{ser-Mg}_{corr} = \text{ser-Mg}_{obs} + 0.007(45 - \text{ser-alb}_{obs})$$

Serum calcium and magnesium are indicated as millimoles per liter, serum albumin as grams per liter.

The incidence of urinary calculi has been estimated from the serum of patients discharged from the hospital under the WHO diagnostic code numbers 592 (nephrolithiasis and ureterolithiasis) and 594 (stones in other parts of the urinary tract). The reports from the chief medical officer in Greenland (4) and from the Danish Public Health Service (5,6) have been searched for the annual number of cases per 1,000 inhabitants over age 15 during the years from 1973 to 1975.

Comparisons have been evaluated by Student's t-test.

RESULTS

Tables 1 and 2 summarize the findings of the calcium and magnesium analyses. Greenlanders living in Greenland demonstrate the lowest serum calcium and the highest serum magnesium of all groups examined. Greenlanders living in Denmark, on the other hand, have the highest serum calcium of all groups, and with regard to serum magnesium they show intermediate values. Danes living in Denmark show the lowest serum magnesium and serum calcium in the upper range, whereas Danes living in Greenland have intermediate values both for calcium and magnesium.

Table 3 gives the absolute and relative number of patients discharged from Greenlandic and Danish hospitals with a main diagnosis of urinary calculi. The inci-

Table 1. Serum calcium in Greenlanders and Danes.

	Number	Mean age	Ser-Ca mmol/l	
Greenlanders				
in Greenland	56	29	2.22 ± 0.01	p < 0.001
in Denmark	25	19	2.37 ± 0.01	p < 0.001
Danes				
in Greenland	16	32	2.29 ± 0.02	NS
in Denmark	32	37	2.32 ± 0.01	NS

Table 2. Serum magnesium in Greenlanders and Danes.

	Number	Mean age	Ser-Mg mmol/l
Greenlanders			
in Greenland	46	29	1.02 ± 0.02 p < 0.001
in Denmark	25	19	0.87 ± 0.01 p < 0.001
Danes			
in Greenland	16	32	0.95 ± 0.02 p < 0.001
in Denmark	32	37	0.84 ± 0.01 p < 0.001

dences in Denmark are nearly double those in Greenland, and the differences for both males and females are highly significant.

DISCUSSION

The low serum calcium and high serum magnesium in Greenlanders living in Greenland compared with the parameters for Greenlanders living in Denmark indicate that serum calcium and serum magnesium are influenced by environmental factors, probably mainly dietary. The low serum calcium may be caused by a low access to calcium-rich dietary items, which may also be the reason for the early onset and rapid rate of age-related bone loss amply documented in adult Eskimos (7,8). Correspondingly, the high serum magnesium in Greenlanders may be due to a magnesium-rich diet. Thus fish and meat of sea mammals have a high content of magnesium. Ordinarily only abut 30% of the dietary intake is absorbed. This percentage to a large extent depends on the calcium content of the food because of the absorptive competition between the calcium and magnesium ions (9). In this context it should, however, be stressed that magnesium

is primarily an intracellular ion, and serum magnesium is not a good guide to body magnesium status. Thus a high serum magnesium may simply be a reflection of altered relations between extra- and intracellular magnesium.

The great majority of cases of urinary calculi are not hospitalized, although the number of hospitalizations may with some reservation serve as a marker in comparisons between different populations as in the present study. It could be argued that the differences observed between incidences in Greenland and Denmark reflect different hospital admission thresholds. However, the number of hospital admissions per population unit under all diagnoses in Greenland is double that in Denmark. This implies that the difference with regard to incidence of urinary calculi may in reality be greater than indicated by the number of hospitalizations.

The incidence of urinary calculi increases with age. Different age composition of the populations compared could therefore invalidate the comparison. However, by disregarding age groups under 15 an acceptable comparability is achieved. Thus

Table 3. Patients over age 15, discharged from hospitals in Greenland and Denmark with a diagnosis of urinary calculi, 1973 to 1975.

	Population > 15 yrs	Number of patients	Annual incidence per 1,000 persons
Males			
in Greenland	17.2×10^3	59	1.1 p < 0.001
in Denmark	1.9×10^6	11,632	2.0 p < 0.001
Females			
in Greenland	13.6×10^3	22	0.5 p < 0.001
in Denmark	2.0×10^6	5,790	1.0 p < 0.001

among males over 15, the average age in Greenlanders is 44 years, in Danes 47 years. Thirty-five and 37% respectively are between 35 and 60 years old.

Because of the low serum calcium and high serum magnesium, the calcium/magnesium ratio of the urine in Greenlanders is low, and may explain the low incidence of stone disorders. The magnesium ion per se is counted among the main inhibitors of formation of calcium oxalate and phosphate crystals (10), and dietary administration of excess magnesium has with some success been used in the prevention of stone formation (11).

Other factors may of course be active as well. A predominantly animal diet, such as the Greenlandic, with a low content of dairy products and vegetables, will lower the pH of the urine. This tends to prevent the precipitation of calcium salts, but at the same time reduces the solubility of uric acid cystine. Finally, the production of urinary calculi is influenced by genetic factors such as the excretion of oxalate and cystine, and the ability to acidify the urine.

REFERENCES

1. Jeppesen BB, Harvald B. Serum calcium in Greenland Eskimos. Acta Med Scand 1983; 412:99-101.
2. Jeppesen BB, Blach A, Bouchelouche PN, Harvald B. Serum magnesium in Greenland Eskimos. Acta Med Scand (in press).
3. Modlin M. The aetiology of renal stone: a new concept arising from studies on a stone-free population. Ann R Coll Surg Engl 1967; 40:155-178.
4. Annual Report from the Chief Medical Officer in Greenland for the years 1973, 1974, 1975, and 1976. Godthåb 1978.
5. Medicinalstatistiske Meddelelser I: Befolkningens forbrug af sygehusydelser 1966-78. Danish National Health Service, Copenhagen, 1981.
6. Statistical tables XIII: Population census 1973. Danish National Statistics 1978.
7. Mazess RB. Bone mineral content of north Alaskan Eskimos. Am J Clin Nutr 1974; 27:916-925.
8. Mazess RB, Mather W. Bone mineral content in Canadian Eskimos. Hum Biol 1975; 47:45-63.
9. Alcock N, MacIntyre I. Interrelation of calcium and magnesium absorption. Clin Sci 1962; 22:185-190.
10. Hammarsten G. On calcium oxalate and its solubility in the presence of inorganic salts with special reference to the occurrence of oxaluria. Carlsberg Research Laboratory, Copenhagen 1927; 17:1-16.
11. Johansson G. Magnesium and renal stone disease. Acta Med Scand 1981; suppl 661:13-18.

Bjarne Bo Jeppesen
Tjørnelundevej 17
DK-4270 Høng
Denmark

Circumpolar Health 84:291-293

HEREDITARY POLYMORPHIC LIGHT ERUPTION IN CANADIAN INUIT

PAMELA H. ORR and A.R. BIRT

The presence of an hereditary form of polymorphous light eruption (HPLE) has been reported among North American Indians by Schenck, Everett et al., and by Birt (1-3). The same condition has been reported by Londono et al. among the Indians of Colombia, South America (4). This paper reports the occurrence of HPLE in 12 Inuit patients from Rankin Inlet in the Canadian Northwest Territories.

Rankin Inlet is a small Inuit community situated on the west coast of Hudson Bay, 475 kilometers north of Churchill, Manitoba (Figure 1). Established in the 1950s, the hamlet was settled by Eskimo people from both coastal and inland areas of the Keewatin District of the N.W.T. Medical care to the area is provided by the Northern Medical Unit of the University of Manitoba, and by the Medical Services Branch of Health and Welfare Canada.

HPLE is a condition affecting the sunlight-exposed areas such as cheeks, nose, lips, dorsal surfaces of the hand, and the lower neck. Those areas not exposed to the sun, such as under the hair, around the eyes, and the anterior surface of the neck just below the chin, are unaffected. The lesions represent an acute eczematous response with erythema, edema, and small papules with exudation and crusting. An acute exudative cheilitis, especially involving the lower lip, may be present alone or in conjunction with other lesions of the face and neck. Vesicles and bullae are not observed, and scarring rarely occurs unless secondary infection develops. In adults the lesions frequently consist of erythematous plaques.

The condition usually appears in childhood, and is seasonally recurrent, with lesions appearing in February and remaining until early fall. Those affected frequently give a positive family history of photodermatitis.

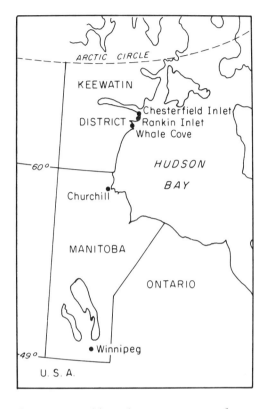

Figure 1. Rankin Inlet, N.W.T., Canada.

MATERIALS AND METHODS

Twelve Inuit patients with the lesions of HPLE were seen by the author (P.H.O.) in Rankin Inlet between July 1981 and February 1983. Two of the patients had previously been diagnosed as having HPLE by a dermatologist (A.R.B.) in Winnipeg, Manitoba. The patients were not on any medication at the time of diagnosis, and had no history of atopic dermatitis. All patients gave an extensive history of "sensitivity" to sunlight.

Data were collected regarding family history, seasonal variation, type and distribution of lesions, and response to treatment. Blood, stool, and urine porphyrins were collected on all patients to exclude abnormalities of porphyrin metabolism. Blood was also analyzed for the presence of the Diego antigen (Di a) in order to test for possible Indian ancestry among our Inuit patients. Skin biopsies were not possible due to isolation of the settlement and problems with air transportation of specimens.

RESULTS AND DISCUSSION

Clinical Manifestations

Of the 12 patients studied, 2 were male and 10 were female, ranging in age from 15 to 56 years old. The average age was 35. Both the average and median age of onset of the condition was 12 years. Seventy-five percent of the subjects indicated that their sunlight sensitivity first occurred prior to the age of 15. This corresponds to previous reports of early age of onset among North American Indians (5,6).

All 12 patients had lesions affecting the sun-exposed areas of the face. Five patients showed involvement of the dorsum of the hands, and two were affected on the sun-exposed areas of the forearms during the summer months. The legs are not exposed and hence were unaffected. An exudative cheilitis, in addition to lesions of the cheeks and nose, was present in only one patient. The latter was the youngest subject (age 15) and the one demonstrating the most severe photosensitivity with secondary infection and scarring.

The observed reaction consisted of erythema in all patients, with papules in 11 subjects. Plaques were noted in 7 patients, all more than 35 years old. Crusting occurred in 2 patients. Vesicles, bullae, and scales were absent, and scarring occurred in only one patient with secondary infection and impetiginization. In general it was noted by both the patients and investigators that the severity of photosensitivity decreased with age.

Eight patients complained of pruritis associated with the condition. A further 2 patients experienced sensations of both pruritis and burning. Two subjects were asymptomatic. They all noted a seasonal recurrence, with lesions first appearing in February and lasting until September.

Laboratory Investigations

In order to exclude photosensitivity secondary to abnormal porphyrin metabolism, blood and urine samples were analyzed from all 12 patients for total blood porphyrin, urine total porphyrin, δ-aminolevulinic acid (ALA), porphobilinogen (PBG). Stool specimens were collected from 10 of the patients and analyzed for total stool porphyrins.

Stool porphyrin levels were all within the normal range. All random urine ALA's and PBG's were normal with respect to creatinine excretion. Urine total porphyrins were normal on all patients except one. Spectral scan on this sample indicated elevated coproporphyrin secondary to documented cirrhosis of the liver.

Seven of the blood porphyrin samples were normal. Five further specimens showed slightly elevated levels ranging from 0.97 to 2.37 μmol/L. Plasma porphyrins were not detected in these specimens. We were unable to relate these abnormalities to either iron deficiency or lead exposure. However, in view of the normal urinary and stool porphyrins in these 5 patients, it is unlikely that these elevated levels represent porphyria. The normal values for blood porphyrins in the Inuit population are not known, and further study in this area is indicated.

Heredity and Distribution

Nine of the 12 patients (75%) indicated a positive family history of photodermatitis, confirmed by clinical examination of the named relatives. This corresponds with previous studies of the inheritance of HPLE among North American Indian and Scandinavian populations (3,7) and suggests an autosomal dominant trait with incomplete penetrance.

The presence of HPLE among North American Indian tribes, including the Cree and Chippewyans, and the absence of previous reports of this condition among the Inuit suggested the possibility of some degree of Indian ancestry in the patients we were studying. Traditionally, the Inuit of the Keewatin and the Cree and Chippewyans of northern Manitoba were hostile peoples who respected their mutual border--the treeline. However, hunting and trading expeditions between the two areas did occur with increasing frequency in the nineteenth and early twentieth centuries.

Pursuing this question of ancestry, blood samples from all patients were analyzed for the presence or absence of the antigen Di a--part of the Diego blood group system. The antigen was first noted in Venezuelan and Brazilian Indians (8,9) and later shown to be present in North American Indian tribes including the Cherokee, Cree, Blood, and Chippewyans (10). The antigen is absent from the Caucasoid and Negroid races, and further studies among the Eskimos of the Eastern and Central Arctic established the absence of Diego factor in the Inuit (10, 11).

Our results also demonstrated the absence of Diego antigen (Di a) in all 12 subjects with HPLE. We thus have no indication of Indian ancestry in these patients. It remains to be seen whether further reports of HPLE in other Inuit populations will appear.

Treatment

The initial treatment of HPLE in North American Indians involved the use of sunscreen lotions, corticosteroid creams, and antimalarials. In 1958, Becker reported the use of psoralen compounds in promoting epidermal changes that provide protection from ultraviolet rays (12). Since then, a successful combination of topical therapy and oral Trisoralen has been used effectively to control HPLE.

Four-5'-8-trimethylpsoralen (Trisoralen) is a furocoumarin that sensitizes the skin to ultraviolet light in the range of 360 nm. Oral ingestion of Trisoralen followed by exposure to ultraviolet light causes a thickening of the stratum corneum and the formation of an eosinophilic homogeneous layer at the base of the stratum corneum similar to the stratum lucidum of the palms and soles. In addition the drug causes increased retention of melanin in the epidermis. The combination of a thickened stratum corneum and increased melanin content in the epidermis is believed to be responsible for increased protection against ultraviolet light.

Trisoralen is given before breakfast in a dosage of 5 mg daily for those 10 years or younger, and 10 mg daily if older. Treatment is usually begun in February when the first signs of photosensitivity appear, and continued until September. Treatment has not been necessary in the winter months. Studies suggest that the spectrum responsible for the lesions of HPLE is in the long ultraviolet range (13,14).

Topical treatment consists of the use of sunscreen lotions and mild steroid creams. Atrophy or telangiectasia in the areas treated did not occur. Secondary infection, which occurred in only one patient, was treated with oral and topical antibiotics.

Six of the 12 patients were treated with oral Trisoralen plus topical therapy. All showed clinical improvement of their dermatitis on this regime. The other 6 patients had mild lesions requiring topical therapy alone. Adverse effects from the use of Trisoralen, such as nausea, vomiting, or vertigo, were not encountered.

CONCLUSION

In conclusion, the presence of hereditary polymorphous light eruption is noted for the first time in Canadian Inuit. We await further reports of this condition in other Inuit populations of Canada, Alaska, Greenland, and the U.S.S.R.

REFERENCES

1. Schenk RR. Controlled trial of methoxsalen in solar dermatitis of Chippewa Indians. JAMA 1960; 172:1134.
2. Everett MA, Crockett W, Lamb JH, Minor D. Light-sensitive eruptions in American Indians. Arch Dermatol 1961; 83: 243.
3. Birt AR, Davis RA. Hereditary polymorphic light eruption of American Indians. Int J Dermatol 1975; 14:105.
4. Londono F, Muvdi F, Giraldo F, Rueda LA, Caputo A. Familial actinic prurigo. Derm Ibero Lat-Am 1968; 111:61.
5. Birt AR. Photodermatitis in Indians of Manitoba. Canad Med Assoc J 1968; 98: 392.
6. Birt AR, Hogg GR. The actinic cheilitis of hereditary polymorphic light eruption. Arch Dermatol 1979; 115:699.
7. Jansen CT. Heredity of chronic polymorphous light eruptions. Arch Dermatol 1978; 114:188.
8. Layrisse M, Arends T, Wilbert J. Peculiar distribution of the Diego factor among the Warrau. Nature 1958; 181: 118.
9. Juqueira PC, Wishart PJ, Ottensooser F, Pasqualin R, Loureiro Fernadez P, Kalmus H. The Diego factor in Brazilian Indians. Nature 1956; 177:41.
10. Chown B, Lewis M. Blood groups in anthropology: with special reference to Canadian Indians and Eskimos. National Museum of Canada Bulletin No. 167, Contributions to Anthropology, 1958.
11. Chown B, Lewis M, Kaita H. The Diego blood group system. Nature 1958; 181: 268.
12. Becker SW. Methods of increasing skin pigmentation. J Soc Cosmet Chem 1958; 9:80.
13. Epstein JH. Polymorphous light eruptions. Phototest Techniques Studies. Arch Dermatol 1962; 85:502.
14. Frain-Bell W, Dickson A, Herd J, Sturrock I. The action spectrum in polymorphic light eruption. Br J Dermatol 1973; 89:243.

Pamela H. Orr
Northern Medical Unit
University of Manitoba
61 Emily Street
Winnipeg, Manitoba R3E 1Y9
Canada

Circumpolar Health 84:294-297

THE ORAL HEALTH OF THE NATIVES OF CANADA: A SURVEY

JOHN T. MAYHALL and JOHN W. STAMM

INTRODUCTION

Although from time to time local and regional assessments of the oral health status of the Native people of Canada have been undertaken, there has been no systematic data gathering on the Indian and Inuit people since the Nutrition Canada survey of 1970-72 (1). This study had severe limitations as an epidemiological survey. First, because of a low participation rate (particularly among Indians), insufficient samples sizes were obtained for both Native groups (1,584 Indians and 346 Inuit). Second, the examination procedures employed were not subject to inter-examiner calibration, leading to severely biased estimates of health status. Third, the fieldwork was insufficiently organized to ensure the collection of consistent data. Finally, problems crept into the data analysis which led to further bias in the reported results.

We have proposed a nationwide survey and have completed a feasibility study (2) as the first step in alleviating this paucity of data on the oral health of the Natives of Canada. The objective of this Native Dental Health Survey is to provide baseline data on the distribution of certain oral conditions and dental health behaviors among the Indian and Inuit populations for whom the Canadian government provides dental services or reimburses for the cost of care.

Specifically, the survey should provide basic, valid, and statistically precise estimates of age- and sex-specific oral health status for each of the 9 Medical Services Branch regions. The oral conditions and dental health behaviors to be assessed are:

Oral conditions

--Dental caries (including classification of carious lesions and the surfaces affected)
--Missing, to be extracted, and filled teeth
--Gingival health
--Periodontal health
--Malocclusion
--Other visible oral pathology
--Dental treatment required

Dental health behaviors

--Oral hygiene practices
--Dental treatment patterns
--Consumption of fluoride supplements or fluoridated water

While this list is not exhaustive, we believe it provides the information needed to allow the Government of Canada to tailor a dental care and prevention program to the specific needs of the Native people of Canada.

We have suggested that in each of the 9 regions of Canada approximately 1,100 Natives be examined. This sample of 8,500 (the Yukon and Atlantic Provinces have small client populations, thus "full" samples will be reduced) will encompass children of ages 5, 11, and 15 and adults in their thirties and over 50 years of age. Since we are mainly interested in circumpolar peoples here, it may be of value to note that there are about 16,000 Inuit and 9,500 Indians in the Northwest Territories and the Yukon (2). Of these, about 1,600 will be included in the study.

While we had hoped to have the first results of the study for presentation, this has not been possible. But, we can use other data, at least, to advance some hypotheses about the anticipated poor level of oral health in Canadian Indians and Inuit.

Previous papers have demonstrated what appears to be a close relationship between dietary change and oral health (3-12). However, dietary change does not seem to provide the complete reasons for the deteriorating dental health of most modern Inuit and Indians (13). To investigate other possible causative factors, such as community isolation, community size, the availability of dental care, and culture differences, we have utilized the results from 5 studies of Canadian arctic and subarctic groups (14-18).

Community Isolation

It has practically become dogma that the more isolated the group in question the lower the dental caries prevalence. Those who have cautioned that isolation is not the complete answer to oral health status have apparently been overlooked. Realizing that "isolation" is not entirely quantifiable, we have attempted to use measures of isolation similar to those in the proposed study, such as the distance from a major supply resource center and the frequency of contact with the "outside" world, to reexamine the results of other Native oral health studies.

A review of 4 studies of the dental caries rates in Indians and Inuit revealed some rather startling results in light of the dogma stated above. Thompson and Gavriloff (18), studying Alberta Indians, demonstrated that the group with the lowest caries rate was the one living in the immediate vicinity of Edmonton, Alberta, while the highest rate was in the group which resided in the most isolated northern district. Among young people, the farther from a large center, the greater the number of caries in teeth.

Myers and Lee (16) demonstrated that the most isolated west coast Indian community had the lowest caries rate of the 4 communities surveyed, while the next most isolated had the highest rate. They concluded that the "degree of isolation from urban centres . . . may not be as much a question of distance as it is of cultural practices or level of income."

Two further studies may help clarify the findings. First, Curzon and Curzon (14) stated that they found that Inuit caries prevalence diminished inversely to the degree of relative isolation. However, this is not apparent from their data for 4 through 8 year olds' deciduous teeth. The community with the fewest airline flights per week had the highest deft scores (decayed, extracted, and filled deciduous teeth) (11.38), while the 2 communities with the most frequent service showed a rate of approximately 10 teeth per affected individual. The other communities had only one flight per week, and their deft rates ranged from 7.18 to 11 teeth involved. Clearly, from their figures, the amount of contact with major centers does not appear to be a factor affecting the caries rates in the susceptible younger age groups.

The same general trends prevail when the distance from a primary trading center is correlated with the deft score. The most distant community had the highest caries rate--a pattern seen already in Alberta. The Pearson's correlation coefficient for the comparison of distance with deft was positive and statistically significant at the 95% level of confidence.

The final study of distance and caries rate is the Sioux Lookout Indian survey (17). Here no trends could be found between distance and caries rate in children.

None of these studies indicates that the greater the distance from the primary centers the lower the caries rates of young people. It is worth emphasizing that we have used the figures for children, adolescents, or young adults because we feel that young people tend to be influenced by cultural changes more quickly than adults and, thus, any effects these might have on oral health are rapidly apparent.

Community Size

Another factor that may have an influence on oral diseases from an epidemiological standpoint is the size of the community.

Presumably, the larger the community, the less the isolation, the greater the availability of cariogenic processed foods, and the chance of contact with different cultures.

In contrast to this line of reasoning, however, the smaller the community, the higher the dental caries rates for Inuit children. The largest community (15) in the Curzons' western Hudson Bay Inuit study (14) was Baker Lake, which had a "moderate" rate of attack, while the next largest was Eskimo Point with the lowest rate.

If, because of the possibility of a differing diet, we exclude Baker Lake from the analysis, there is an almost perfect inverse relationship between community size and the deft score in children. The correlation coefficient is -0.81, which is statistically significant at the 95% level of confidence.

The results from the northern Ontario Indian study (17) are based on approximately 20 communities ranging in size from 74 to 1,100 persons. For children up to age 11, the correlation coefficient for population versus deft score was 0.29, not a statistically significant correlation. The same comparisons for the permanent teeth of individuals up to age 18 again produced a statistically nonsignificant correlation.

Thus, these 2 studies produce results that are not entirely clear, although there is the suggestion that the smaller the community, the greater the caries rate in young people.

Dental Care Availability

Another factor that should be considered is the availability of dental care to residents of the communities and its effect on oral disease. To test the hypothesis that increased availability of dentists to a community will prevent increases in oral disease, we have taken oral health data from 20 northern Ontario Indian communities, as well as the number of days the dentist was in the community for comparison. To equalize the number of days spent in communities that differed in population, we used the ratio of population divided by the days spent by the dentist in each community for a 3-year period before the oral health levels were determined. The measures of dental caries prevalence were the deft score for children up to age 12 and the DMFT (decayed, missing, and filled permanent teeth) score of individuals up to 18 years.

The population per dentist per day for the 3-year period ranged from 2.28 to 12 with a mean of 4.9 people per dentist-day. For the under 12 years of age group the mean deft score was 7.6 carious teeth. The correlation coefficient for the comparisons of population by dentist-days and deft score was 0.04. The same magnitude of correlation was evident if the DMFT rate was substituted for the deciduous attack rate.

At least two explanations of this low correlation are possible. First, the use of number of dentist days in a community tells little about the availability of the dentist to the population during his visits or about the response of potential patients to the presence of the dentist.

The other explanation is, we feel, the more important one. The activities of the dentist while in the community are not specified by the dentist-day index. While treatment of pain has a high priority and may occupy a large amount of time initially, many dentists in remote situations tend to spend large amounts of time treating disease rather than attempting to provide preventive measures. Because of the transient nature of these positions, the dentist probably won't see the results of his attempts at prevention and will concentrate on those procedures such as extractions and restorations that give both the dentist and patient an immediate sense of improving oral health. Thus, preventive measures are sometimes inadvertently assigned a low priority.

Cultural Differences

There is one other factor we would like to invoke now which eludes measurement: a cultural factor. As we noted earlier, Myers and Lee (16) suggested that differing cultural attitudes affected caries and periodontal disease rates. Gavriloff and Thompson (18) also make the same general observation when they note that the residents of some of the areas of Alberta appeared apathetic when it came to availing themselves of dental care. Certainly, this is a factor in many communities of northern Ontario.

Unfortunately, many of the dentists working in isolated areas are apparently unaware of the differences in the cultures and attitudes of their patients and assume that what is effective in the dentist's culture will be so in the new environment in which they are now operating. The value of dental care may not be of a high priority in many cultures and, therefore, the level of cooperation between the dentist and the patient may be low.

Bedford (10), writing for practitioners venturing into isolated areas, notes that cultural differences, along with other "problems" not seen in the south, may inhibit the level of care provided. He reminds the dentist, "Many of these communities have had several different dentists visit them in the past--some good and some otherwise. Bear this in mind as you will be considered to be on trial until a few people have been treated and the word filters through the community." (11)

We suggest, therefore, that two of the primary factors affecting oral health are diet and culture as reflected in awareness of preventive dental hygiene measures rather than the ignoring of the dentition until it becomes painful. These two factors are ones which are difficult to regulate but must be given more emphasis in planning future programs for oral health maintenance.

REFERENCES

1. Nutrition Canada. Dental Report. Ottawa: Minister of National Health and Welfare, Canada, 1977.

2. Stamm JW, Waller MI, Mayhall JT. Native Dental Health Baseline Survey Feasibility Study. Unpublished, 1984.

3. Bang G, Kristoffersen T. Dental caries and diet in an Alaskan Eskimo population. Scand J Dent Res 1972; 80:440-444.

4. Hargreaves JA. Changes in diet and dental health of children living in the Scottish island of Lewis. Caries Res 1972; 6:355-376.

5. Kristoffersen T, Bang G. Periodontal disease and oral hygiene in an Alaskan Eskimo population. J Dent Res 1973; 52:791-796.

6. Mayhall JT. The effect of culture change on the Eskimo dentition. Arctic Anthro 1970; 5:117-121.

7. Mayhall JT. Canadian Inuit caries experience. J Dent Res 1975; 54:1245.

8. Mayhall JT. Inuit culture change and oral health: A four-year study. In: Shephard R, Itoh S, eds. Proceedings of the Third International Symposium on Circumpolar Health. Toronto: University of Toronto Press, 1976:414-420.

9. Mayhall JT. The oral health of a Canadian Inuit community: an anthropological approach. J Dent Res 1977; 56:C55-61.

10. Mayhall JT, Dahlberg AA, Owen DR. Dental caries in the Eskimos of Wainwright, Alaska. J Dent Res 1970; 48:886.

11. Moller RJ, Poulsen S, Orholm Nielsen V. The prevalence of dental caries in Godhavn and Scoresby and districts, Greenland. Scand J Dent Res 1972; 80:169-180.

12. Russell AL, Consolazio CF, White CL. Dental caries and nutrition in Eskimo Scouts of the Alaska National Guard. J Dent Res 1961; 40:594-603.

13. Jenny J, Frazier PJ, Bagramian RA, Proshek TM. Explaining variability in caries experience using an ecological model. J Dent Res 1974; 53:554-564.

14. Curzon MEJ, Curzon J. Dental caries in Eskimo children of the Keewatin district in the Northwest Territories. J Canad Dent Assn 1970; 36:342-345.

15. McPhail CWB, Curry TM, Hazelton RD, Paynter KJ, Williamson RG. The geographic pathology of dental disease in Canadian central Arctic's populations. J Canad Dent Assn 1972; 38:288-296.

16. Myers GS, Lee M. Comparison of oral health in four Canadian Indian communities. J Dent Res 1974; 53:385-392.

17. Titley KC, Mayhall JT, Beagrie GS. The Sioux Lookout caries experience 1973. Unpublished, 1973.

18. Thompson GW, Gavriloff TJ. Dental survey of the registered Indian school population of Alberta. Edmonton: Medical Services, Alberta Region, Health and Welfare Canada, 1975.

19. Bedford WR. Look before you leap. J Canad Dent Assn 1982; 48:96-97.

John T. Mayhall
Faculty of Dentistry
University of Toronto
124 Edward Street
Toronto, Ontario M5G 1G6
Canada

Circumpolar Health 84:298-300

DENTAL CARIES PREVALENCE IN SCHOOL CHILDREN FROM TWO ETHNIC GROUPS IN LABRADOR: 1969 AND 1984 SURVEYS

JAMES G. MESSER

The communities of Nain, Hopedale, and Makkovik are located on the northeast coast of Labrador. Their populations consist of both Labrador Inuit and settlers who have co-existed there since the early 18th century. The Inuit population of each community was further increased in the late 1950s when the Government of Newfoundland initiated a resettlement program. This led to the predominantly Inuit communities of Hebron and Nutak further north being merged with the existing communities at Nain, Hopedale, and Makkovik. Figure 1 gives the location of the communities and their total populations.

Grenfell Regional Health Services (formerly the International Grenfell Association) provides dental care for the communities. In this study 2 dental surveys are compared. They were conducted in 1969 and 1984 using DMFT (damaged, missing, and filled teeth) and deft (decayed, extracted, and filled deciduous teeth) scores in 7, 12, and 15 year old school children. The purpose in comparing these 2 surveys was to find out if there had been any improvement in dental health.

In common with many areas of northern Canada, the provision of comprehensive dental care is beset by many problems. Pelton (1) in 1975 noted that attempts to attract dentists to work in northern and rural communities in Manitoba were only partially successful. In a study of Keewatin Inuit in 1972, high caries levels were reported by McPhail (2). These authors felt this dispelled the notion that the Inuit has a "built-in" resistance to decay.

In an epidemiological baseline investigation involving West Greenland settlements, Vangsted (3) noted that the children in these settlements exhibited twice the number of decayed, missing, and filled tooth surfaces when compared to Danish children in Denmark. Also, it was noted that the frequency of extracted surfaces exceeded the filled surfaces whereas the reverse was the case in Denmark. The West Greenland communities also compared unfavorably with larger Greenland townships. Inappropriate dietary habits were mentioned as an important factor in the high incidence of caries recorded, as was a limited interest in dental health by the people themselves.

The correlation between sugar availability, consumption, and dental caries was investigated by Sreebny (4), who found a positive relationship between caries prevalence and sugar availability. In a study of the epidemiology of oral disease, differ-

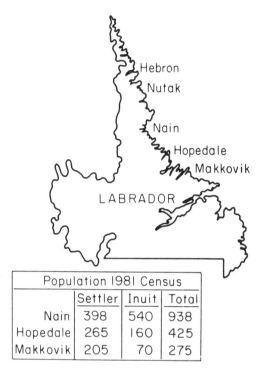

Population 1981 Census			
	Settler	Inuit	Total
Nain	398	540	938
Hopedale	265	160	425
Makkovik	205	70	275

Figure 1. The locations of the Labrador communities involved in the 1969 and 1984 dental surveys.

ences in national problems were described by Sardo Infirri and Barmes (5). They concluded that in countries with traditionally low caries levels the caries incidence is increasing, whereas the caries incidence appears to be leveling off and even declining in countries with traditionally high levels.

While the communities in this study are in one of the more advanced countries, in many ways the communities are similar to developing areas. On the one hand, the people have easy access to the harmful excesses of modern dietary habits and on the other, limited access to comprehensive dental care and persistent oral hygiene teaching on a regular basis. This combination of circumstances was also recorded by Jakobsen (6) in a report of dental health care in Greenland in 1982.

Since 1969 there have been many improvements in the dental service offered to the communities involved in this study. Well-equipped facilities have made portable

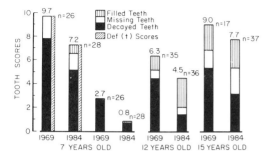

Figure 2. Caries prevalence by age; the results of dental surveys carried out in three Labrador communities in 1969 and 1984.

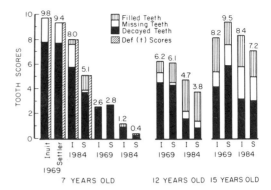

Figure 3. Caries prevalence by age and ethnic group; the results of dental surveys carried out in three labrador communities in 1969 and 1984.

equipment redundant and visits by traveling dentists are more frequent. For the last 5 years a 0.2% sodium fluoride mouthrinse program has been available for all school children from kindergarten to grade six.

RESULTS

Figure 2 shows the DMFT and deft scores for the 7, 12, and 15 year old children in the 1969 and 1984 surveys. There has been a significant reduction in the total DMFT and deft scores over the period, most noticeable in the 7 year-old permanent dentition. In all age groups there is an increase in the number of filled and missing teeth, especially in the dentition of 12 year olds. It can also be seen that in 1984 filled tooth scores for the deciduous and permanent teeth of 7 year olds are evident, albeit small. Perhaps the most striking feature is the lower incidence of caries in 7 year old and 12 year old permanent dentitions.

Figure 3 compares the DMFT and deft scores by age and ethnic group from the 1969 and 1984 surveys. Again there is an overall reduction in DMFT and deft scores for both groups over the period.

In 1969 the untreated caries condition for Inuit and settler children in the 7 and 12 year old age groups was remarkably similar. Also in 1969, 15 year old settler children exhibited a higher level of untreated caries than the Inuit. In the 1984 survey there was an overall higher level of untreated disease among the Inuit children of all ages. In the 7 year old deciduous dentition, the settler children had a higher proportion of filled teeth compared to missing teeth than the Inuit. In the permanent dentition there was slightly more evidence of fillings in the Inuit groups in the 12 and 15 year old age groups.

In 1984 the 12 year old settler and Inuit children show similar proportions of missing and filled teeth in both groups but again the overall DMFT score is higher in Inuit mainly due to the higher decayed scores.

DISCUSSION

The purpose of this study was to examine dental health changes measured by DMFT and deft scores between 1969 and 1984 by age and ethnic group. The number of subjects studied is probably too small to permit definite conclusions, even though all available subjects were examined.

While noting improvements in dental health measured by DMFT and deft scores, there are other less salubrious factors which should be considered. In common with other northern areas older nutritional patterns are being eroded. The level of sugar intake, particularly in the form of softdrinks, candy bars, and processed foods, has increased dramatically in recent years. This point was also noted by Jakobsen in the Greenland Study.

It was recently reported in a Labrador newspaper that 270 people in one Labrador community each consumed 92 liters of softdrinks over a 7 month period (7). By personal communication the author was further informed that in another Labrador community the consumption of softdrinks was 43 liters per person per year.

This level of sugar intake from only one of many sources makes it possible to exceed the "safe limit" of 50 grams per day mentioned by Sreebny in 1982. While it would be imprudent and an oversimplification to assume that sugar intake alone is responsible for a deft of 7.2 in the 1984 survey of 7 year olds, it could surely be a significant etiological factor.

Sugar intake was considered by Bradford and Crabb (8) in 1961 and again by MacDonald et al. (9) in 1981 when they investigated the dental health of dentists' children. Not only did the dentists' children have a lower caries prevalence but they also had less evidence of traditional dental treatment as expressed by missing, extracted, or filled teeth compared with peer groups. They concluded that of all the methods used by dentists to prevent dental caries in their own children the single most important method was a persistent and conscious effort to restrict sugar consumption.

It also appears that there is a connection between the degree of isolation which is pertinent to this study and caries experience in more urbanized areas such as was noted by Vangsted in West Greenland (3).

In another example, Stamm et al. (10) in a report of the dental health status of Alberta school children in 1980 noted a difference in caries prevalence between urban and rural 6 and 7 year old children. Rural dwellers had a mean deft of 4.3 compared to 3.8 for urban residents. In the Labrador study in 1984 a deft score of 7.2 was recorded for the 7 year old children, considerably more than for the Alberta children. However, for the 12 year old Labrador children with DMFT of 4.5 the caries prevalence was similar to that of Alberta 13 year old children with 4.74. In a study of Quebec 13 and 14 year old school children in 1980 Stamm and his co-authors (11) recorded a mean DMFT of 8.9. This is a higher score than was found in the Labrador 15 year olds which was 7.7 in 1984.

These comparisons suggest that the caries prevalence in 7 year old primary dentitions is higher in Labrador than in Alberta, whereas the caries prevalence of 15 year olds in Labrador is lower than in Quebec.

Caries prevalence in this Labrador study by ethnic status is far higher in 7 year old Inuit children with a deft of 8.0 than in the settler children where the deft score was 5.1. It might be that genetic differences such as tooth emergence times and crown and root morphology may offer a partial explanation. These differences were reported in a study of 600 Inuit in Igloolik and Hall Beach by Mayhall (12) in 1977. Without further research, however, these factors may not be applicable to this study.

CONCLUSION AND SUMMARY

Despite the difficulty experienced providing comprehensive dental health care and attempting to modify dietary habits, dental health is improving when measured by DMFT and deft scores in these Labrador communities. However, any complacency would be ill-advised. It is obvious that greater efforts are required, especially for the deciduous dentition of younger children, if current caries levels and their ramifications are to be treated, or preferably reduced, by preventive measures.

The pursuit of further improvements by a greater emphasis toward restorative and replacement dentistry remains a formidable challenge. Great efforts must also be directed toward reducing the level of disease by education and prevention. For these measures to be successful, a reassessment of priorities by the people themselves may be the most important factor.

REFERENCES

1. Pelton AJ. Public health dental auxiliary training program at The Pas, Manitoba. J Canad Dent Assn 1975; 6:347-348.
2. McPhail CWB, Curry TM, Hazelton RD, Paynter KJ, Williamson RG. The geographic pathology of dental disease in Canadian Central Arctic populations. J Canad Dent Assn 1972; 8:288-296.
3. Vangsted T. Dental caries in children from West-Greenland settlement. Nordic Council Arct Med Res Rep 1982; 31:42-42.
4. Sreebny LM. Sugar availability, sugar consumption and dental caries. Community Dent Oral Epidemiol 1982; 10:1-7.
5. Sardo Infirri J, Barmes DE. Epidemiology of oral diseases: differences in national problems. Int Dent J 1979; 29:183-189.
6. Jakobsen J, Senderovitz F. The caries situation and the organization of dental health care in Greenland. Nordic Council Arct Med Res Rep 1982; 31:31-32.
7. The Northern Reporter. October 26, 1983:9.
8. Bradford EW, Crabb HSM. Carbohydrate restriction and caries incidence. Brit Dent J 1961; 111:273-279.
9. MacDonald SP, Cowell CR, Sheiham A. Methods of preventing dental caries used by dentists for their own children. Brit Dent J 1981; 151:118-121.
10. Stamm JW, Lizaire A, Fedori, Finnigan P, Taylor G, Willey J. J Canad Dent Assn 1980; 2:98-107.
11. Stamm JW, Dixter CT, Langlais RP. Principal dental · health indices for 13-14 year old Quebec children. J Canad Dent Assn 1980; 2:125-136.
12. Mayhall JT. The oral health of a Canadian Inuit community: an anthropological approach. J Dent Res Special Issue C 1977; 56:55-61.

James G. Messer
Grenfell Regional Health Services
St. Anthony, Newfoundland A0K 4S0
Canada

Circumpolar Health 84:301-302

A REPORT OF A CONFERENCE ON HEARING IMPAIRMENT IN THE BAFFIN ZONE

HENRY J. ILECKI, JAMES D. BAXTER and F. O'DONOGHUE

While the problem of hearing loss (typically secondary to chronic otitis media and noise exposure) in the eastern Canadian Arctic has been documented for several years, a permanent and continuing approach to its northern management had not been effectively instituted until recently with the establishment, in October 1983, of an audiologic test facility in Frobisher Bay. The evolutionary process which culminated in the present situation was often multi-faceted (and, at times, contradictory) in direction and uneven in growth. Even now, the process continues and a final program has yet to emerge.

Within the last several years, a new sense of cooperation has slowly evolved among agencies and individuals directly or indirectly involved in the identification and management of hearing loss. This new direction was perhaps best symbolized by the collaborative effort made in the organization of the conference: "Hearing Impairment in the Baffin Region" held in the fall of 1983 in Frobisher Bay. The conference was organized by the educators in the region and was sponsored by the Northwest Territories Council for the Disabled, the Baffin Inter-agency Committee, and the Secretary of State, Canada. Over 100 doctors, nurses, teachers, social workers, and the general public met for 3 days to discuss the problems of hearing loss in the Baffin Zone. Fifteen speakers covered such topics as: the history of otitis media and hearing impairment in the Baffin Zone, public awareness and resource development, cultural considerations in hearing impairment, early identification of hearing impairment, etc.

As suggested, the delivery of hearing health care in the North had not always enjoyed the currency (either professionally or with the general public) as it now appears. Although stimulated by educators' frustrations in dealing with hearing-impaired children in the general classroom, the basic investigative work in the area was initiated by teams of physicians and audiologists from McGill University beginning in the 1970s. Those initial visits revealed that over one-third of 200 Inuit students studied suffered from chronic otitis media and that many of the students with learning problems had significant hearing loss. In one special class for children with behavioral problems, for example, all students were found to have significant hearing loss secondary to chronic otitis media.

As a reaction to such findings, the Nakasuk Project was born. It was an effort by physicians, audiologists, and educators to resolve hearing problems in the Nakasuk Elementary School. Modalities of medical treatment of chronic otitis media in Inuit children were explored and a hearing aid program was expanded. Every hard-of-hearing pupil was seen on a daily basis by a special teacher for instruction in basic areas of the school program. This teaching was carried out in a room outfitted with an induction loop system and a variety of audiovisual equipment. Instruction was generally designed to stimulate improvement in speech and reading. During the course of the project most of the hard-of-hearing pupils caught up to their peers and in some cases achieved beyond the academic means. The amount and severity of pupil behavioral problems also decreased in the school.

The original intent was to extend the Nakasuk Project as a model for service throughout the schools in the Baffin Zone. There were 2 reasons that this did not happen. The first was a lack of understanding of the nature of the problem by various levels of government. This was particularly the case in education. In 1977, for example, educators in the Nakasuk School were convinced that the hearing and learning problems associated with chronic otitis media had been resolved and they sought unilaterally to terminate the Project. This situation was aggravated by the high rate of turnover of decision-making personnel.

The second reason that information and implications from the Nakasuk Project were not propagated throughout the Baffin Zone's school system was the lack of direct involvement by the Inuit in the early and middle 1970s in decisions being made about their well-being. Experience over the years has shown the importance of enlisting the active cooperation of the Inuit in the design and implementation of health care programs.

Given time and the right combination of ingredients, mistakes can be corrected and old problems redressed. We believe that this is now happening in the Baffin Zone. A year following termination of the Nakasuk Project, the first coordinator of Special Education for the Northwest Territories was appointed. A special committee of the legislature on education (1980-1981) ultimately led to the appointments of special education consultants to each of the regions of the Northwest Territories in 1982. In the Baffin Zone, the action was highly successful in re-sensitizing educators to the persistent problems in the schools.

Concurrently, the Inuit have become more involved in decision-making processes affecting their lives. Each settlement now has a community health committee which is composed of Inuit and which serves to advance public health within the Zone. Recently, the control of the Frobisher Bay General Hospital transferred from the federal government to the Northwest Territorial Government. The renamed Baffin Regional Hospital now has Inuit representation on the hospital board. At a board meeting we (H.J.I., J.D.B.) were invited to attend, the Inuit participated in a spirited discussion of their hearing problems.

It appears, then, that the problems which contributed to the lack of continuance of the Nakasuk Project have come to an end. The Inuit are taking a greater share of responsibility in their own destiny, and the Education Department appears very intent on ensuring that hearing-impaired students receive the specialized assistance they require. The organization of the 1983 conference on hearing impairment needed, and received, input and expertise from a wide variety of interested parties. The Inuit played a large factor in this regard.

The conference has been described as a symbol of a new start in providing hearing health care, and there have been some practical achievements from the conference as well. There has been a definite surge of enthusiasm to do something positive about the hearing problems in northern Canada. Public and professional awareness of the problem has increased by virtue of media coverage of the conference. There has been an increased cooperation among agencies either directly or indirectly providing services to the hearing impaired. The conference helped to contribute to the development of an expanded commitment in the McGill-Baffin Zone Project to provide on-site and remote professional support in the management of the hearing impaired based on the recently opened audiology unit in Frobisher Bay. Finally, it inspired an extension of the McGill Study of Deaf Children in Canada to include the problems of hearing impairment in the Canadian North (through a grant by the Donner Canadian Foundation).

During the conference, the audiology unit at Frobisher Bay was officially opened. This is a well-equipped facility comparable to any such unit in a major teaching hospital in the country. Its role is to function as an audiological facility to serve the Baffin Zone. It is planned that it will cooperate with the various nursing stations in the region providing screening audiometry. The center will aid substantially in the identification and management of school age children and others with hearing defects and will alleviate the need for these Inuit to commute south for specialized audiological service. The unit is supervised by the Division of Speech and Hearing, Institute of Otolaryngology of the Royal Victoria Hospital and McGill University, through the McGill-Baffin Zone Project.

Although there are outstanding problems still to be solved in providing services to the North, it is felt that the major hurdles are in the past. The program appears to have community acceptance, and support from allied professionals. A plan for the systematic delivery of hearing health care for the long-term is now in place.

Henry J. Ilecki
Royal Victoria Hospital
Room E.471
687 Pine Ave. West
Montreal, Quebec H3A 1A1
Canada

SECTION 6. ACCULTURATION, MENTAL HEALTH, AND SUBSTANCE ABUSE

Circumpolar Health 84:305-311

ACCULTURATION AND MENTAL HEALTH AMONG CIRCUMPOLAR PEOPLES

J.W. BERRY

Recently the World Health Organization expressed the need for "health for all by the year 2000." Recognizing that for many of the world's peoples a high-tech medicine might be difficult and costly to deliver, WHO approached a group of behavioral and social scientists to find out what we know that may help them attain their goal. In addition to such areas as a group's customary behavior concerning sanitation, and food production and preparation, one of the more obvious areas of relevance is that of the impact of social and cultural change on the mental health status of individuals. Without much doubt, the circumpolar peoples have been major recipients of, and adaptors to such change.

The relationship between acculturation and mental health is one of long-standing interest and controversy. Simply put, is it the case that acculturation alters the mental health status of individuals? To answer such a question, it is first necessary to define the concepts, then to organize a framework for an answer, and finally to examine the empirical evidence.

THE CONCEPTS

Acculturation is a term which has been defined as culture change which results from continuous, first-hand contact between two distinct cultural groups (1). While originally proposed as a group-level phenomenon, it is now also widely recognized as an individual-level phenomenon, and is termed psychological acculturation (2). At this level, acculturation refers to changes in an individual who is experiencing acculturation.

The broader concept of culture change refers to changes in a culture which come about as a result not only of culture contact (as in the case of acculturation), but also as a result of other factors such as natural disaster, innovation within the culture, or diffusion of a single cultural feature (such as the use of the plow or of firearms) over broad geographic ranges.

What kinds of changes may occur as a result of acculturation? The range is very large, and some of them will only receive brief mention in this review. First, physical changes may occur: a new place to live, a new type of housing, increased population density, more pollution, etc., are all common with acculturation. Second, biological changes may occur: new food and nutritional status, new diseases (often devastating in force), interbreeding yielding mixed (Métis, Mestizo, etc.) populations are all common. Third, cultural changes,

which are at the heart of the definition, necessarily occur: original political, economic, technical, linguistic, religious, and social institutions become altered, or new ones take their place. Finally, as we noted above, psychological changes, including changes in mental health status, almost always occur as individuals attempt to adapt to their new milieu. Of these four categories of change, it is the latter two on which we will be focusing in this review.

A typical acculturation situation with which we are concerned in the North involves an individual of a particular (often non-dominant) cultural background being in contact with another cultural group (usually dominant) which leads to that individual having to adapt to his new situation, using a variety of strategies. The acculturation situations occur during colonial expansion, military invasion, international development; group and individual strategies can vary from readily and easily adopting the changes, to resisting them, or collapsing under their weight.

Mental Health

Just as there is tremendous variation in forms of acculturative experience, there is also a wide range of psychological characteristics which can be (and have been) used to indicate one's mental health. Despite this heterogeneous set of indicators there is still the possibility of arriving at a core definition of mental health which includes the notions of effective functioning in daily life and the ability to deal with new situations. The first is a key element in virtually all conceptions of mental health, while the second is a particularly important characteristic in the situations of cultural change with which we are most concerned here. Implicit in both of these notions is a positive quality, one which is currently widely emphasized: mental health is more than just the absence of illness, disease or dysfunction--it is the presence of psychological well being, however that may be defined in a particular culture.

A concept which has been employed to refer to these negative consequences when they result from acculturation is acculturative stress (3). Of course stress is a widely used construct, not only in psychology and psychiatry, but also more widely in the physical, biological and social sciences. As the term is employed here, while stress may be present in all (including unchanging) situations, culture contact often brings stressors to bear on the group and on the individual, including tension in the group and in the individual. Acculturative stress is thus limited to those reactions which can be theoretically or empirically linked to the acculturation process.

STUDYING ACCULTURATION AND MENTAL HEALTH

A widespread view formerly held was that the experience of acculturation inevitably brings about a decline in the mental health status of individuals (i.e. induces acculturative stress). However, since the work of Murphy (4) and Chance (5) such a broad general relationship is now no longer supported. The relationship depends on a variety of factors which govern it. The following framework is an attempt to identify and systematize these governing factors. Since most of them have been proposed by numerous authors, there is no attempt in this section to trace origins or to give credit; specific references will be given in the later empirical review section.

Phases of Acculturation

As a process which takes place over time, acculturation may be considered as a series of phases. In the pre-contact phase, there are two independent cultural groups with sets of characteristic customs, and each composed of individuals with a variety of psychological characteristics; it is presumed that mental health is present to varying degrees in the society across individuals. In the contact phase, the groups meet, interact and new stressors appear. Cultural and behavioral exchange and change also begin; in principle, the notion of acculturation allows for cultural exchange in either, or both, directions, but in practice, the balance of flow is usually from one (the larger donor or dominant society) to the other (the receptor or acculturating group), placing more and more serious stressors on the non-dominant group. In this review we will be concerned with what happens in this non-dominant group only. Usually, but not inevitably, a conflict phase appears, in which tension builds up and pressures are experienced by the non-dominant group to change their way of life; stress is induced here, particularly when there is less than complete willingness to change. If conflict and tension do appear, a highly stressful crisis phase may then occur, where the conflict comes to a head, and a resolution is required. Finally, an adaptation phase may take place, in which the group relations are stabilized in one form or another (see next section). These varieties of adaptation may or may not bring about an adequate solution to the conflict and crisis, or a reduction in stress.

The implications of this phase analysis for mental health are numerous. First, in the pre-contact phase, there may be varying mental health statuses in the two groups; the very impetus toward contact may itself be the result of stressors (e.g. overpopulation, famine, warfare) in one of the groups. Thus the initial mental health status, prior to contact, is one factor of importance in understanding the relationship between acculturation and mental health. Second, at contact, the purpose or goal of contact needs to be understood; if the intent is to take over, either territorially (by warfare), spiritually (by conversion), or intellectually (by schooling), then the consequences for mental health are different from those in situations where the goals are more benign (e.g. trade, tourism, controlled immigration). Third, whether conflict does or does not occur is a crucial issue. Here we should distinguish between intergroup and psychological conflict, but both imply lowered mental health status. Intergroup conflict creates threats to person and property, while psychological conflict (even without social conflict) creates uncertainty and confusion. Fourth, the crisis point (if it follows the conflict) is the culmination of the difficulty, and is associated with the overt behaviors so often noted in acculturating peoples, such as homicide, suicide, family and substance abuse, etc. Finally which kind of adaptation is achieved also has consequences for mental health status; those which perpetuate the conflict and crisis in one form or another are likely to be associated with lower mental health status than those which relieve it or manage it in some way.

We may see at the onset, then, that any relationship between acculturation and mental health will depend on the phase of acculturation, and also on a number of specific features of each phase.

Modes of Acculturation

Acculturation has sometimes been used to mean assimilation, where it is assumed that an acculturating individual will inevitably lose his original pre-contact culture, and be absorbed into the larger society. While this often happens (especially in societies where there is an assimilationist ideology), it is not inevitable. Viewing acculturation as varieties of adaptation, it is possible to identify four different modes of acculturation according to how individuals and groups deal with the two central issues which arise in all acculturation arenas. The first issue is "Is my cultural identity of value and to be retained?", and the second is "Are positive relations with the larger (dominant) society to be sought?" In this manner, four distinct varieties of acccultur-

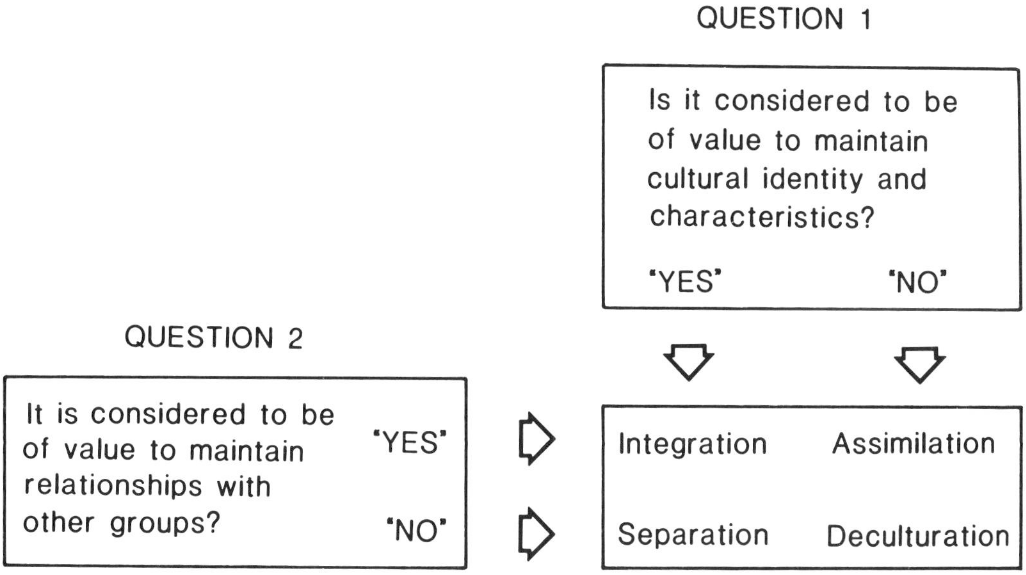

QUESTION 1

Is it considered to be of value to maintain cultural identity and characteristics?

"YES"   "NO"

QUESTION 2

It is considered to be of value to maintain relationships with other groups?

"YES"

"NO"

Integration   Assimilation

Separation   Deculturation

Figure 1. Four modes of acculturation as a function of orientation to two issues.

ation may be identified: assimilation, integration, separation, and deculturation (Figure 1).

In assimilation, relinquishing cultural identity and moving into the larger society is the option taken. This can take place by way of the absorption of a non-dominant group into an established "main-stream," or it can be by way of the merging of many groups to form a new society (the "melting pot").

Integration, by contrast, implies the maintenance of cultural integrity as well as the movement to become an integral part of a larger societal framework. Therefore, in the case of integration, the option taken is to retain cultural identity and move to join with others in the larger society. In this case there are many ethnic groups, all cooperating within a larger social system (the "mosaic"). Such an arrangement may occur where there is some degree of "structural assimilation," but little "cultural and behavioral assimilation," to use Gordon's terms.

Let us consider the types of acculturation that are identified by answering "no" to the question of establishing or maintaining positive relations with the larger society. Separation refers to self-imposed withdrawal from the larger society. When imposed by the larger society, however, it becomes one of the classical forms of segregation. Thus, the maintenance of one's traditional way of life outside full participation in the larger society may be due to a desire on the part of the group to lead an independent existence (as in the case of

"separatist" movements), or it may be due to power exercised by the larger society to keep people in "their place" (as in slavery or apartheid situations).

Finally, there is an option which is accompanied by a good deal of collective and individual confusion and anxiety. It is characterized by having lost essential features of one's culture, but not having replaced them by entering the larger society. There are often feelings of alienation and loss of identity. This option is deculturation, in which groups are out of cultural and psychological contact with both their traditional culture and the larger society.

The point of this analysis is to illustrate the various ways in which groups and individuals may acculturate; all result in cultural and psychological changes following culture contact, but the extent and nature of the changes are likely to vary greatly. In particular, change in the mental health status of individuals may be expected to vary across these four modes, both as a function of the mode itself, and as a function of the congruence between an individual's preferred mode and that of the majority of his group. For example, we may reasonably expect that those who are in a situation of deculturation will have poorer mental health than an individual who is integrated, and that a person who seeks separation while most members of his group seek assimilation will also suffer poor mental health. In essence, because not all peoples acculturate in the same way, we cannot expect the relationship between

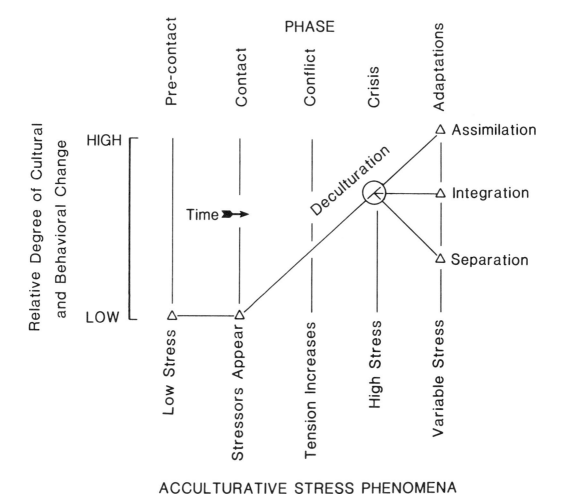

Figure 2. *Variations in acculturative stress as a function of phase and mode of acculturation.*

acculturation and mental health to be independent of these variations.

Putting these first two analyses
together, we can produce a schematic diagram
(Figure 2) which illustrates the relationship between phase (on the horizontal axis),
mode, and the relative amount of cultural
and psychological change experienced by an
individual (on the vertical axis); variations in acculturative stress are also
suggested (below the horizontal axis).

Three modes represent various forms of
adaptation, while one (deculturation) tends
to suspend the individual in a highly
stressful crisis; it is here that poorest
mental health might be expected. Of the
other three, separation tends to maintain
the resistance to intergroup relations, and
thus maintain the conflict to some extent,
suggesting that mental health may be rela-

tively poor in this mode as well. And since
assimilation represents cultural loss,
mental health may be less there than in the
integration mode, where selective involvement in two cultural systems may provide the
most supportive sociocultural base for the
mental health of the individual. The point
here is not to make exact predictions about
the mental health status of individuals who
are to be found at various places in the
diagram, but to suggest that it is reasonable to expect mental health variations
during acculturation which are a function of
the phase and mode variables.

Type of Acculturating Group

Not all people experience acculturation
for the same reasons. Some voluntarily seek
out culture contact experiences, while

others have it forced upon them. Some remain in their ancestral areas (initially surrounded by an intact society and traditional resources), while others experience their contact far from home. And some are in a temporary acculturation situation, while others are locked in for life. These distinctions are all likely to have an effect on the relationship between acculturation and mental health. At least five distinct groups may be identified on the basis of these distinctions: immigrants, refugees, Native peoples, ethnic groups, and sojourners. Our interest here is primarily on the Native peoples category, although newly-arrived groups in the North would qualify as immigrants, while short-term workers would be classed as sojourners. The point of these distinctions is that Native peoples have largely experienced involuntary acculturation; their land and their lives have generally been taken over by others, without their seeking the resulting culture contact. In contrast to other types, (such as immigrants and established ethnic groups), this involuntary acculturation may predispose Native peoples to experience greater acculturative stress.

Nature of the Larger Society

The society which exerts the acculturative influences may do so in a variety of ways. One important distinction is the degree of pluralism extant (4). Culturally plural societies, in contrast to culturally monistic ones, are likely to be characterized by two important factors: one is the availability of a network of social and cultural groups which may provide support for those entering into the experience of acculturation; and the other is a greater tolerance for or acceptance of cultural diversity, termed "multicultural ideology" (6). Taken together, one might reasonably expect the mental health status of persons experiencing acculturation in plural societies to be better than those in monistic societies who pursue a forced inclusion or assimilationist ideology.

A second factor, paradoxically, is the existence of policies which are designed to exclude acculturating groups from full participation in the larger society; to the extent that acculturating people wish to participate in the desirable features of the larger society (such as adequate housing, medical care, political rights) the denial of these may be cause for lower mental health status.

A third factor, one we have already encountered, is that of the reasons for the culture contact, from the point of view of the larger society. Reasons which imply some threat to acculturating groups (e.g.

military, colonial, evangelical goals) are likely to create conditions for poor mental health.

The point of these comments, once again, is not to provide a comprehensive list of features of the larger society, but to suggest some variables which are likely to affect the relationship between acculturation and mental health.

Characteristics of Acculturating Group

What socio-cultural qualities of the acculturating group may affect the mental health status of their members during acculturation? The list of possible factors identified in the literature is extremely long; thus we attempt here only a selective overview. It is useful to distinguish between original (pre-contact) cultural characteristics, and those which evolve during the process of acculturation. Some factors, however, involve the interaction of variables from these two sets (pre- and post-contact).

One basic cultural factor which appears in the literature is the traditional settlement pattern of the group: nomadic peoples, who are usually hunters, gatherers, or pastoralists, may suffer more negative consequences of acculturation than peoples who were sedentary prior to contact. A complex of factors has been suggested to account for this proposal: nomadic peoples are used to relatively large territories, small population densities, and unstructured socio-political systems; during acculturation, sedentarization into relatively dense communities with new authority systems is typically required, and this induces relatively greater tension among nomadic peoples than among others.

Status is also a factor even when one's origin is in a relatively stratified society. For example, "entry status" into the larger society is often lower than "departure status"; this relative loss of status may result in stress and poor mental health. One's status mobility in the larger society, whether to regain one's original status, or just to keep up with other groups, may also be a factor. In addition, some specific features of status (such as education and employment) provide one with resources to deal with the larger society, and these likely affect one's ability to function effectively in the new circumstances.

Some standard indicators, such as age and gender, may also play a role: relatively older persons, and often females, have frequently been noted to have poorer mental health, as have those who are without a partner (unmarried, because of loss or unavailability).

Perhaps the most comprehensive variable in the literature is that of social supports; this refers to the presence of social and cultural institutions for the support of the acculturating individual. Included here are such factors as ethnic associations (national or local), residential enclaves (e.g. reservations), extended families (including endogamy), availability of one's original cultural group (visits to, vitality of, alienation from the culture), and more formal institutions such as agencies and clinics devoted to providing support.

A final set of variables refers to the acceptance or prestige of one's groups in the acculturation setting. Some groups are more acceptable for reasons of ethnicity, race, or religion than others; those less acceptable run into barriers (prejudice, discrimination, exclusion) which may lead to marginalization of the group and which are likely to induce greater stress. The point here is that even in plural societies, (those societies which may be generally more tolerant of differences) there are still relative degrees of social acceptability of the various acculturating groups.

Table 1. Framework: Variables which may affect relationship between acculturation and mental health.

Category	Variable affecting relationship
Phase of acculturation	Pre-contact Contact Conflict Crisis Adaptation
Modes of acculturation	Assimilation Integration Separation Deculturation
Type of acculturating group	Immigrants Refugees Native peoples Ethnic groups Sojourners
Nature of larger society	Pluralism Tolerance/prejudice Multicultural ideology
Sociocultural characteristics of acculturating group	Settlement pattern Stratification Entry status Status mobility Size of groups Rapidity of change Social support network Group acceptability
Psychological characteristics of acculturating individual	Prior knowledge Prior intercultural encounters Prior motives and attitudes Education Employment Age Gender Marital status Contact experiences Identity confusion/consolidation Attitudes to modes of acculturation Acquisition of knowledge and skills Cognitive control Cognitive style Congruity between expectations and actualities

Characteristics of Individuals

What kinds of psychological variables may play a role in the mental health status of persons experiencing acculturation? Here again a distinction is useful between those characteristics which were present prior to contact, and those which developed during acculturation. In the pre-contact set of variables are included certain experiences which may predispose one to function more effectively under acculturative pressures. There are: prior knowledge of the new language and culture, prior intercultural encounters of any kind, motives for the contact (see the earlier distinction between voluntary versus involuntary contact), and attitudes toward acculturation (positive or negative). Other prior attributes which have been suggested in the literature are achievement motivation, rigidity versus flexibility, and cognitive style.

Contact experiences may also account for variations in mental health. Whether one has many contacts with the larger society (or few of them), whether they are pleasant (or unpleasant), whether they meet the current needs of the individual (or not), and in particular, whether the first encounters are viewed positively (or not) may set the stage for all subsequent ones, and affect mental health.

Among factors which appear during acculturation are the attitudes towards the various modes of acculturation: individuals within a group do vary in their preference for assimilating, integrating or rejecting; and these variations, along with experiences of deculturation, are likely to affect one's mental health status. Another variable, the sense of cognitive control which an individual has over the acculturation process, also seems to play a role; those who perceive that the changes are opportunities which they can manage may have better mental health than those who feel overwhelmed by them. In essence, then, the attitudinal and cognitive perspectives propose that it is not the acculturative changes themselves which are important, but how one sees them and what one makes of them.

Finally, a recurring idea is that the congruity between expectations and actualities will affect mental health. Individuals for whom there is a discrepancy, such that they expect more than they actually obtain during acculturation, may have poorer mental health than those who achieve some reasonable match.

The point of these observations is that there are likely to be individual differences in how a person actually engages in the acculturation process, how he perceives them, how he values them, and whether they satisfy him, and that these are all likely to be factors in the mental health status of the individual.

To summarize this section, Table 1 lays out some of the factors which have been identified in this excursion through the literature. While not intended to be a complete list, it will serve to organize the review of empirical studies which follow.

CONCLUSIONS

From this brief overview, it is possible to see that circumpolar peoples are likely to be experiencing variable mental health statuses, depending on the various factors outlined. While some groups in some places are experiencing serious difficulties (indexed by substance abuse, suicide, homicide, and social disintegration), others are adapting rather well to acculturation. Moreover, simple-minded assertions about the relationship between acculturation and mental health can (and should) be avoided when we are armed with a knowledge of these moderating factors. Finally, periods and places of problematic behavior might be anticipated on the basis of this type of analysis, and preventive policies and programs can be developed in advance.

REFERENCES

1. Redfield R, Linton R and Herskovits MJ. Memorandum on the study of acculturation. Amer Anthropol 1936; 38:149-152.
2. Graves T. Psychological acculturation in a tri-ethnic community. Southwestern Jour Anthropol 1967; 23:337-350.
3. Berry J. Acculturative stress in Northern Canada: ecological, cultural and psychological factors. In: Shephard R, Itoh S, eds. Proceedings of the Third International Symposium on Circumpolar Health. Toronto: University of Toronto Press, 1976: 490-497.
4. Murphy HBM. Migration and the major mental disorders: a reappraisal. In: Kantor MB, ed. Mobility and mental health. Springfield: Thomas, 1965: 5-29.
5. Chance NA. Acculturation, self-identification and personality adjustment. Amer Anthropol 1965; 67:372-393.
6. Berry JW, Kalin R, Taylor D. Multiculturalism and ethnic attitudes in Canada. Ottawa: Supply and Services, 1977.

J.W. Berry
Psychology Department
Queen's University
Kingston, Ontario K7L 3N6
Canada

Circumpolar Health 84:312-315

SEASONAL VARIATION IN SUICIDE AND MENTAL DEPRESSION IN FINLAND

SIMO NÄYHÄ

INTRODUCTION

Since the early part of the nineteenth century it has been clear that most suicides in the north occur in the light period of the year (1). The reasons underlying this phenomenon have remained obscure. One assumption seems to be that suicides follow the annual variation in social interaction (2), a view originally put forward by Emile Durkheim (3), but no conclusive evidence has been presented to support this argument. The seasonal variation in mental depression seems to offer another explanation, but this issue has not been examined in depth. The main reason for this is the obvious diffi-culty entailed in measuring temporal varia-tions in psychiatric disturbances in a population. The introduction of the psychi-atric aspect into this field has not been very popular due to the common belief that only a certain proportion of suicides suffer from mental illness (1,4).

The seasonal variation in suicides since 1851 is well established in Finland (1,4,6). Suicides are most numerous in spring or early summer, but a secondary peak in autumn has been noted in periods of rapid urbanization, i.e. in the 1920s and 1950s. The present study was carried out in order to compare the seasonal patterns of suicides and mental depressions. Mental disorders were screened in 831 males living in a country district of northern Finland (Figure 1), and national data on suicides were used for comparison. The findings strongly suggest that depression may have a seasonal variation essentially similar to that found in suicides.

MATERIAL AND METHODS

The material consisted of individual data from the death certificates of all those who committed suicide in Finland during the period from 1961 to 1976. The total number of suicides was 16,312, of which 1,328 were committed in the province of Oulu and 717 in Lapland. Determination of the cause of death was based on autopsy in 73% of cases, and on autopsy or external inspection of the corpse in an average of 81% of cases. A detailed description of the material is given elsewhere (1,5,6).

Comparative data on variations of mental illness were obtained using a sample of 849 males. Invitations were made to 1,073 war veterans of age 50 years and older from a country district of 13,000 inhabi-tants (Figure 1) to participate in a routine medical examination, of the kind performed on this sector of the population from time

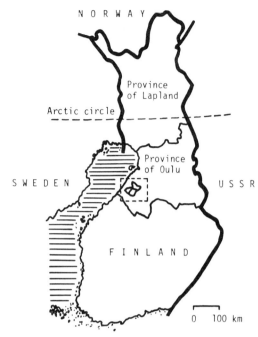

Figure 1. The study area in Oulu, Finland. Sample communes (framed) from left to right: Merijärvi, Oulainen and Vihanti.

to time. The invitations were sent out in 1976 through 1979 and were accepted by 849 persons, or 79.1% of the original sample. Those examined represented 53% of the male population of the same age living in this area, and were considered representative of the local male population as to age struc-ture, occupation, and social status.

As the medical examinations were extended over all months of the year in an essentially random way, it was possible to investigate how mental states within the sample varied from month to month. Mental disturbance was measured using a 12-item questionnaire devised by Goldberg (7). This test focuses on non-psychotic morbidity of a depressive character, and has been shown to correlate well with the severity of the underlying disorder. The test result was scaled so that the total yield ranged from 0 to 12, a high score indicating pathological findings.

RESULTS

Seasonal Variation in Suicides

Figure 2 presents monthly suicides in Finland during the period 1961 through 1976 in the form of refined mortality indices.

INDEX

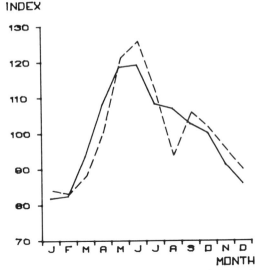

Figure 2. Seasonal variation in suicides in Finland (solid line) and northern Finland (province of Oulu and Lapland) (broken line), 1961-1978.

Each index has been adjusted for long-term and other non-seasonal effects and is taken to represent the seasonal effect alone. A detailed description of the method is given elsewhere (1). It is seen that suicides in Finland reach their peak in May-June, with the low trough occurring in January. Suicides in northern Finland alone seem to increase more steeply in late winter to early spring and to have a peak somewhat higher than for the whole of the country. Suicides decrease fairly slowly during the

latter part of the year, and even show a minor secondary rise in September-October in northern Finland taken separately.

The seasonal patterns of suicides are broken down into broad social classes in Figure 3. The classes are defined according to the usage of the Central Statistical Office of Finland (8), and restricted to males aged 15 to 64 years, since determination of social class is most reliable in this group. It emerges most clearly that the standard May-June peak in suicides is typical of the middle social classes (II through V), while the two extreme classes, i.e. the first and sixth (students, or social class indeterminate or unknown), show a bimodal incidence with peaks in spring and autumn.

Seasonal Variation in Mental Illness

Questionnaires were completed by 831 persons (97.9%) of the total 849. Since different age groups were somewhat unevenly distributed over the months, an allowance was made for age by the use of the analysis of covariance (9), employing a logarithmic transformation of age as an independent variable. It emerges from Figure 4 that the severity of mental disturbance is highest in spring and lowest in autumn. When an adjustment is made for age, the seasonal pattern becomes slightly less pronounced, but remains essentially similar. The variance test based on monthly figures gave a significant result ($p\sim0.208$ for the difference between adjusted means).

Table 1 attempts to analyze the test score with a division by social class, defined as in the case of suicides except that the farmers (59% of the sample) were

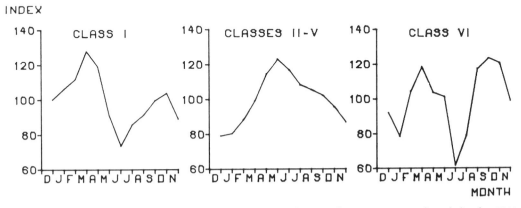

Figure 3. Seasonal variation in suicides among males aged 15-64 years in Finland, 1961-1972, classified by broad social classes. Class I = higher administrative (N=368), classes II-V = lower administrative, skilled and unskilled workers and farmers (N=7,227), class VI = students, indeterminate or unknown (N=316). Smoothed using a 2-point moving average.

MEAN
SCORE

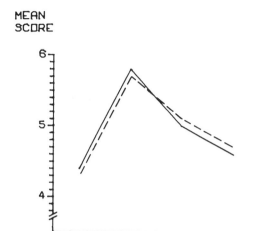

Figure 4. Seasonal variation in mental disturbance. 3-month averages of the test scores. Crude score (broken line); adjusted for age (solid line).

assigned to classes I through IV using the area of cultivated land as the criterion (8), and excluding class VI which contained only 44 cases. Comparison is made between the two extreme classes and the others, which were sufficiently homogeneous. The observation is that the spring peak in depressions is typical of the two middle classes, while in the extreme classes the score is very low in spring and the peak tends to be focused on the latter part of the year. A two-way analysis of variance (using month and social class as factors) showed the month of examination ($p \sim 0.001$) and the month times social class interactions ($p \sim 0.019$) to exercise significant effects, suggesting a real difference in the seasonal patterns between the two social categories in Table 1.

DISCUSSION

The present results suggest that the seasonal variation in affective mental illness may be strikingly similar to that established for suicides. This similarity is corroborated when the data are carefully screened for anomalous seasonal patterns. Given an agricultural society, suicides followed a consistent unimodal variation with the peak in early summer, but with advancing industrialization the pattern has changed to a bimodal one with the peaks in spring and autumn (1). Recent work has shown that this anomalous bimodal cycle exists in those subgroups of the population, which are characteristic of modern life, e.g. among higher administrative staff, unskilled laborers in industry and modern types of occupation (5). In northern Finland, which has suffered from the drawbacks attached to rapid modernization (6), the autumn peak in suicides is quite prominent (Figure 2). It now seems that the seasonal patterns in mental depression may differ by social class in a similar way to those for suicides. Differing seasonal variations associated with the various occupations suggest different etiologies. One may hypothesize that suicides and depression were originally linked with the annual cycle of daylight, which is most intensive in early summer, while the secondary rise in the autumn period is more indirect and may be ascribed to changes in social conditions that occur in autumn in modern society (e.g. unemployment and readjustment to work after the summer vacations).

REFERENCES

1. Näyhä S. Short and medium-term variations in mortality in Finland. Scand J Soc Med 1980:suppl 21.
2. Lester D. Seasonal variation in suicidal deaths. Br J Psychiatry 1971; 118:627-628.

Table 1. Mean test score for mental disturbance by season and social class.

Social class	Winter (Dec–Feb)	Spring (Mar–May)	Summer (Jun–Aug)	Autumn (Sept–Oct)	Total
Classes I and IV					
Mean score	4.3	3.5	5.0	4.7	4.6
S.E.	0.7	1.4	0.6	0.5	0.3
N	34	12	55	58	159
Classes II and III					
Mean score	4.9	5.3	5.1	4.3	4.8
S.E.	0.4	0.4	0.3	0.3	0.2
N	115	106	211	196	628

3. Durkheim E. Suicide. A study in sociology. London: Routledge and Kegan Paul, 1970:104-122.
4. Silverman C. The epidemiology of depression. Baltimore: Johns Hopkins University Press, 1968:62-66.
5. Näyhä S. Autumn incidence of suicides re-examined: data from Finland by age, sex and occupation. Br J Psychiatry 1982; 141:512-517.
6. Näyhä S. Autumn and suicide in northern Finland. Arct Med Res Rep 1984; 37:25-29.
7. Goldberg DP. The detection of psychiatric illness by questionnaire. London: Oxford University Press, 1972.
8. Central Statistical Office of Finland: Population Census 1970: Occupation and social position. Official statistics of Finland VI C:104, vol. IX. Helsinki: State Printing Office, 1974.
9. Guenther WC. Analysis of variance. New Jersey: Prentice Hall, 1964:143-166.

Simo Näyhä
Department of Public Health Science
University of Oulu
Kajanintie 46E
SF-90220 Oulu 22
Finland

Circumpolar Health 84:316-319

PSYCHOLOGICAL AND CULTURAL PERSPECTIVES ON ARCTIC HYSTERIA AMONG THE SKOLT LAPPS

LEILA SEITAMO

INTRODUCTION

In the course of my studies among Skolt Lapp children and their parents in the years 1967-70, parents occasionally reported behavior among older people of their society that suggested the condition known as arctic hysteria. Some of the parents, for example, told of the grandmother in the family who "was the sort of person who is easily startled." The phenomenon seemed important for many reasons: it was interesting in itself, it had an impact on child development and could be used as an indicator of frustrations and behavior patterns typical of the traditional Skolt culture. Thus my basis for studying "startle-behavior" arose from field work among a normal population, not from clinical practice. This source has influenced my approach to study of arctic hysteria.

Little attention has been given in the literature to detailed description or analysis of the immediate stimuli which evoke hysteric attacks or to verbal interpretations of these factors offered by the affected person. Foulks' (1) review of the literature illustrates my point. The occasional reports by Skolt parents that I received and the more intensive interviews that I made about Skolt culture directed my attention to the significance of these factors:

- the typical traits of arctic hysteria attacks among the Skolt Lapps;
- typical events and stimuli which evoke hysteric attacks, and perception and interpretation of these stimuli; and
- psychological and cultural aspects in the development of arctic hysteria.

The theoretical context is based on integration of cognitive-behavioral and dynamic theories. The biological aspects of arctic hysteria are not considered here.

The Skolt Lapps

The Skolt Lapps are one of the three Lappish tribes living in northern Finland. After the Second World War the Skolts living in the western part of the Kola Peninsula were evacuated and later resettled by the Finnish government in the Sevettijärvi and Nellim area of Finland, the others remaining in the Kola Peninsula in the Soviet Union. These changes divided the Skolt tribe between two nations, about 700 of them in Finland (500 in Sevettijärvi, 200 in Nellim)

and the majority (about 2,000) remaining in the Soviet Union.

The traditional economy of the Skolt Lapps was fishing, hunting, gathering, and raising reindeer. This tradition sent the man into the woods but tied the woman to her home with the main responsibility for the household and the children. The women also participated in the raising of reindeer, and looked after fishing near the home. After the Second World War, the economic basis of the community changed such that traditional means of livelihood no longer assured a decent living. Temporary employment, frequently at a distance from the homes has become necessary for the men. During the main study (1967-74) both men and women appeared dissatisfied with being Skolts, the least prestigious minority group in northern Finland, characterized by old traditions and a different language. In recent years acculturation has progressed, leading to major changes in the Skolts' lifestyles (2,3).

METHODS

The data are based on semi-structured interviews about Skolt culture carried out among nearly all adult Skolt Lapps living in Finland in the years 1970-74, and in part again in 1980-84, and on participant observation. The most important data were interviews of those suffering from arctic hysteria and their family members. In the interviews I tried to elicit the Skolts' own spontaneous views and their interpretations of events and their causes (2,3).

In the years 1970-74, six women and one man living in Sevettijärvi and three women in the Nellim area were reported as being easily startled. Because the most severely disturbed Skolts were considered to need permanent hospital care, and are not included here, this sample is the non-clinical segment of the group. Five of the women in Sevettijärvi themselves explained their startle experiences, although some of them did so only briefly. Family members or other Skolts added accounts of their own or others' experiences in the startle situations.

RESULTS

In the interviews the Skolts described the attacks of arctic hysteria, "startling" --in the Skolt Lappish language "keavmus" --as follows: When suddenly startled by a precipitate event, if a person is sitting, he or she jumps up, hopping, dancing, and prancing on the spot, being in an hypnosis-like state, with a piercing but unseeing look, talking so fast that it is hard to understand, often uttering erotic or obscene words, or cursing. He or she may attack those present or the person causing the startle reaction, grabbing whatever happens to be at hand and striking with it. Such an individual possesses unbelievable strength. The person may run in the wilds for hours and imitate birds until exhausted, or may tear off clothing. The attack lasts from a few minutes to an hour or more. Some may experience an attack every day or two, and in one day there may be several seizures. Usually the attack ends with a cough; the person then commonly laughs and asks what he or she has been babbling about and says that he or she remembers nothing, or has a bizarre perception of what has happened. Others present may have an influence on the duration of the attack, for example, by directing the person's attention upward and saying "look at that," or by throwing something for the person to catch. The affected person often remembers what the triggering event or object was, but the explanation which he or she offers is most often "an interpretation."

Arctic hysteria occurs in Skolt females more often than in males, especially during the late teens. Both Skolt men and women believed that there were both genuine attacks and attack-like behavior used intentionally in social situations. The men often doubted whether some of the attacks in the women were genuine. In interviews, women were angered by men's suspicions, saying that it was just men's nonsense to doubt the authenticity of women's attacks. During participant observation it became clear that for the boys and young men, startling those who were supposedly prone to startle reactions was often an amusement which they exploited when there was nothing better to do.

In comparing the traits of arctic hysteria among the Skolt Lapps to the imitative and frenzied types of arctic hysteria among the Eskimos and other Arctic people reviewed by Foulks (1), Parker (4), and Yap (5), we can find many similarities between them.

Case Examples

-- A widow, aged 70 years, is startled daily or more often by quite minor happenings. If something falls to the floor or if a needle pricks her finger, she jumps up, with piercing eyes, utters erotic words and obscenities, then coughs and the attack is over. She often asks, ashamed, what she has been babbling about. Few other Skolts know that she startles, because she doesn't run outdoors. The grandchildren deplore her

behavior and often ask her why she talks so rudely. She says that she doesn't remember what she has said and cannot help talking as she does. When I was interviewing her in the health center she accidentally kicked a pail, was startled by it, jumped up, and was on the point of saying something but then looked at me and laughed. I conclude that her attacks are at least sometimes partly conscious. She has lost many of her closest family and began to be startled since that time. She is a very intelligent woman.

-- A married woman, about 60 years old, is often severely startled. Once in the woods she was frightened by a white ptarmigan that suddenly took off in flight. She threw down her knapsack, ran after the bird, flapping her arms like its wings and imitating its noises and in that way fleeing far into the woods until she was exhausted. Afterwards her husband told her (while she was in a startled state) not to shed her knapsack when she is startled. Since then she has not done so. This family represents the traditional lifestyle. Some old Skolt men have suspected that her husband is a shaman, coming to this conclusion from the fact that "he is able to eat so much: a whole kettle of fish; a normal man can't do that".

-- A widow, about 70 years of age, was frightened by a bear. She ripped off all her clothing and her rings and earrings and threw them one after another onto the moorland towards the bear, then ran home saying that she had met a gentlemen on the moor and though she had thrown him everything she had, the man had not gone away. The woman could not remember where her clothing was. Family members startled her again, and made her show them where her startle had happened. In that state she was able to recover her possessions.

-- A woman, about 60 years old, was in a small boat on a lake, when thunder and lightning broke out. The woman was startled, agitated, and began furiously to hew at the boat with an axe.

-- A woman of about 60 years was cooking when a man with sunglasses entered the house. The woman, startled, took a knife and ran after him trying to seize him. Afterwards, she told her family that a devil had come there but that she had succeeded in driving it away.

DISCUSSION - INTERPRETATION

In the attacks described, and also in many other cases, perception and discrimination of the events and objects which evoked the attacks were diffuse. The expressed or obvious interpretations of these events and the related behavior were thoroughly inadequate at first glance. An analysis of their content, however, reveals possible cultural

meaning in situations of fright or frustration. In some cases mastery of the startle
situation may also reflect traditional
beliefs of the culture.

A bird had an important meaning in the
traditional beliefs of the Skolt Lapps. It
could be a shaman or his assistant. In the
old culture, a shaman was both valued and
feared. "Fleeing like a bird" was naturally
a suggestive behavior pattern typical of the
startled states, imitation of a powerful
model in a hypnotic state. According to the
hypotheses of Parker (4) and Foulks (1),
attacks of arctic hysteria may have their
roots in the shamanistic behavior tradition.
Imitative behavior of this kind could imply
a shamanistic component, and mastery of the
fear of a powerful shaman by identification
with it and behaving accordingly.

Thunder was a heathen god, "Tiermes" or
"Ilias Morovits" who drove his wagon across
the sky, the sparks from the wheels being
the lightning. A traditional Skolt belief
says that you are safe if you have a piece
of wood while it is thundering. Hewing at
the little wooden boat in the case above
could be understood, despite its hysterical
nature, as adequate behavior in the reality
of this traditional world. A devil, who was
extremely feared, had an important role in
the Skolts' belief system. A bear was the
totem animal in the traditional nature-
religion of the Skolt Lapps and is the
subject of beliefs and stories. A bear
could be a man, and a man could take the
form of a bear by carrying out some ceremo-
nial movements. Seeing the bear as a man
links these stories and beliefs in the sense
that either one may represent the other.
Confusion of the feared objects becomes
still more complicated by the fact that in
the wilds strangers may pose a sexual
threat.

In spite of the changes taking place in
the Skolt traditions, belief in old traditions was still alive at the time of the
main study. Fear of the supernatural was
still high among both the adults and the
children, reflected also in people's night-
mares (2,3). On the basis of the cognitive
-behavioral theories (6) we can assume that
anticipation of a threat by supernatural
beings affected the intensity of becoming
frightened, on confusion of the perception,
and on the interpretation of the images of
the anticipated threat. In the cases
described, the content of the perceptions
and interpretations of the stimuli could
have some of the same qualities as those of
the objective immediate stimuli: generalization caused these stimuli to work as conditioned stimuli for becoming frightened. On
the basis of content analysis, behavior in
the startled state could be understood as
implying elements of mastery of the threat
learned in the Skolt culture.

Social Nature of Arctic Hysteria

In interviews of the Skolt Lapps I
learned how the startle attacks developed,
and may have been reinforced. Some claimed
that this behavior is learned. At first a
person may act startled on purpose when
getting very angry with someone. Over time
the startle response becomes both more
intensive, deeper, and finally "real."
Therefore, people used to warn others not to
begin to get startled. The following
aspects were emphasized as the most important antecedent factors in startle behavior:

- the importance of traditional
  beliefs, startling, and affectionate teasing in upbringing and
  social life, including sexual
  stimulation and play;
- ambivalence of female status and
  role; and
- periods of high sensitivity to
  psychic disturbances.

The explanations of the Skolts about
their upbringing were in accordance with my
earlier studies (2,3); although love and
indulgence had traditionally been the basis
of child-rearing among the Skolt Lapps,
control over aggressive behavior had been
and still was quite severe. At around the
age of 5 years, traditional beliefs and
traditional stories were used as a means of
controlling the child's behavior. In the
years 1967-74 this practice was partly
conscious and intentional and partly based
on the parents' genuine beliefs. It is
evident that fear of traditional beliefs was
instilled in this period of childhood.
Startling and affectionate teasing has been
very common in social intercourse. Warm
emotion, joking, and merry-making have been
the basis for social communication and also
for startling and affectionate teasing of
the women. Coming up behind a woman and
suddenly jabbing her in the sides with one's
fingers is very common. Some of the Skolts
were of the opinion that this kind of
behavior was very important for the development of startling and of uttering erotic
words during a startling attack. The lower
status and value of women and the sanctions
connected with sexuality restricted and
bound the woman more than the man (3). In
the traditional culture the only occasion
when a woman was allowed to speak about
sexual matters would be during an attack, at
which time she was not responsible for her
behavior. It is clear that part of the
frenzied behavior toward men during an
attack has had its roots in the imbalance
between the male and female roles. At the
same time it may represent the expression of
a sexual wish and the prohibitions against
this wish as Foulks (1) has also suggested

(p. 116). In this sense startling seems to have a functional meaning.

The Skolts were wary of the serious consequences of startling during periods of high sensitivity caused by accidents, losses, or other drastic occurrences. Friends will often protect an especially vulnerable person, by warning others not to startle or tease him or her during a crisis period. They believe that this protection can prevent serious cases of mental disturbance.

In summary, it seems that startling behavior among the Skolt Lapps may be regarded as a social institution having both positive and negative qualities and consequences, with roots deep in the traditional culture. As the Skolts' lifestyles change, the startling phenomenon seems to be disappearing.

REFERENCES

1. Foulks EF. The arctic hysterics of the north Alaskan Eskimo. Anthropological Studies. No 10. Maybury-Lewis D. ed. Washington, DC: Amer Anthrop Ass'n, 1972.

2. Seitamo L. Vulnerability of children from minority groups: scholastic learning problems of Skolt Lapp children. In: Anthony EJ, Koupernik C, Chiland C, eds. The child in his family. Vulnerable children, vol 4. New York, Wiley: 1978.

3. Seitamo L. Development of the role of Skolt women. In: Harvald B, Hart Hansen JP, eds. Circumpolar Health 81. Nordic Council Arct Med Res Rep 1982; 33:464-466.

4. Parker S. Eskimo psychopathology. Amer Anthr 1962; 64:74-76.

5. Yap P. The Latah reaction: Its psychodynamics and nosological position. J Ment Sci 1952; 98:515-562.

6. Bandura A. Self-efficacy: Toward unifying theory of behavioral change. Psych Rev 1977; 84:191-215.

Leila Seitamo
Sepänkatu 6 as 12
90100 Oulu 10
Finland

Circumpolar Health 84:320-321

SOCIAL ENVIRONMENT, PERSONALITY STRUCTURE AND SCHOOL AVOIDANCE:
A STUDY IN A NORTH FINNISH RURAL DISTRICT

HARRIET FORSIUS, EEVA-RIITTA KOKKONEN and PAIVI HIRVONEN

School avoidance either in the form of real school phobia or of truancy has been a problem of increasing frequency in northern Finland.

The purpose of this study is to assess the frequency of school absence without physical disease, to get a picture of the student who has difficulties in attending school regularly, his personality characteristics and his social background. Factors generally affecting a child's school attendance are shown in Figure 1.

METHODS

A rural district about 20 km northeast of the university town of Oulu was chosen for this investigation because the school system there consists of four small isolated schools and two larger ones (Figure 2).

Together with the teachers, all of the 1,023 pupils in these six schools were considered. Those pupils who had many absentee days or many scattered absentee hours without any signs of somatic disease formed the study group. For each pupil in the study group, the child following in alphabetical order who was of the same sex and in the same class, was chosen as a control. In both the study group and

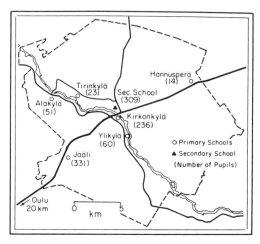

Figure 2. Map of Kiiminki Commune, Finland, showing school locations.

control group there were 21 boys and 10 girls. The ages ranged from 8.3-16.3 years, with a mean age of 12.8 years.

The absentee percentage in the large secondary school was 5.2%, in the large primary school with classes I-VI it was 1.6% and in the small schools it was 4.0%, for an

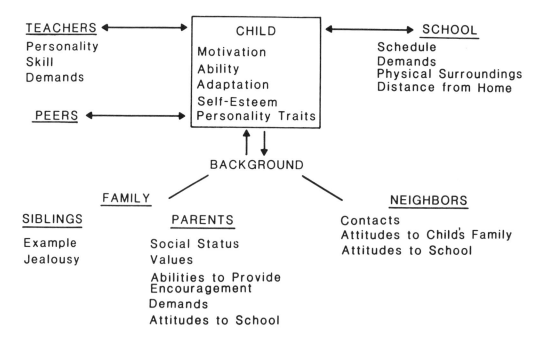

Figure 1. Factors generally affecting the child's school attendance.

average of 3.0%. The parents were personally interviewed by a physician with child-psychiatry experience.

The children were physically examined and for evaluation of their personality traits they were given the Rorschach Personality Test, the Ego-Picture Invention and the Sentence Completion Test. For assessment of their IQ capacity they were asked to perform the verbal part of the WISC test, the Bender Test and to draw a man according to Goodenough. The teachers' assessment of the children was included by questionnaire. The school, teachers, and the peers were the same for the children in the study group and the control group. Thus the reasons for absence from school were found in the family background and in the personality characteristics and abilities of the child.

RESULTS AND DISCUSSION

The family background of the children in the study group was significantly more unstable and there were more problems within the family (for example, chronic illness, alcohol problems, economic problems, child neglect) than in the families of the control group (Table 1). The differences in the family's abilities to interact in cooperative actions is shown in Table 2.

Table 1. Comparison of family conditions between students (study group) and controls.

	Study(%)	Control(%)	P
"Biological" family	64.5	80.6	
Parents divorced	32.3	9.7	<0.05
Severe problems in family	74.2	29.0	<0.001

Table 2. Comparison of family interactions between frequently absent students (study group) and controls.

	Study(%)	Control(%)	P
Disagreements often:			
on economic matters	25.9	6.5	<0.05
on other subjects	16.1	-	<0.02
Disagreements often solved	51.6	80.6	<0.05

Table 3. Comparison of progress in school and IQ between frequently absent students (study group) and controls.

	Study(%)	Control(%)	P
Average grade	7.0	7.2	NS
Time spent on homework:			
half hour	29.0	9.7	<0.01
one hour	29.0	42.0	<0.01
IQ (WISC, verbal part)	105.8	103.0	NS

There were no differences between the study group and the control group concerning signs of minimal brain dysfunction or other neurological disorders, nor in school records or IQ (Table 3).

Rated by teachers and parents, however, the study group was found to be more bad-tempered, aggressive, "nervous," depressed, listless, untidy, having more difficulties in making friends, and having less motivation for schoolwork, than the controls.

The psychological tests revealed that the children in the study group had weak self-esteem. They also had difficulties in making contacts with others and had signs of high anxiety. Every child in the study group was in need of supportive psychotherapy and in 30% of the cases there was a need for intensive psychotherapy. Thus it can be concluded that sociocultural factors, above all a stable family background which supports the child's self esteem and provides motivation for schoolwork, are important for the child's regular school attendance. To find the potential "risk families" and intensify the cooperation between the school and the home in such cases, ought to be one of the most important preventive tasks in the mental health care of schoolchildren.

Harriet Forsius
University of Oulu
Department of Pediatrics
90220 Oulu
Finland

Circumpolar Health 84:322-326

ALCOHOL-RELATED HEALTH PROBLEMS IN ALASKA--PREVENTIVE STRATEGIES

BILL RICHARDS

INTRODUCTION

A national plan for prevention of alcohol misuse has been developed in the U.S. over the past 5 years. In 1979, the first Surgeon General's report on health promotion and disease prevention, entitled "Healthy People," was issued (1). It set broad national goals for a number of conditions, including alcohol misuse, calling for reductions in overall death rates and in days of disability. In 1980, a follow-up report, titled "Promoting Health/Preventing Disease-Objectives for the nation" set out specific objectives to be reached by the year 1990 for high priority health problems, including alcohol misuse (2). Progress on the national alcohol misuse prevention objectives has recently been summarized (3).

This paper presents a brief overview of emerging trends in Alaska in alcohol misuse prevention programming. This may be of interest to other circumpolar countries facing high rates of alcohol-related problems.

INDICATOR CONDITIONS AND SPECIFIC TARGETS

How best to prevent alcohol misuse has been a subject of considerable debate. Is the problem basically a legal one, educational, or a social and health problem? Which agency should play the lead? How can one measure results?

The basic strategy proposed in the national plan, which is beginning to be incorporated into Alaska programming, involves the selection of a number of target indicator conditions for monitoring. Rather than selecting a single type of indicator that might measure only one dimension to the problem, several indicators are used. Baseline rates for these indicators are then established, as well as target rates to be reached by 1990. Multiple agencies are involved.

The indicators include measures of:

1. Per capita alcohol consumption
2. Drinking behavior of particular target groups such as adolescents and women of child-bearing age.
3. Mortality from cirrhosis, and from alcohol-related motor vehicle accidents.
4. Education of adults on the risk of head and neck cancers associated with excessive alcohol consumption.
5. Availability of employee assistance programs.

These particular indicators were chosen because available evidence suggests that prevention programs may have a better chance of demonstrating success on these specific types of problems. (For example, fetal alcohol syndrome can be prevented if mothers do not drink during their pregnancies, etc.) Table 1 summarizes the national prevention objectives for alcohol misuse, U.S. baseline rates, and 1990 targets (3).

Alaska's rate of per capita alcohol consumption has fluctuated in a range of 3.72 to 4.64 gallons of absolute alcohol per year over the past 10 years (for those 14 years and older). This is about double the national average. The rate as of 1982 was 4.58 gallons per capita (4).

Going along with these high consumption rates are more severe alcohol-related problems as measured by the national prevention indicators. For example, national high school surveys indicate the proportion of adolescents age 12 to 17 who abstain to be 68.8% (3). A school survey in Alaska showed that for grades 7-9, (ages 12-14), 45% of a sample of 639 reported abstaining from any drink in the past year (9). For grades 10-12 (ages 15-17), only 22.5% of a sample of 701 reported abstaining. For the total sample of 1,340 students aged 12-17, 447 or 33% were abstainers. Motor vehicle fatalities, as another example, run about 10 to 20 per 100,000 for alcohol-related accidents, compared to the national rate of 11.5 per 100,000 (5,8). Between 48 and 73% of fatal driving accidents in Alaska over the past 5 years have involved alcohol, according to figures from the Highway Traffic Safety Agency (5). Detailed information is being assembled to monitor each of the national indicators for Alaska. Considerable work remains to be done, however, to establish reasons for apparent differences in indicator rates for different sub-populations within Alaska, and to set up systematic procedures for collecting data.

ALASKA'S PREVENTION STRATEGIES

Measures to decrease alcohol availability and consumption, as well as measures to reach specific target groups such as adolescents, mothers of child-bearing age, and drunk drivers, have evolved. There have also been many attempts to promote alternatives to drinking, and build support systems to encourage non-drinking behavior. These will be discussed under the headings of legislative and regulatory measures, public information and education programs, and community and cultural programs. In addition, measures to increase early intervention and improve direct services will be mentioned. Since a number of interventions are being made simultaneously, it is difficult to pinpoint the effectiveness of any single intervention. Assuming the overall approach works, however, documentation of success by monitoring progress towards the 1990 target objectives should be possible.

Table 2 summarizes in outline form some of the major efforts to prevent alcohol misuse currently taking place in Alaska. Brief comments about some of the more innovative efforts follow, with some key references for readers interested in details about particular projects.

Legislative and Regulatory Measures

Alaska has taken a number of legal steps to make access to alcohol more difficult, and to affect specific target groups such as adolescent drinkers and drunk drivers. As Table 2 indicates, these have included limiting bar hours, raising the legal drinking age from 19 to 21, tougher penalties for drunk drivers etc.

One of the more interesting developments has been enactment of a state-wide "local law option," which began in 1981. This allows unincorporated communities, of which there are many in rural Alaska, three

Table 1. National prevention objectives for alcohol misuse: U.S. baseline data and 1990 targets.

Objective	U.S. Baseline	1990 Target
1. Stabilize per capita consumption of alcohol	2.82 gallons of alcohol per capita per year (for those aged 14 or older)	2.82 gallons of alcohol per capita per year
2. Maintain proportion of adolescents 12 to 17 years old who abstain	68.8%	68.8%
3. Increase education of women of child-bearing age regarding fetal alcohol syndrome (FAS)	73%	90%
4. Reduce incidence of FAS births	1/2,000	1/2,500
5. Reduce cirrhosis mortality	13.8/100,000	12/100,000
6. Reduce fatalities from alcohol-related motor vehicle accidents	11.5/100,000	9.5/100,000
7. Educate adults of risk of head and neck cancers associated with excessive alcohol consumption	unavailable	75%
8. Expand employee assistance programs	57%	70%
9. Establish comprehensive data capability for monitoring and evaluating status and effects of alcohol misuse	-	-

options: selling liquor only with a selected liquor license, stopping sale of alcoholic beverages, and stopping both sale and
importation of alcoholic beverages. Municipalities have an additional option under the
law of selling liquor only with a community
liquor license. Over 60 rural villages have
voted to ban both the sale and import of
alcoholic beverages under this law. Evaluation of the longer range effects of this
form of prohibition will be interesting,
since the isolation of some of the villages
allows for enforcement of the law in a way
that would be difficult in communities where
alcohol could be smuggled in more easily
(7).

Public Information and Education Programs

Besides the ordinary kinds of public
awareness campaigns, there are several
special projects being undertaken in Alaska
to influence adolescent drinking behavior
that might be unfamiliar to readers from
other circumpolar countries and thus worthy
of special mention.

A special school curriculum called
"Here's Looking At You" began in 1976, and
was implemented statewide in 1979 (9). This
includes a formal curriculum for grades
kindergarten through 12 and an in-service
teacher training workshop. The curriculum
consists of a teacher's instructional guide
and accompanying kits for teacher aides.
The guide is a specific manual of teaching
activities and projects covering 15 hours of
class work at each grade level. The kits
include films, charts, instructional games,
and puppets.

"The Chemical People" project is
another major public education effort.
Alaska has held over 150 town meetings
during the past year in various communities,
to listen to materials developed nationally
dealing with school age alcohol and drug
abuse, and then form local task forces to
work on prevention projects. Projects
include alternatives to drinking such as
building of youth recreation centers.

Special health education kits for
pregnant women have been developed to
promote the idea that "Your Baby Deserves
The Best" and therefore that the mother
should avoid drinking. Regional workshops
on fetal alcohol syndrome are raising
awareness of this condition.

Table 2. Summary of strategies used in Alaska for prevention of alcohol misuse.

I. Measures to decrease alcohol availability and consumption and promote alternatives

    A. Legislative and regulatory measures

"Local Option" laws, decreasing hours that bars are open, limiting new liquor licenses,
restricted advertising for alcohol products, toughening drunk driving laws with increased
jail sentences, fines, and period of driver's license revocation for persons convicted of
driving while intoxicated by alcohol safety action program, pre-arrest breath-taking
devices, stricter enforcement of laws on serving minors, raising drinking age from 19 to
21.

    B. Public information and education programs

"Here's Looking At You" school curriculum, community based public education programs
developed by Alaska Council on Prevention of Alcoholism and Drug Abuse, "Chemical People"
projects, teleconferences.

    C. Community and cultural programs

Citizen activist groups (Mothers Against Drunk Driving, Students Against Driving Drunk,
parent groups), Town Meetings, "Youth Centers" and other alternative recreation projects
including village level, village elders' projects, promotion of traditional cultural
values.

II. Measures To Increase Early Intervention and Improve Quantity, Quality, and Availability of Direct Services

Increasing use of Village Counselors and regionalized, decentralized community programs,
statewide management information system to improve program monitoring used by federal as
well as state programs training certification system including regional trainers, more
systematic use of program standards and evaluations, programs targeted for specific groups,
jointly funded state-federal-regional health corporation coordinated projects.

Remote communities are also making increasing use of teleconferencing for health education and alcohol program planning activities, to decrease the high costs of travel to distant meeting sites.

Community and Cultural Programs

A variety of interesting approaches are being developed. Citizen activist groups such as "Mothers Against Drunk Driving" (MADD) have been influential in getting tougher legislation against drunk drivers. Alaska Native communities are making active use of village elders as role models for younger Natives, promoting traditional cultural values in a variety of ways. It is believed that a more positive self-image will make problem drinking less likely. Efforts along these lines include Elders' Workshops on traditional ways of coping with problems and traditional values considered still useful today; special days in schools where Native dancing, games, and foods are studied; tribal doctors programs; documenting of successes of older Native people by biographies; and promotion of continued use of Native languages. Reference 10 gives a review of one regional health organization's program where there is an emphasis on cultural values of this type. Another development has been the spread of programs similar to Alcoholics Anonymous but adapted for rural areas and different cultural groups such as the "Villager to Villager" self help program (11).

Measures to Improve Direct Services

Efforts to upgrade secondary and tertiary prevention services are also developing, as outlined in Table 2. An especially interesting one is the "village counselor." There are approximately 200 communities in Alaska, widely scattered geographically, many with small populations of fewer than 300 people. It is often a considerable distance to the nearest larger community where a fuller range of alcohol treatment services is available. There has been a village Community Health Aide program in Alaska for some time (12). Primary care is given by these village health workers, who receive training in how to handle common medical problems, and have a back-up system with itinerant public health nurses, and call-in procedures to reach the nearest hospital. In the past few years a new role seems to be evolving, that of a village worker in addition to the Health Aide who focuses more on behavioral problems. About 100 communities now have Village Alcohol Counselors, and a statewide certification system, with regional trainers, is developing. These counselors carry out brief counseling and aftercare services for problem drinkers, and serve as staff for community prevention activities developed by the village.

SUMMARY

This brief overview of Alaska's prevention programs for alcohol misuse may aid readers from other circumpolar countries who wish to become familiar with the overall context when reading reports on specific Alaska projects.

Emerging trends which have been reviewed include:

1. Development of a national plan with specific long-range prevention objectives for alcohol misuse,
2. Monitoring of rates for indicator conditions associated with each objective,
3. More precise targeting of specific high risk groups for prevention efforts, such as drinking women of child-bearing age and adolescents,
4. Multi-agency approaches including a mixture of legislative and regulatory reforms, public information and education programs, community and cultural programs, and improvements in existing direct services.

REFERENCES

1. Healthy people. The Surgeon General's report on health promotion and disease prevention 1979. U.S. Department of Health, Education, and Welfare, Public Health Service, DHEW (PHS) Publication No. 79-55071.
2. Promoting health/preventing disease. Objectives for the nation. U.S. Department of Health and Human Services, Washington Government Printing Office, 1980.
3. Segal M, Palsgrove G, Sevy T, Collins T. The 1990 prevention objectives for alcohol and drug misuse: Progress report. Public Health Reports 1983; 98:426-435.
4. Malin HJ, Munch NE, Archer LD. A national surveillance system of alcoholism and drug abuse. 32nd International Congress on Alcoholism and Drug Dependence. Warsaw, Poland. September 1978.
5. The Alaska State Alcoholism and Drug Abuse Plan, 1981-1983. Juneau: State of Alaska Office of Alcoholism and Drug Abuse.
6. Alaska Area Native Health Service long range objectives FY 1984. Anchorage, Alaska.
7. Lonner TD, Duff JK. Village alcohol control and the Local Option Law. A

report to the State Legislature. Center for Alcohol and Addiction Studies. University of Alaska, Anchorage, 1983.

8. Kelso D. Anchorage alcohol safety action program: client outcome evaluation. Alaska Highway Safety Planning Agency, Department of Public Safety, 1980.

9. Pieper, L. An evaluation of the statewide alcohol education project, effectiveness of the "Here's Looking At You" alcohol education curriculum. Alaska Council of Prevention of Alcohol and Drug Abuse, 1983.

10. 1983 Annual report and directory of services. Kotzebue, Alaska: The Maniilaq Association, 1983.

11. Mendenhall N, Thomas D. Self-help manual for organization, development, and operation of a rural Alaskan village alcohol action committee. Nome, Alaska: Norton Sound Health Corporation, April 1983. (Mimeo.)

12. Guidelines for primary health care in rural Alaska. U.S. Department of Health, Education and Welfare, Health Services Administration, Indian Health Service, Alaska Area Native Health Service, 1976.

Bill Richards
Alaska Area Native Health Service
P.O. Box 7-741
Anchorage, Alaska 99510
U.S.A.

Circumpolar Health 84:327-331

ALCOHOL: AVAILABILITY AND ABUSE

C. EARL ALBRECHT

Easy access to alcohol followed by a high per capita consumption usually leads to drunkenness, abusiveness, violence, crime, and premature death. Alcohol when used excessively also creates social, health, law enforcement, and judicial problems that in combination are extraordinarily costly. Beyond this, those associated with the alcohol abuser suffer personally to a marked degree. Alcohol also continues to be a major contributing factor in traffic accidents and highway-related fatalities.

For these reasons much attention is being and should be devoted to measures that will control these serious problems. They should include education, counselling, prevention, intervention, and treatment.

The most immediate and certainly long-range means of reversing all the problems associated with the abuse of alcohol is reducing its availability to the consumer. Nine approaches will be suggested, each of which if implemented could reduce the ready availability of alcohol to some degree. Certain approaches are more effective than others in different settings over Alaska as well as in other circumpolar regions; therefore, each region and community must implement the control measure that would be most useful.

Probably the most obvious control measure is to decrease the number of retail outlets and convenience liquor stores. Outlets are places where alcohol can be bought by the general public. Alaska is a "license" state (1,2). That is, there are privately owned liquor stores licensed by the state for distribution of alcoholic beverages, rather than a "control" state in which there are government-owned liquor stores. This has led to the licensing of a great many outlets to such an extent that in Alaska there is one outlet for every 330 people, or roughly double the U.S. average. This availability has certainly contributed to Alaska's relatively high per capita consumption of alcohol beverages (3,4) which is 45.8 U.S. gallons (166 liters) annually including beer, wine, and spirits, or 5.1 gallons (18.5 liters) of absolute ethyl alcohol. This level of intake is roughly twice the per capita intake of the rest of the United States. This high ratio of outlets, according to authorities, increases the alcohol-related problems. Thus a reduction in the number of outlets can, to some degree, reduce the ready availability.

A second step to lower the high per capita consumption is to reduce the total hours of retail sales. Alaska law permits outlets to be open for the public 21 hours daily, thus making alcoholic beverages available for very long periods of time. This contributes to drinking in excessive amounts since it not only permits the alcoholic to drink early in the day, but also for many hours into the night. It is during these hours that most alcohol-related crime takes place and traffic violations occur. Fortunately, Alaska Statutes permit municipalities to set bar hours and several have reduced the hours during which bars can be open. Juneau police found their alcohol-related police calls decreased 27% from 7 p.m. to 7 a.m. after open hours were reduced. Anchorage recently by a 3 to 2 popular vote shortened the hours of open bars.

A controversial means for controlling alcohol abuse that has been advocated is to place a legal responsibility upon the bartender or retailer who sells alcoholic beverages to already intoxicated individuals. In fact, efforts have been made to sue those who made the sale to persons who later were arrested for "driving under the influence" and who were involved in a fatal highway accident. How effective this approach can be will be determined by the courts and by societal attitudes, one of which too commonly is that it's acceptable to drink and get drunk. At cocktail parties, hosts take no responsibility for consequences which may result from guests drinking too much.

Many of us can look to the successful Scandinavian example for attitudes about drinking and driving. There the hosts literally determine if a drinking person is driving home. If he is, the host will either gently take the drink away and arrange another way home, or take the person's car keys away. There the societal value is for the host and friends to assume some responsibility when a person drinks too much. Furthermore, Scandinavian laws are very strict and the police and courts effectively use them. The use of law can help reduce the irresponsible use of alcohol and is an important tool in its control.

The people of the circumpolar areas of the world have some distinctly special situations when drinking leads to severe intoxication. The most serious of these is the harsh freezing climate that has often destroyed the life of an inebriated person. Here then, the sale of alcohol to an inebriated person becomes all the more reason for a legal responsibility to be placed on the bartender for the death of such persons.

Another significant change occurring among northern populations is the migration into larger centers where they must make many adjustments. This marked change in environment and way of life is a cultural shock for many and results in difficult societal change. Not only is there migration into the municipalities, but in the rural areas there is increasing travel to the "rural cities" or "hubs" for many good purposes. While most Native people find this useful and helpful, there are those who drink excessively because alcoholic beverages are readily available. This creates more problems for these centers, since drunkenness often leads to serious incidents, crime, and prison. It has been said that when villages have used the local option law to ban importation of alcohol, the rural city for the area gets more problems because some persons go there to drink and often do so to "get drunk." Here again a responsibility seems to rest upon the retailer of alcoholic beverages.

With the migration to the larger communities such as Anchorage, Fairbanks, Godthåb, and Copenhagen, problems often arise. In Anchorage, for example, records show that many crimes and accidents occur as a result of excessive alcohol consumption.

Copenhagen has also experienced many problems with Greenlanders who have migrated 2,500 miles. They experienced for many reasons a jolting cultural shock and as Lars Petersen of the Greenland House in Copenhagen explained, "The reality was that the young people couldn't handle the shock of the culture, the climate and the freedom of a modern city." Many of them fell into alcoholism and drug abuse. Another authority, Nils Grann, who heads the Greenlander section of Kofoed-Hus, a clinic that offers social services and treatment to alcoholics, said, "In fact Greenlanders are not genuine alcoholics, but more like situational alcoholics. If we can get them back to Greenland, the drinkers may stop completely."

Some communities recognize responsibility to the alcoholic who becomes intoxicated and have arranged for such persons to be placed in protective custody to prevent their consuming amounts that will lead to acts of violence, crime, or greater injury to themselves. This plan reduces the total amount consumed and at least for the incident, prevents a bad situation from developing. In Bethel, Alaska, a group of citizens concerned originally about inebriated citizens in the coming winter months have incorporated as the "Helping Hand" to open a 24 hour walk-in human shelter. Such facilities are essential because they not only provide physical protection but also prevent the intoxicated person from consuming excessive amounts. Some communities have patrols that pick up intoxicated individuals from bars or from public places and streets to forestall excessive drinking and for self-protection. This service not only saves lives but curbs the development of crime and behavioral problems.

Increasingly, a greater responsibility will be placed upon the retailer and the bartender in controlling the availability of alcohol to intoxicated customers, habitual drunkards, and to persons under the legal age of drinking. Violations need to be enforced by prosecuting the underaged who make purchases and the retail dealer involved. In Alaska the new law establishes the legal drinking age at 21 but permits those presently at age 19 and 20 to make purchases. The identification of youth becomes very important and certainly gives all retailers a difficult task but one that legally must be met.

Establishing the legal age for purchase and consumption of alcoholic beverages at 21 has gained momentum in recent years because of the great number of drinking young people that are involved in driving while intoxicated. Although most of Alaska is rural, the urban areas with more automobile traffic have experienced many fatal accidents when the driver was found to be operating the vehicle while intoxicated. The smaller municipalities surveyed urged that the legal purchase and drinking age be raised to 21 years. They all stressed the desirability for the Alaska State Legislature to enact such a law. As a result, this was achieved in 1983, providing one more tool toward reducing the ease of obtaining alcoholic beverages by the young.

Nationally, the President's Commission on Drunk Driving has proposed that Congress set a minimum legal drinking age of 21. They also recommended that a person with 0.08% alcohol concentration would be presumed to be driving under the influence, and would be found illegally drunk if tests showed a concentration of 0.10%. Whether this will become a national law is not known, but by December 1983, 19 states had enacted laws setting a minimum drinking age of 21.

Although there is some opposition to a minimum drinking age of 21 and there are complaints that it is difficult to enforce, it reduces the ease and permissiveness of drinking before age 21. There is evidence that drinking early in life frequently leads to abuse and development of health problems from alcoholism. In a recent editorial appearing in the New England Journal of Medicine (5), some very significant statements appear. For example:

Throughout the history of humanity, alcoholic beverages have been widely used for their pleasing taste and their mood-altering effects. However, the use of alcohol has evoked strong opposition, because of the potential for abuse and the associated adverse effects on safety and health. In large urban areas, one of the complications of alcohol abuse--cirrhosis. of the liver--is now the second most common of all deaths in the age group of 25 to 44 years and the third in the group 45 to 64.

Within the United States each state has the power to adopt laws concerning drunk drivers; therefore, there are no standard penalties for convictions. This creates some problems, particularly in communities near state borders where the two states have different legal age restrictions. Because of the great public outcry against the carnage on the highways in which drunk drivers frequently were involved, President Reagan established the Commission on Drunk Driving. The Commission's recommendations for uniform strict national penalties for drunken driving may be adopted, but in the meantime many states have put new or stricter laws on their books to discourage those under the influence of liquor from getting behind the wheel. In 1982, 33\states took such action and by 1983 all but 10 states had enacted measures. There is considerable variation in their content, as the following illustrations suggest: 1) mandatory 48-hour lock-up of drunk drivers upon their first arrest, 2) license revocation for different periods of time depending on several factors, 3) a 45-day sentence for second-time offenders in one state, 4) fines ranging from $500 to $2,500 and two-year license loss for second offenders, 5) third and subsequent drunken driving convictions, penalties not less than 120 days in jail, a $1,000 to $5,000 fine and three year license revocation.

Alaska has enacted state legislation which requires upon conviction for driving while legally intoxicated a mandatory jail sentence of varying lengths depending upon its being the first or second offense; license loss of different lengths; mandatory screening or treatment for first offenders; as well as other penalties depending upon the circumstances of the arrest.

That such measures are effective is shown by the evidence submitted by the national Highway Traffic Safety Administration which found that eight states which had raised their drinking age showed an average 28% annual reduction in night time fatal accidents involving drivers between the ages of 18 and 21.

Raising the excise tax on alcoholic beverages is not popular, but alcohol prices do affect how much people drink. The cheaper alcohol is, the more it is consumed. Alcohol prices nearly everywhere have increased at a slower rate than wages or the cost of living. Alaska had not raised the state excise tax in 25 years until recently; even then it was a very modest increase. Tax increases must be considered by state legislators and members of Congress as a means, though admittedly small, to curb

excessive drinking and simultaneously to increase revenue to help pay for the costs of alcohol education, treatment, and rehabilitation.

In 1981 the Alaska State Government passed an Alcohol Local Option Law for municipalities and unincorporated communities (villages) (6). The options for villages are: 1) to sell liquor only with a selected liquor license, 2) to stop the sale of alcoholic beverages, 3) to stop the sale and importation of alcoholic beverages. Municipalities had one more option, namely 4) to sell liquor only with a community liquor license. The latest statistics reveal that 68 communities have held location option elections, and 65 voted to ban the sale and importation of alcoholic beverages. Three villages have held second elections to reverse their first action.

With the enactment of the local option law, efforts have been made to measure the progress, influence, and effectiveness of the law in areas of Alaska. One report appeared in the Tundra Drums (weekly, Bethel, Alaska) during May and June, 1983, under the title, "The local option ordinance: two years later" by Richard Goldstein. Lt. Glenn Godfrey, Commander of the State Troopers having jurisdiction over an area encompassing the Yukon-Kuskokwim Delta in the south and the Kotzebue region in the north has categorically stated that the advent of local option elections has had a positive impact. According to the article,

> Godfrey said that the alcohol sale and importation ban adopted by 28 villages in the Delta has made liquor that much harder to obtain. He indicated that if villagers don't have easy access to liquor, they are much less likely to engage in the violent anti-social behavior that occasionally characterizes life in the Bush. He said that the fact that Bethel is a "dry" town has reinforced the village local option laws by making liquor even harder to get.

Two judges having jurisdiction over a large area of Alaska stated that the local option law adopted by a majority of the villages within their judicial areas is a mixed blessing. Each judge has noticed a marked decrease in the violent alcohol-related crimes that have plagued Bush Alaska. At the same time, however, each man has noted that the crime rate in their population centers--Nome and Kotzebue--has greatly increased.

"We're as wet as they get," said Judge Tunley about his hometown, Nome. He said that like Kotzebue, Nome has a number of bars and package liquor stores. As a consequence, he said, "there is no question that police contacts in Nome are up dramatically." Judge Tunley explained that those contacts are for the domestic violence and harassment offenses that very often accompany drunken behavior. "We do have bootlegging offenses in a lot of our dry villages," said Judge Jones, who added that the Troopers "have made pretty effective arrests...[but] it's still getting in."

Asked about their attitude to the local option law, both Judge Jones and Judge Tunley indicated that it was a village-based decision to go "dry." "It's the villages themselves that have made this determination," said Judge Tunley, and whether the law is effective or not is for each affected village to answer, he said.

Judge Jones noted that "people are trying to achieve something. The long range answer," he said, "is for people to deal with alcohol in a reasonable and not excessive manner."

Mr. Goldstein also interviewed the Director of the Phillips Alcoholism Treatment Center in Bethel who made several significant comments on the effect of communities voting no importation and no sale. He stated that it's giving the people a chance to take a breath so that local agencies can take advantage of the breathing spell and mobilize their forces at the local level to develop further alcoholism education and continuing counselling in the villages. Director Flood said that it is his understanding that the crime rate in villages which have adopted local option liquor laws has been reduced. But caution must be taken because this does not mean it will remain low. He warned that a problem that could develop in that people who wanted liquor will get it elsewhere, so they migrate to the transportation centers where liquor is readily available.

Others interviewed were personnel working in the alcohol field at Kotzebue and Nome. The Director of the Northwest Regional alcoholism Program in Kotzebue expressed a similar view of the local option situation. Mr. Green said "...in fact they come in here (Kotzebue) to drink and sneak drinks to dry villages." He did indicate, however, that in the villages that have adopted local option laws, the rate of apparent alcoholism is less, because it made liquor hard to get. "You have to do a lot of footwork to get it." He emphasized that local option "is a very good first step."

In the Nome area Sharon Bullock heard from villages about the decrease in crime since local option laws have been adopted. Connie Hollenbeck, Director of the Comprehensive Alcoholism Program in Nome agreed that "things are definitely quieter in the villages (with) less temptation to drink because it's less available." She believed that alcohol-related crimes have increased in Nome as villagers came from dry communi-

ties to Nome. But she conceded that the impact in Nome was not as great as everyone expected. Those who desire alcoholic beverages visit the trading and transportation centers where alcohol is readily available.

In another study done by David Marshall he found the annual rate of "incidents" showed a 48% decline after banning importation and sale. After one village had voted to discontinue the ban of alcohol importation, Trooper Tim Litera reported that the rate of arrests increased greatly, going from one every five days to 1.7 each day. He stated the reasons for the arrests have also changed since alcoholic beverages were again allowed in the village.

A comprehensive study (7) gives deep insight into the many ramifications of the local option law. Since the report was made in June 1983, the period of time after local options were adopted is relatively short, and the full influence on village health, safety, crime and behavioral changes could not be measured. Its real value, as the report states, makes it possible "to compare the local option to the purposes, history, culture and social and political organization of the villages for when the law was provided." The thoroughness and comprehensive detail in the report make it most useful for the reader to grasp the complex aspects of village problems and their solution.

It seems from the available data and reports that local option in Alaska villages has become a valuable method to control the use of alcohol. It certainly has had a beneficial effect in this short period. Whether it will be beneficial in the long term remains to be seen. This method of control deserves trial and further study since it was the intent of the legislature to devise a legal and administrative solution to assist local communities to exercise greater control over the availability of alcohol.

Nine controls have been discussed which if implemented can contribute to a reduction in the per capita absolute alcohol consumption. 1) Decrease the number of retail outlets and convenience liquor stores. 2) Lower the total hours of retail sales. 3) Enforce laws, regulations or ordinances that prohibit sales to intoxicated individuals. 4) Pick up intoxicated individuals and place them in protective custody. 5) Rigidly enforce legal age purchase and consumption with prosecution of violators, both the underaged and the retail dealer involved. 6) Establish 21 as the minimum legal age. 7) Strictly prosecute and sentence violators who drive while intoxicated (DWI). 8) Increase excise tax on alcoholic beverages. 9) Grant authority to local governments enabling them to enact control measures.

REFERENCES

1. Albrecht CE. Alcohol abuse in Alaska. Nutrition Today 1982; 17(3):6-15.
2. Kelso D. Impact of alcoholism and alcohol abuse in Alaska. Final report 1977; Altam Associates, Anchorage, Alaska.
3. Albrecht CE. Alcohol abuse in Alaska. Polar Record 1983; 135:601-603.
4. ACPADA. Facts about alcohol consumption in Alaska. Annual report 1982; Alaska Council on Prevention of Alcohol and Drug Abuse. Anchorage, Alaska.
5. Lieber C. To drink (moderately) or not to drink. N Engl J Med 1984; 310:846-848.
6. Alaska Statutes, 1981. Local Option Election, Title 4-11: 490-501. Juneau: Alaska State Legislature.
7. Lonner T, Duff J. Village alcohol control and the local option law. A report to the Alaska State Legislature 1983.

C. Earl Albrecht
Drawer L
Advance, North Carolina   27006
U.S.A.

Circumpolar Health 84:332-334

ALCOHOLISM AND MENTAL HEALTH TREATMENT IN CIRCUMPOLAR AREAS: TRADITIONAL AND NON-TRADITIONAL APPROACHES

THEODORE A. MALA

Throughout the circumpolar world there seems to be increasing concern by national governments and health professionals at the rising rate of accidents and and preventable health problems related to alcohol and substance use and abuse. I was especially made aware of this on recent travels to Canada, Finland, Denmark, and the Soviet Union, where I had the opportunity to discuss the matter with other public health specialists in their home environment.

Numerous foundations have been established to examine this problem. In Finland, researchers have examined everything from alcohol consumption and mortality in Nordic countries to theories of set and psychological effects of alcohol (1). In Canada, the government has established a special office under the Minister of Health to review alcohol-related problems and most recently has established a special board examining alcohol abuse in Canadian Natives. In the Soviet Union, I was able to see a number of clinics devoted to the care of the worker with an alcohol problem and his program of rehabilitation back into society. Dr. Lidiya N. Lezhepekova has done some excellent work in this area and has published several books in Russian on the subject (2).

Within the United States, there are extensive studies done by a number of state and federal agencies looking at these problems. A number of statistical studies have been done in Alaska on the subject of substance abuse, including a definitive baseline study of Alaskan schools and communities by the University of Alaska Center for Alcohol and Addiction Studies, released in the summer of 1983 (3).

With all of this sophistication, the problems relating to alcoholism and mental health in the circumpolar countries seem to be worsening despite our efforts. Of special concern is the alarming rate of increase of alcoholism and mental health-related problems in Native communities. The continual concern expressed in circumpolar countries is that the established agencies overseeing these problems cannot seem to reach indigenous populations despite all their good intentions and expertise in the field.

Let us examine this problem a bit further. I have divided circumpolar inhabitants into three groups for the sake of simplicity: a) the "transient newcomer", b) the resident, and c) the Native resident. I believe that each of these groups has its own special needs and considerations that should be further explained and addressed.

The "transient newcomer" is one who has come to a circumpolar area for a job opportunity, for adventure, or quite possibly is running away from a situation and just wants to get as far away as possible from everyone. This individual has no roots or support system to fall back on. He is considered "away from home" and tends to act differently from the way he would if this were his true home community. We see this in Alaska in his carefree attitude toward the state as the "Last Frontier" where "anything goes," a subculture which seems to encourage alcohol abuse and a sense of individualism which sometimes includes breaking the law. If you ask a member of this group where he is from, he will always name another city or state as "home," never Alaska.

The "resident" group is made up of non-Native people who have adopted the circumpolar area as their home and have invested something in their place of residence either in the form of being quite involved in the community and its future or of closely identifying with it as "home." Members of the group have lived in the area for several years and intend to stay there in the future.

The Native or indigenous population is one whose members' roots extend into the area since pre-historic times. In Alaska this includes a number of groups we call "Alaska Natives" made up of Eskimo, Indian, and Aleut individuals. Alaska is further divided into 12 regions through the Alaska Native Claims Settlement Act of 1971, according to custom, language, and traditional habitation areas. Alaska Natives include two groups of Inuit (Eskimo groups), speaking Inupiaq and Yupik dialects, Athapaskan, Tlingit, Haida, and Tsimpsian Indians and Aleut tribes. Native groups have nowhere to call home other than where they are living. With the rapid rate of change that is being experienced in the developing circumpolar areas, it is this group of individuals that I believe is most adversely affected by alcohol and to whom I plan to address the balance of this work. The first two groups seem to respond to conventional treatment but the Native group does not.

To address Native problems one must consider history and the role it has played in the lives of indigenous peoples. Natives of circumpolar regions have survived for centuries in some of the harshest environments known to man, yet they have managed to live through cold and even starvation situations and have been able to adapt their lifestyles accordingly. There is, however, an element of change that is entering their lives that they have never had to face before. It is a result of a number of outside influences from dominant cultures seeking to bring change into the community either for the good or bad effects they might achieve.

In Alaska, the first non-Native contact was with a combination of missionaries and traders. The impact was mild to dramatic depending on the area under consideration. A change of language and customs was introduced together with alcohol and tobacco, not to mention new diseases and new genetic pools. Eventually, with the settlement of land claims and the extraction of petroleum reserves from the North Slope, a tremendous cash infusion was injected into the State. Swarms of bureaucrats and consultants covered the state selling either wares or programs to the Native people.

New homes were built according to the non-Native community's standards, and electricity and telephones were introduced into rural communities. Changes that had taken the rest of the United States decades to adjust to, were brought into rural communities in a very few years. Survival in this new world no longer meant success in subsistence ways of life (e.g. hunting and fishing), but rather success in a cash-based economy. With the introduction of all these modern appliances came a change-over from a subsistence economy to a cash economy. One had to pay for goods in cash to have them.

Local schools were built in each village, including high schools, where students literally step in and out of the twentieth century each day. They go from a high school loaded with computer technology and advanced methods of teaching right back into a subsistence-based economy in transition. Parents cannot relate to what their children are learning in school and a division begins to take place between an old way of life and a new one.

After traveling to numerous circumpolar communities and observing how many approaches have not been effective in these target groups, I was surprised and pleased that the most effective answer and approach I have seen is that being taken in the Kotzebue region of Alaska by the Northwest Alaska Native Association (NANA) known as the "Spirit Movement."

The Spirit Movement is basically a philosophy which stresses self responsibility and concern for those around us. It is a resurrection of basic human values which seem to have gone by the wayside in this period of transition. Using basic Inupiaq (Eskimo) values and having its roots in the community itself, it is a movement from within this Native society to improve itself and bring itself closer together in response to the increasing rates of alcoholism, suicide, and mental health problems that are facing the society. This philosophy came out of a sense of frustration of these individuals that they were indeed losing control of their lives by numerous outside influences that were being introduced to their villages and way of life. They observed that if they have a problem in their village today with a child, they call a social worker. If someone has an alcohol problem they call a medical worker. If someone is not behaving, they call the police. If money or assistance is needed, they call some agency. They found themselves looking outside of the community whenever a need arose and that outside intervention slowly took the control they had over their lives away from them. In essence, each helping agency took a little bit more of the responsibility for their own lives out of their hands and put it into someone else's. What others had done in the name of religion, charity, or government (either federal or state), although it appeared helpful and good from the outside, really was harmful in the long run.

And so my proposal for the treatment of alcoholism and mental problems in Native peoples is based on the idea that "true change must come from within." Change will not occur with governments throwing money on problems and hoping that they will go away.

The Spirit Movement has a set of basic values for Native people that include sharing, caring for others, responsibility for self, knowledge of language and traditions, pride in one's heritage, respect for elders and an inclusion of them in daily lives. They feel that although persons may be biologically ready to bear children, they are not prepared enough in life to raise and teach them because the parents are too young and have not lived enough life. It is here that the elders come in, passing on traditional values and teachings to those younger so that they can pass them on in turn to their children one day. A "spirit camp" has been established where there are no telephones or modern conveniences and where young people can go back to traditional hunting and fishing methods as passed on there by the elders. Pride and knowledge of heritage and culture are stressed.

Native healers are employed to work with modern-day medical personnel. Traditional methods of healing such as body manipulation, massage, use of hot springs, Native herbs, and community support are stressed. It is in joining the modern-day approaches to medicine with the traditional values of the Spirit Movement that true change is beginning to be noticed.

I believe that this system can easily be adapted to other circumpolar countries and cultures, and deserves more examination.

Elements of this type of community response are used on American Indian Reservations in Indian Health Service Hospitals where the medicine man is used side-by-side with the modern physician in seeking holistic medical care of their target populations.

The Spirit Movement program does not support an unrealistic "going back" to an earlier time of life when satellites, television, telephones, and computers did not exist. It does advocate looking towards the elements of strength and spirituality that have sustained these peoples throughout the centuries as a way of surviving this cultural shock and combatting the trend toward cultural assimilation, by being proud of who Native peoples are and of the heritage that makes them special and unique.

There is a way of providing health and social services to Native communities without alienating them or imposing non-traditional, threatening ways of treatment on them. It is by being aware of their historical roots and cultural differences and bringing the awareness into the type of medicine we practice.

REFERENCES

1. Report on activities. Finnish Foundation for Alcohol Studies, Helsinki, 1981.
2. Lezhepekova, LN. Treatment of Alcoholism. (in Russian) Leningrad, USSR.
3. Segal B, Mala T, Bowman JD, McKelvy JG. Substance use and abuse in Alaska: School and communities surveys. Alaska State Office on Alcoholism and Drug Abuse through University of Alaska, Center for Alcohol and Addiction Studies, Anchorage, 1983.

Theodore A. Mala
Department of Biological Sciences
University of Alaska, Anchorage
Anchorage, Alaska 99508
U.S.A.

Circumpolar Health 84:335-339

VILLAGE ALCOHOL CONTROL: TRADITIONAL METHODS AND THE "LOCAL OPTION LAW"

THOMAS D. LONNER

The primary immediate cause of death and significant injury in rural Alaska is alcohol-related behavior resulting in homicides, suicides, and accidents. This paper reports on the early implementation and consequences of a modern legal solution to this public health problem--the "local option law." Alaska's is one of many efforts to combat the loss of village residents due to abusive and problem drinking. Although too recent a law to evaluate its outcomes on village health and safety statistics, it is not too early to compare the law to purposes, history, culture, and social and political organization of the villages for whom the law was provided.

Alaska's local option law is a legal solution devised to assist villages in the exercise of greater local control over the availability of alcohol. The law provides an opportunity for villages to elect one of the following mutually exclusive "options": 1) prohibit the sale of alcohol unless sold under a single community liquor license, 2) prohibit the sale of alcohol with the exception of specific types of retailing, 3) prohibit the sale of alcohol, or 4) prohibit the sale and importation of alcohol. Due to the magnitude of the public health problem, the state government, through the local option law, granted to villages certain powers usually reserved to larger municipal powers; it also reinforced village options with the threat of state police enforcement.

The problems stemming from the use of alcohol in villages affect not only the drinking individual but the entire community. Due to their cultural, social, and economic origins, Alaska villages operate as large family units. Village populations are so small, interrelated, and interdependent that they become vulnerable to the entire array of negative effects associated with excessive drinking, including interpersonal violence, child neglect, loss of economic opportunity, demoralization, and physical deterioration. Therefore, the alcohol-related social impacts severely impair family and community morale, perpetuate a cycle of negative, even disastrous, events, and jeopardize the physical and cultural survival of the village.

Many villagers consider that the future of their culture is dependent solely on the traditional values and caliber of the future community leaders, that is, the young people of the community. The villagers' concern with alcohol is less a preoccupation with the personal health or moral implications of ingesting alcohol than with the death of village members, particularly death among the young men. The deaths of young men, while terrible personal and family tragedies, also constitute a major cultural concern.

Banning alcohol importation and sale was justified in arguments for the local option law which suggested that the public health problem posed by alcohol was quite great and that there is a close and substantial relationship between the means (the local option law) and the ends (limiting the magnitude and tragedy of the public health problem). The prohibition of sale and importation becomes potentially more powerful under the local option law than under the limited prior authority available to villages in that:

1) the local option law extends village authority over all residents and visitors, who previously may have denied the authority of the village governing bodies to constrain the sale and importation;

2) the local option law extends village authority to a five mile boundary around the village;

3) the local option law requires compliance by commercial carriers, under severe penalty for violations;

4) the local option law requires compliance by all state-wide and regional alcohol distributors; and

5) the local option law implies some state law enforcement and judiciary response to violations.

In practice, the option banning sale and importation is by far the most popular choice, given village desires to limit severely, if not prohibit, access to alcohol. Many have translated their option to mean "prohibition." They (and many government agency personnel) talk about voting "dry" and having "dry" communities. To villagers, "dry" means no more alcohol, no more drinking, and no more drunks in the villages. Were it possible for village law to prohibit totally the manufacture or possession of alcohol and to search and seize persons and property for evidence, many villages would have chosen to do so. The fact that the United States Constitution denies villages these powers is inexplicable and frustrating to them, since their motive is to save human lives, entire communities, and entire cultures.

The new state law did not provide for: 1) real increases in police effort; 2) the cultural, social, and situational variety among villages; 3) the village-desired prohibition of the manufacture, possession, or use of alcohol; or 4) alternative flexibilities of enactment or enforcement desired by villages in order to have the least intrusive law to solve their particular problems. Thus, in many villages, the law is and must be supplemented by the use of more traditional, ingenious, sensitive, extra-legal, culturally appropriate, and sovereign means to achieve desired ends. These supplemental means suggest that untapped self-controls are still available in villages or may be re-learned to enhance public health and safety while maintaining cultural integrity and continuity.

If power is known primarily through its exercise, then villages retain powers via extra-legal, unsanctioned elections and ordinances as well as local enforcement and adjudication; that is, the consequences of the exercise of power are real, even if the authority of the village is only apparent or achieved through the consent of the governed. There appears to be some implied consent to or support of village extra-legal methods by external authorities to accomplish ends desired by both the village and external authorities, as long as these methods become neither publicized nor challenged.

Some villages, having adopted an option under the local option law, find it necessary to pass implementing and supplementary ordinances dealing with public drunkenness, alcohol possession, search and seizure, involuntary commitment, and jail and financial penalties. These villages see the local option law as merely a back-up to other forms of local control, and an external threat to be used if local authority is violated. In some instances, these ordinances have been used to modify the terms of the elected option, even though they do not have the legal power to do so.

Some village cultures find the local option law inconsistent with their accepted modes of community problem-solving. Differences occur in the arena of who makes decision, how decisions are made, how interventions are made in the behaviors of others, the role of informing as a form of social control, the range of acceptable control mechanisms (e.g., embarrassment, isolation, exile, jail, internal versus external policing), and the degree of rigidity or flexibility that is desired in community-wide laws, enforcement, penalty, and rehabilitation.

The local option law, while empowering villages to control aspects of their own lives, still remains a Western law. It was not designed or written by rural people, and its purpose, intent, powers, procedures, language, limitations, and relationships to other parts of Western law and law enforce-

ment remain unclear to many rural people. Villagers also see that other, vaguely understood aspects of Western law formally prohibit villages from taking actions which would solve the very problems for which they are turning to the local option law. In order for them to utilize fully the local option law, they may wittingly or unwittingly violate other laws.

In effect, villages using the local option law are not writing their own law, consistent with the underlying elements that make aggregations of individuals and families into "communities." The writing of law comes from receiving or assuming generalized powers, then convening to draft, adopt, implement, and revise one's own laws to deal directly with self-perceived problems. The use of the local option law is less an exercise in the writing of law than in trying to solve a most difficult problem through the adoption of a pre-formulated and externally-designed option.

Given these conditions, the enactment of a new law facilitating local control over alcohol raises many questions. The most obvious question is whether the various legal options will significantly help communities over time, to reduce the incidence of negative and dangerous events. A less obvious but potentially more significant product may be the growth of local and indigenous management of problems and the personal internalization of community values and rules. In addition to the process of extra-legal modification of the law, some villages initiated a reinvestment of authority in more traditional local governance and in those social control methods which had proved acceptable and effective in the past. Thus, these villages appear to pursue their local objectives by relying on the threat of external force, the enhancement of local control authority, and the flexibility of action afforded by their remoteness and the consent of the governed.

Communities which believe that they have retained sovereign powers to control their internal affairs and their relationships with the outside world tend to expend more energy than other communities in the construction and enforcement of local laws. Since they do not derive their authority from larger governments or bodies of law, nor do they feel they can depend on outside law enforcement supports, they must exercise their authority continuously; it is likely that continuous exercise of authority makes it easier to continue. Characteristics of continuous law-making and enforcement in these communities include some of the following:

-- signed commitment by each community member to support community laws and the actions of council

members;
-- commitment by each community member to support physically and psychologically the law enforcement effort;
-- annual review, reconsideration, amendment, specification, rejection, and re-enactment of the law by the entire community;
-- creation and maintenance of local law on a wide range of daily life matters, such as loose dogs, curfews, speed limits, truancy, drug use, drunken behavior, theft, threatening behavior, family neglect, gambling, fish and game salvage, and others;
-- no assignment of enforcement to specific individuals, so that responsibility rests with each and every community member;
-- enforcement by large numbers of persons (men, women, children, elders, council members) at the same time and place, creating mutual pride and support and re-individualization of the burden;
-- formal investigation, trial, and punishment methods;
-- no record kept of violators except in community memory, so that there is no long-term permanent reduction of future opportunities for individuals;
-- formal methods of exile with hoped-for and encouraged returns and re-integrations;
-- semi-permanent exile of consistent violators, particularly violent persons and substance distributors;
-- increased, rather than decreased, enforcement of alcohol restrictions during major celebrations;
-- extensive monitoring of luggage and freight at points of entry into the community;
-- immediate destruction of prohibited substances at point of entry, as the basic fine (rather than later trial) for attempted importation and as the basic social embarrassment;
-- more intensive enforcement of repeated violators' activities within and without the village (through villages' or relatives' reporting systems in other, particularly hub, communities);
-- conviction of violators on the grounds of possession and use or using possession and use as *prima facie* evidence of illegal importation;

-- exercise of controls over visitors as well as residents;
-- illegal search, seizure, and destruction of alcohol from private homes based on observed and reported possession and use;
-- unaltered policy of prohibition, but methods and penalties of enforcement renewed or otherwise modified to meet new needs; for example, penalties may be stiffened by reducing the amount of basic physical support provided by peers;
-- non-reliance on outside enforcement entities or procedures, since these commonly result in after-the-fact actions; the village desires and achieves immediate behavior intervention and modification.

Thus, the local option law is only one mechanism of many which encourage more community self control.

There are communities which view the local option law as an unnecessary, redundant, and useless tool to reduce access to alcohol. These communities have had a long tradition of controlling access through internal formal governance (i.e., each community member sharing some of the active responsibility for controlling access and use). Some of the means used by these communities are legitimized by community consensus but may be illegal in that they violate the constitutional rights of residents; lack of complaint about violations is due, in large measure, to shared cultural community values, respect for traditional and community authority, and a desire to live within the protected confines of a conservative but healthy community.

The supports for the continuing tradition of enforced "dryness" appear limited in number:

-- geographic remoteness;
-- late contact with the outside world;
-- strong religious values from the origins of the community;
-- consensus about 1) the authority of the elected or traditional government and the community itself, 2) legal and/or traditional local sovereignty, 3) the merits of a conservative range of tolerated behaviors, and 4) absolute restrictions and strict enforcement being the only means to maintain the healthy lifestyle;
-- remoteness from state-supplied law enforcement agencies;

-- no tradition of extensive alcohol use, related problems, or tolerance of use;
-- a tradition of local law-making, continuous law enforcement, and verified attachment to the substance and pre-eminence of the law;
-- pride in having a good community reputation;
-- ability to control or maintain distance to nearby industrial development;
-- ability to control the behaviors of new Native and non-Native residents;
-- a healthy continuing subsistence resource base;
-- maintenance of distant relationships with government programs, resulting in reduced contact, few negotiated compromises, and greater self-determination;
-- family and cultural obligations which require extensive visiting and, thus, close uniform scrutiny of private lives as a form of social control and support;
-- members who cannot tolerate such close restriction emigrating or exporting their activities;
-- members who refuse to abide strictly by community rules being closely watched, counselled, penalized, or exiled;
-- members who violate the rules but whose behavior is not found troublesome being watched closely but not unduly punished;
-- persons who wish a retreat from more permissive communities being allowed to immigrate and settle in the village;
-- continuous discussion of, voting on, and enforcement of local restrictions;
-- continuous monitoring of the bad events in other communities.

Some villages appear too divided or demoralized, at present, to organize themselves to utilize any of the options provided under state law or take other actions to control alcohol use and behaviors.

It appears that those communities that desire greater self-determination over aspects of their quality of life and whose traditional systems no longer suffice (for a variety of reasons) to meet these objectives are the most likely to look to the local option law and other tools to achieve their goals. In other words, the communities that are most likely to avail themselves of the local option law are those that are in a transition, returning to a healthier, self-controlling state; these may be communities that have experienced a twenty-year decline in quality of life due to factors mentioned earlier. Thus, it is suggested that the local option law does not create healthier communities but that healthier communities or communities that are becoming healthier are the ones most attracted to the local option law as an additional support. In general, the village attributes which are most likely to be predictive of successful local option law outcomes are:

-- a secure, activist, and strong village or city council;
-- a village council which is not itself typified by abusive use of alcohol;
-- consolidation of or unanimity among all village power bases;
-- a population marked by stability, in terms of racial composition, migration, economy, goals, and problem rates;
-- a community desire and ability to identify problems, set goals, establish priorities, establish solutions, and take action as a community;
-- other difficult goal-directed actions taken by the community which indicate that the community can exercise self-control.

Even in the most positively responding villages, the use of Western legal tools to meet community objectives is highly problematic. The contrasts which exist in the introduction of Western legal solutions to problems in the daily lives of geographically and culturally remote villages are predictive of unresolvable tensions, if not direct conflict. These contrasts are summarized in Table 1.

Given these complexities, it is worthwhile to ask, how well has the local option law served village public health and safety objectives? The immediate objective was to reduce the incidence of alcohol-related public behavior (such as violence and public drunkenness) and the community fear which accompanies it. Since the local option law elections, many villages have perceived a steep decline in visible drunken behavior. Whether or not this perception is correct (and it is likely to be correct), whether or not there is less actual drinking or drunkenness as distinct from visible or public drinking or drunkenness, are probably not relevant distinctions in the villagers' assessment of the quality of their daily lives.

There is no indication that the overall rates and volume of alcohol consumption have declined since the inception of the local option law. What, then, accounts for the perceived steep decline in alcohol-related

Table 1. Contrasts between local option law and Western legal system (non-local) in controlling alcohol in Alaska's villages.

Local	Non-local
community power	state power
Native	non-Native
traditional	modern and Western
protective solutions	punishing solutions
preventive solutions	punishing solutions
person-oriented	law-oriented
rule by consensus	rule by constitution
decentralized solutions	centralized solutions
flexible solutions	inflexible solutions
pre-eminent rights of the community	pre-eminent rights of the individual

problems and behaviors in the village? Findings suggest these changes are due to altered patterns of use by the using population, including:
 a) increased "privatization" of alcohol use and behaviors,
 b) altered and intermittent patterns of distribution and consumption,
 c) substitution of other substances, and
 d) externalization of the behaviors and problems from the villages to regional hubs and larger communities with large health care and public safety services.

What, then, is the benefit of the local option law? Some villagers are under the illusion that the law is self-executing, that by passing the law, the reality of daily life will automatically change. This illusion is not totally without foundation. What appears to happen in some villages is that the vote on the local option constitutes an elaborate reaffirmation of village authority and rules. The threat of external force appears to support and mobilize the internal control mechanisms of the village and thereby produce modified behaviors among residents, including reduced drinking and improved morale. The longevity of these positive social health changes will depend, ultimately, on the continuing development of greater internal village controls and corresponding improvements in the perceived quality of life. What is achieved, ultimately, by the local option law may be less some formal control over alcohol than enhanced village self-control over vital aspects of community life, health, safety, and morale.

Thomas D. Lonner
Center for Alcohol and Addiction
  Studies
University of Alaska, Anchorage
Anchorage, Alaska 99508
U.S.A.

Circumpolar Health 84:340-343

COMMUNITY CONTROL OVER HEALTH PROBLEMS: ALCOHOL PROHIBITION
IN A CANADIAN INUIT VILLAGE

JOHN D. O'NEIL

In this paper I will describe the process whereby a Canadian Inuit community brought about alcohol prohibition and its general effects on the community over a four-year period. The paper is based on ethnographic research carried out during two years: the first in 1978 when the village voted to prohibit alcohol and the second in 1982. Standard epidemiological methods were considered inappropriate due to the small size of the community and the very low incidence rates for health indicators such as suicide, accidental deaths, and family violence. In-depth interviewing with community leaders, elders, and administrators provided a descriptive social history of processes leading up to prohibition and the general response of both non-drinkers and drinkers to the new restriction. Participant-observation with both White and Inuit illegal drinkers provided an understanding of changing drinking styles, associated health problems, and community reaction to bylaw violations. The paper concludes that alcohol prohibition contributed to an increase in family integrity and respect between genders and generations, an increase in youthful interest in traditional values and lifestyles, a decrease in abuse of other destructive substances, and an increase in hostility between Inuit and White ethnic groups where Whites were perceived as flagrant violators of a locally constituted bylaw.

While many observers have noted the alarming rise of alcohol-related health problems among Canadian Inuit, there have as yet been no evaluations made of the primary Inuit initiative to control alcohol abuse, namely, prohibition. Prohibition for most Westerners conjures up many negative and offensive images. As I have argued elsewhere, however, prohibition in Canadian Inuit villages is a regulatory option made available by the territorial government, and its selection and support by Inuit in the villages is a product of decidedly Inuit negotiations occurring within locally controlled institutions such as the Hamlet Council and churches (1). It has not been forced onto Inuit by Whites (as was the case with prohibition on Canadian Indian reserves) and in fact, most Whites in the "alcohol abuse business" would probably prefer a less authoritarian alternative (2). Since 8 of 25 Inuit villages with populations of between 200 and 1,000 now prohibit alcohol completely (all since 1978), research into the effects of prohibition on community life should be a high priority. This paper represents a preliminary attempt

to evaluate this tactic for the primary prevention of alcohol abuse.

Prior to the shift to a sedentary village society, alcohol use was unknown among Inuit in the central Canadian Arctic. Although a trading post and religious missions had been active in the area since 1930, it was not until 1965, with the opening of the public school and the start of the Northern Rental Housing Program, that settled life began on a year-round basis. The first residents came from a quite diverse range of "tribal" backgrounds covering a large geographic region; as a result, there was little initial sense of community. As subsistence strategies changed to include wage labor, families competed for access to these scarce new resources. Jealousy, envy, and suspicion increased. The new religious institutions created factional conflict which overlay traditional band rivalry. Problems and conflicts had been traditionally resolved within extended family groups and since indigenous procedures for dealing with community-wide problems were non-existent, authority was largely assumed by Whites (3,4). For a people who considered self-reliance and individual autonomy as paramount virtues, these new conditions were intolerable. When alcohol was introduced by Whites and Inuit from other regions into these stressful conditions, problems were exacerbated. Inuit feel that by brooding or worrying about a problem, a person can make himself ill. Emotional management is an important preventive health strategy; by avoiding "bad feelings" or depression, sadness, or guilt, a person also avoids physical illness. Many Inuit indicated that they initially thought of alcohol as a medicine. Village life seemed to provide more sources of worry, and alcohol seemed to provide an antidote similar to other White remedies for other new diseases.

Other anthropologists have written about Canadian Inuit alcohol use during the late 1960s and early 1970s (5,6,7). They argue for an approach that recognizes variation in the role and effects of drinking and situates alcohol use within Inuit understandings of social structure and kinship obligations. Brody (7) warns that if economic development in the North continues without meaningful Inuit involvement, more and more Inuit communities will become "skid rows."

By the late 1970s, Brody's warning had been realized in some of the larger Inuit communities particularly. Health statistics since the mid 1970s have shown an alarming increase in alcohol-related morbidity and mortality. Many Inuit have expressed concern for this growing problem and a variety of solutions have been discussed. The first attempt to control the problem was in Frobisher Bay in 1976 when the liquor store was closed. Since then, 8 Inuit communities have voted for total prohibition, 2 have a system of interdiction for problem drinkers, 2 have rationing system, 2 have closed their liquor outlets, and 10 have set up alcohol committees and hired counsellors.

The perception of alcohol abuse as a local problem was determined largely by the village elders and religious leaders. Various informants in 1977 expressed concerns that alcohol was contributing to a drastic increase in family violence and a breakdown in moral codes for behavior. Although the number of individuals involved was low, extended families were often called in to mediate conflicts. Cases were cited where brothers fought with each other, husbands beat their wives, adulterous behavior increased, and children were afraid to go home. For those who found these situations abhorrent, but who were nonetheless involved when mediation was required, alcohol abuse seemed to constitute a major threat to community life.

The incidence rate for alcohol-related problems remained low in comparison to other settlements in the North. Whites and Inuit alike commented that this village was friendly, peaceful and quiet. Many local Inuit expressed concern about visiting or travelling through other towns and villages where alcohol use was more widespread and violence more prevalent. Nonetheless, people expressed concern that they were losing control over their own lives and the future of their community. Old people argued that alcohol made a person lose his reason. They worried that if adults continued to act like children, their very survival would be compromised.

To deal with the problem, the community had to reach consensus on a new level of decision-making. Creating a community out of the groups of previously separate family groups occurred largely through the efforts of Inuit leaders in the Anglican and Catholic church. Both churches had been administered since the early 1970s by Inuit lay preachers and elders, and they had attracted large congregations. While there had been some factional rivalry between the two congregations earlier in the village's history, by the mid-1970s relations were less strained. Traditional messages of morality and ethics were reinterpreted through Christian doctrine and people were looking increasingly to the churches for moral guidance.

The village council, established in 1970 and initially an advisory body to White bureaucrats, eventually became the village's main political force. Councillors were elected largely from the leadership in the two churches and council activities expanded quickly beyond routine municipal affairs to include both inter- and intrafamilial conflict resolution. Together, these two institutions have been the major forums for the generation of communal values and supra-familial obligations; ideas foreign to the emphasis on seniority and kindred loyalty which characterized traditional Inuit society.

Another important historical factor was the absence of a police detachment in the village. Consequently, instead of directing aggression towards this symbol of White society, social offenses such as theft and vandalism continued to be understood as internal transgressions rather than acts against a foreign institution.

Several alcohol-related violent deaths involving young people sparked the movement which culminated in prohibition. Church leaders had been warning the community that continued adulterous behavior and intra-familial squabbles under the influence of alcohol would not go unpunished, and they were now able to invoke supernatural restitution as a factor in these accidental deaths. People began to accept the interpretation that drunkenness was akin to possession by an evil spirit. While this explanation absolved individuals from responsibility for their actions, it also fueled the religious arguments to banish alcohol from the community.

These arguments preceded the awareness that prohibition was a legal possibility. Church sermons advocated prohibition months before the council was advised regarding appropriate strategies for holding a plebiscite. White advisors from the various health, social, and corrective service agencies usually argued against prohibition and for a research and education solution at council meetings. However, when the plebiscite was finally held, there was an 83% voter turnout and a 96% vote in favor of prohibition, at a time when roughly a third of local Inuit were drinking alcohol regularly. Many individuals who enjoyed drinking indicated that they voted in favor of prohibition because they felt it was in the best interests of their children and in the long-term interests of the community.

When prohibition came into effect, two families decided to move to wet towns; their decision to move in part related to their desire to continue drinking. One of these families has since returned, and reported that they were unable to endure the alcohol-related problems in the other village.

In the spring of 1982, nine new families from wet villages relocated to the dry town, despite its reputation for high unemployment and a heavy welfare load. No one moved away, although several middle-aged men indicate they make occasional trips to wet villages in order to "party."

For a year or so immediately after prohibition, alcohol consumption virtually disappeared. Now, illegal drinking does occur, but offenses are rare and drinkers take care to camouflage their activities. During the three years of prohibition, there have been five charges brought against people for illegal possession of alcohol in a restricted area, four of them arising from the same incident in 1981. In each of these cases, the offenders provided alcohol to other local people and the parties became public knowledge.

These arrests, however, do not represent the total incidence of drinking that actually occurs. Most illegal drinking takes place in the company of one or two trusted friends (who may or may not be related) and rarely progresses beyond moderate use. Clandestine drinking is complicated by the patterns of Inuit visiting which make it difficult to lock doors or drink unobserved by non-drinkers in the village. Visitors often walk in unannounced and must be soberly offered tea. Aggressive behavior has virtually disappeared. Despite these attempts by drinkers to disguise their drinking, most people in town are generally aware of who is drinking illegally. There seems to be a tacit agreement in the community that as long as drinkers keep their activity private and do not cause public disruptions, no action will be taken. The prevalence of illegal drinking is difficult to estimate but my guess is that about 10 Inuit households (out of approximately 80) and 4 White households (out of 14) are involved. For Inuit, however, supplies are difficult to obtain and even the "heaviest" drinkers rarely consume more than three or four 40 oz. bottles in a year.

Illegal drinking in the White community has as yet gone unpunished. Whites are very adept at camouflaging their drinking activities. They are able to lock their doors to visitors and spend entire weekends isolated from the community. Knowledge within the White community of who is drinking is widespread, but those who do not drink protect those who do. Whites find it much easier to secure supplies from sympathetic colleagues visiting from wet towns who will exchange a bottle for hospitality. White heavy drinkers are sometimes drunk every weekend.

Because of the concern for anonymity and fear of the consequences of exposure (for Whites, probably dismissal from their jobs), inter-ethnic drinking has virtually

disappeared. As a result, White involvement in underage drinking and sexual exploitation, a major problem in the early 1970s, has also largely disappeared, and contributed to a slight reduction in inter-ethnic tension.

Enforcement of the prohibition bylaw has relied primarily on community pressure. For the reasons described above, it is very difficult to drink unobserved, and those who risk it are fully aware that the penalty may be social ostracism. The threat of police action is reserved for those who flagrantly disregard community standards. (In the arrest cases mentioned above, the council requested the Royal Canadian Mounted Police to come to the village and charge the offenders.) Whites however, stand outside this system by avoiding any alcohol-related social interaction with Inuit. However, Inuit generally know which Whites are drinking and many resent their disregard for a local bylaw. The young Inuk bylaw officer, whose task it was to report liquor infractions to Council, was advised by one local White that he ran the risk of libel action if he made any unsubstantiated allegations (i.e., no empty bottles with fingerprints).

Aside from these general changes in drinking patterns, what specific effects has prohibition had on the town's youth, the group most at risk in situations of high substance abuse? Young people in this dry town appear to be better off than their counterparts in wet villages. They are generally in superb physical condition, emotional problems are minimal, and they are relatively well-integrated into the social life of the community. Those people who do experience difficulty are not pushed to the extremes that so often end in tragedy elsewhere.

Although most young people are familiar with "getting high," few youth now show any exaggerated interest in drinking or the use of other drugs. Many expressed views that they felt fortunate to be living in a dry town. On two occasions, I travelled with a group of teenagers to wet towns, and was surprised at how many avoided parties and showed no interest in drinking. In several instances, young men selectively chose to stay with relatives known to be abstainers when visiting wet towns. Many also indicated they got homesick easily for their own village's quiet, peaceful atmosphere, and had little interest in going elsewhere for education or employment.

The absence of alcohol also seems to decrease the opportunities and temptation to use other substances; a finding in contrast to some professional expectations that abuse of more dangerous substances may increase if alcohol is not available. Most youth indicated that although they had experimented with marijuana when the town was wet, both it and gasoline sniffing, which was once fairly prevalent among young teenagers, had virtually disappeared. Where use of these substances did occur, it was almost always provoked by teenagers visiting from other towns. It seemed that without the adult example of "getting high," using other substances had little appeal.

For those people in their late teens and twenties who once had drinking problems (as indicated by arrest records, alienated families, etc.), prohibition has had a profound impact. In wet contexts, the continual round of parties leads to fighting and bouts of depression. Although problem drinkers talked about parties and about ways to smuggle booze into the village, in actuality they rarely drank and in fact avoided travel to wet villages. Many admitted that they were happy to live in a dry town because they considered it the best way to control their drinking.

To conclude, I have described a situation where the prohibition of alcohol was initiated by the Inuit leaders in a community to cope with the locally perceived problem of alcohol abuse. It has "worked" extremely well in the sense that alcohol-related problems have virtually disappeared. It has been successful in part because enforcement of the by-law is through local social pressure without reliance on White law enforcement officers. For particularly stressed groups such as youth, the dry town provides an environment where young people can cope constructively with other problems with more confidence and self assurance. How long these effects will last can be expressed best in the words of one of the town's elders:

> Before White people came into the North we knew nothing about alcohol. We had good lives and were happy without alcohol. Our ancestors survived for many, many years without alcohol. What use is alcohol then? It has only caused problems.

> Our lives are better now that we no longer have alcohol to worry about. I hope we never have alcohol here in the future. I would like to see alcohol banned forever.

ACKNOWLEDGMENTS

I acknowledge the financial support of the National Health Research and Development Program, Health and Welfare Canada, and the Arctic Institute of North America.

REFERENCES

1. O'Neil JD. Beyond healers and patients: the emergence of local responsibility in Inuit health care. Etudes/Inuit/Studies 1981; 5:17-27.
2. Bruce D. Alcohol in the Northwest Territories: The Canadian enigma. Northern Social Research Information Service. Ottawa, 1978.
3. Brody H. The people's land: Eskimos and Whites in the eastern Arctic. Aylesbury: Penguin Books, 1975.
4. Pain R, ed. The white Arctic: Anthropological essays on tutelage and ethnicity. Newfoundland Social and Economic Papers No. 7. Toronto: Univ Toronto Press, 1977.
5. Matthiasson JS. You scratch my back and I'll scratch yours: continuities in Inuit social relationships. Arctic Anthrop 1975; 12:31-37.
6. Riches D. Alcohol abuse and the problem of social control in a modern Eskimo settlement. In: Holy L, ed. Knowledge and behaviour. The Queen's University Papers on Social Anthropology 1976; 1:65-80.
7. Brody H. Alcohol, change and the industrial frontier. Etudes/Inuit/Studies 1977; 1(2):31-45.

John D. O'Neil
Department of Social and Preventive Medicine
University of Manitoba
750 Bannatyne Avenue
Winnipeg, Manitoba R3E OW3
Canada

Circumpolar Health 84:344-347

DRUGS IN ALASKA: PATTERNS OF USE BY ADULTS AND SCHOOL AGE YOUTH

BERNARD SEGAL

INTRODUCTION

Alaska, with its youthful population and its "last frontier" mentality, represents a place where drugs are purportedly used at a higher level than in the other states. Additionally, the prevalence of a "macho" ethic in the state, particularly among younger white men and women, also allegedly contributes to drug-taking behavior. Linked to these phenomena is the fact that Alaska is a developing entity, or a place in transition, and as such it is still struggling to develop a sense of identity and purpose. This unique situation is manifested by such phenomena as migration linked to a boom-bust economy; an upheaval in the life of Alaska Native people who are having to deal with the health, social, and economic influences on their traditional cultures and life styles; new arrivals having to adjust to living in arctic and subarctic environments; and high rates of violent crimes and suicides. These are but a few of the factors that contribute to placing people in Alaska at high risk for both alcohol and drug abuse. Although significant achievements have been made in gaining a perspective on the nature and extent of alcohol abuse in the state, efforts have only recently begun to acquire a similar perspective on the problem of drug abuse. The purpose of this research was to help obtain an understanding of how prevalent drug-taking behavior is in the state, and to determine how drug use may be related to some of the unique aspects of living in Alaska. The specific research objectives were:

1. To assess the nature and extent of drug-taking behavior in Alaska;
2. To examine age-cohort differences with respect to drug-taking behavior;
3. To identify psychosocial correlates of drug use that may contribute to, mediate, or prevent drug use, and to explore some of the implications that such phenomena have for treatment and prevention programs.

This paper presents some of the major findings from this study that pertain to the prevalence of drug use, and briefly review some of their implications.

METHOD

During 1982-83 an extensive state-wide survey was undertaken to assess the incidence and prevalence of drug-taking behavior among adolescents and adults in Alaska (1,2). Briefly, 3,609 school age youth ranging in age from 12 to 19, of whom 49% were male and 51% female, were surveyed by direct questionnaires in eight different locations of the state. Additionally, 1,007 persons 18 years and older, whom 44% were female and 56% male, were surveyed by means of telephone and face-to-face interviews from the general population in seven different communities around the state.

RESULTS

Table 1 provides the statistics for lifetime experiences (ever having tried a drug one or more times) with psychoactive drugs in Alaska, together with confidence limits that define the interval within which the true value for population may lie. Inspection of the data reveals that over half the sample (51.1%) have tried marijuana, and that over a quarter of the sample have had experiences with stimulant-type drugs. Just under one-fifth of the sample (19.6%) have tried cocaine. Experiences with the remaining drugs range from a high of nearly 15% for experiences with inhalants, to a low 2.1% for heroin. It should be noted that the nature of the three most prevalent drugs that respondents reported experiencing, marijuana, stimulants, and cocaine, share the psychopharmacological characteristic of being able to induce a feeling of pleasantness or euphoria, and both cocaine and stimulants have the additional capacity to induce a "rush," which is a feeling of euphoria and physical well-being experienced immediately after a drug has been taken. Marijuana, which also induces a "rush," albeit less intense than that of

Table 1. Prevalence of experiences with psychoactive drugs in Alaska (N=4,616).

Drug	Lower 95% limit	Ever tried (mean)	Upper 95% limit
Marijuana	49.4	51.1%	52.8
Stimulants	25.7	27.3%	28.9
Cocaine	18.3	19.6%	21.0
Inhalants	13.5	14.7%	15.9
Depressants	14.8	13.8%	14.8
Tranquilizers	10.2	11.2%	12.2
Hallucinogens	9.4	10.4%	11.4
Heroin	1.7	2.1%	2.6

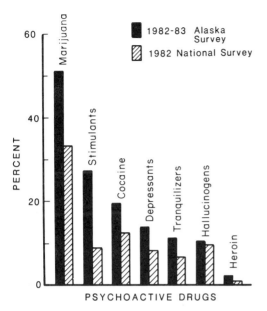

Figure 1. *Lifetime experiences with psycho-active drugs: comparison between Alaska and national survey data.*

Table 2. *Lifetime experiences with psychoactive drugs: comparison of Alaska and national survey data by age groups.*

	12-17 year olds	
	Alaska (N=3,103)	National survey (N=1,581)
Marijuana	47.4%	26.7%
Stimulants	25.9%	6.7%
Cocaine	16.6%	6.5%
Depressants	14.0%	5.8%
Tranquilizers	11.1%	4.9%
Hallucinogens	7.9%	5.2%
Heroin	2.3%	<0.1%

	18-25 year olds	
	Alaska (N=483)	National survey (N=1,283)
Marijuana	76.8%	64.1%
Stimulants	43.9%	18.0%
Cocaine	41.0%	28.3%
Depressants	21.5%	18.7%
Tranquilizers	15.3%	15.1%
Hallucinogens	21.7%	21.1%
Heroin	1.0%	1.2%

	26 and over	
	Alaska (N=790)	National survey (N=2,760)
Marijuana	56.3%	23.0%
Stimulants	25.3%	6.2%
Cocaine	20.3%	8.5%
Depressants	10.4%	4.8%
Tranquilizers	10.5%	3.6%
Hallucinogens	14.9%	6.4%
Heroin	2.7%	1.1%

cocaine or stimulants, provides more of a sustained "high," which is the continuing state of relaxation and well-being experienced while the drug remains active in one's body. It thus appears that the pattern of drug use that has emerged tends to center around experiences with drugs that help one to achieve a high, that is, to "feel good."

Figure 1 provides a comparison of the Alaska data with findings compiled from the 1982 National Survey on Drug Abuse (3). The comparisons show that the prevalence rates for lifetime experience with drugs among Alaskans exceed the rates for each drug obtained in the national sample, and the magnitude of the differences range from a low of 2:1 to a high of 3:1. It is apparent that drug-taking behavior occurs at a higher prevalence rate among Alaskans than among those residing in the other states.

Contained within Table 2 are comparisons of drug use between Alaskans and respondents in other states, grouped by age brackets that were defined within the national survey. Except for a slightly higher prevalence rate (1.2 to 1.0%) for heroin among 18-25 year olds in the national sample, the prevalence rates for experiences with psychoactive drugs among Alaskans within all the age groups are higher than those reported within the national survey.

Table 3 contains a comparison of the prevalence rates among school age youth, young adults, and adults. Although there are some variations, the young adult group

(ages 18-25) tended to show the highest prevalence rates, but the school age group, surprisingly, reported a higher prevalence rate for experiences with heroin; experiences with inhalants and tranquilizers were generally comparable. In all, the findings indicate that although drug-taking behavior tends to be most prevalent in the young, such behavior is nevertheless distributed across age groups, particularly the use of marijuana, stimulants, and cocaine.

Figure 2 depicts the relationship between age of first experience with the three drugs most tried by the school sample: marijuana, stimulants, and cocaine. Inspection of the curves for these three drugs reveals bimodal peaks for all three drugs. There is sharp rise in first experience beginning after age 10, with the first peak

Table 3. Prevalence of lifetime experiences with psychoactive drugs among three Alaska sample groups: youth (students), young adults and adults.

Drugs	Youth 11-19 (N=3,609)	Young adults 18-25 (N=212)	Adults >26 (N̄=795)
Marijuana	49.5%	82.5%	49.9%
Stimulants	27.2%	43.9%	22.8%
Cocaine	18.3%	43.4%	18.1%
Inhalants	16.5%	16.0%	6.2%
Depressants	14.3%	20.8%	9.4%
Tranquilizers	11.5%	12.3%	9.4%
Hallucinogens	8.7%	26.9%	13.6%
Heroin	2.2%	0.5%	2.5%

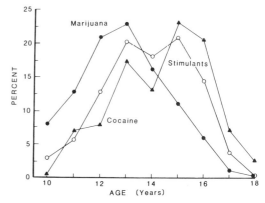

Figure 2. Age at first trial of psychoactive drugs in Alaska school age youth.

occurring at age 13, after which there is a steady decline in new experiences with marijuana, while first experiences with stimulants and cocaine re-peak at age 15, and then both curves decline rather sharply. It thus appears that as experiences with marijuana begin to decline, new experiences with other drugs may start, and that first experience, as a whole, begin to decline after age 15. In all, the configuration indicates that age and first experiences appear to be non-linear, that is, one does not change as a direct function of the other. It should be noted that 13 represents the age when transition to junior high school generally occurs (7th grade), while 15 generally corresponds to the age of transition to senior high school (10th grade).

DISCUSSION

The results of the study indicate a clear pattern of drug-taking behavior that is consistent across age groups throughout the state. Additionally, the overall prevalence levels of lifetime experiences for all segments of the Alaska sample exceed those reported in the national survey.

The high rate of apparent drug use in Alaska from this study raises two questions: 1) whether to believe those data, and 2) how to explain the prevalence of drug use in Alaska.

Although there was no way to check that all self-reporters had had experience with genuine drugs (not substitutes or look-alike substances) this problem is inherent in all forms of survey research. Moreover sufficient research has been conducted on this problem to conclude that self-reports are generally free from systematic bias (4).

Part of the explanation for prevalence of drug use in Alaska seems to be its incorporation into the lifestyle of many people. As such, it tends to be more of a social phenomenon than it is deviant behavior. Consistent with the "last frontier" or "macho" mentality of much of the state's population of young adults, drug-taking behavior may represent breaking away from conformity with the traditional establishment, and a search for excitement and stimulation. Adolescents may largely be emulating this social behavior of young adults, as well as satisfying their own curiosity and seeking excitement. These factors may not account for all drug-taking behavior, but previous research (4) has established a strong relationship between these motives and drug use.

This study has several implications for prevention programs. One implication, for example, is that different prevention goals should be devised in consideration of the prevalence curves for age of first experience with drugs (Figure 2). Prior to the ages of positive acceleration in exposure, delay or prevention of exposure may be the most logical strategy. After these ages of peak first exposure, efforts would probably be best spent on reducing use rates, such as redirecting behavior and developing meaningful behavioral alternatives to drug-taking.

Prevention programs should also be designed to incorporate information on developmental trends in drug-taking behavior and the psychosocial factors that influence the use and non-use of drugs. If drug use prevention programs take into account that drug-taking behavior may have become a social norm, that such behavior is not necessarily deviant or pathological, and that social drug-users may not need in-depth treatment, the programs seem more likely to succeed.

In summary, drug use is high in Alaska, and may be increasing, in contrast to use in other states. We are just beginning to learn of the factors contributing to high rates of drug use in Alaska. Exchanges of information among circumpolar nations on this subject should be rewarding.

REFERENCES

1. Segal B, McKelvy J, Bowman D and Mala T. Patterns of drug use in Alaska: School survey. Juneau, Alaska: Department of Health and Social Services, 1983.
2. Segal B., McKelvy J, Bowman D, Mala T. Patterns of drug use in Alaska: Community survey. Juneau, Alaska: Department of Health and Social Services, 1983.
3. Miller JD, Cisin I. Highlights from the National Survey on Drug Abuse, 1983.
4. Segal B. Confirmatory analyses of reasons for try/taking psychoactive chemicals during adolescence. Int J Addict (In Press.)

Bernard Segal
Center for Alcohol and Addiction Studies
University of Alaska, Anchorage
3211 Providence Drive
Anchorage, Alaska 99508
U.S.A.

Circumpolar Health 84:348-351

RECREATIONAL DRUG USE BY ALASKA'S YOUTH: A REPORT ON SECONDARY SCHOOL STUDENTS IN TWO REGIONS

JANICE DANI BOWMAN, THEODORE A. MALA, BERNARD SEGAL and JILL G. McKELVY

This paper is a report of some of the findings from the first major, systematic study of the recreational use of various psychoactive drugs by the secondary school-age youth of Alaska. The project obtained information on the use of a broad spectrum of chemical substances ranging from legally and socially sanctioned drugs such as alcohol and tobacco, to illegal or unsanctioned use of drugs such as marijuana, cocaine, and stimulants.

The entire study includes data for over 3,600 students across the state. In order to focus the findings from such a large study around the theme of "circumpolar health," the current paper reports results from only two regions of the state: 1) a "rural" region, consisting of data aggregated from Kotzebue, Barrow, and Nome, and 2) an urban region, the city of Anchorage.

The use, and at times the abuse, of psychoactive chemical substances continues to be a fact of life in the contemporary cultures of the United States. Both accepted "conventional wisdom" and published figures on per capita alcohol consumption (1) suggest that usage rates for adults are probably higher in Alaska than in other parts of the U.S. Until now, few data have been available on whether this higher than average usage rate of a psychoactive drug extends to any substance other than alcohol.

In recent years, American society in general has experienced a sizable increase in the frequency and intensity of the use of psychoactive substances other than alcohol for recreational purposes. This increased rate of usage has shown itself to be quite strong among the younger segments of the population, especially those between the ages of 18 and 25.

Of special concern to our society is the use of psychoactive drugs by school-age youth, and judging by national survey figures the secondary school-age youth of America have participated in some degree in this increasing recreational use of psycho-active substances (2). Reports from two recent national surveys (2,3) suggest a decline for the first time in many years of the use of some psychoactive drugs by secondary school students. The current survey allows a first-time comparison of some of the secondary school youth of Alaska with their counterparts in the other states and in a province of Canada in terms of their recreational use of psychoactive drugs.

METHODS

The survey instruments were developed in cooperation with each school district and are included at the end of the paper. The instrument used in Anchorage differed slightly from that used in the rural areas mainly because of additional questions added at the request of the Anchorage School District. The survey was conducted during regular school hours by research team members and classroom teachers. Every effort was made to insure the confidentiality of the information given by students, and at no time was access to the individual completed questionnaires allowed to any personnel other than research team members.

Questions included in the survey instruments addressed the use/non-use of drugs for recreational purposes, specifically: marijuana, hallucinogens, cocaine, heroin, inhalants, stimulants, depressants, tranquilizers, alcohol, and cigarettes. Reasons for taking/not taking these drugs were explored along with questions about frequency and recency of use. All students filled out the forms in groups, either in classroom or auditorium settings, the entire process taking approximately half an hour. It was carefully explained that the purpose of the study was to gain an understanding of drug use in Alaska and not to identify individuals who use or have used drugs. Students' names were not requested in any phase of the research; the only identifying information was age, grade, and gender. In the Anchorage sample the procedure was "representative" sampling based on the judgment of school district officials, thus, only certain classes were surveyed at each school. In the rural areas, the type of sample was "total population"; thus, every secondary school student in attendance on the day of the survey filled out a questionnaire. Table 1 indicates the number of respondents in each area, and the percentage of the total population of students participating in the survey.

Table 1. Number and percent of student sample and type of sample.

Area	Students surveyed	Percent of students present
Kotzebue	203	100
Barrow	154	100
Anchorage	1,588	10.4
Nome	243	100

Table 2. Proportion (%) of secondary students having the opportunity to try, and who have ever tried various drugs.

	Barrow-Kotzebue-Nome (N=600)		Anchorage (N=1,588)		1982 National survey (N=1,581)	
	Chance to try	Ever tried	Chance to try	Ever tried	Chance to try	Ever tried
Marijuana	72.2	58.5	64.5	51.4	50.5	26.7
Cocaine	29.3	18.0	27.0	23.5	19.6	6.5
Hallucinogens	17.7	9.2	12.2	9.5	14.6	5.2
Stimulants	33.3	25.8	32.6	28.6	na	6.7
Inhalants	22.3	15.0	27.7	18.4	na	na
Depressants	14.5	10.5	23.0	19.9	na	7.4
Tranquilizers	9.0	6.3	19.7	17.9	na	4.9
Heroin	8.3	2.2	5.7	3.2	6.8	<0.5
Alcohol	na	68.0	83.9	82.1	na	65.5
Cigarettes	na	72.2	64.9	64.9	na	49.5

RESULTS

As expected, alcohol and tobacco, the two legally and socially sanctioned drugs for adults in our society, are the psychoactive substances which the most students have encountered and tried. Table 2 indicates that the proportion of students ever trying alcohol was 68% for the rural sample, 82.1% for Anchorage, and 65.5% nationally. The proportion trying cigarettes for the rural sample was 52.0%, Anchorage 64.9%, and nationally 49.5%. The figures on marijuana indicate that it has been tried by about the same number of students as tobacco cigarettes have been here in Alaska. The proportion of students who have tried marijuana was 51.4% for Anchorage, 58.5% for the rural sample, and 26.7% nationally.

After alcohol, cigarettes, and marijuana, more students had not tried the other substances than had tried them. Of those tried, stimulants (rural 25.8%; Anchorage 28.6%; nationally 6.7%) and cocaine were the most often cited (rural 18.0%; Anchorage 23.5%, nationally 6.5%). These were followed closely by depressants (rural 10.5%; Anchorage 19.9%; nationally 7.4%), inhalants (rural 15.0%; Anchorage 18.4%; nationally no figures available), and tranquilizers (rural 6.3%; Anchorage 17.9%; nationally 4.9%). Of all the drugs surveyed, hallucinogens (rural 9.2%; Anchorage 9.5%; nationally 5.2%) and heroin (rural 2.2%; Anchorage 3.2%; nationally less than 0.5%) have been tried by the smallest number of students.

The opportunity to try the drugs surveyed varied appreciably between the Alaska samples and the national sample as illustrated in Table 2. This is especially

Table 3. Past year (1983) frequency of students in Barrow-Kotzebue-Nome district taking various drugs expressed as percent of total sample. Total sample, N=600. Frequency columns rounded to nearest integer.

		Frequency of use			
	% of sample taking in past year	Once a month or less	2-4 times a month	2-5 times a week	Once a day or more
Marijuana	50.7	20	15	7	8
Cocaine	11.2	7	3	1	1
Hallucinogens	4.1	3	1	1	<1
Stimulants	14.7	10	4	1	1
Inhalants	7.3	5	2	<1	<1
Depressants	6.3	4	2	<1	<1
Tranquilizers	3.2	2	1	<1	1
Heroin	2.5	2	<1	<1	<1
Alcohol	43.0	18	21	3	2
Cigarettes	22.0	<1	7	<1	16

Table 4.   Past year (1983) frequency of students in Anchorage district sample taking various drugs expressed as percent of total sample.   Total sample, N=1,588. Frequency columns rounded to nearest integer.

	% of sample taking in past year	Frequency of use			
		Once a month or less	2-4 times a month	2-5 times a week	Once a day or more
Marijuana	45.5	21	12	7	6
Cocaine	21.5	15	4	<1	<1
Hallucinogens	8.1	6	<1	<1	<1
Stimulants	26.2	15	7	2	1
Inhalants	14.0	11	2	<1	1
Depresssants	17.1	11	4	1	1
Tranquilizers	14.9	10	3	1	<1
Heroin	4.1	1	1	1	<1
Alcohol	74.8	30	30	10	4
Cigarettes	50.2	23	6	4	17

true for the opportunity to try marijuana (rural 72.2%; Anchorage 64.5%; nationally 50.5%) and cocaine (rural 29.9%; Anchorage 27.0%; nationally 19.6%).

Tables 3 and 4 indicate that in Alaska, alcohol, cigarettes, and marijuana have been used during the past year (1983) by at least half the students surveyed. Alcohol was used during the past year by three-fourths of the Anchorage sample (74.8%) and by almost half of the rural sample (43.0%). Cigarettes have been used by half of the Anchorage students (50.2%) but by only about one-fifth of the rural students (22.0%; the use of tobacco products in this area is probably higher than this figure indicates, since it is commonly used in forms other than cigarettes in rural Alaska). Marijuana had been used in the year by about half of both the rural (50.7%) and the Anchorage (45.5%) samples. The use of cocaine (rural 11.2%; Anchorage 21.5%) and stimulants

(rural 14.7%; Anchorage 26.2%) in the past year was appreciable in both samples. The frequency of using the rest of the drugs surveyed was much lower, as the Tables indicate.

Daily use of cigarettes was highest of any drug surveyed, with about one-fifth of both Alaska samples using this drug daily. Daily use of alcohol and marijuana were approximately the same, ranging from 2 to 8% of the sample. Daily use of any of the other drugs was 1% or less.

Comparisons of the percent of students using the various drugs in some amount over the past year is illustrated in Table 5 for the Alaska samples, the U.S. national sample, and for a 1981 sample of secondary students in the province of Ontario, Canada (5). Table 5 clearly indicates a higher usage during the last year for Alaskan students for a number of drugs. The difference is particularly evident for marijuana

Table 5.   Comparison of four surveys: Percent of secondary students who have taken various drugs in the past year (1983).

Drug	Barrow-Kotzebue-Nome (N=600)	Anchorage (N=1,588)	1982 National Survey(3) (N=1,581)	1981 Survey, Province of Ontario (5) (N=1,300)
Marijuana	50.7	45.5	21.0	29.9
Hallucinogens	4.1	8.1	3.6	14.9
Cocaine	11.2	21.5	4.0	4.8
Heroin	2.5	4.1	<0.5	1.5
Inhalants	7.3	14.1	na	5.5
Stimulants	14.7	26.2	5.6	21.5
Depressants	6.3	17.1	7.4	20.6
Tranquilizers	3.2	14.9	3.3	12.4
Alcohol	43.0	74.8	47.3	75.3
Cigarettes	22.0	50.2	24.9	30.3

(rural 50.7%; Anchorage 45.5%; nationally 21%; Ontario 29.9%) and for cocaine (rural 11.2%; Anchorage 21.5%; nationally 4.0%; Ontario 4.8%). On the other hand, reading the table from stimulants on down through cigarettes, the rural Alaska sample and the U.S. national sample look similar, and the usage rates are quite a bit lower than those for the Anchorage and the Ontario samples.

DISCUSSION

Over two-thirds of secondary school students in Alaska have had the opportunity to try at least one illicit drug other than alcohol and tobacco. One-half of all those surveyed have tried marijuana at least once in their lives. Cocaine is relatively available to students and about one-fifth of those surveyed have tried this drug. These are high levels of substance use, whether considered alone or in comparison to the rest of the United States or to a part of Canada. In the case of marijuana, the figures are twice the national average, for cocaine, three times the national average. When past year experiences with these drugs are considered, the rural Alaska sample cannot be distinguished from the national sample except for the marijuana and cocaine categories. Specifically, the use of alcohol was no different over the past year for the rural and national samples. The past year alcohol use for the Anchorage sample is about one and one-half times the national average, and is nearly identical to the Canadian sample.

The question of why Alaska students should be trying drugs like cocaine and marijuana, and for the Anchorage sample,

alcohol, at these rates cannot be addressed by the parametric data reported here. One obvious hypothesis for future work is that the increased availability of many drugs in Alaska leads directly to increased experimentation.

There is some good news in the results. The daily use of alcohol and cigarettes is somewhat lower in Alaska than nationally, especially in the rural areas. But on the whole, the current results send a clear message to all who care to address themselves to the future adults of Alaska. The drug problem is both real and immediate.

REFERENCES

1. Mala TA. The status of substance use and abuse in Alaska: 1982. Paper presented at World Assembly of First Nations, Regina, Saskatchewan, Canada, 1982.
2. Johnston L, Bachman J, O'Mally P. Student drug use: attitudes and beliefs. Rockville, MD: National Institute of Drug Abuse, 1982.
3. Miller JD, Cisin IH. National survey on drug abuse: main findings. Rockville, MD: National Institute of Drug Abuse, 1982.
4. Segal BG, McKelvy JG, Bowman JD, Mala TA. Patterns of drug use: School survey. Center for Alcohol and Addiction Studies, University of Alaska, Anchorage, 1983.
5. Smart et al. Addiction Research Foundation, Toronto, 1981. Reprinted in U.S. Public Health Service Research Monograph 43, 1982.

Janice Dani Bowman
1005 Potlatch Circle
Anchorage, Alaska 99503
U.S.A.

Circumpolar Health 84:352-356

A MODEL FOR THE DELIVERY OF ALCOHOL AND DRUG ABUSE TREATMENT IN ALASKA

VERNER STILLNER

INTRODUCTION

Alcoholism and drug abuse are serious problems in Alaska. Environmental conditions are so extreme that the state's inhabitants are subjected to unusual degrees of stress, with the result that many become dependent on alcohol or drugs. This paper focuses on the treatment of such alcohol and drug dependency. First, however, an overview of the nature and extent of the problem is necessary.

Alaska's land mass is one-fifth the size of the continental United States. About one-quarter of that land mass is above the Arctic Circle, where permafrost keeps two-thirds of these arctic lands in perpetual ice. This rugged terrain experiences temperatures ranging from 38°C to -62°C, with precipitation varying from 508 cm in the southeast to desert-like dry conditions in the high Arctic. The northern and western diurnal changes alternate between complete darkness in the winter to complete sunlight in the summer.

As of 1980, Alaska's population was estimated at over 400,000, an increase of 100,000 since the 1970 census. This population is young and ethnically diverse. In short, Alaska has an extreme environment that challenges a young, rapidly growing population to adjust constantly to a changing climate and to diurnal variation.

Alcohol consumption in Alaska is quite high and rising. The per capita sales of absolute alcohol in Alaska increased from 11.01 liters (2.91 gallons) in 1960 to 14.95 liters (3.95 gallons) in 1970, to 16.65 liters (4.4 gallons) in 1978. By contrast, per capita sales of absolute alcohol in the United States between 1960 and 1977 increased from 3.79 liters (2.0 gallons) to 10.83 liters (2.86 gallons) (1). Alaskans also report a much higher rate of lifetime experiences with drugs other than alcohol; in some instances, they report a rate two to three times higher than the national average, as indicated by the most recent National Survey on Drug Use (1982) (2,3). Although the discussion that follows concentrates on the problems of alcohol abuse, the treatment techniques and procedures described here will apply to the problems of drug abuse as well.

The rate of alcoholism in Alaska is alarmingly high; in 1975 it was 418% above the national average. The state's alcoholism mortality rate rose by a dramatic 153% between 1959 and 1975; during this period, the rate of death from cirrhosis of the liver alone increased by 142% (1). These increases in death rates due to alcoholism and cirrhosis of the liver correspond

closely to the increases in the average annual consumption of beverage alcohol (4). Since 1960, the rate of death from alcoholism in Alaska has consistently exceeded the national death rate for this disease (5).

The economic impact of alcoholism and alcohol abuse has been enormous. To Alaska's health and medical delivery system, the cost of the utilization of excess hospital services only was determined to be $13.3 million in 1975. Productivity is lowered through absenteeism, injuries, premature death, and associated industrial costs, since workers with alcohol problems produce less and are prone to more occupational injuries; in 1975, the economic cost of this lost production amounted to $86.4 million. The total economic cost to Alaska of alcoholism and alcohol abuse amounted to $131.2 million in 1975 (1).

Clearly, alcoholism and its consequences present the state of Alaska with growing problems, and not enough is being done. For example, although the number of problem drinkers in Alaska was estimated at 30,000 in 1975, only about 3,600 persons were admitted to local alcoholism treatment programs in fiscal year 1976 (1). Obviously, a large percentage of problem drinkers are not receiving treatment.

The situation, however, is far from hopeless. For one thing, the problem of alcoholism presents great similarities with Alaska's tuberculosis epidemic in the 1950s and 1960s. Like tuberculosis, alcoholism and other chemical dependencies are chronic illnesses that are progressive and disposed toward relapse, affecting to some extent the entire family. So, presumably, we can learn something about treatment from this past experience with a somewhat similar problem. Also encouraging is the knowledge that alcoholism and chemical dependencies are tractable illnesses, and that treatment is cost-effective. Once an alcoholic receives treatment for his drinking, there is a median reduction of other health care services by 40% (6).

To respond effectively to these encouraging signs, Alaska needs a comprehensive treatment network within its borders that will accommodate varying regional needs. Such a network would have to provide specialized services to accommodate different needs for delivery of treatment. Coordination of treatment modalities would be essential, since Alaska's health care delivery system is a pluralistic one, involving the private sector, the Alaska Area Native Health Service, Native health corporations, military hospitals, and state and locally supported programs.

General Phases of Treatment

This paper will deal only with the treatment aspects of alcoholism and substance abuse. The state of the art in the treatment of alcohol and substance abuse, following diagnosis, involves three phases: (1) medical detoxification, (2) treatment, and (3) aftercare (Table 1).

The medical detoxification phase is designed to rid the body of the noxious chemical or chemicals, while minimizing the withdrawal symptoms by using decreasing doses of a similar, longer-acting chemical over a 5-14 day period. The length of this phase depends on the half-life of the patient's drug of choice and on the overall physical and mental condition of the pa-

Table 1. Treatment phases for alcohol and drug abuse.

I. Detoxification Phase (4-14 days); Place: Hospital

   A. Provide warm, safe, and supportive environment

   B. Obtain history

   C. Evaluate physical status

   D. Begin treatment of physical condition.

   E. Begin mental status and psychological assessment

   F. Begin social assessment

   G. Prepare patient for participation in treatment

   H. Prepare family or significant other for participation in treatment

II. Treatment Phase (14-17 days); Place: Hospital or Outpatient

   A. Establish physical assessment

   B. Establish a comprehensive nursing or counseling assessment

   C. Establish a psychosocial assessment

   D. Establish a psychological assessment

   E. Establish a comprehensive treatment plan

   F. Orient and facilitate patient's participation in self-help group (Alcoholics Anonymous, Narcotics Anonymous) and activities

   G. Provide a comprehensive education program for the patient about addictive diseases

   H. Facilitate the recovery process through group therapies

Table 1. (continued)

   I. Facilitate the recovery process through individual therapies

   J. Facilitate the recovery process through the learning practice of adaptive activities, such as meditation and relaxation techniques

   K. Facilitate the recovery process through unit community milieu

   L. Facilitate the recovery process through activity therapies, such as recreational therapy, occupational therapy, and movement therapy

   M. Provide the opportunity for personal spiritual counseling and religious services

   N. Facilitate the recovery process through family participation in educational groups, therapeutic groups, self-help groups, and couples counseling

   O. Prepare the patient for re-entry into the community through therapeutic trial visits and discharge planning

III. Aftercare Phase (One Year After Hospitalization); Place: Outpatient/Community

   A. Establish a coherent system of support for patient recovery

   B. Provide a weekly support group for former patients

   C. Provide telephone access to hospital staff on a 24-hour basis for former patients

   D. Maintain contact on a monthly basis with former patients by phone and/or mail

   E. Evaluate the effectiveness of the patient and aftercare program

tient. For example, the detoxification of alcoholics takes approximately 3-5 days, depending on the individual's age. Sedative-hypnotic and opiate drugs, on the other hand, require approximately 10-14 days for detoxification, depending on the dosage and duration of dependence. This treatment should ideally take place in a hospital environment. During the hospital stay, other physical conditions should be identified and treated simultaneously, such as infections, fractures, burns, metabolic disorders, and neuropsychiatric problems.

The treatment phase has as its goal total abstinence from the drug or drugs of choice and from similarly acting chemicals; this goal can be achieved by a well-designed educational program that teaches the patient about chemical dependencies, new coping mechanisms, and self-help groups. The patient can be treated either in a hospital or in an outpatient setting, but regardless of the setting, this phase of treatment is most effective when the patient's family is involved. Addictive diseases lead to pathological patterns of familial interactions; therefore, a change in the patient requires changes in the entire family system surrounding that patient.

Finally, the aftercare phase of treatment should take place in the home community, with the involvement of self-help groups, therapists and counselors where indicated, employee assistance programs, and aftercare personnel. The aftercare phase lasts for a year after the patient's release from the hospital and is designed to insure his or her health readjustment to everyday life.

An individual undergoing treatment should progress sequentially through all three phases of treatment; he or she can be treated in a hospital, as an outpatient, or in a community setting, depending on the availability of resources and the severity of the individual's chemical dependency.

MODEL ADDICTIVE DISEASE TREATMENT PROGRAM

The ideal center for this Alaska treatment network would be approximately 48 beds, located in an urban hospital. This model program should be situated near Alaska's major hospitals (where health care professionals are concentrated), universities, and communication and transportation networks. The program could operate through either public or private monies, but the private-for-profit model would generate funds more quickly for capital construction and would make possible greater versatility in programming (Figure 1).

In the ideal model treatment program, specialized care to special population groups, such as adolescents and the elderly, would be deliverable. Those individuals who have multiple relapses in treatment needs

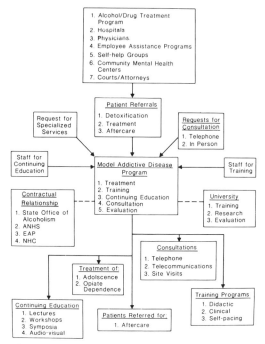

Figure 1. Model Addictive Disease Treatment Program.

outside of the urban area and have special further treatment problems, such as opiate and cocaine dependency, could also be referred to the model treatment center's program staff.

Mission

The mission of this model program would be: (1) treatment of addictive diseases; (2) training of clinicians to work in hospital and community programs throughout Alaska; (3) continuing education for personnel in Alaska's alcohol and drug abuse treatment facilities; (4) consultation to all of Alaska's treatment facilities; and (5) evaluation of treatment outcome.

The treatment of patients would follow the steps outlined in Table 1, with the average treatment lasting 21 days for alcohol and 28 days for substance dependence.

The training and continuing education needs of Alaska's urban and rural addictive disease clinicians would be delivered through didactic programs, clinical settings, and self-paced learning methods. An important component of training and continuing education would be a library of literature, audio tapes, audio-visual tapes, and films to supplement the training needs of the visiting professional. This same library could offer professional assistance in answering questions raised by personnel from all of Alaska's alcohol and drug treatment programs.

Educational programs for the treatment of addictive disease patients would be conducted on a three or four week cycle. The entire series would be taped, and these audio-visual materials could then be used by all treatment programs in Alaska. Telecommunications would also allow the transmission of this educational program from the model center to all other Alaska treatment sites. This didactic training curriculum in addictive disease treatment should ideally be certified by the universities for all of the professionals involved. The participation of the universities in the treatment aspects of this model program would ensure a high standard of training and would legitimatize this training for future certification and licensing.

The continuing education needs of personnel outside Alaska's chosen urban center could also be met through the use of newsletters, audio-visual tapes, and scheduled telecommunications programming. Such a training and continuing education program in the treatment of addictive diseases would provide physicians, nurses, counselors, social workers, and psychologists with the opportunity to be trained throughout Alaska in a program that addresses the unique needs of Alaska's population.

The specialized staff of the model treatment program could provide consultation upon request to all of Alaska's treatment programs. These consultations could be delivered by telephone, telecommunication, face-to-face consultation in the model treatment program, and by model treatment program staff visits to programs outside the urban area.

Finally, standards should be developed at the outset of the program to evaluate outcome and training. Since development of such standards requires objectivity and some neutrality, it could best be done by the state's university.

Personnel

Staffing for the model treatment program should include nurses, physicians (psychiatrists, internists, pediatricians), addictive disease counselors, social workers, and psychologists with special training, experience, and interest in the treatment of alcoholism and substance abuse.

The staff of the model program involved in treatment and training should all subscribe to the treatment orientation: that alcoholism and substance abuse are addictive diseases arising out of multiple causes with serious bio-psychosocial, cultural, and spiritual consequences. Most important, the staff members must believe that they are dealing with treatable diseases. Staff members working in addictive disease treatment should have specific training and experience in the phase of treatment in which they are involved. Recovering staff, those who have had personal experience with alcoholism or drug dependence, could provide good role models for patients and could help to develop a good therapeutic bridge with self-help groups.

Training of staff in detoxification, treatment manuals, educational sessions at the site of the program, through experience at a central model program, or through on-going telecommunications. After finishing an initial orientation program designed for the particular phase of treatment, all staff members would complete a core curriculum involving the three phases of treatment. The common core curriculum would provide a skeleton upon which all programs in Alaska could build and add their own particular regional variations. The core curriculum would also provide continuity of programming for all three phases of treatment; trainees would learn to use a common treatment vocabulary, and thus patients would be assured a good, smooth flow from one phase of treatment to another, even though the treatment may be rendered by different staff in several Alaska locations.

Economics

If developed as a private-for-profit or non-profit hospital, this model treatment facility might be too concerned about the patient's ability to pay. Therefore, the costs of treatment rendered should be covered by the major third-party payors in Alaska. Also, if the facility is licensed, certified, and accredited by the Joint Commission on Accreditation of Hospitals, it becomes eligible to receive payment from Medicaid, Medicare, and CHAMPUS (a government-paid supplementary health insurance plan for military personnel and dependents). For those individuals not covered by the third-party payors, including Medicaid/Medicare, and are unable to pay fees for services, contractual relationships could be developed. For example, the State Office on Alcoholism and Drug Abuse, the Alaska Area Native Health Service, Native Health Corporations, and Employee Assistance Programs, could contract with the model treatment program for inpatient, outpatient, training, continuing education, and consultative services.

Because of its statewide linkages through treatment, training, continuing education, and consultative services, the model treatment program would receive patient referrals from throughout Alaska. For this to happen, however, the quality of staff and treatment at the model program must hold the respect of Alaska's population, health professionals, self-help groups, and agencies.

Linkages

The presence in Alaska of this program for the specialized care of addictive disease patients would give Alaska's students in the medical sciences an opportunity to be trained in Alaska. An Alaska-based program would help to address Alaska's future manpower needs in the treatment of alcoholism and substance abuse. At the beginning, training could be conducted under the auspices of the University of Alaska and the WAMI (Washington, Alaska, Montana, Idaho) Medical Program's component of the University of Washington Medical School.

Furthermore, this university network could arrange to have the beds and patients available for applied research relating to one of Alaska's major public health problems. Much could be learned from studying treatment outcome among Alaska's diverse population.

DISCUSSION

The type of treatment program discussed here has several advantages. First of all, developing a model treatment program for alcoholism and substance abuse within Alaska will help meet the need for solutions to a major public health problem in Alaska. Such a specialized health service and training center within Alaska's borders would further develop Alaska's increasing sophistication in its own health care delivery system. It would allow Alaskans to address their own needs within the state near their communities of origin. Developing such a model program centered in Anchorage, for example would allow for locating regional programs in Fairbanks and Juneau, which would provide even greater opportunities to address regional and cultural differences, while keeping both patients and trainees closer to their home communities.

This treatment program also has economic advantages. The utilization of a private model does not require state or federal monies for initial capital expenditures, nor does it require additional public employees. The advantage to the private sector is that such a model treatment program would attract patients from all over the state through its intimate contact with clinicians in Alaska's rural and urban alcohol and drug treatment facilities; as a result, the facility would not lack sufficient numbers of patients.

The program described here is a comprehensive one, designed not only to treat individuals with alcohol and drug dependency problems, but also to train the health care professionals responsible for that treatment. Given Alaska's rapidly growing population and the state's serious problems with alcoholism and drug dependence, the need for such a comprehensive approach is clear. This model program would give Alaska an ideal treatment and training center capable of addressing the needs of the whole state.

REFERENCES

1. The Alaska state alcoholism and drug abuse plan, 1981-1983. Juneau: State of Alaska Office of Alcoholism and Drug Abuse.
2. Miller JD, Cisin IH. National survey on drug use: Main findings. Washington: National Institute on Drug Abuse, 1983.
3. Segal B, McKelvy J, Bowman D, Mala TA. Patterns of Drug Use: Community Survey. Anchorage: University of Alaska Center for Alcohol and Addiction Studies, 1983.
4. De Lint J, Schmidt W. Consumption averages and alcoholism prevalence: A brief review of epidemiological investigations. Br J Addiction 1971; 66: 97-107.
5. Kraus RF, Buffler PA. Sociocultural stress and the American Native in Alaska: An analysis of changing patterns of psychiatric illness and alcohol abuse among Alaska Natives. Cult Med Psychiat 1979; 3:111-151.
6. Doves KR, Vischi TR. Impact of alcohol, drug abuse and mental health treatment on medical care utilization. Med Care 1979; 17:3-5.

Verner Stillner
Charter Ridge Hospital
3050 Rio Dosa Drive
Lexington, Kentucky 40509
U.S.A.

Circumpolar Health 84:357-360

THE EFFECTS OF A SMOKING PREVENTION PROGRAM FOR ALASKA YOUTH

JOHN F. LEE

Concerned about the apparent high prevalence of smoking among rural Alaska school children and its deleterious effect on health, the Alaska Native Health Board and the Maniilaq Association, both Native consumer advocacy groups, decided to conduct jointly a survey in five Northwest Alaska communities to determine the extent of smoking, and the smoking practices and attitudes of its residents. The information was then used to design an educational program to help dissuade Alaska youth from smoking. This report gives the highlights of the initial survey findings, a description of the smoking prevention program and its short-term efficacy as measured by post-intervention testing.

Setting

The Northwest Alaska Native Association Region (NANA) was selected as the area in which to carry out the project. The Maniilaq and Native Health Board staff, with the cooperation and participation of the teachers of the Northwest Arctic School District, performed the work. This beautiful NANA Region is bisected by the Arctic Circle. It lies on the south slope of the Brooks Range, and touches the Chukchi Sea. The 5,300 inhabitants live in 11 villages situated on the sea or on one of the rivers running into it. The culture is a blend of ancient Eskimo and modern ways because of mineral, oil, and tourist development, along with acceleration of change due to the Alaska Native Claims Settlement Act. Preservation of culture and language is high priority for the people; they take pride in being Eskimo in their traditions, skills as artisans, hunters, whalers, and in their prowess in mastering the elements by their fitness and endurance. These ways are vital to their spirit.

Table 1. Initial survey participants, 1981.

Grade group	Number	% of regional population at risk
Children K-3	216	52
Children 4-6	161	40
Youth 7-12	319	61
Subtotal	696	52
Adult	435	14
Total	1,131	21

METHODS

Five villages--Kotzebue, the largest, plus Ambler, Shungnak, Buckland and Noatak-- participated in the project. All school children from kindergarden (K) through the 12th grade took part in the initial survey, as did representative samples of adults. Table 1 shows the distribution of the participants by group. Standard self-report questionnaires modified for age were used, and administered in the classroom. Adults were personally interviewed. Over 50% of children and 14% of adults at risk were tested (Table 1).

RESULTS

Adult smoking was very prevalent. In this group, 56% smoked, 46% on a daily basis, 24% using at least a pack (20 cigarettes) per day. Prevalence was highest in the 40 to 49 year old group (69%). Next highest was the 19 to 29 group (60%), the youngest of the adults. Slightly more men than women smoked (59% vs. 55%). Most smokers did not know why they smoked, and wanted to quit. Smoking was perceived by 93% to be harmful. Prevalence ranged from 50% to 74% in the five communities. Obviously this type of environment results in high pressure on children and teenagers to smoke.

Of the K through 3 grades, 8.4% have tried smoking, about one-third of them often. Of these, 38% thought it harmless.

In grades 4 to 6, 9.6% claimed to smoke and almost all of them often, with girls smoking as much as boys. Knowledge of smoking effects was high, with 98% scoring correctly. Attitude was highly favorable. Some 20.6% chewed tobacco or used snuff, apparently a carryover of traditional practices.

This group of students in grades 7 to 12 included 319 students; 203 from Kotzebue, 25 from Ambler, 27 from Shungnak, 25 from Buckland and 35 from Noatak. Of the total, 54% were boys and 46% girls.

Ambler and Shungnak had smoking rates of 79% and 69% respectively, while rates for Buckland and Noatak were 32% and 21%. The prevalence at Kotzebue was 37%. These wide variations among communities reflect significant factors influencing smoking behavior of the residents.

The age at which smoking began peaked at 12 to 13 years when 13% of youngsters said they started smoking, and coincident with reaching the 6th and 7th grades. By this time the great majority had tried tobacco. Smokers by grade increased strikingly from 16% to 42% from grade 7 to 8, progressing to 63% in the 12th grade. This is an extremely high level compared to the national average of 23% for the 12th grade. An analysis by sex showed that 49% of the girls were smokers versus 29% of the boys.

Of the 319 group members, 124 or 41.4% were cigarette smokers; 79% smoked daily. Among the daily smokers 58% were girls, as were 59% of the total smokers. Tobacco-chewing and taking snuff were practiced by 28% of the students, nearly all of them boys.

Over 95% knew that smoking can cause heart attacks and lung cancer, but awareness of the lesser known and immediate effects was in the 60 to 70% range. Ninety-three percent believed most teenagers smoke (true in this group but not so generally). High pressures from friends and family by example alone was indicated because of the high prevalence of smoking in these close associates. There was moderate favorable pressure from parents in that they frowned on smoking, but 85% of those in grades 7 to 12 lived with a household smoker.

Findings from the Initial Survey

Tobacco use, especially cigarette smoking, among adults and school-age children in the NANA Region is much higher than in the general U.S. population, and approximates that of Inuit youth of the Northwest Territories of Canada (NWT), as shown in Table 2.

Smoking rates as related to sex and age parallel each other in the different groups in that men smoke somewhat more than women, while the opposite is true for youth--more girls tend to smoke than boys. The alarming thing is the high rates in both the Canadian and Alaskan Inuit or Eskimos. NANA girls smoke almost four times as much as U.S. girls, and their older counterparts twice as much as U.S. women as a whole (2-5).

These patterns were essentially the same in each of the five communities except for a very high prevalence among the youth in Ambler and Shungnak compared to Buckland and Noatak, with Kotzebue in an intermediate

position. Undoubtedly these differences were due to unique local values not revealed in the survey.

Correlation analysis was performed to determine the relationships among attitude, health knowledge, social pressures, smoking behavior, and smoking frequency based on the test scores. From the results it appeared that the most important factor influencing youth to smoke or not to smoke is pressure from family, friends, or environment. How friends behave, one's attitude on sports, and belief about what others say all factor into the complex process of making a choice about smoking. Knowledge of adverse effects on health was a common denominator, and could not be singled out as a factor exerting a definite influence on smoking behavior. The significance of the survey results was that patterns of response were the same for the youth of Northwest Alaska as for those in other parts of the U.S., and for that matter, the world.

The Smoking Prevention Program

In designing a suitable smoking prevention program, our prime concern was sensitivity to the culture, and how the children would receive such a program. It had to fit the environmental and cultural setting and relate to their values and activities as much as possible. Based on analysis of the survey findings, the objectives set for the prevention program were to provide to students a better awareness of:

- the immediate effects of smoking and how it can interfere with what they like to do (i.e., sports, hunting).
- how others influence them to smoke or not to smoke.
- how to cope with pressures to smoke.

After literature search, and contact with those involved in applying successful programs, two models were selected--The Biofeedback program, as implemented by the New Hampshire Lung Association (5), and the

Table 2.   Comparison of NANA, U.S., Alaska, and NWT smoking prevalences.

Group	NANA	U.S.	Alaska Native	Non	Canada Native	Non	NANA/U.S. Ratio
Adults	56.4%	33.2%	47%	36%			1.7
Women	54.8	29.6		35			1.9
Men	59.0	37.5		40	(ages 15-19)		1.6
Youth 12-18	41.4	11.7			58%	42%	3.5
Girls	49.3	12.7			61	47	3.9
Boys	28.8	10.7			55	36	2.7

Peer Led Social Consequences program designed by the University of Minnesota (6). The content of these programs was modified to fit the local setting, and curriculum guides prepared for use by teachers.

Teacher training was conducted by a trained health educator with initial involvement of the Minnesota director; continuous support was provided the teachers throughout the program (7).

The elements selected to constitute the program were:

1. Smoking prevention school curriculum, Grades 4-6: biofeedback program to be linked with "Here's Looking at You" (a substance abuse curriculum), Grades 7-12: peer-led classes on smoking pressures.
2. Local film production to reinforce learning.
3. Teen-sponsored "Feeling Good" fair on smoking.
4. Smoking cessation resources.
5. Apply the intervention program.
6. A post-intervention evaluation.

The Biofeedback Module

The basis of the biofeedback module concept is the use of measurement instruments to feed back information immediately to the subject on what happens to the body as a result of smoking cigarettes. The use of a carboximeter to measure the carbon monoxide level in the breath, a digital heart rate monitor to measure pulse rate, a digital thermometer to measure skin temperature and a tremor tester to measure hand steadiness vividly demonstrate the effect of cigarette smoking on body physiology. Adolescents can relate this to their ability to perform in sports, a matter of great pride to almost all youth, and especially to the students involved in this study. This program has a good record of acceptance and success in the short term (6).

The peer leadership technique is based on the premise that adolescents are more likely to be influenced by peers whom they respect or admire than adults delivering the same message. A second premise of this program is that most adolescents begin smoking as a result of pressure brought to bear by their friends, family members, or the advertising media. By the use of peer opinion leaders selected by their own classmates, fellow students become aware of the ways in which pressure is exerted, learn coping skills to resist them, and more about the immediate effects of smoking (7).

The production of a culturally relevant film/videotape to be used as part of the curriculum content and available for public use for health education, was judged to be an important program component. Consequent-

ly, theme and story were developed by the Native staff, set locally, acted by the students and produced in Kotzebue. Health information messages were conveyed using biofeedback equipment and other verbal and visual techniques. In addition, messages demonstrating peer pressure, coping methods, and the need to make decisions based on preferred values were transmitted through the story acted out by the players (1).

To publicize the smoking prevention program, we helped organize a region-wide Health Day (known as "Feeling Good Day") to promote a healthy lifestyle. It was given strong support by community associations and the school district, and sponsored chiefly by the Maniilaq Association. A smoking prevention exhibit featuring movies, literature, posters, biofeedback testing and discussion was held. Many other health activities occurred.

As a result of participating in the smoking prevention course, many students inquired about assistance to help quit smoking. Existing resources, such as the Alaska Lung Association and Seventh Day Adventist materials were recommended, and a network in the region established for obtaining services.

With the help of the classroom guides the five lessons of the biofeedback module were given by the teachers at Ambler, Shungnak, and Kotzebue elementary schools, in the spring of 1982. Peer-led classes consisting of six lessons were conducted in the high school grades in the same communities during the winter and spring months.

Effect of the Smoking Prevention Program

A post-intervention survey was carried out at the end of April 1982 on all students in grades 4 to 6 and grades 7 to 12, including those who received the program (study group), and those who did not receive the program (control group). Pre- and post-intervention scores were compared for the same grade groups, combined and separated according to study or control group. Additionally, groups which received the program (Ambler and Shungnak, one-half of Kotzebue) were compared with those who did not (Buckland, Noatak, one-half of Kotzebue). Table 3 summarizes those finding (1).

DISCUSSION

The term "attributes" refers to the chief characteristics tested for in the questionnaires, namely attitude, social pressure, smoking behavior and frequency, and health knowledge. All questions fell into one of these categories and received a negative or positive value.

Significance testing was done by employing the "t" test for this part of the

Table 3.   Pre- and post-intervention survey results compared.

Group	Effects
All schools combined and by study and control groups, grades 4-6	No significant change
All schools combined, grades 7-12	No significant change
Study and control groups Ambler and Shungnak, grades 7-12 (study)	Significantly improved knowledge, Improved trend in all attributes
Buckland and Noatak, grades 7-12 (control)	No significant change, Declining trend in 4 attributes
Kotzebue, grades 7-12 received program (study)	Significantly improved knowledge, Improved in 2 other attributes
Did not receive program (control)	Scored less favorably than participant group

analysis; significance was determined to be at the 0.05 level.

No significant alteration in the status of smoking attitudes, social pressures, behavior, or knowledge was demonstrated on the total population of each of the two cohorts, grades 4 to 6 and grades 7 to 12. On the other hand those students who received the program did better than those who did not. For example, Ambler and Shungnak significantly improved their knowledge of health, as did Kotzebue students. Moreover these groups showed improved trends in the other attributes. The opposite was true for Buckland and Noatak, and the Kotzebue students not receiving the program. The achievement is all the more remarkable, since Ambler's smoking rates (79%) are highest followed by those in Shungnak (69%).

Heavy smoking by parents and other householders acts as a constant opposing force to any youth wanting to make a choice against smoking. Programs to help parents, and campaigns to influence adults are needed to support attempts to help youth.

Since the program was new and untried, there were expected difficulties and delays in starting up. Most teachers and students rated the program favorably. The techniques require training and practice. The smoking prevention program created additional work for the school.

The smoking prevention program, containing the latest innovative concepts and methods, was successfully conducted in a rural Native Alaska region, with good measurable results obtained in its first year of operation. Its feasibility has been demonstrated, and its effectiveness should increase with experience. It is a sound model to use in similar settings.

REFERENCES

1. Evaluation of medical care provided to Alaska Natives, Volume 7. A smoking prevention program for Alaskan youth. Alaska Native Health Board, Anchorage, Alaska, May 1982; 1-78.
2. Lee JF. Smoking among Alaska Native youth. A profile of smoking patterns in five northwest arctic communities. Proceedings of the 5th World Conference on Smoking and Health, Winnipeg, Canada, July 1983; 1-4.
3. The health of Alaskans. An assessment of the prevalence of behaviors posing health risks. The Alaska Department of Health and Social Services Health Education and Risk Reduction Project, Juneau, 1983; 6-7.
4. Tobacco use among students in the Northwest Territories 1982. Published by the Minister of Health, Government of the Northwest Territories, 1983; 5-9.
5. Smoking programs for youth. U.S. Department of Health and Human Services, National Institutes of Health, Washington 1980; 2, 41, 47.
6. Biofeedback Program. New Hampshire Lung Association, Manchester, 1980.
7. Roemhild HF, Murray DM. Minnesota smoking prevention program. A teacher's guide to the peer led social consequences curriculum. Minneapolis: University of Minnesota, 1980:1-62.

John F. Lee
3214 Wesleyan Drive
Anchorage, Alaska 99508
U.S.A.

SECTION 7. HEALTH PROGRAMS AND MANPOWER

Circumpolar Health 84:363-368

EXPERIENCES IN MATERNAL AND CHILD HEALTH SERVICES IN A NORDIC COUNTRY

HOLGER HULTIN

The maternal and child health (MCH) service is part of primary health care and thus a multidisciplinary branch of social medicine. Such services must be closely linked with and carried out as part of total family health care. School health services are in turn viewed as an integral part of maternal and child health services. Finally, the linkage of all MCH services, expressed in a cumulative system of records, is essential for a successful outcome.

In practically all countries MCH services are regarded as basic health programs, and therefore given high priority. From a humanitarian as well as from a purely national economic viewpoint, it is more rewarding to spend funds on the growing generation than on other groups of the population. The priority given to MCH varies from country to country, depending on the known health hazards among mothers and children.

In some countries MCH services have long since established a very high coverage of those groups. These services have been regarded as extremely important prerequisites for general social development. In some of these countries, such as Finland and Sweden, practically 100% of all deliveries take place in hospitals. There remain however, highly developed countries where a large percentage of deliveries still take place at home. In these countries one can reach an obstetrician and a hospital within 15 to 30 minutes from any part of the country. Distances play an important role in all discussions regarding delivery services (1,2).

In Finland, the Maternal and Child Health Centers Act was passed on March 31, 1944. This act placed responsibility for establishing MCH centers upon the 464 local communes, emphasizing the objectives and aims of such centers, rather than the methods for creating them. It contained guidelines for combining prenatal and child health services, thus for the first time creating both linkage and continuity of health care provided by physicians, midwives, and public health nurses. From its inception in 1944 until 1972, the basic provisions of the Act provided the framework for MCH services. Central to these purposes was a concentrated team effort to decrease health risks connected with pregnancy, childbirth, and the postpartum period. All expectant mothers received free pregnancy and childbirth education, supervision, and counseling in the promotion of good physical and mental health. Fathers-to-be also participated in the family training program (3).

The year 1944 was thus a turning point for health care in Finland. Two other important acts were passed that year: the Midwives in Rural Communes Act and the Public Health Nurses in Rural Communes Act. Preventive aspects were clearly expressed. The midwives act stated that communal midwives were appointed for prenatal care and for home deliveries only, and that they were not allowed to work in the local lying-in hospitals, except as stand-ins for short periods of time, and then only with approval of the provincial health officer. The work of the public health nurse was stated to be family centered and to cover both child health and curative medicine in the homes. The idea of preventing complications through health education and anticipatory guidance was stressed.

The recommendations were that all pregnant women visit maternity clinics at least 14 times during their pregnancies, 10 to 12 appointments with a midwife, and 2 to 4 appointments with a physician. In addition, all mothers are scheduled to visit their physician 5 to 12 weeks after delivery for postpartum check-ups. When a high risk pregnancy is evident or suspected, the above prenatal examination schedule is, of course, altered accordingly (4).

Table 1 shows the 1975 and 1979 attendance figures for pregnant women in Finland. It can be seen that in 1975, 93% of pregnant mothers had their first examination before the end of the fourth month of pregnancy.

Table 1. Percent of mothers examined at different stages of pregnancy, and percent examined by total number of examinations at maternity centers in 1975 (64,369) and 1979 (63,080).

	1975	1979
Stage of pregnancy		
<3 months	24.0	30.0
3-4 "	69.0	65.4
5-6 "	5.3	3.6
7-8 "	1.0	0.5
9-10 "	0.4	0.2
post partum	0.3	0.3
No. of examinations		
1-5	2.2	1.4
6-10	13.1	11.8
11-15	47.3	52.5
16-20	29.2	28.7
21-	8.2	5.5
no contact	(ca 18)	(ca 24)

In 1979 the corresponding figure was 95.4%. In 1975, 47.3% of expectant mothers had 11 to 15 examinations, and in 1979 the figure was 52.5%. In 1975, 37.4% of the mothers had 16 or more examinations during pregnancy, whereas in 1979 the corresponding figure was 34.2%.

In 1972 a new Primary Health Care Act was passed by the Finnish Parliament. In general the Act conforms to the principle of communal autonomy where services are organized by the communes with State assistance. Accordingly, the MCH service became part of basic health services rendered by the 213 local health centers. The minimal population base was set at 10,000 to 15,000, and so communes had to "federate" into districts when establishing a center. Out of these 213 health centers, 100 cover a single commune, and the rest two or more. Most health centers have at least 4 physicians, and other personnel, among them midwives and public health nurses, in the ratio of roughly 12 to a physician. In principle there is an MCH clinic within short distance of every family.

For regional administration, the country is divided into 12 provinces. Under each provincial governor's authority is a department of social affairs and health, which includes 2 provincial health officers (physicians), and provincial midwives and public health nurses who form the regional stronghold of MCH supervision.

On the national level, there is the National Board of Health, under the Ministry of Social Affairs and Health. The Department of Public Health at the National Board of Health administers MCH as a part of primary health care at the national level.

A substantial achievement of national planning has been the shift of emphasis in the distribution of resources between primary health care and hospital treatment,

Table 3. Fetal indications for sending mother to maternity outpatient department.

Slow growth of fetus
Abnormal heart sounds of fetus
Slowing down of fetal movements
Malposition of fetus
  - breech presentation
  - oblique presentation
  - transverse presentation
Multiple gestation
Unusually big fetus
Fetus mortus

in favor of the former. Another major goal has been regional equity. After 1972 the entire health care system showed a remarkable improvement, especially in isolated regions (5).

In order to improve consultation services between the specialized hospitals and maternity clinics, and thus form information links, maternity outpatient departments were established in university hospitals and later in other central hospitals as well. Upon certain standardized indications, pregnant women are referred to these hospitals for consultation and, in some instances, for observation and treatment in an obstetrical ward. Thus the central hospital, where the expectant mother eventually will deliver her child, will have all the pertinent information regarding the at-risk mother or fetus before the mother delivers, which is reassuring to both the mother and her family. The pregnant woman is still considered a client of her local maternity clinic, however, and is referred back to it when possible.

Standardized indications for referring pregnant women to the maternity outpatient departments are shown in Tables 2 and 3. The

Table 2. Indications for sending mother to maternity outpatient department.

Chronic hypertension	Diabetes
Heart conditions	Renal diseases
Other chronic conditions	
Age over 40	Hereditary diseases in family
Menstrual cycles irregular	
Estimated date of delivery unsure	Abnormalities of uterus

Mothers who in previous pregnancies had:

- stillbirth	- prematurity
- delayed growth of fetus	- congenital malformed fetus
- hereditary disease of child	- recurrent abortions
- early toxemia (from 24th-30th preg. week)	

Mothers whose pregnancy is result of sterility treatment
Rubeola or toxoplasma infection (or suspicion) during pregnancy

Table 4. Factors related to an increased risk of having a malformed child.

1. Maternal age over 35 years
2. Mother not married
3. Previous abortions
4. Previous defective children
5. Threatened abortion
6. "Influenza" during early pregnancy
7. Plentiful use of salicylates
8. Placenta <400g

former lists the indications for the mother, the latter for the fetus (6,7).

The Finnish Register of Malformations was established in 1963 by the National Board of Health. During the last 20 years the Register has functioned well and collected data on more than 17,000 congenital malformations. Primary information is collected from compulsory reporting and from copies of death certificates on which a malformation is recorded (8).

In Table 4 eight factors are listed which increase the risk of malformations in the central nervous system and skeletal bones (9).

In order to improve the linkage of records in MCH, and to secure the continuity of child health services, a cumulative health record was introduced in 1962. This record follows the children from birth throughout the compulsory school years (to age 16) wherever the health service may be delivered. This highly structured record provides space to record all relevant observations. In addition to this master record, a small health booklet was introduced for each child, and later on a similar one for the school child. the booklet is kept by the child's guardian, and the entries are made by practitioners, hospital physicians, outpatient clinic staff, and of course by health center personnel. The same year, a health booklet was also issued for pregnant women, with space provided for recording maternity services received. Information in this booklet includes delivery data and pertinent facts concerning the newborn (i.e. Apgar score etc.). The booklet remains with the mother, and is an important link to the child health service. The mother's master record with analogous data is on file at the maternity clinic, where the mother is registered. The delivery hospital makes entries in the record booklet, but also sends a copy of the delivery record upon request to the health center. This recording system has been adapted for data processing units at the health centers (10).

Finland was one of the first countries in which the MCH service was brought together with the school health service under the same administrative body, namely, the Department of Public Health at the National Board of Health. This merger took place in 1954, and has proven to be very profitable indeed for the linkage of these 3 services.

In Finland, maternity clinics are almost always combined with child health clinics in the more than 2,000 health stations throughout the entire country. This facilitates the linkage of services and ensures continuity of care for mother and baby. Teamwork of the midwife, public health nurse, and physician is easier to establish in this setting, and this has beneficial effects in family contacts.

With the legislation of 1972, the child health service, among others, was staffed with a team of various professionals such as a dentist, a dental nurse, a psychologist, a nutritionist, a physiotherapist, a speech therapist and a number of consulting physicians specialized in different fields. The two-way consultation of these experts is of utmost importance, even if they do not work regularly in the child health clinics at the health centers. The 22 central hospitals, with 5 university hospitals among them, are responsible for the consultation service.

The aim of child health care is that each infant should be examined at the child health clinic at least 3 times during the first year of life, and then once a year or every other year. The number of visits to the public health nurse (or contacts with her on home visits) should be at least twice as many as visits to the physician. Medical examinations of preschool children should be arranged annually, since many problems of the school child stem from the preschool period.

The vital statistics of MCH in Finland are presented in Table 5. The infant mortality rate, which was 7.6 per 1,000 live births in 1980, was 6.5 in 1981, and by 1982 it had decreased to 5.8, the lowest figure in the world. It may be said in this connection, that since the Oulu University Central Hospital was completed in the mid-1960s, and the Departments of Obstetrics and Pediatrics of the medical faculty came into full activity, the infant mortality rate of northern Finland decreased rapidly, and was in 1969 even below the figure for the whole country.

Infant mortality rates in certain countries where the rate has been low are presented in Table 6. Japan was in this respect ahead of Finland in 1980, when Sweden had the lowest figure. In 1981 Finland had surpassed both Japan and Sweden, and in 1982 the order was Finland, Japan, Sweden (11,12).

An important preventive activity at the child health clinic is immunization. According to the law of 1951, all immunizations became voluntary. In spite of this,

Table 5. Vital statistics of MCH in Finland (1975-1982).

Year	1975	1976	1977	1978	1979	1980	1981	1982
Birth rate	13.9	14.1	13.9	13.5	13.3	13.2	13.2	13.7
Infant mortality	10.0	9.1	8.8	7.7	7.6	7.6	6.5	5.8
Perinatal mortality	12.0	11.8	11.2	9.5	8.4	7.9		
Stillbirths	5.8	5.7	5.1	4.9	4.2	4.2	4.1	
Maternal mortality	0.11	0.09	0.08	0.08	0.03	0.02		

the vaccination and immunization program has been excellently carried out, as can be seen from Table 7. By the beginning of school, Finnish children have been immunized at the child health clinics to a very high degree. This result is an indicator of the successful health education and immunization activities performed by the health nurses.

The decrease in signs of rickets diagnosed by physicians in infants has been remarkable from 7.1% of the infants in 1962 to 0.6% in 1972. The credit for this achievement also belongs to the health nurses (13).

Table 8 illustrates that the prevalence of chronically ill school children in Finland in 1975 was 17.5 per 1,000. Because of the crippling effect of traffic accidents among children, it may be stressed in this connection that according to investigations in Finland and elsewhere, only 12% of 7 year old normal children can grasp the abstract notion of right and left. This concept forms the basic message in all traffic safety education (14).

To summarize, the following factors have contributed to the popularity and success of MCH services in Finland:

1. Pregnant women, infants, and children are not obliged to attend communal (free) services. They can elect private health care if they wish, or they can choose to use both services simultaneously with no strings attached. Thus, the MCH service in Finland has never been looked upon as something for the poor, as it has, unfortunately, in many countries.

2. Pregnant women and infants and children may choose to attend any health center in Finland ("open house policy"). Clients are thus not restricted to the center closest to their homes, or in a certain district, even if everyone is registered at her own "basic" center, where her master-record is on file. This ambulatory possibility is working successfully, thanks to the maternal and child health booklets, introduced in 1962. Mothers and mothers-to-be simply carry those health record documents with them when travelling.

3. The services of midwives or public health nurses are not restricted to preventive activities; social work and care of the sick in the home are also considered an integral part of the job. The midwife and public health nurse together forming the backbone of the MCH service, are therefore real helpers for families in difficulty and accordingly welcome everywhere.

4. At times of physician shortage, the midwife and public health nurse have been provided with extensive rights to

Table 6. Infant mortality rates in different countries 1960-1982.

	1960	1970	1979	1980	1981	1982
Sweden	16.6	11.0	7.5	6.9	6.9	6.8
Finland	21.0	13.2	7.6	7.6	6.5	5.8
Japan	30.7	13.1	7.9	7.5	7.1	6.6
Denmark	21.5	14.2	8.8	8.4	7.9	8.2
Netherlands	16.5	12.7	8.7	8.6	8.3	8.2
Switzerland	21.1	15.1	8.5	9.0	7.6	7.7
Norway	18.9	12.7	8.8	8.1	7.5	8.1
Iceland	13.0	13.2	5.4	7.7	6.0	7.1

Table 7. Percent children vaccinated at child health centers in Finland.

Vaccinated against:	%
Pertussis	97.6
Tetanus	97.6
Diphtheria	97.6
Polio	96.6
Variola	71.1
BCG	99.4

make health decisions, based upon their training and examinations. This has naturally increased their reputation among the public.

5. The policy has been to appoint health workers, if possible, to health centers in their own native province. This promotes communication and contact with families.

6. To stimulate pregnant women to use the maternity service facilities, a maternity aid package was introduced in 1938. This baby clothing package was presented to every mother upon delivery, if she had visited a physician or the midwife at the maternity clinic before the end of the fourth month of pregnancy, and followed the suggestions and guidance given to her. The value of the package is roughly $75.

7. Home visits by the midwife to every newborn in her district, and home visits at regular intervals by the public health nurse, are crucial in establishing good contacts and a sound health care plan for every client. Without knowing the living environment of the family, adequate advice cannot be given and confusion between real need and demand will easily occur.

Table 8. Chronically ill school children in Finland 1975 (total number of pupils was 791,148).

Diagnosis	No. of pupils	Per 1,000 pupils
Crippled	1,482	1.9
Brain injury	1,705	2.2
Asthma	4,502	5.7
Diabetes	2,519	3.2
Heart defect	1,676	2.1
Rheumatic	621	0.8
Kidney disorder	1,267	1.6
Total	13,772	17.5

8. The MCH service is a voluntary one in the proper sense of the word. The service must not deteriorate to a control system of any kind. In other words the less knowledgeable the client, the greater her right to consult with the service. The problem family and problem child have priority in using the MCH service.

9. No attempt is made to distribute the services evenly to everybody; the result usually would be that no one gets anything really substantial. Beyond a certain basic health service, efforts should be directed to benefit those most in need of help and encouragement, whether called "risk groups," "problem families" or "social cases." Tasks should be delegated, whenever possible, to less expensive professions.

10. Continuous in-service training, guidance, supervision, and encouragement of the health personnel will change even the most depressing and seemingly hopeless work situation, and thus bring about surprisingly good results.

REFERENCES

1. Hultin H. Infant health services at child health centers in Finland in the 1960s. National Board of Health, Helsinki, 1973.
2. Haraldson S. Personal communication.
3. Hultin H. Child health care in Finland. Paediatrician 1980; 9:35-40.
4. Finland. Instruction for maternal and child health centres and their function. National Board of Health, Helsinki, 1962.
5. Hultin H. Role of the midwife: The Finland experience. Prevention of perinatal mortality and morbidity. Child Health in the Community 1984; 3 (in press).
6. Castren O. Prevention of complications in pregnancy (In Finnish) Gummerus, Jyvaskyla 1980:14-18.
7. Timonen S, Widholm O. Recommendations for referrals to maternity outpatient clinic in Finnish maternity services. National Board of Health, Helsinki, 1977.
8. Saxen L. The Finnish register of congenital malformations and its application in epidemiological studies (In Finnish). Duodecim 1980; 96:1390-1399.
9. Klemetti A. Relationship of selected environmental factors to pregnancy outcome and congenital malformations. Ann Paediat Fenn 1966. 12, suppl 26.
10. Finland: Health and health services in Finland. Official statistics of Finland 1982. National Board of Health, Helsinki, 1984.

11. Health statistics in the Nordic coun-
    tries Copenhagen: Nomesko, 1980.
12. Annus Medicus 1983. The health situa-
    tion in Nordic countries; (Hälsositu-
    ationen i Norden, Nordiska Minister-
    ådet, Oslo), Helsinki 1983.

13. Hultin H, Opas R, Sarna S. Infant
    health services in Finland, 1972-1973.
    National Board of Health, Helsinki,
    1977.
14. Hultin H. Traffic accidents in chil-
    dren (In Finnish). Duodecim 1966;
    82:465.

Holger Hultin
Department of Public Health Science
University of Helsinki
02110 Espoo 11
Finland

Circumpolar Health 84:369-372

REFERRAL PATTERN STUDY IN NORTHERN NEWFOUNDLAND AND LABRADOR

JAMES H. WILLIAMS [1] and ALISON C. EDWARDS

Epidemiological studies for recognizing problems in health care delivery are well established in the remote areas of Canada and appropriate control methods have been developed. Some specific services are, however, only available outside the community. It is important to recognize those items of service which are the most common reason for referral from the primary health care facility in the home community, when present facilities are being reviewed or new centers developed.

In order to determine the effectiveness and weakness of the present system, a study was undertaken by the Grenfell Regional Health Services (GRHS) to establish a baseline concerning the present pattern of referral. For the purposes of the study, the region was divided into 4 geographic areas with differing socioeconomic backgrounds (Figure 1).

Northern Labrador: An area with small fishing communities and a predominance of Native people.

Southern Labrador: The area from Cartwright to Mary's Harbour, predominantly Caucasian in origin.

Central Labrador: Associated with the airport at Goose Bay and hydroelectric development at Churchill Falls.

Northern Newfoundland: Caucasian, including the Forteau area of Southern Labrador, as well as the Northern Peninsula of Newfoundland.

The annual number of visits per member of the population to the local health care facility was considerably higher in the coastal region than in the recently developed area of Central Labrador or the Northern Peninsula (Table 1). The highest referral rate was from the coastal Labrador area (i.e. Northern and Southern Labrador)

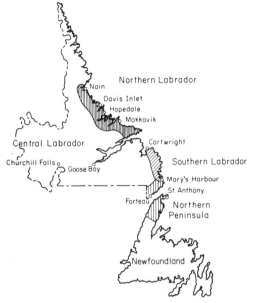

Figure 1. Grenfell Regional Health Services geographic areas, Labrador and Northern Newfoundland.

where the nursing stations are staffed by outpost nurses with support from a travelling physician. The lowest rate of referral was from Central Labrador where physicians, some with specialist training, are in practice. The hospitals at Goose Bay and St. Anthony are the referral centers for obstetric patients so, in contrast with other areas, few obstetric patients are referred out of Central Labrador or St. Anthony.

Table 1. Regional use of local health care facilities (1981-1982).

	Northern Labrador	Southern Labrador	Central Labrador	Northern Peninsula
Total population	2,444	2,809	9,129	10,991
Patient visits	17,430	17,519	30,428	33,269
Visits per capita	7.14	6.24	3.33	3.03
Total number of referrals	691	561	432	996
Referral rate per 1,000 population per year	283	200	47	91

---

[1] Deceased

The overall pattern of referral (Table 2) indicates the majority of patients went to the nearest facility where the appropriate service was available. The choice of location was not always dependent on the geographic location. Physician preference or previous consultation experience, patient preference or family associations often influenced the choice of referral center in non-emergency situations. Weather conditions may have influenced the choice of referral centers in an emergency.

The rates of referrals from Coastal Labrador and the Northern Peninsula areas, to the tertiary care center in St. John's, were similar (3 to 5%); whereas half the patients referred from the Central Labrador area went directly to St. John's.

The age and sex pattern of referrals (Figure 2) shows that the majority of referrals are either children under the age of 10 years or females of child-bearing age. Seasonal variation was not particularly marked, although there was a tendency for more referrals in winter months from Coastal Labrador.

Personal transportation costs (Table 3) reflect the impact of the referral on the individual and the community. Of the total number of patients referred, 80% gave information on transportation costs. Forty-seven percent of these had no personal travel expense, the cost being borne by the provincial government, insurance and other employee benefit schemes. In Central Labrador, a high percentage of referrals were to centers outside the GRHS area, thus incurring a considerably higher air fare.

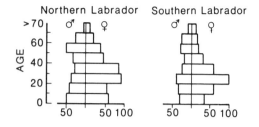

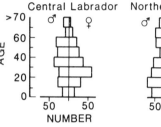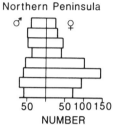

Figure 2. Age and sex distribution of health care referrals from home communities in Labrador and Northern Newfoundland, 1981-1982.

An International Classification of Disease (ICD) group diagnosis was made on all responses received (Table 4). "Pregnancy/birth" was one of the largest group of system-related referrals. The recent policy of advising delivery in a modern, well-equipped hospital is one of the main factors responsible for the fall of the infant mortality rate, from 27.8 in 1972-1973 to

Table 2. Referral sites utilized "within and outside" the GRHS area, expressed as percent (1981-1982).

	Northern Labrador	Southern Labrador	Central Labrador	Northern Peninsula
"Within" GRHS	94.6	97.0	49.1	86.2
Sites:				
Northwest River	44.4	5.5	0.7	0
Goose Bay	34.4	11.4	18.1	0.4
St. Anthony	15.1	79.3	30.3	85.0
Community Health				
Centre	0.6	0.7	0	0.8
"Outside" GRHS	5.4	3.0	50.9	13.8
Sites:				
St. John's	4.8	2.9	45.6	3.6
Corner Brook	0.1	0.2	1.4	3.2
Gander/Grand Falls	0	0	0.9	0
Blanc Sablon, Quebec	0	0	0	6.9
Other	0.4	0	3.0	0
Total referrals (100%)	691	561	432	996

Table 3. Transportation costs of referred patients (1981-1982).

	Northern Labrador	Southern Labrador	Central Labrador	Northern Peninsula
Total number of referrals	691	561	432	996
Number of responses re expenses	464	404	412	858
Number with expenses (percent)	88 (19)	152 (38)	108 (26)	784 (91)
Mean cost	$74	$60	$204	$46
Range of cost	$7-380	$2-800	$50-700	$2-400
Total costs	$6,543.00	$9,099.00	$25,962.00	$36,338.00

12.5 in 1982-1983, in the GRHS area. The injury rates are high, especially in Northern Labrador communities. Specific programs are being developed to try to reduce this problem.

The ICD group diagnoses were subdivided to give an indication of the proportion of cases which could be regarded as "medical emergencies" compared to "non-emergency" referrals (Table 5). For the Labrador region, only 25% of the patients in all 3 areas fell into one of five recognized groups of medical emergencies, while on the Northern Peninsula, 44% of the referrals were of an emergency nature. The number of patients referred from Coastal Labrador for

procedures and investigations, where facilities are limited at the nursing stations, is much greater than in Central Labrador where dental, radiological, and laboratory departments have been developed.

The study provides useful information for planning and development within a Regional Health Service so that optimal use of a facility can be achieved, with a reasonable availability of frequently used services to the vast majority of patients. It is important that cost effectiveness, to both the individual and the health care system, should be correlated with an improvement in health care delivery. The advantages of regionalization of obstetric

Table 4. Referral diagnoses expressed as percent of total responses (1981-1982).

Diagnosis	Northern Labrador	Southern Labrador	Central Labrador	Northern Peninsula
Infectious/Parasitic	1.4	1.0	2.2	0.7
Neoplasms	1.6	1.0	3.2	2.6
Endocrine/Metabolic	1.1	1.0	1.0	1.0
Blood	0.4	0.3	0.6	0.4
Mental	2.5	1.7	2.2	2.0
CNS/Sense Organs	6.4	2.2	7.9	4.2
Circulatory system	3.2	4.4	3.6	5.1
Respiratory system	4.3	2.9	5.4	4.9
Digestive system	4.6	7.5	8.7	7.7
Genitourinary system	5.5	8.6	6.3	7.1
Pregnancy/Birth	7.7	6.8	4.6	5.6
Skin/Subcutaneous	1.4	1.0	1.8	1.5
Musculoskeletal/ Connective	4.2	6.2	9.7	7.0
Congenital	0.7	0.4	1.4	0.7
Perinatal period	1.2	0.4	1.0	0.9
Ill defined condition	9.6	12.9	11.7	22.9
Injury/Poisoning	12.9	8.7	9.7	10.9
External causes	0.8	0.9	0.8	1.3
Procedures, etc.	30.5	31.9	18.1	13.4
Total referrals (100%)	691	561	432	996

Table 5.   Number (and percent) of referrals for the five most common emergency and non-emergency referrals (1981-1982).

	Northern Labrador	Southern Labrador	Central Labrador	Northern Peninsula
Emergency				
Abdominal pain	30 (4.3)	37 (6.6)	20 (4.6)	175 (17.6)
Chest pain	45 (6.5)	49 (8.7)	¹31 (7.2)	118 (11.8)
Injuries	81 (11.7)	43 (7.7)	33 (.76)	85 (8.5)
Vaginal bleeding	14 (2.0	17 (3.0)	3 (0.7)	31 (3.1)
Haematemesis	8 (1.2)	15 (2.7)	11 (2.5)	31 (3.1)
Non-emergency				
Procedures	108 (15.6)	95 (16.9)	20 (4.6)	76 (7.6)
Investigations	62 (9.0)	58 (10.3)	27 (6.3)	32 (3.2)
Antenatal Care	45 (6.5)	25 (4.5)	26 (6.0)	32 (3.2)
Normal delivery	47 (6.8)	34 (6.1)	13 (3.0)	44 (4.4)
Backache	19 (2.7)	15 (2.7)	26 (6.0)	55 (5.5)
Total referrals (100%)	691	561	432	996

services appear to outweigh the disadvantages. A similar advantage to the patient, when centralization or decentralization of a particular item of service is planned, should be demonstrable.

ACKNOWLEDGMENTS

We thank Ms. Cora Snow and Ms. Mary Murphy for their secretarial assistance, Ms. Sue Rideout, R.T., Clinical Clerk, Memorial University of Newfoundland (Canada) Medical School for her field work, and the staff of the Department of Community Medicine, GRHS, for their cooperation with the collection of survey data.

Alison C. Edwards
Memorial University of Newfoundland
St. John's, Newfoundland A1B 3V6
Canada

Circumpolar Health 84:373-376

ALASKA'S APPROACH TO PLANNING AN EMERGENCY MEDICAL SERVICES SYSTEM: HOW IS IT WORKING THREE YEARS LATER?

GLORIA HOUSTON WAY and MARK S. JOHNSON

A brief review of Alaska's approaches to planning an emergency medical services system may be of interest to others in arctic areas faced with similar tasks. While the political contexts are different, the geographic factors dictating these approaches are the same, as are other practical considerations.

Role of the Federal Government

In the United States, little national attention was given to improving pre-hospital emergency care until the early 1970s. By the mid-1970s a Federal program had been launched to facilitate development of regional emergency medical services systems (or EMS systems). Annual grants were made available to applicant agencies to carry out a sequence of planning and implementation steps set out by the Federal program guidelines (1).

The Federal program was rather rigid in dictating the components which must be addressed by grantees in developing their EMS systems. There were 15 components in all:

> Manpower
> Critical care
> Coordinated recordkeeping
> Training
> Public safety agencies
> Public education and information
> Communications
> Consumer participation
> Evaluation
> Transportation
> Accessibility to care
> Disaster response
> Facilities
> Transfer of patients
> Mutual aid agreements

It was considered essential that all these components work together in order for a total system to function effectively.

Within the general area of "critical care" the Federal guidelines required that each region address seven critical conditions which should receive priority attention:

> Cardiac emergencies
> Neonatal emergencies
> Burn emergencies
> Head and spinal injuries
> Poisonings
> Behavioral emergencies
> Trauma

While these requirements were logical starting points for planning, they didn't quite fit Alaska's needs; and the special projects required annually by the Federal program were clearly not appropriate for Alaska's rural and wilderness orientation.

Fortunately, at about the time political priorities changed and Federal funding for the program was greatly diminished, Alaska's oil revenues started flowing, and the State of Alaska was willing to continue funding the EMS program. Free from Federal constraints, the state coordinating agency, which is the EMS Section of the Division of Public Health, was able to build upon the basically sound foundation that the Federal program had laid, and plan for a system truly realistic for Alaskans.

An Inherited Infrastructure

The State of Alaska continued to grant funds to regional non-profit corporations to continue the work of facilitating EMS systems development, provide training and technical assistance to local emergency services, and to carry out annual planning and evaluation at regional levels. These agencies have strong advisory councils that take an active part in planning and setting priorities for program activities and expenditures.

The EMS Section itself works with an active 15-member State Advisory Council on Emergency Medical Services appointed by the Governor. A State EMS Medical Director, who is an emergency physician, provides medical consultation and technical assistance to the EMS Section on a contractual basis. He also provides liaison with the medical community, and provides leadership for local and regional EMS medical directors, who provide medical supervision at those levels either on a contractual or volunteer basis.

Involved in the actual delivery of emergency medical care at the "front line" are a wide range of personnel and agencies whose roles have evolved historically in response to needs as they were perceived. These include: village public safety officers, police and State Troopers, firefighters, and volunteer search and rescue teams who all function as first responders in time of medical emergency; certified emergency medical technicians and paramedics who work on local ambulance services and rescue squads (70% of whom are volunteers); the Community Health Aides who provide daily primary care to the hundreds of isolated Native villages scattered throughout Alaska; physician assistants and nurse practitioners who staff clinics in the larger rural communities; six small regional Alaska Area Native Health Service hospitals--a few of these now run by Native health corporations; and finally, 13 community hospitals, only six of which are connected by road to Fairbanks or Anchorage where there are several fairly large hospitals. The nearest major medical center is in Seattle, hundreds of miles south of our southern panhandle. In addition, the State is dependent upon a wide variety of air services for emergency transport of the sick and injured: private air taxis, large commercial airliners, air ambulances, and military air rescue services.

In short, Alaskans depend on a mixture of Federal, State, regional and local health, military and public safety agencies; as well as public, private, and volunteer pre-hospital and hospital providers in time of medical emergency.

The goal of the EMS program has been to work with all of these inherited elements to "establish a comprehensive, coordinated system of emergency medical services which assures that citizens and visitors gain easy access to services; that initial response is expeditious; that appropriate life-saving and stabilization measures are rendered at the scene and that patients are transported or transferred in a timely and efficient manner to facilities capable of effecting maximum recovery and rehabilitation" (2).

Partly because of the involvement of so many elements responsible for delivery of EMS, there was a great disparity around the state in ability to meet this overall goal. On the other hand, with the advent of oil money, the state was presented with the very real challenge of determining just how much service it could afford to maintain.

The Planning Process

A formal process of planning began in the fall of 1979 at the state-wide level and continued for over a year, resulting in the document titled Alaska's EMS Goals: A Guide for Planning Alaska's Emergency Medical Services System, published in 1981 (2). This document is not a plan, but a guide for further planning at local and regional levels, and was intended to provide a consistent approach to planning throughout the state.

It was recognized that in order for this document to be useful, i.e., truly used, it would have to be acceptable to the many elements responsible for delivery of EMS. One key factor in acceptance is always ownership. Not only was a democratic process considered necessary to insure this ownership, but it reflected our inherent belief that a more realistic product would emerge, even though efficiency would be sacrificed.

The State Advisory Council provided overall direction, review and comment on all details of the planning guide throughout the process. The real work of drafting it fell to a small group of state and regional representatives. Local and regional advisory councils (which are made up of representatives of all agencies involved in EMS) provided input and review all along the way, as did medical specialists who reviewed the critical care section. The State EMS Medical Director played a key role throughout. In Alaska this kind of participation is time-consuming and expensive--dependent on air travel, telephone, and mail.

Models

The model utilized for the basic format was adapted from one conceptualized for the Alaska State Health Plan, first completed in 1979 (3). In order to describe the current distribution of population within the state, as well as to place the elements necessary for a continuum of services, a "levels of care" model was developed. The State Health Plan describes five community "levels of care," and every community in the state is placed in one of these categories:

Level I   Villages
Level II   Sub-Regional Centers
Level III Regional Centers (by definition each has a hospital)
Level IV   Urban Centers
Level V   Metropolis (none in Alaska)

These categories are based on population, proximity to higher levels of care (expressed in minimum time required by surface transportation, i.e., degree of isolation), accessibility from a lower level community (again expressed in time), transportation, and communications services available. These parameters describe what exists. Then general guidelines are listed for what health services and facilities are in place or ought to be in place for each level.

Utilizing this model, the EMS planning guide sets out for each level of community a set of minimum conditions that should exist in order to provide an appropriate level of emergency response as well as a continuum of care with higher or lower level communities. The recommendations, or "goals," are loosely organized around those 15 components recognized by the national guidelines as essential. However, the Alaska guidelines also include "administration" as an essential component.

Since emergencies do not always occur in communities, in addition to the community categories utilized by the State Health Plan, the EMS planning guide also lists recommendations for highways between communities, high risk occupation work sites, schools, and even smaller settlements like fish camps.

The list of "critical care" priorities outlined by the national guidelines was augmented to address cold injuries, cold water near-drowning and hypothermia.

Acceptability Considerations

In addition to striving to maintain a democratic process of development, many other features were incorporated into the planning guide to insure acceptability and usability.

1. Format--The document is designed for local use. It summarizes overall state goals and general standards for services, outlines roles for state and regional agencies, then devotes the remainder of its pages to goals for each community level.

All communities are listed alphabetically and assigned a color and a category. Each community level is a different color, and that section starts by listing all communities of that level by region. A community can easily find material that is appropriate for its level. Each section can also be reproduced and used by itself.

2. Ease of Reading--A sincere attempt was made to produce a document that has a consistent format, is succinct (it is in outline form), and that is easy to read, with a minimum of jargon and technical wording except when discussing hospital capabilities. A glossary is included.

3. Realistic Goals for Alaska--This planning guide attempts to outline a system that is realistic for Alaska, not an ideal system impossible to attain in such a vast land with harsh conditions and sparse population. It describes a set of minimum conditions that should exist. Communities deciding to exceed those minimums are advised to consider seriously the issues of cost-effectiveness, skills retention, and community resource priorities.

On the other hand, capabilities recommended for hospitals and clinics in the smaller communities, most of which are totally isolated, exceed those which would be considered essential in areas with large medical centers easily accessible by road.

4. Avoiding Rigid Standards--The document makes a point of insisting that the standards or goals set out are not to be interpreted as regulations. While this possibility did not even occur to the planning committee, more conservative physicians on the advisory council insisted that a disclaimer be added to every page, and it was. The wisdom of this was confirmed very early after its publication when an initial attempt was made to use these goals as legal evidence in a court of law. In addition, there is great resistance to over-regulation in this state, by both

volunteers and by the private medical community.

The introduction stresses that the goals are a list of "shoulds" toward which communities can work, not a set of "musts." And it points out that no list is totally appropriate for any one community.

5. Flexible Time Frame--The standard requirement of most plans, a time schedule, was deliberately avoided. This is no "five year plan" or "ten year plan"; it is a guide for communities to set their own goals and priorities within their own time frames. The document sets out to systematize a process that was already underway. Many communities had already achieved most of these goals; others had barely begun. It was recognized, too, that the status of some of these goals would change from year to year, especially manpower and training goals. It was also rationalized that other state and local planning mechanisms, mainly budget documents, are in place for translating these goals into time-specific objectives.

6. An Evolving Document--Upon completion, it was recognized that the document was incomplete and subject to change; and indeed, after three year's use, it has just undergone major revisions.

The Plan in Use

The document has proven to be useful, and actually used, in at least six ways:

1. Regional coordinators have found it to be extremely useful in assisting small communities that are just starting to organize a local EMS system but don't know how to get started. They find the document easy to understand. It tells them what capabilities they need to have, and serves as a starting point for assessing specific needs and setting priorities for action. Most are surprised to find that the majority of goals don't require money; they call for local responsibilities and procedures to be defined.

2. Regional agencies are still required to submit annual grant applications to the state for funding regional EMS systems development. This planning guide is now used as the basis for their regional planning. Their priorities are based on assisting the communities in their region to meet these goals and are determined by evaluating the progress of communities throughout the region. Limited money is usually available through these grants for some capital expenditures as well, and this kind of assistance is granted if requests are consistent with these goals.

3. Local communities and regional EMS agencies also submit requests for special appropriations to the state legislature for capital funds. The state and regional

advisory councils do not endorse requests which are not consistent with the goals.

4. To assist in assessing the status of communities toward meeting these goals, simple yes-no checklists were developed reflecting each recommended goal. These have been very helpful to regional coordinators in working with communities and local EMS councils to determine annually what they need to work on in the coming year.

5. At the state level, annual development of budget and action priorities have been given a clear rationale through this planning guide. It has also been an extremely useful tool in explaining to legislators and administration officials our program goals. Again, its relative simplicity has been a real asset in this endeavor.

6. In 1983 an attempt was made for the first time to have the community checklists filled out by every community in Alaska. The resulting information has been valuable in assessing statewide status and needs in one consistent quantifiable format, and forms the baseline for annual statewide assessment.

The tabulation of these checklists also revealed a number of goals in the original document that needed to be modified or deleted because they turned out to be unrealistic after all. This summary became one of the tools used for the current revision.

Revisions Required

Some major revisions have included the following:

1. Villages and sub-regional centers (Levels I and II) have each been divided into two sub-groups: communities which are totally isolated from a higher level community; and those which have road access to a higher level community.

2. The goals for highways have been incorporated into the goals for the communities responsible for serving those highways.

3. There has been an even greater attempt to simplify wording and format, which has resulted in combining some of the components addressed.

4. Another component has been added: "medical control," which more clearly spells out the minimum mechanisms which should be in place for adequate medical supervision of pre-hospital providers.

5. Numerous changes have been incorporated to make the plan more realistic. goals which are clearly unattainable for small communities have been modified or deleted. Other changes reflect upgraded expectations in response to rapidly changing technology, rapid expansion of Alaska's service infrastructure, or in some cases, greater community capabilities than had once been realized.

6. The critical care categories receiving attention have increased in number.

7. Detailed lists of recommended equipment for first responders, ambulances, clinics, hospitals, medical evacuations, work sites, and training courses have been added in response to the need for a consolidated approach by the regions in seeking capital appropriations from the legislature.

8. And finally, these revisions reflect other program efforts which have been achieved during the intervening years, for example: adoption of state-wide certification and standardized training for EMS personnel and for ambulance services; near completion of basic state-wide treatment and transfer guidelines for major critical care categories; initiation of standardized medical evacuation escort training and procedures.

CONCLUSION

The basic format of the original planning guide, as well as the conceptual models used, have proven to be sound, adaptable and flexible. We expect the document to be even more useful in its revised form.

REFERENCES

1. U.S. Dept. of Health, Education and Welfare, Health Services Administration. EMS systems program guidelines. Hyattsville, MD: Bureau of Medical Services, Division of Emergency Medical Services, 1976.
2. EMS Section, Div. of Public Health, Alaska Dept. of Health and Social Services: Alaska's EMS goals: a Guide for planning Alaska's emergency medical services, Juneau. 1981.
3. Statewide Health Coordinating Council, and Div. of Planning, Policy and Program Evaluation, Alaska Department of Health and Social Services: Alaska State Health Plan, Juneau, 1979.

Gloria Houston Way
Emergency Medical Services Section
Alaska Department of Health and Social
   Services
Pouch H-06C
Juneau, Alaska 99811
U.S.A.

Circumpolar Health 84:377-380

ADMINISTRATION AND MAINTENANCE OF A LONG TERM SODIUM FLUORIDE MOUTHRINSE PROGRAM IN NORTHERN NEWFOUNDLAND AND LABRADOR

JAMES G. MESSER

In 1976 high levels of dental decay were being observed in school children by dentists, physicians, and other health professionals working with the Grenfell Regional Health Services in northern Newfoundland and Labrador. This was confirmed by selected school dental examination. There are 54 elementary schools in the region located in urban, rural and isolated communities (Figure 1). The schools range in size from one- and two-room buildings to large urban schools with over 200 students.

Dental services have been available for the last 20 years; however, only in the last 8 or 10 years have facilities or manpower permitted more than an emergency service in the more isolated communities. In an attempt to improve dental health with a preventive program, the dental coordinator and public health director sought approval from the school boards and set about designing a suitable preventive program.

Reports in the literature provided evidence of the beneficial effects of weekly rinsing with sodium fluoride in schools (1,2). Guidelines for implementing such programs were available (3), but at that time there were few reports on long-term administrative aspects of such programs.

In 1977 a decision was made to implement a weekly mouthrinse program to include all school children from kindergarten to grade six. Since dental staff were under considerable pressure coping with the demand for clinical treatment, the program was organized to use non-dental manpower. The program began in the fall of 1978.

The structure and organization of the program are illustrated in Figure 2. It soon became obvious that the bureaucracy involved was progressively more complex as the number of schools, funding, personnel training, lines of communication, poison control, and supply distribution aspects were organized. Although this complexity was regrettable, a reasonable degree of control over these and other variables was deemed essential in order to satisfy safety requirements and to ensure that delivery and feedback were consistent.

Funding

The International Grenfell Association provided a loan to purchase supplies and was repaid when parental fees were collected.

Personnel Training

Workshops for the public health nurses were arranged at which they were familiarized with all aspects of the program. They then instructed the teachers using movies

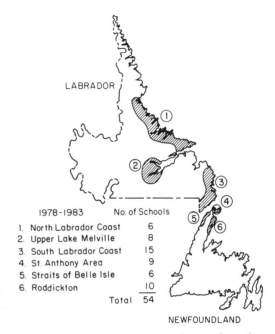

LABRADOR

1978-1983	No. of Schools
1. North Labrador Coast	6
2. Upper Lake Melville	8
3. South Labrador Coast	15
4. St. Anthony Area	9
5. Straits of Belle Isle	6
6. Roddickton	10
Total	54

NEWFOUNDLAND

Figure 1. Regional distribution and number of schools participating in the 0.2% sodium fluoride mouthrinse program.

and practical demonstrations. The nurses also supervised the initial rinsing sessions in the schools, using water. Newspapers, radio, and letters accompanying the consent forms were used to announce the program in 1978 and subsequently at the beginning of each year.

Delivery of the Programs in Schools

The teachers were instructed to dispense 10 ml of the 0.2% sodium fluoride solution into a cup. Each child who had parental consent would rinse his mouth with the solution for one minute. The children then expectorated the used rinse into the cup using the napkin to dry their lips and then to absorb the contents of the cup, which was then discarded. Children who were unable to rinse or who were observed swallowing the solution after three attempts were withdrawn from the program. Plain water was used at the initial rinse for the kindergarten children.

Poison Control

All health centers, nursing stations, and hospitals in the area were supplied with

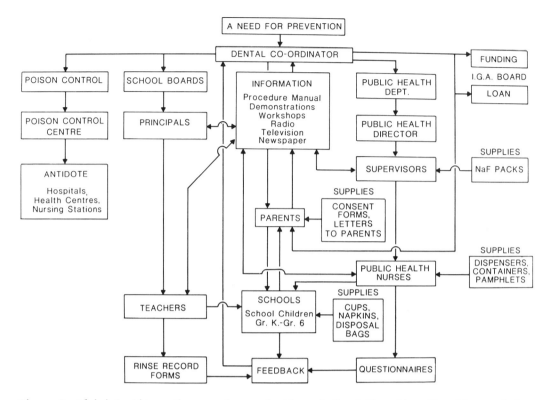

Figure 2. Administrative pathways and organization of the 0.2% sodium fluoride mouthrinse program in northern Newfoundland and Labrador.

the antidote. The concentrated sodium fluoride packs were controlled by the coordinator and distributed to the public health nurses through their supervisors. The solutions were prepared by the public health nurses prior to being delivered to the schools. The teachers were instructed to keep them in a safe place when not in use. Despite a wide safety margin, these precautions were considered necessary.

Feedback of Information

Information about the progress of the program was obtained by using questionnaires distributed to the teachers and public health nurses in 1978 and 1983. Formal and informal meetings were held between the dental coordinator, public health director, the nurses, their supervisors, and the school principals.

The teachers were provided with forms to record the number of rinses carried out by each child. Using non-participants as a control, it will be possible to evaluate the benefits from the 1979 and 1984 dental examinations.

RESULTS

Table 1 shows the results of the questionnaires. The 1983 results revealed few problems with the implementation of the program. Eighty-eight percent of eligible children were participating and 94% of the teachers approved of the program. Only 2% of the teachers reported classroom disruption related to the program. Despite this excellent start, complaints about the taste of the solutions were noted by 79% of the teachers and 70% of the nurses.

The responses in the 1983 questionnaire revealed that the participation rate had fallen from 88% in 1978 to 52% in 1983. Complaints about taste were still being observed by 82% of the teachers, but only by 21% of the public health nurses. The number of teachers who said the rinsing session caused classroom disruption had risen from 2% to 11%. When specifically asked if this was due to the drop in participation rate 72% replied affirmatively. By 1983, only 66% of the teachers approved of the program, compared to 94% after the first year.

To explain the 36% drop in the participation rate there was obviously a need to

evaluate the program. This fall in participation was not evenly spread. In many
schools there was still a 100% compliance by
the children.

Table 2 tabulates the reasons given by
the 82 teachers and 24 public health nurses
for the drop in participation.

The difference between the responses
was striking. Ninety-two percent of the
teachers had serious reservations about its
effectiveness and 63% felt there was a
general lack of enthusiasm. Sixty percent
felt a lack of follow-up and not enough
publicity were significant factors. The
cost and resistance from children and
parents were also mentioned but considered
less important.

The public health nurses, on the other
hand, felt that parental apathy and resistance from the children were significant.
They also reported a low priority for dental
health. In sharp contrast to the teachers,

the public health nurses did not feel that a
need for proof of effectiveness was necessary.

DISCUSSION

Complaints about the taste of the
solution was and has remained a persistent
problem noted by other researchers (4,5).
Attempts to overcome this problem by introducing flavored solution in 1982 were
difficult to evaluate. One public health
nurse noted in one school that teachers felt
the flavored solutions were more acceptable
to the children although, in fact, they were
still using unflavored solutions. This
problem may simply provide an excuse for the
children to withdraw. Such a phenomenon was
also noted by De Paola (6), particularly
among older children.

The reasons given in 1983 for the drop
in participation rate are more difficult to

Table 1. *Answers to the mouthrinse program questionnaires in 1979 and 1983. Responses from the teachers and public health nurses.*

A. Teacher Questionnaire		1978 N=123	1983 N=82
1) Participation Rate	88%	max 100 min 60	52% max 100 min 15
2) How long does the rinsing session take?		5.7 minutes	5 minutes
3) Do you approve of the program?		Yes 94%	Yes 66%
4) If you disapprove is it because you			
a) Disapprove of flouride		1	2
b) It takes up too much time		3	1
c) You doubt its effectiveness		7	10
d) It should be done by hygienists		13	6
5) Does it cause significant class disruption?		Yes 2%	Yes 11%
6) Did you have complaints about			
a) Taste		Yes 79%	Yes 82%
b) Post-rinse taste		Yes 45%	Yes 56%
c) Laughing or spitting out		Yes 48%	Yes 56%
7) Was fee collection a problem?		Yes 13%	Yes 7%
8) Do you receive adequate instructions?		Yes 97%	Yes 92%
9) Would you be interested in OHI programs?		Yes 92%	Yes 92%
10) Would you be interested in other Dental Programs?		Yes 96%	Yes 98%
B. Public Health Nurse Questionnaire		1978 N=19	1983 N=24
1) What is the participation rate in your area?			55%
2) Did you encounter resistance from the teachers?		Yes 17%	Yes 37%
3) Did you encounter resistance from the parents?		Yes 10%	Yes 4%
4) Is fee collection a problem?		Yes 63%	Yes 41%
5) How long do you spend mixing and dispensing solution?		57 minutes	32 minutes
6) Have you received complaints about taste?		Yes 70%	Yes 21%

Table 2. Reasons given by the teachers and public health nurses for the drop in participation rate from 88% in 1978 to 52% in 1983.

A. Teachers (N=82)

1) Doubt about the program's value	92%
2) Waning enthusiasm and apathy	63%
3) Lack of publicity and follow-up	60%
4) Cost: $2.00/child/year 1983	44%
5) Resistance from children	29%
6) Resistance from parents	15%

B. Public Health Nurses (N=24)

1) Parental apathy	66%
2) Resistance from children	50%
3) General lack of enthusiasm	50%
4) Low priority of dental health	45%
5) Resistance from teachers	21%
6) Insufficient publicity	21%
7) Need to prove effectiveness	21%

interpret. The need for proof of effectiveness expressed by the teachers may simply reflect a feeling that the program was too "experimental." This attitude, also noted by Bissell (5), was hard to explain because each year updated information about the effectiveness of similar programs is made available to the teachers via the public health nurses. In 1983 only half of the teachers were interested in reading this information, according to the public health nurses. This seeming indifference by teachers was also noted by Mutter (7) in a program offering preventive dental techniques to elementary schools in Ottawa.

One disturbing finding reported by 3 out of 24 public health nurses was carelessness about keeping the solutions in a safe place when not in use. This reinforced the need for close supervision and poison control. Despite a wide safety margin, it has been suggested that as little as 150 ml of the solution would be toxic to a 22 kg (five year old) child (8).

SUMMARY AND RECOMMENDATIONS

1) Initial collaboration and subsequent cooperation between all long-term parties involved in the program is vital.
2) Initial assessment of dental caries experience with follow-up evaluations demonstrating improvements are necessary.
3) It is essential to establish the cost-effectiveness of mouthrinse programs as an accepted and proven method of reducing the caries incidence in permanent teeth.

4) The problem of maintaining enthusiasm over a long period should not be underestimated and will require concerted efforts by all concerned. Reward systems should be developed.

Despite the problems which have appeared during the six years it has been in effect, this program sill remains a worthwhile venture. Over 2,500 children are participating and receiving the rinse and the majority of teachers and nearly all the public health nurses feel it should continue.

Therefore, action taken now to deal with the snags encountered thus far will help to ensure the continuation of this program on a sound basis.

REFERENCES

1. Horowitz HS, Creighton WE, McClendon BJ. The effect on human dental caries of weekly oral rinsing with sodium fluoride mouthwash: A final report. Arch Oral Biol 1971; 16:609-616.
2. Ripa LW, Leske GS, Lowey WG. Fluoride rinsing: A school-based preventive program. J Prev Dent 1977; 5:25-30.
3. U.S. Dept. of Health, Education and Welfare. Preventing tooth decay. A guide for implementing self-applied fluoride in schools. Public Health Service Publication No. (NIH) 77-1196, 1977.
4. Gross SG. Acceptance of a weekly 0.2% sodium fluoride mouthrinse program in the Regional School District No. 10 elementary system. J Conn State Dent Assn 1977; 2:67-71.
5. Bissell GD, O'Shea RM, Mann J. Recruitment and participation in a school mouthrinse program. J Pub Health Dent 1980; 1:57-63.
6. De Paola PF, Soparkar P, Jauron SK. Considerations of supervised weekly sodium fluoride rinsing: Result from a demonstration program after two school years. J Prev Dent 1980; 6:95-100.
7. Mutter G. Barriers to the establishment of a regular dental program for elementary schools. J Canad Dent Assn 1978; 7:316-319.
8. Spoerke DG, Bennett DL, Gullekson DJK. Toxicity related to acute low dose sodium fluoride injections. J Fam Pract 1980; 10:139-140.

James G. Messer
Dental Services
Grenfell Regional Health Services
St. Anthony, Newfoundland A0K 4S0
Canada

Circumpolar Health 84:381-383

ASSESSMENT OF PRENATAL RISK FACTORS AND PREGNANCY OUTCOMES FOR ALASKA NATIVE WOMEN, 1979, 1982, 1983

JACKIE PFLAUM, NANCY SANDERS, TERESA WOLBER and JACQUELINE A. GREENMAN

With the region served by the prenatal program of the Anchorage Service Unit of the Alaska Area Native Health Service (AANHS), no method has existed for accurate and consistent data collection for reporting prenatal risk factors and pregnancy outcomes. A risk assessment procedure was initiated in 1982 in Anchorage and throughout the service unit to identify clients at risk. The effectiveness of the risk assessment procedure in increasing identification and treatment of high risk clients was yet to be examined.

The purpose of the study was to compare data collected regarding pregnancy risks and pregnancy outcomes of Alaska Native women in the Anchorage Service Unit for the years 1979, 1982, and 1983 with statistics for Alaska and the United States. It is hoped that these data and this analysis will be applied directly to continued program planning.

DESCRIPTION

The overall goal of the Women's Health Program at the Alaska Native Medical Center (ANMC) is to provide comprehensive reproductive health services to Alaska Native women within the Anchorage Service Unit (ASU). The Anchorage Service Unit spans a geographical area from Anchorage to the Aleutians, including Kodiak Island and the Kenai Peninsula. The population is diverse, primarily Aleut but also includes Athapaskans and Eskimos. Urban Anchorage and 46 villages are included in the service unit.

The program provides prenatal, gynecological, and family planning services to this diverse and scattered population. The goal of the prenatal component of the program is to provide optimal prenatal care, safeguarding the well-being of mother, child, and family. In the village, early pregnancies are identified and initially assessed by the Community Health Aides. Nurse practitioners at the Alaska Native Medical Center then assign risk factors and outline a management plan for the pregnancies. The Community Health Aide submits monthly progress reports which are used to monitor each pregnancy. If there is any evidence of problems or complications, the pregnant woman is brought to ANMC for an evaluation by a physician. Women with uncomplicated pregnancies are transferred from the village to a prematernal home in Anchorage at 37 weeks gestation to await delivery by a nurse midwife or physician. In Anchorage, women are seen in a prenatal clinic on a monthly basis by nurse practi-

tioners and physicians who follow similar procedures for the more urban population. These individuals also deliver at ANMC.

This program has undergone several changes within the past three years. The major changes have addressed problems identified in past program evaluations. One of these changes involved the development and implementation of a data collection form to provide accurate risk assessment information and target those clients at greatest risk.

METHODOLOGY

In order to evaluate the impact of the new data collection system during the years 1982 and 1983, a data base for 1979 was established. A total case chart review for all three years was initiated and data collected. The data included place of residence, age, parity, gravidity, the trimester the patient sought care, number of prenatal visits, hemoglobin, prenatal risks, labor risks, maternal complications, Apgars at 1 and 5 minutes, birth weight, and infant complications.

Data were obtained from the prenatal risk assessment forms, delivery records, nurses' notes, and hospital discharge summaries. The prenatal risk category was determined from the risk forms instituted in 1982. Numbers were assigned to identify those patients at risk as outlined by the high risk factors and guidelines (AANHS) (1). Patients were identified as no risk, low, high, and social risk. Labor risks, maternal complications, and infant complications were also identified by the standards developed by the AANHS guidelines. Four hundred fifty-eight cases were reviewed for 1979, 485 for 1982, and 541 for 1983.

Using the Statistical Package for the Social Sciences (SPSS), frequencies were determined to describe the Anchorage Service Unit population that delivered during the years 1979, 1982, and 1983.

RESULTS

Fertility rates decreased significantly during the 1970s for all Alaska Natives (2). These rates increased, however, during 1979 to 1982 from 94.4 to 100 live births per 1,000 women ages 15 to 45. The overall U.S. fertility rate in 1980 was 68.4 live births per 1,000 women. The fertility rates for the population studied increased in 1982 to 1983 from 100 to 110 live births per 1,000 women (10% increase in 1 year).

Trimester of First Prenatal Visit

Women from the Anchorage Service Unit sought prenatal care later in their pregnancies than the national rate of prenatal care. Nationally, 74.1% of the women received care in the first trimester of pregnancy and 18% in the second trimester (3). As illustrated, Alaska Native women sought care later, approximately 45% in the first trimester and 39% in the second (Table 1).

Number of Visits

The average number of visits by year were: 1979--9.2 visits; 1982--9.4 visits; and 1983--9.7 visits. The trend indicates that clients are being seen more frequently during their pregnancies. However, these averages fall below the national average of 11.1 visits in 1980 as well as being below the number of visits for all racial groups (3). Seeking prenatal care later in the pregnancy is one explanation for this lower number of encounters.

In this population, 51% of all clients were found to have at least one prenatal risk factor. The three most frequent risk categories were consistent for all three study years. These were: hemoglobin 11 grams or less, gravida 5 or more, smoking (10 or more cigarettes per day). The three most frequent risk categories were comparable for all age groups (Table 2). It appears that the most frequently occurring prenatal risks were preventable and related to lifestyle.

Summary of Risk Factors

The incidence of prenatal clients at risk increased from 1979 (51%) to 1982 (62.1%) and 1983 (73.5%). Figure 1 summarizes the data by year broken down into risk category. Whether the increased number of women at low and high risk is indicative of a real increase in the total number of clients at risk or a reflection of the

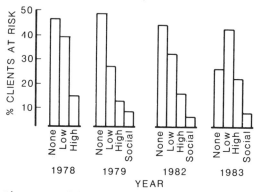

Figure 1. *Risk summary percentages for 1979, 1982, and 1983 for the Anchorage Service Unit.*

better data collection system is impossible to determine. The authors believe it is a reflection of the improved data collection system.

Cesarean Section Rates

The rates of cesarean sections is very low for this sample. The rate has increased during the period studied. Still, the rate of cesarean sections is 2.5 times greater in the private hospitals in Anchorage than the rate for the prenatal patients from the Anchorage Service Unit who delivered at the Alaska Native Medical Center (4)(Table 3).

Birthweights

The median birthweight for ASU babies was 3,373 g in 1983, a figure similar to the national average, which was 3,360 g in 1983. The incidence of low birthweight infants (less than 2,500 g) decreased over the years studied (6.8% to 6.5%) but was still higher than the incidence reported in the State of Alaska for all races (5.4%).

Table 1. *Percentages of women initiating prenatal care by trimester for the Anchorage Service Unit.*

| Trimester | ANMC | | | U.S. |
	1979	1982	1983	1980
First	47.8	42.4	46.7	74.1
Second	34.9	41.6	40.5	18.0
Third	9.8	15.3	10.8	6.7
No Care	1.7	0.7	2.0	1.2

Table 2. *Combined prenatal risk factors for 1979, 1982 and 1983 for the Anchorage Service Unit.*

	1979	1982	1983
Hemoglobin 11 g or less	16.4	22.4	13.8
Gravida 5 or more	11.1	13.8	11.8
Smoking 10 or more cigarettes per day	5.7	14.1	14.5
50 lbs. over/20 lbs. under ideal weight	8.8	4.8	4.3
Weight gain high/low	4.3	3.0	4.2
2 or more spontaneous abortions	4.3	3.0	5.6

Table 3. Cesarean section percentages for the Anchorage Service Unit and other Anchorage hospitals.

Cesarean Sections	ANMC			Anchorage
	1979	1982	1983	1983
Primary	4.0	5.6	5.6	
Repeat	3.1	3.1	3.9	
Total	7.1	8.7	9.5	23-24

Adolescent Pregnancy

The incidence of adolescent pregnancy was very low. Adolescents sought prenatal care later in their pregnancies and had fewer prenatal visits than other age groups. During the years 1979, 1982 and 1983, 1.5% of all adolescents younger than 15 delivered low birthweight infants. This group consistently had a higher rate of anemia than any other age group during 1979, 1982 and 1983. Of note, only one cesarean section was performed among the 100 clients 16 years and less during this 3-year period.

Residence

Village women had a higher incidence of low hemoglobin (less than 11 g) among all age categories. These were 45% for 1979, 32% for 1982, and 27% for 1983. The incidence decreased in 1983 as compared to 1979 and 1982. Village and urban clients had comparable pregnancy risks and outcomes. The system of risk assessment and initiation of prenatal care in the village setting may have contributed to the declining incidence of low hemoglobin.

RECOMMENDATIONS

The initiation of the risk management data system appears to have contributed to better reporting and monitoring of prenatal risks within this population. The authors would like to recommend that the following be considered in further program planning efforts:

1. Decrease through educational programs those risks identified as preventable, such as smoking, number of pregnancies, and anemia.
2. Investigate further why these clients seek prenatal care later in pregnancy.
3. Observe whether fertility rates continue to increase through continued monitoring.

REFERENCES

1. Goals, objectives and action plans. Prenatal Program, Alaska Area Native Health Service. 1978.
2. Public Health Service, U.S. Dept. of Health, Education and Welfare. Trend in fertility among Alaska Natives. Prepared by Larry Blackwood, January 1980.
3. U.S. Dept of Health and Human Services. NCH Monthly Vital Statistics Report, Nov. 30, 1982, Vol. 31(8), suppl.
4. Chandonnet A. Caesarean sections increase in Anchorage, nation. The Anchorage Times, April 27, 1984:E1-3.

Jackie Pflaum
School of Nursing
University of Alaska
3211 Providence Drive
Anchorage, Alaska 99508
U.S.A.

Circumpolar Health 84:384-387

ALASKA'S IMPROVED PREGNANCY OUTCOME PROJECT: AN EVALUATION

MARTI DILLEY

The Improved Pregnancy Outcome (IPO) project was initiated in Alaska at the Fairbanks Health Center in 1980. The goal of the project was healthier babies through increasing accessibility of prenatal care to high risk women, especially teenagers. Assessment of risk was based on medical, social, and economic criteria.

Staffed by a full-time public health nurse and a half-time Community Health Aide, IPO services included: 1) financial assistance for prenatal visits to the doctor, 2) prenatal education classes, 3) teen pregnancy support groups, 4) individual counseling, 5) referral to other agencies, including the woman-infant-children nutrition program, and 6) coordination of care and services.

An evaluation of the program was conducted in 1983. After an extensive literature review (available upon request), of both the measures of and factors affecting pregnancy outcomes, especially among teenagers, three indicators were chosen as outcome measures: infant's birth weight, gestational age, and 5-minute Apgar score. Prematurity, low Apgar score, and especially low birth weight have all been consistently linked to higher rates of infant mortality.

Factors influencing pregnancy outcomes were divided into two categories: sociodemographic (mother's age, race, education, and marital status; father's race and education; family size; annual income; and amount of IPO financial assistance), and medical-obstetric (mother's risk score, gravidity, and parity; timing and frequency of prenatal care; complications of pregnancy, labor, and delivery; and specific risk factors such as use of tobacco, alcohol, and drugs).

Data on these explanatory variables were gathered for the 309 women enrolled in the IPO program during 1981, 1982, to mid-1983. A random control group of 275, stratified by age, race, and marital status, was selected from women who delivered in Fairbanks during the 20 months immediately preceding the initiation of the IPO program. The second phase of the study, not included here, assessed the level of satisfaction with the IPO program by clients, providers, and staff.

RESULTS

The average monthly enrollment in IPO was 72 in 1981, 71 in 1982, and 45 in 1983 as a result of funding reductions. Over half of the women were in their 20s at delivery; over one-third were teenagers (15% were 17 years of age or younger); one-tenth were in their 30s. Over 80% were white.

Table 1. Birth weight for IPO babies in grams.

	N	%
Very low BW (≤1,499 grams)	7	2.6
Low BW (1,500-2,499)	12	4.5
Normal BW (2,500-4,499)	238	88.8
High BW (≥4,500)	11	4.1
Total	268	100.0

Alaska Natives and Blacks each constituted about 8%, with 2% Asian. At delivery, 54% were married. Two out of 3 mothers and almost 9 of 10 fathers had completed at least high school, while 9% and 12% respectively had completed at least 4 years of college. Over half (55%) of the IPO women were assessed as medical high risk, 38% as social high risk.

The percentage of IPO financial assistance for doctor visits was determined by a sliding scale based on the client's income. Of 254 annual incomes reported, 82% were less than $10,000; half were under $5,070. Two out of every three enrollees (201 in all) were assisted with IPO funds at some level, IPO paying 100% for 154. The amount per client ranged from $13 to $954, with half receiving $152 or less. Other sources of financial aid included Medicaid (11%), Alaska Area Native Health Service (9%), military (4%), and private means (8%).

Of IPO women, 71% initiated prenatal care in the first trimester, 24% in the second, and 5% in the third. The number of prenatal visits to the physician ranged from 0 to 28; half had 10 or more. It was the first pregnancy for 45% of the IPO clients; the first child for 68%. In all, 268 of the 309 clients (87%) delivered babies while enrolled. Of the 41 who did not deliver, 31 had either moved out of town or were lost to follow-up. Ten women, 4 of them teenagers, had spontaneous abortions, half before 14 weeks gestation. Of all deliveries, 21% were by cesarean section; 96% of all deliveries occurred in a hospital.

As the data in Table 1 reveal, nearly 90% of the IPO mothers delivered babies of normal birth weight. The median birth weight of infants born to IPO women was 3,387 grams. The tiniest baby that survived weighed 870 grams; the heaviest baby weighed 4,918 grams.

Table 2 shows that over 87% of the IPO babies were term, 10% were pre-term, with nearly 3% post-term. The range of gesta-

Table 2. *Gestational age for IPO babies in weeks.*

	N	%
Pre-term (<38)	27	10.1
Term (38-42)	234	87.3
Post-term (>42)	7	2.6
Total	268	100.0

Table 4. *Means for IPO group and control group.*

	IPO	Control	
Birth weight	3,351.1	3,327.5	p>.05
Gestational weight	39.5	39.8	p>.05
Apgar score	8.6	8.7	p>.05

tional age was 28 to 43 weeks, the median being 40. All seven of the very low body weight (VLBW) babies were premature, as were six of the 12 LBW babies. The data in Table 3 show that nearly 94% of IPO infants had high Apgars, fully half having scores of 9 or 10.

Nearly three out of four VLBW babies had low Apgars, as did over one-fourth of the HBW babies. However, all 12 LBW babies had Apgars of 7 or above. High Apgars characterized 80% of the premature babies, nearly 86% of the post-term babies as well as over 95% of term babies.

Table 4 compares the measures of the 3 outcome variables for the IPO and control groups. The mean birth weight for IPO babies was 3,351.1 grams, compared to 3,327.5 grams for the controls, a difference which was not statistically significant as determined by the difference of means t-test. Neither did the groups differ significantly on gestational age or Apgar score.

The data in Table 5 show, however, that the birth weight of babies born to IPO women age 18 years of age or less (3,473.0 grams) was significantly higher than that for the babies of control group women of the same age (3,209.3 grams).

Thus, for the teenagers, who were the real focus of the program, IPO services did in fact result in healthier babies, as measured by birth weight.

The IPO data were examined in greater detail in order to determine which explanatory variables were highly associated with pregnancy outcomes. Pearson product-moment correlation coefficients between each

variable and each of the three outcome measures were calculated, and then tested for statistical significance. Table 6 presents the result of that analysis for only those variables which were found to be significantly correlated with one or more of the three outcome measures.

DISCUSSION

Of the socio-demographic variables studied, three were significant: mother's age, mother's race, and father's education. Research studies have consistently reported that adolescents are more likely than older women to deliver premature babies. In this study, however, younger mothers were less likely to have premature infants. Women under 15 years of age delivered babies with a mean gestational age of 40.3 weeks, while women 25 to 29 years old, generally considered to be the prime age for childbearing, delivered babies with a mean gestation of 38.9 weeks. Teenagers made up nearly 40% of the entire IPO group, yet delivered only 19% of the premature babies. The results for Apgar scores are similar. In general, babies of younger mothers had higher Apgars. It appears that the IPO program was successful in promoting healthier babies among teenagers.

The mean birth weight of infants born to Black women (2,670 grams) was significantly lower than for Whites (3,386 grams), Natives (3,728), and Asians (3,156). Blacks accounted for about 8% of the entire IPO group, yet delivered nearly 43% of the very low birth weight babies. Similarly, infants of Black women had shorter gestations on the average than others. These findings of less

Table 3. *Apgar scores for IPO babies.*

	N	%
Low (<7)	16	6.2
High (7-10)	244	93.8
Total	260	100.0

Table 5. *Birth weight of babies of IPO and control groups born to women age 18 years or less (p<0.05).*

	IPO	Control
Mean birth weight	3,473.0	3,209.3
Standard deviation	469.9	584.9
N	65	122

successful pregnancy outcomes for Black women are consistent with the research literature.

The level of father's educational attainment was positively correlated with the baby's Apgar score. Fifty-five of 56 babies born to fathers who had had some college had high Apgar scores, while nearly 9 of 10 low Apgar babies were born to men who had a high school education or less.

While differences in birth weight between IPO women actually financially assisted with IPO funds as compared to IPO women whose prenatal expenses were paid by other sources were not statistically significant, the mean birth weight for IPO-assisted babies was 3,367.5 grams, which was within 60 grams of the mean birth weight of babies born to mothers using insurance and private means for prenatal expenses, a group generally characterized by lower risk pregnancies. The IPO babies' average birth weight was 350 grams higher than that for Medicaid patients. Perhaps the education and counseling components of the IPO program resulted in higher birth weights than a program such as Medicaid that gives financial assistance only.

The medical-obstetric variables which were significantly related to one or more of the outcome measures included mother's gravidity, parity, and risk score; number of prenatal doctor and health center visits, home visits, and telephone contacts; whether or not there had been pregnancy complications; and type of delivery.

Gravidity refers to the total number of pregnancies which a woman has had. The results of this study showed that the Apgar score of the baby decreased as the number of pregnancies increased. The mean Apgar for babies of first pregnancies was 8.6, but dropped to 5.3 for sixth through tenth pregnancies. Parity is the total number of live births a woman has had. The baby's birth weight increased as parity increased. Higher birth weight infants were more likely to be born to women with a greater number of previous live births. The mean birth weight of women giving birth to a first child was 3,327.4 grams, compared to a mean of 3,532.8 grams for mothers having a third, fourth, fifth, or sixth child, a difference of over 200 grams. It is unclear why Apgar scores were negatively correlated with number of pregnancies, while birth weight was positively correlated with number of live births. A suggestion is the increasing evidence that multiple abortions have a negative impact on subsequent births.

The risk assessment, an evaluation of the woman's risk regarding favorable birth outcome, was completed at enrollment or first prenatal visit, and was based on her prenatal history and current health status. An assessment of social high risk indicated potential problems during the pregnancy or after the baby's birth, such as unmarried mother, maternal age under 16, use of alcohol or drugs, or psychiatric problems. A woman was assessed as financial high risk if her annual income would be insufficient

Table 6. Pearson product-moment correlation coefficients.

		Outcome measures	
Explanatory variables	Birth weight	Gestational age	Apgar score
Socio-demographic:			
Mother's age	-0.05	-0.17**	-0.14*
Mother's race	-0.16*	-0.14*	0.00
Father's education	0.06	-0.02	0.15*
Medical-obstetric:			
Gravidity	0.01	0.00	-0.14*
Parity	0.13*	0.07	-0.04
Risk score	0.01	-0.06	-0.17*
Number of prenatal visits	0.23**	0.22**	0.06
Number of health center visits	0.07	0.14*	0.02
Number of home visits	-0.20**	-0.20**	-0.19**
Number of phone contacts	-0.16*	-0.11	-0.18**
Complications of pregnancy	-0.04	0.09	0.17**
Illness or condition affecting pregnancy	-0.12	-0.05	0.18**
Type of delivery	-0.07	-0.14*	-0.05

$* \ p<0.05 \ ** \ p<0.01$

to pay for adequate prenatal care. IPO was of the most help to that group of women caught in the gap between eligibility for welfare and economic solvency. Over 93% of the IPO women were assessed as high risk on one or more of these three dimensions.

The data revealed that lower risk scores were related to higher Apgar scores. The women whose risk assessment scores of 6 to 9, indicating the highest risk, constituted less than 20% of the total enrollment, yet accounted for over 36% of the low Apgar infants. Every one of the low Apgar babies was born to a high risk mother. As for specific risk factors, non-smokers delivered babies that were on the average 232 grams heavier than those of smokers, although this difference was not statistically significant. Birth outcomes did not differ significantly between users and non-users of either alcohol or street drugs.

Better birth outcomes were associated with a higher number both of prenatal doctor visits and prenatal health center visits, the latter occurring as the client picked up a voucher prior to each doctor's appointment, attended prenatal education classes or teen pregnancy support group meetings, or received nutritional counseling. Better birth outcomes were also associated with fewer home visits by the public health nurse and with fewer telephone contacts with the health center. Women with problem pregnancies or premature, low birth weight babies prompted more intensive staff follow-up.

Mothers with pregnancy complications of any kind delivered babies with significantly lower mean Apgar scores (8.0) than mothers having no complications (8.7). The mean number of weeks of gestation for babies of mothers having vaginal deliveries was significantly greater than that for cesarean section deliveries (39.8 versus 39.0 weeks).

Multiple stepwise regression analysis showed that variables which in combination explained the greatest amount of the variance in each of the 3 outcome measures were essentially the same ones discussed above.

CONCLUSION

In summary, the babies of IPO teens had significantly higher birth weights than did the babies of the control teens. Healthier babies did in fact result from IPO intervention for the targeted group, the high-risk teenager.

ACKNOWLEDGMENT

The IPO project was funded by a federal grant (Health and Human Services MCJ-023119-02-0), and was administered by the Alaska Department of Health and Social Services.

Marti Dilley
Alaska Department of Health
  and Social Services
Pouch H-01A
Juneau, Alaska 99801
U.S.A.

Circumpolar Health 84:388-389

HALF A LOAF IS BETTER THAN NONE OR MINIBACTERIOLOGY FOR MINIFACILITIES

ANNE GILLAN

INTRODUCTION

For the past four years the Stanton Yellowknife Hospital laboratory, the only regional laboratory in the Mackenzie Zone, has provided service to two budget hospitals and 12 nursing stations. Over this time, we have become increasingly frustrated with our inability to give a satisfactory bacteriological service to the nursing stations. We are many air miles and erratic plane schedules away from these places. The time lapse between the collection of a specimen and its arrival in the laboratory varies between 3 and 14 days, the specimen possibly having been exposed to the extremes of arctic weather. After that time interval, the organisms have either been overgrown by a non-causative contaminant, or more likely, and almost definitely in the case of the gonococcus (G.C.), the organisms are no longer viable. In our early work we were particularly interested in the diagnosis of G.C. and were reduced to diagnosing a positive G.C. by gram stain of the smear made in the nursing station. It has long been accepted that this method is a very poor way of diagnosing the disease, especially in women where the gram stain provides us with a large number of false positives and false negatives. There would also be no means of confirming the diagnosis.

How then, if we cannot help the nursing stations within a clinically significant time period for most organisms, and in the case of G.C. not at all, can they help themselves? For that reason we became interested in a product called the ISOCULT System (trademark of SmithKline Diagnostics), introduced into Canada two years ago. This system basically is a culture system similar to that used in all laboratories, but with the major advantage that it can be used by relatively untrained personnel because it standardizes inoculation procedures and enables interpretation with the aid of a very detailed color chart. It is a simplified system which uses specially prepared culture media to provide a rapid, convenient way of culturing certain medically important organisms as an aid to diagnosis. The media are selective, encouraging the growth of specific microorganisms, while inhibiting others, and making visual diagnosis earlier by color changes.

A number of publications have confirmed that under laboratory conditions these media are just as successful, for identifying the organisms they are designed for, as conventional media.

COMPONENTS AND PROCEDURES

The two basic components of this system will be briefly reviewed. The ISOCULT culture tube has a paddle which holds the culture medium. The collar has built-in tines which streak the specimen along the medium to separate organisms and isolate colonies. A slit in the top of the paddle is provided for the insertion of a carbon dioxide tablet for culturing organisms which require a carbon dioxide atmosphere, such as G.C. and throat streptococci. The specimen is collected and inoculated on the paddle, inserted into the tube and incubated. After 24 to 48 hours incubation, the growth on the ISOCULT paddle is compared to color photographs on an ISOCULT organism identification chart. Such comparison is sufficient for all organisms except G.C., which requires a further test.

G.C. organisms produce an enzyme called oxidase, which can be detected by adding a drop of solution called detectase (supplied) to the colonies. A purple/black stain which appears between 10 and 60 seconds indicates a positive result. At this stage one can be reasonably sure that the organism is G.C. For further confirmation of the diagnosis, however, the specimen has to be sent to the nearest laboratory which will then carry out their confirmation routine, usually by biochemical tests. The laboratory may, of course, not be able to confirm due to the death of the organism and that is exactly the reason why we should go as far as we can in the nursing station.

Inuvik Study

We decided to try this system by running a controlled study in Inuvik, N.W.T. The results, which are reported elsewhere will be summarized here. Sixty-four patients were investigated by taking two swabs and processing one by ISOCULTs put up by public health nurses, and the other in the hospital by conventional methods. Sixty-three percent of these specimens were negative by both methods, and 23% were positive by both methods. Fourteen percent (9 specimens) were negative by ISOCULT and positive in the laboratory. Why was the error so large? G.C. is a fastidious organism and it is well known in all quality control programs that even under the best conditions, many laboratories have difficulty in culturing it. Even if we accept the fact that ISOCULT, if used by relatively untrained personnel, may miss growing some G.C. organisms, the alternative is no confirmation whatsoever. However, we found that our greatest problem was the fact that staff were inadequately trained. We have remedied the situation by giving one hour's training and discussion to staff passing through Yellowknife, and demanding that the provided literature is studied carefully. This seems to have greatly improved our chances of growing positive cultures.

Present Use

This system can be used for investigating a number of other organisms. Presently the ISOCULTs are used routinely for throat streptococci, bacteriuria and *Candida*. We have not run any more controlled studies, but I have had positive comments from Dr. Sarsfield in Cambridge Bay, who has been able to diagnose some throat infections as streptococcal which he might otherwise have though to be viral. Positive comments have also come from the nursing stations stressing their ability to determine by the bacteriuria method whether a urinary tract infection was present, and if so, whether it was caused by gram positive or gram negative organisms. Similar positive comments have been made about the differential diagnosis of *Candida*.

Cost Effectiveness

Is this system cost effective? In 1982-83 Stanton Yellowknife Hospital supplied three nursing stations, Fort Simpson, Coppermine, and Cambridge Bay, with a very limited supply of ISOCULTSs. For all three communities there was a considerable drop in cost of processing bacteriological specimens during the time ISOCULTs were available. As soon as the supply stopped, the cost went back up again. The cost represents only charges paid to Stanton Yellowknife Hospital for processing the specimens. The additional and frequently very high costs of transporting specimens from nursing station to hospital have not been considered.

Problem of Supply

There is sometimes a problem getting the supplies in good condition. It is necessary to use a supplier who has mastered the intricacies of northern transportation systems. In Bio-Pacific of Vancouver, B.C., we have found such a supplier.

CONCLUSION

This brief report shows what the ISOCULT system can do; now, in conclusion I will describe what it cannot do.

It cannot replace a regional laboratory. It is not capable of finding unsuspected organisms. It is not even capable of growing or identifying an organism other than the one the particular medium is designed for.

The user will have to ask the question, "Is this such-and-such an organism?" The answer will be "yes" or "no." I feel that, in isolated places, to be able to get this kind of answer within a clinically significant time period, will be helpful.

REFERENCES

1. U.S. Public Health Service Center for Disease Control, Venereal Disease Branch, Criteria and techniques for the diagnosis of gonorrhea. Atlanta, 1971.
2. Beilstein HR. Comparative studies of media for the identification of *Neisseria gonorrhoeae*. II. Public Health Laboratory 1973; 31:126-136.
3. Schaad Urs B, Wuilloud AH. Simple and reliable detection of beta-hemolytic streptococci in throat swabs with the ISOCULT system. Switzerland, Schweiz Med Wschr 1981; 111:892-897.
4. Gillan A. 3/4 of a loaf is better than none. Paper presented at Can. Pub. Health Assn. Conf., Yellowknife, N.W.T. 1982. (In press).

Anne Gillan
Laboratory Services
Stanton Yellowknife Hospital
P.O. Box 10
Yellowknife, Northwest Territories X1A 2N1
Canada

Circumpolar Health 84:390-393

AN ECONOMIC PERSPECTIVE ON TELERADIOLOGY FOR REMOTE COMMUNITIES

JOHN HORNE

INTRODUCTION

The delivery of radiographic diagnostic and consulting services to remote communities via telecommunications technology has been shown to be feasible in several field trials (1-5). There are, however, some significant obstacles to the implementation of teleradiology systems on a wider non-experimental scale. Technical problems of image quality and speed of transmission continue to plague several variants of the technology and until these are overcome clinicians will remain restrained in their enthusiasm. Once solutions to these problems are found, economic considerations will inevitably assume major importance, especially in a publicly-financed health care system like Canada's where health planners and policy-makers have a responsibility to assess the cost-effectiveness of new medical technologies.

In studies published to date there has been a dearth of evidence on the cost-effectiveness of teleradiology. The purpose of this paper is to explore the prospects for cost-effective teleradiology using the limited information from previous studies, and more revealingly, some estimates of potential costs and benefits specific to Norway House, a remote community in Manitoba which illustrates the relevant economic challenge. In this particular setting, the conditions under which teleradiology would be a cost-effective alternative to the present system of "mail-order" radiology and "fly-in" consultant services are identified and discussed. Data on the utilization and cost of the present system are analyzed to determine the extent to which teleradiology might yield significant savings via reduced incidence of travel by both patients and physicians.

MATERIALS AND METHODS

Norway House is located at the top of Lake Winnipeg 560 kilometers north of Winnipeg. In the 1981 census, the resident population numbered 2,785 and included 2,331 Cree Indians with treaty status, 300 non-treaty Indians (Métis) and 154 Euro-Canadians. Medical facilities include a 16-bed primary care hospital operated and staffed by the federal government with an outpatient clinic and emergency department. The Northern Medical Unit of the University of Manitoba provides the services of four resident general practitioners, one resident social worker, three public health nurses and 53 consultant days on a contractual basis.

On-site radiological services are currently provided by one x-ray technician and by radiologists-in-training who visit Norway House for two days 5 to 6 times per year, thereby providing the expertise to perform barium-related procedures. Films taken between radiologists' visits are initially read by the resident general practitioners and then mailed to Winnipeg for more formal interpretation. Reports are mailed or phoned back to Norway House. Typical turnaround time is one week.

Assessment of the potential costs and benefits of a teleradiology system between Norway House and Winnipeg entailed a variety of steps. First, the literature was reviewed unsuccessfully for any evidence of cost-effectiveness in either experimental or operational teleradiology systems. Second, data on the utilization and costs of the present radiological service in Norway House were obtained from administrative records on file at the hospital and the Northern Medical Unit. These data, and supplementary statistics from the same sources on the incidence of patient evacuations from Norway House to Winnipeg, defined the "baseline" against which the incremental costs and benefits of teleradiology were subsequently compared. Third, persistent problems of image quality and speed of transmission peculiar to existing slow-scan (narrowband) teleradiology in which single images are sent over phone lines were deliberately sidestepped in order to shift attention away from purely technical matters to the hitherto ignored issue of cost-effectiveness. This was accomplished not simply by assuming these problems away, but by accepting as potentially feasible a hypothetical variant of slow-scan teleradiology in which these problems are overcome. Termed "Rapid Digital Narrowband Teleradiology" by its architects, the system would employ a variety of new technologies and software to preserve image quality and, simultaneously, to achieve unprecedentedly fast transmission times using ordinary phone lines (6). The capital and operating costs of such a system were roughly estimated based on consultations with knowledgeable specialists in radiology, image processing and telecommunications. Key parameters such as the long-distance telephone rate were specified on the basis of current charges levied by the Manitoba Telephone System (MTS). Equally rough estimates of the system's potential benefits were based on alternative and rather arbitrary assumptions concerning its effectiveness in reducing the incidence of travel by patients and physicians, an admittedly stringent measure of benefit, but

Table 1. Utilization and costs of radiological services, Norway House
1982-83.

Number of radiologic examinations	2,107
Number of radiographic films	4,367
Estimated operating costs*	$70,000

* Includes radiologists' remuneration,
employee remuneration and all of the non-
capital expenses; based on cost of $27 per
exam in rural Manitoba hospitals as estimated by MacEwan et. al. (7) using 1979 data;
adjusted for inflation, equivalent unit cost
in 1982-83 is $33.

one that has unambiguous policy relevance
and can be confidently expected to figure
prominently in any future official assessment of the technology. Finally, the
assumed conditions yielding benefit-cost
ratios greater than one (indicating the
system to be a cost-effective alternative to
present arrangements) were further analyzed
using selected baseline data on patient and
physician travel to determine whether the
assumed reductions in transportation costs
were consistent with the clinical reality.

RESULTS AND DISCUSSION

Information on the utilization and
costs of the existing radiological service
in Norway House is shown in Table 1. For
the twelve month period ending March 1983 a
total of 2,107 radiologic exams were performed, of which over half (54%) were bone
and extremity exams, one-third were chest
exams and the remainder (13%) abdominal
exams. Excluding barium-related procedures,
a total of 4,367 films were taken; these
constitute the subset of "teleradiology
eligible" films. In the absence of a detailed cost analysis, operating costs were
estimated at $70,000 based on radiological
cost data for rural Manitoba hospitals
reported by MacEwan et al. (7).

Table 2 shows the rough estimates of
potential annual costs of the rapid digital
teleradiology system. Central to this hypothetical system is an assumed transmission
time of five minutes per chest radiograph
using four phone lines simultaneously.
Hence, total phone time is 20 minutes per
film with an associated long-distance charge
of $8.40, based on the current MTS daytime
business rate of $25 per hour for lines over
the 560 km distance between Norway House and
Winnipeg. Operating costs are shown to vary
between $23,000 and $41,500 depending on
whether 50% or 100% of the roughly 4,400
"teleradiology eligible" films are transmitted. Annualized capital costs to finance a
teleradiology station in Norway House and an
appropriate share of a required reading

Table 2. Rough estimates of potential
annual costs of teleradiology,
Norway House.

Operating costs*	$23,000-41,500
Capital costs**	$20,000
Total	$43,000-61,500

* Includes data phone line estimated at
$2,160/year, Telidon charges estimated at
$2,400/year, and long-distance charges of
$8.40/radiograph transmitted; lower figure
assumes transmission of 2,200 radio-
graphs/year (50% of current workload);
higher figure assumes transmission of 4,400
radiographs/year (100% of current workload).

** Includes assumed amortization at 12% over
5 years of teleradiology station in Norway
House estimated at $50,000 and central
computer and reading station in Winnipeg to
serve 50 remote sites estimated at
$1,300,000.

station and central computer in Winnipeg
(designed to serve 50 remote sites) are
estimated at $20,000. Total operating and
capital costs are thus estimated to range
from $43,000 to $61,500.

Table 3 presents rough estimates of
potential benefits, restrictively defined to
include readily quantifiable savings via
elimination of "mail order" radiology,
reduction in "fly-in" visits by radiolo-

Table 3. Rough estimates of potential
annual benefits of teleradiology
for Norway House.

Elimination of "mail order" radiology*	$ 4,400
Reduction in "fly-in" visits by radiologists**	$ 2,000- 4,200
Reduction in elective air evacuations***	$18,800-36,000
Total	$24,500-44,600

* Assumes mailing of all radiographic
films (4400/yr) at average postage cost of
$1 per film.

** Assumes $700 per two-day trip; lower
figure assumes 50% reduction in trip frequency to 3 per year; higher figure assumes
elimination of all 6 trips.

*** Assumes $400 per elective air evacua-
tion; lower figure assumes 45 fewer evacuations per year (10% reduction); higher
figure assumes 90 fewer evacuations per year
(20% reduction).

Table 4.   Rough estimates of potential benefit/cost ratios for teleradiology, Norway House.

Benefits defined to include:	Costs defined to include: Operating and capital		Operating only	
	($43,000)	($61,500)	($23,000)	($41,500)
"Moderate" transportation savings ($24,500)	0.57	0.40	1.07	0.59
"Substantial" transportation savings ($44,600)	1.04	0.73	1.94	1.07

gists, and reduction in elective air evacuations of patients. The latter category generates by far the greatest benefit, with savings ranging from $18,000 to $36,000, depending on whether evacuations are reduced by 10% or 20% respectively. Total benefits are thus estimated to range from $24,500 to $44,600.

Table 4 combines the estimated costs and benefits of the system for various pairing of assumptions concerning system utilization and transportation activity. As well, costs are alternatively defined to include and exclude capital items in order to gauge the sensitivity of the results to arguments that capital costs can be substantially reduced by making use of the system to transmit other medical data (e.g., EKG's, dermatological, and pathological images) and hence spread the cost over several programs. It is evident that the system is provisionally cost-effective (i.e., generates a benefit-cost ratio greater than one) in four of the eight situations. In only one instance is this achieved on the assumption of "moderate" transportation savings; the corresponding cost condition requires transmission of only 50% of the "teleradiology eligible" films and omission of all capital costs. In the other three instances where the benefit-cost ratio exceeds one, "substantial" transportation savings must be assumed and, in the most compelling case, where the ratio is 1.94, capital costs must be omitted.

The crucial importance of the assumption regarding transportation savings and, in particular, savings from reduced numbers of elective air evacuations prompted questioning whether such an assumption was reasonable. Results of a detailed chart review (8) of 101 evacuations from Norway House over a four month period in 1979 are presented in Table 5. It is evident that two-thirds of the evacuations were in the elective category; in slightly more than one-half (53%) of these cases, evacuation was for "initial investigation" where a diagnostic technology such as teleradiology might be presumed to have some impact. In point of fact, however, in none of these cases was the evacuation for radiological investigation. On such evidence the assumption of "substantial" transportation savings from teleradiology must be regarded as highly unrealistic. Indeed, the assumption of even "moderate" savings must be seriously challenged.

Table 5.   Analysis of patient evacuations for all causes from Norway House to Winnipeg, by category and by reason for evacuation, September-December 1978.

Category	Reasons for Evacuation Initial investigation	Surgery, delivery, etc.	Total
Emergency	1	4	5
Urgent	12	14	26
Elective	35	31	66
Sympathetic	n/a	4	4
Total	48	53	101

CONCLUSIONS

The literature on teleradiology has long evidenced a preoccupation with the technical issues of image quality and speed of transmission, and an almost total absence of interest in the economics of the technology. This paper has attempted to redress this imbalance by sidestepping the technical issues and focusing on the economics of a recently proposed system of rapid digital narrowband teleradiology with the theoretical capability of transmitting radiographs without loss of image quality in a matter of five minutes. To achieve the same image quality from existing systems using standard video equipment and a single phone line would apparently require almost 35 hours!

Having "stacked the deck" in favor of a technology which could dramatically reduce the long-distance telephone charges per transmitted image, a "rough" assessment of its costs and benefits produced disappointing results. Based on the Norway House experience, the scope for tangible benefits in the form of savings from reduced travel by patients and physicians was shown to be very limited. Moreover, since the clinical efficacy of more timely radiographic data in remote communities remains to be firmly demonstrated, it is apparent that teleradiology lacks the compelling cost-effectiveness necessary for wide-scale implementation.

Advocates of teleradiology are wont to assume rather than analyze its cost-effectiveness (9). Their optimism that technical progress will dramatically increase its benefits may well be ultimately justified, but it will never be a substitute for careful economic evaluation based on well-controlled demonstrations. Obviously, rough assessments of the sort presented in this paper are themselves no substitute for rigorous evaluation. They can however provide a useful point of departure for the long overdue discussion on the economics of the technology. Even more to the point they can force the advocates to entertain the more pessimistic prognosis that teleradiol-

ogy is destined to be an expensive "add-on," quite capable, as here suggested, of increasing the cost of a radiographic exam by 50%. In that too rarely recognized "worse case," teleradiology reduces to an elaborate "video game"!

REFERENCES

1. Curtis DJ, Gayler BW, Gitlin JN, Harrington MB. Teleradiology: results of a field trial. Radio 1983; 149: 415-418.
2. Dunn E, Conrath D, Acton H, Higgins-Bain H. Telemedicine links patients in Sioux Lookout with doctors in Toronto. Can Med Assoc J 1980; 122:484-487.
3. Carey LS, Russell ES, Johnson EE, Wilkins WW. Radiologic consultation to a remote Canadian hospital using Hermes spacecraft. J Can Assoc Radiol 1979; 30:12-20.
4. Page J, Grégoire A, Galand C, Sylvestre J, Chalaoui J, Fauteux P, Dussault R, Séguin R, Roberge F. Teleradiology in northern Quebec. Radio 1981; 140: 361-366.
5. Page J, Sylvestre J. Roberge F, Grégoire A, Chalaoui J, Galand C, Laperrière J, Séguin R. Narrowband teleradiology. J Can Assoc Radiol 1982; 33:221-226.
6. Gordon R, Rangayyan R, Wardrop D, MacEwan D. Preservation of image quality in rapid digital narrowband teleradiology. (To be published).
7. MacEwan DW, Gelsky DE, Lock JR, Popoff J, Sourkes AM. 1979 diagnostic radiology services in the Province of Manitoba. J Can Assoc Radiol 1982; 33:246-254.
8. DuVal L. A four month review of evacuations from Norway House. Department of Social and Preventive Medicine report. Winnipeg, Manitoba, University of Manitoba, 1979.
9. Carey LS. A perspective for teleradiology in Canada in the 80's. J Can Assoc Radiol 1983; 33:257-259.

John M. Horne
Department of Social and Preventive Medicine
Faculty of Medicine
University of Manitoba
750 Bannatyne Avenue
Winnipeg, Manitoba R3E 0W3
Canada

Circumpolar Health 84:394-397

THE SPECIAL PREMEDICAL STUDIES PROGRAM TO PREPARE NATIVE STUDENTS FOR THE MEDICAL PROFESSION

M.C. STEPHENS and J.D. SILVER

The Special Premedical Studies Program (SPSP) is an extended science program for Canadian students of Native ancestry who wish to apply to the Faculties of Medicine and Dentistry at the University of Manitoba. This program was established because Indian and Inuit people are severely underrepresented in these professions. It is hoped also that eventually these professionals will help correct the imbalance that now exists between the number of urban versus rural health professionals. It is the only program presently available in Canada for this purpose. There is a similar program in the U.S.A. at the University of North Dakota, Faculty of Medicine, which has been in existence for approximately 10 years.

The main differences between these two are that our program sets a three year limit for premedical studies, and that there is no allotment of a fixed number of places in medical/dental schools for these students. SPSP is not an affirmative action program because students are not guaranteed entry into medicine/dentistry, but must compete for positions.

The SPSP was established in 1979 when the Northern Medical Unit (Faculty of Medicine, University of Manitoba), the Division of Continuing Education and the Department of Education of the Government of Manitoba recognized that there were no Native Canadians sufficiently prepared for immediate application to medical or dental schools. The Program Director reports to the Dean of Continuing Education. Program staff includes academic (teaching) personnel from the Faculties of Science and Medicine and academic and administrative support staff in Continuing Education and Medicine. An advisory committee composed of representatives from Continuing Education, Science, Medicine, Dentistry, the Manitoba Indian Education Association, Government of Manitoba, and Native Studies meet twice a year to review program policy. Funding for the program is secured through contractual agreement with the Government of Manitoba. Financial supports provided the students include living allowances, housing, day care, tuition fees, books, tutors, etc.

Eligible students must be born in or considered residents of Manitoba. Twenty-six different communities and reserves are represented by students accepted into SPSP, and include remote northern communities, reservations, small towns, and a few applicants from Winnipeg. Communities can be as distant as 1,000 kilometers from the University, with many accessible only by air.

Table 1. Outline of courses in SPSP, September through May.

Year I	Year II	Year III
Chemistry	Chemistry	Org. chem.
Physics	Physics	Biochemistry
English	Biology	2-3 Opt courses
Noncredit	Noncredit	Noncredit
"Med I"	"Med II"	"Med III"
Opt course (spring)	Opt course (spring)	Open
12 credits*	24 credits	24 credits

*Total credits required for medical/dental schools = 60

Applicants enter with very diverse levels of academic training (from 10th grade education to some postsecondary training). The vast majority have an insufficient science background. Most students are not aware of the commitment required for university studies, particularly in medicine or dentistry.

It is for the above reasons that this program was developed to extend over three years, instead of the regular two years necessary for entrance into medicine or dentistry at the University of Manitoba. It is designed to build as strong a background as possible in the sciences, particularly chemistry and physics. This is done by expanding these first year courses over a two year period (from 8 months to 18 months), as Table 1 indicates. Final examinations in these and other courses are written with the main university student population. By the third year all courses are taken with regular students. Additional courses (mathematics, English) are taken as needed in the first two years; workshops in chemistry and physics have been added, and extra tutoring is available.

Because this is a program of "premedical" studies, a substantial connection to medicine is included. Although the program might also be a stepping stone to other health-related careers, the primary thrust is to prepare and motivate students for medicine or dentistry. To enhance this, the student must feel a tangible link with the Faculty of Medicine. Therefore a "medical" component has been included for each one of the three years, taking about one-half a day per week throughout the school year.

Table 2. Medical component of SPSP.

Year admitted	"Med I"	"Med II"	"Med III"

1979	Physiology
	4 visits
		Clinical biochemistry
		4 visits
			Reading skills
			MCAT/DAT
			  preparation
			  (21 hr)+
			Practicum interview

1980	Physiology
	4 visits
		Medical specialty
		  seminars
			Reading skills
			MCAT/DAT preparation
			  (60 hr) +
			Practicum interview

1981	Physiology 4 visits	Medical specialty seminars Reading skills	MCAT/DAT preparation (60 hr)+ Practicum interview

1982	Medical specialty
	  seminars
	Visits 1/2 yr.
		Physiology
		4 medical specialty seminars
		Reading skills
		MCAT/DAT preparation +
			MCAT/DAT preparation
			  (60 hr)+
			Community medical
			  seminars
			Practicum interview

1983	Medical specialty
	  seminars as above
	  (Full yr.)
	Reading skills
		Physiology
		4 medical specialty seminars
		MCAT/DAT preparation +
			As above

Table 2 describes this component of the program. It has changed with time, as our perception of needs and students' suggestions were taken into consideration. It is to be noted that the physiology course was transferred to the second year, and the medical specialty seminars and visits to hospitals and clinics transferred to first year. In this way interest and motivation have been increased considerably. Also, students were better prepared in the second year to accept a human physiology course.

The reading and study skills were introduced at first where they were immediately needed, and were progressively anticipated and expanded. The Medical College Aptitude Test/Dental Aptitude Test (MCAT/DAT) training has been expanded; in addition, second year students are encouraged to attend these sessions. The MCAT/DAT training component is composed of science reviews, multiple choice exam training, and the perceptual/motor ability training for dentistry applicants. Practice interviews with staff from the Northern Medical Unit and other members of the Faculty of Medicine are also provided.

Another important component of the "medical" program is a summer practicum lasting six weeks between the first-second and second-third years. The objective of the practicum is to provide an opportunity for the students to observe and take part in some aspect of the health care field. Table 3 shows the range of placements utilized.

Table 3. SPSP summer practicum experiences, 6 weeks minimum.

1. Clinical aides/rotating clerkships in nursing stations, clinics, rural hospitals.
2. Interpreters in nursing stations, hospitals.
3. Laboratory aides in basic sciences, Faculty of Medicine, Faculty of Dentistry.
4. Aides in clinical departments: Faculty of Medicine, psychiatry, out-patient, pediatrics, emergency.
5. Aides in city clinics.
6. Aides in hospital pharmacies, X-ray, laboratories.
7. Administration position at Northern Medical Unit.
8. Accompany dentists in trips to north.

Table 4. Distribution of SPSP students according to age, sex, and location.

Year admitted	No.accepted/No. applied	Mean age (Range)	F/M	Rural/urban
1979	11/31 (17-30)	25	8/3	10/1
1980	11/42 (18-30)	24.4	5/6	11/0
1981	9/27 (20-29)	24.8	5/4	8/1
1982	13/37 (17-29)	21	9/4	11/2
1983	13/40 (17-35)	20.5	9/4	11/2

The number of students and some data about them are shown in Table 4. There are many more applicants eligible than students accepted, and more female than male (and this is also true in the applicants pool). The mean age has been decreasing in successive new classes, although the range is still the same. There are more rural than urban students; the recruitment emphasizes remote communities because they are thought to have less access to university education.

The retention rate of students is shown in Table 5. Retention rate appears to be higher in more recent years. The reason for this is not known, but at least two factors could account for it: a younger student population, or changes in curriculum to suit the perceived needs. It must be pointed out that the students who have completed the SPSP program and were accepted in medicine or dentistry are all in the upper age range.

Table 6 shows the increasing number of summer placements for each year. This rate is indicative of the increased retention rate of the program, and greatly increased interest on the part of the students.

In conclusion, it appears that this program has achieved, at least in part, the goal it had set. Many modifications were made in course structure, to supplement gaps in the students' academic backgrounds. In general, a well-structured program appears to result in better attendance, and to increase motivation. An intensive and extensive communication network between students and staff results in better compliance.

With our increased experience, more suitable positions and programs for the summer experiences have resulted in quite a good compliance.

Table 5. Number and fate of students admitted to SPSP.

Year admitted	1st yr.	2nd yr.	3rd yr.	Medicine	Dentistry
1979	11	6 1*	3 2*	2 1982	1 1982
1980	11	8	4 4*	1** 1983	
1981	9	4 1**	4		
1982	13	8 (1)	8		
1983	13	11 (1)			

*   Students continuing university education outside SPSP.
**   Students who did university work in 2 years.

Table 6. *Number of SPSP placements for summer practicum.*

1979-1980	6
1980-1981	10
1981-1982	8
1982-1983	12
1983-1984	21

Students who have completed the program have been of great help in encouraging and orienting other SPSP students, and in giving us a better insight into their difficulties.

REFERENCES

1. Poonwassie DH. The Special Premedical Studies Program at the University of Manitoba. (Unpublished.)
2. Special Premedical Studies Program student handbook. University of Manitoba, 1980.

M.C. Stephens
Northern Medical Unit
University of Manitoba
61 Emily Street
Winnipeg, Manitoba R3E 1Y9
Canada

Circumpolar Health 84:398-401

MEDICAL RECRUITMENT FOR THE AUSTRALIAN NATIONAL ANTARCTIC RESEARCH EXPEDITIONS

DESMOND LUGG

Australia has an active medical work force of some 27,500 practitioners with an annual increase of 1,400 new graduates from Australian universities. A doctor:population ratio of 1:543, projected for 1991 (1), was reached in 1981. Despite this medical manpower oversupply and a serious exacerbation of the position as indicated by a recent report (1), the Antarctic Division has great difficulty in recruiting four satisfactory doctors to winter for 12 to 15 months with each Australian National Antarctic Research Expedition (ANARE).

ANARE was established in 1947 and for the first two years there were ample applicants for this new, exciting, well-publicized venture. From 1950 to 1960 problems occurred, and after 1960 there were frequent crises. In 1962, 1964, 1972 and 1975, five medical officers spent a second consecutive wintering year to avert closure of a station with repatriation of expedition staff to Australia. On several occasions recruits were found with only days to spare before the last ship sailed; frequently, most extraordinary measures were taken to engage medical staff.

Currently, during summer, one medical officer is on each relief ship, field operation (including diving programs) or marine science cruise; and one medical officer winters at Mawson, Casey, Davis or Macquarie Island (Figure 1). The total health care service provided, which has been described (2), is unique in Australian medical practice. The Antarctic stations do not have all-weather airfields nor permanently based aircraft, so no direct intercontinental flights are possible. The only access is by ship during 12 weeks of the austral summer, when the sea ice can be

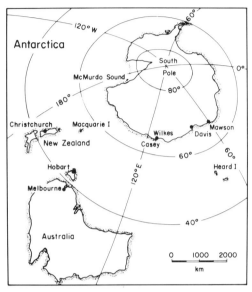

Figure 1. Map showing Australian Antarctic stations.

penetrated, and there is no physical contact with other national expeditions during winter.

The total inaccessibility for most of a year means that the recruited doctor must have a suitable temperament to survive in a small, isolated group of 4 to 35 persons for this time. In addition, he or she must have the ability to conduct a solo practice capable of dealing with any medical, dental, or surgical emergency that may arise. The only contact with Head Office medical staff is by voice radio, telex or satellite telephone, and the only assistance available

Table 1. Medical position, qualifications and university of graduation of doctors recruited, ANARE, 1947 to 1984.

	Winter ANARE	Summer ANARE
Number of medical positions	122	60
Qualifications of recruits		
Basic medical degree only	87%	59%
Specialist	13%	41%
Additional non-medical degree	9%	7%
University of graduation		
Australia	59%	75%
Overseas	41%	25%
Number of doctors employed*	97	36

* Total number employed 112, 59% summer doctors having also wintered.

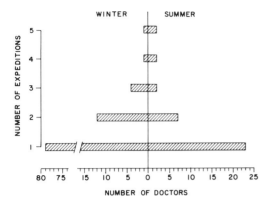

Figure 2. Frequency of doctor's service on ANARE.

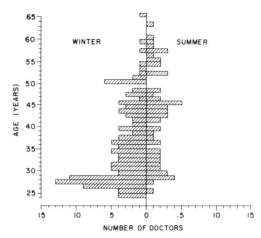

Figure 3. Distribution by age of doctors recruited by ANARE.

is from selected station personnel who have had limited training in the elementary administration of anesthetics and in operating room techniques.

As research initiatives by Australia and a multi-million dollar rebuilding program have been in jeopardy due to lack of medical support, a survey was made of the medical practitioners who have worked on ANARE in the period 1947 to 1984. Data such as age on joining, university of graduation, qualifications, and experience were assessed for changes in the recruitment pattern in an effort to predict the most likely source of recruits in the future.

Table 1 shows the medical positions on ANARE, qualifications, and university graduation of doctors recruited since 1947. One hundred twelve practitioners have filled 182 posts with 21 of these having wintered in addition to serving with summer expeditions. Although 70% of the 112 were Australian graduates, such graduates have only staffed 59% of winter expeditions. This fact indicates the large number of overseas graduates who have returned to ANARE after their first winter. Figure 2 illustrates the importance of returning doctors to the ANARE medical services. It should be noted that no serving defense doctor has ever been recruited for ANARE and it seems inevitable that doctors for the Antarctic must be recruited from civilian practice. Recruiting from Australian medical schools was not uniform across the country but the reason for this was unclear.

The distribution of age (Figure 3), experience (Figure 4), and practice category (Figure 5) revealed some surprises. ANARE folklore has suggested that most doctors were under 30 years of age: 30% of the 112 were under 30, but there was a wide distribution of ages, with a mean of 35 years. The number of years since graduation were also greater than anecdote had suggested.

Trends in recruiting patterns are observed when ANARE data are represented in four equal time periods. In the first period there were 4:3 overseas graduates but since then the ratio has been 2:1 in favor of Australian graduates. Increases in both age and years since graduation, over the four periods, reflect a number of factors: older practitioners applying, younger doctors not having the skills of their earlier counterparts, skills generally taking longer to acquire, and more ability being expected of ANARE doctors. This factor of increased ability has been brought about by community expectations over the past decade: ANARE must no longer have primitive equipment or only simple techniques. There has been a dramatic change in the work value of Antarctic doctors; the complexity of operations adds to the pressures on the isolated doctor in his decision-making and deters many potential recruits.

Examination of the practice distribution demonstrates poor recruiting for wintering groups from general practice and specialist categories. It is practitioners from these that have the best skills and experience for ANARE. Figure 5 shows that 58% of medical officers come from 30% of the Australian medical work force--the salaried. As this category includes top-salaried administrators who often lack clinical skills, and junior residents who in recent years are not being recruited because of decreasing practical skills, the small pool of potential first class practitioners is clearly shown. The high number of specialists on summer ANARE reflects the influence the 12 to 15 month winter term has on recruiting: many are prepared to go for short periods only.

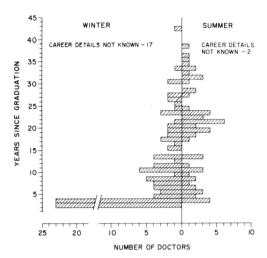

Figure 4. Distribution by years since graduation of doctors recruited by ANARE.

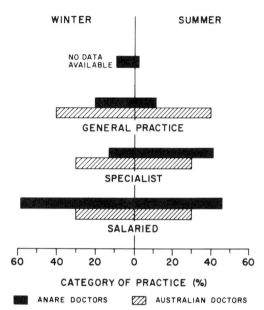

Figure 5. Distribution by practice category of all Australian doctors and of those recruited for ANARE.

The most positive factor in recent recruitment has been the employment of women doctors for ANARE. Since 1976 when the first female surgeon wintered, 21% of wintering doctors have been women. This initiative of the Medical Branch has provided a great boost but it is doubtful if it can be improved upon.

In reviewing medical recruiting a number of practices were questioned. The policy of "no doctor means no expedition" has existed for many years, and has been agreed to by successive ministers; public statements have reflected this. It is considered that in our operations paramedical care is no substitute for well-trained doctors, so while the stations remain inaccessible for most of the year and families and expeditioners expect a medical service which meets Australian standards, no change is foreseen. Practices of some Antarctic nations in not wintering a doctor have been carefully assessed and taken into account.

Medical advertising and public relations are considered excellent by review groups from outside the Antarctic Division. Great care and attention is paid to recruiting through personal contact, lecture tours, press, radio, TV, documentaries, posters, exhibitions at conferences, and articles, reports and scientific papers.

Current selection criteria for ANARE include registration in Australia, several years' postgraduate experience with desirable surgical skills: emergency appendectomy, laparotomy, craniotomy, splenectomy, oversewing of a perforated ulcer, enucleation of an eye and tracheostomy. Experience in occupational, industrial and public

health, and operational research is desirable. As a higher rate of appendicitis exists on ANARE than is found in Australia (3), a prophylactic appendectomy is mandatory for medical officers. All of the above practices are endorsed by experts.

Table 2 lists a number of factors identified as having a negative influence on recruiting. Some of these, such as the small pool of potentially satisfactory doctors, cannot be remedied overnight. Other factors, however, would not be hard to change. Conditions of service, which include an anomalous salary structure that pays more to salaried practitioners in Australian cities and remote areas than Antarctica are in this category. A change here would also counter the better conditions given to doctors for foreign service. Long and bitter industrial cases over salaries have been fought in the Australian Conciliation and Arbitration Commission. These battles cause adverse publicity and obstacles to successful recruitment. Cases of ANARE doctors having difficulty regaining employment or losing their practices because of poor *locum tenens* or financial problems, have also provided poor publicity.

The current practice of allowing doctors one month in Australia at the conclusion of their terms in Antarctica to complete studies is unrealistic and does not make the best use of the excellent opportunities for human biological studies. Further, this deters the polar-oriented

Table 2. Factors having negative influence on recruiting for ANARE.

Availability of doctors with skills to cope with breadth and isolation of practice
Conditions of employment
Adverse publicity
Failure to utilize medical research potential
Competition from commercial agencies recruiting for foreign service
Lack of medical care for doctors becoming ill
Isolation from families, colleagues and continuing medical education

medical practitioner who has research ability in addition to clinical skills.

The negative influence of the professional isolation could be alleviated by the provision of two doctor teams which would also provide a better health care service including that to the doctors themselves. The health problems a doctor may suffer are real: cases of appendicitis (before prophylactic appendectomy was mandatory), acute abdomen, amebiasis, and severe frostbite of the hands.

A review of the medical area of the Antarctic Division was concluded three months ago, many years after its initiation was publicly announced. Present indications are that it may suffer the fate of many other reviews and not improve recruiting. Over the last 16 years a plethora of reports and representations have been made with no resolution of the recruitment problems. The survey reported in this paper has identified some factors, removal of which might assist ANARE medical staffing. However, special and significant steps are needed to ensure recruitment and to support adequately polar medical practice if all services to future expeditions are to remain acceptable and be maintained with any degree of certainty.

REFERENCES

1. Anonymous. New report shows serious worsening of oversupply. Med Prac 1983; 12:8-9.
2. Lugg DJ. Australian medical services in Antarctica. In: Harvald B, Hart Hansen JP, eds. Circumpolar Health 81. Nordic Council for Arct Med Res Rep 1982. 33:71-3.
3. Lugg DJ. Appendicitis in polar regions. Thesis, Cambridge, England: University of Cambridge, 1973.

D.J. Lugg
Antarctic Division
Department of Science and Technology
Kingston, Tasmania 7150
Australia

Circumpolar Health 84:402-405

TRAVELLING PHYSICIANS IN NORTHERN CANADA

PETER SARSFIELD and KATHRYN A. WOTTON

Physicians who travel from community to community continue to play an important role in health care delivery in northern Canada. In some areas the physicians are hospital-based, visiting the remote communities from "outside" on a regular basis. This is the pattern of service, for example, from Inuvik, Northwest Territories (N.W.T.) to the Mackenzie Delta region; from Frobisher Bay, N.W.T., to the Baffin Island communities; from Churchill, Manitoba, to part of the Keewatin Region of the N.W.T.; from Moose Factory, Ontario, to the James Bay region; and from Sioux Lookout, Ontario, to northwestern Ontario. Travelling to the remote communities in all of these practices is the shared responsibility of several physicians.

In a few areas the physicians reside in small and isolated communities and travel regularly to other villages in the same area. Examples of these practices are Nain in northern Labrador (1,6), Cartwright in southern Labrador (2), Cambridge Bay in the Kitikmeot (Central Arctic) Region of the N.W.T., Fort Simpson in the lower Mackenzie region of the N.W.T., and Rankin Inlet in the Keewatin Region of the N.W.T.

In most of these practices the travelling physicians provide support and consultant services to the nurse practitioners who are the primary care providers, the "general practitioner," in the remote communities (3). Local non-professional health workers also provide a vital part of the service (4,5).

These travelling positions have practical, historical, and philosophical origins, including increasing population and political voice in remote areas, an increasing recognition of the right of all Canadians to have "reasonable access" to a physician, a recognition of the need for nurse practitioners to have more immediate physician support, a recognition that health workers do not deliver health but are a vital part of any adequate health care service, and concomitantly the willingness of some physicians to live and work in remote areas and become involved in community health problems.

METHODS

There are very few data available documenting the activities of travelling physicians, making the questions of cost-effectiveness, travel time, numbers of patients seen, clinical problems dealt with, and community health-related activity all relative unknowns.

We have individually worked as travelling physicians in northern Labrador, southern Labrador, northern Manitoba, and the Keewatin and Kitikmeot Regions of the N.W.T. In our practices daily records of physician work have been kept. These included information on each patient seen, on the frequency and method of travel, telephone consultations, and health education activities. Another paper in these Proceedings (Sarsfield, following paper) deals with the data collected in some of these practices. This paper will discuss the foundations and implications of such practices.

Health Services

A major demand of these positions lies in the frequency and difficulty of travel, a challenge accentuated by the absence of roads and the varying reliability of air transport. There is considerable variation across the north of Canada in the frequency of visits made to the remote communities by travelling physicians, ranging from weekly to every several months, with the average being one visit each month. For example, travel by the physicians in north and south Labrador and in the Kitikmeot Region of the N.W.T. led to their being away from the home community about half the time, visiting each village every four to six weeks. About 15% of physician work time in these practices is spent en route from community to community. The average length of stay was 48 to 72 hours in the places with nursing stations.

Public health/preventive medicine is the most difficult, and over the long run the most influential to the health of the community, of the various roles that a travelling physician must fill (7,8). The very fact that the job is a mobile one prevents rapid development of an adequate knowledge of the communities' health needs unless the physician is willing to stay at least two years in the area and spend considerable time in each community talking with local councils, doing home visits, investigating water/sewage/garbage options, visiting schools, and continually acting as a resource for the community as well as for the nursing station staff. Visits made by physicians to remote communities which do not include attempts to influence the overall health of the community are incomplete (9).

Clinical work is the part of the travelling physician's job which is the most visible, and often the dominant one (10), taking from 50% to 60% of the physician's time in the Labrador and Kitikmeot practices. Although this is often a "loss leader," because nurse practitioners handle most cases of primary patient care as capably as physicians (11,12), the public and the nurses feel more secure in their medical interactions if a physician is available. Occasionally in person and always by telephone, physicians serve to offer advice and support. For a minority of cases the physician input is crucial. The line between cases which can be handled competently by nurse practitioners and those which need a physician's input is unfortunately an indistinct and shifting one, varying from community to community, practitioner to practitioner, and even fluctuating with the time of day, the season of the year, and the availability of transport. In Canada the training of nurse practitioners is still primarily done by the apprenticeship (on-the-job) method, with the exception of the Outpost Nursing courses at Dalhousie University, Halifax, Nova Scotia, and Memorial University, St. John's, Newfoundland. The result is that the clinical community health abilities of the nurses practicing in remote areas vary widely. This varying and fluctuating capability of the local practitioners can only be defined and managed by the travelling physician to the benefit of the communities if she/he stays in the area for years.

The clinical portion of the visits should have a predictable style and content. Scheduling of the clinic should allow adequate time and privacy for contact with each patient. At least 15 minutes per patient, not interrupted by phones and other staff, and preferably with one of the referring nurses present, is ideal. The physician should primarily see referrals from nurse practitioners. If the communities have the impression that they are receiving second-rate care when the physician is not in town, resulting in a "saving up" of problems by the local population for the next physician visit, then either the community needs to be educated regarding the realities of the nurses' skills, and/or the nurses' training and capabilities need to be increased. Often talks with local representatives will relieve some of the concerns, especially when the formal and apprentice training of the nurses is spelled out.

From 15% to 20% of the travelling physician's time is spent in telephone and radio-telephone consultations with nurse practitioners and hospital consultants, a time-consuming and important part of the service.

Chart reviews and careful (legible) documentation of each patient contact are essential parts of the job. Detailed records, including possible alternative approaches, are necessary.

Home visits should be part of every trip, as there is no other way to glimpse the social reality of a community. These visits are usually appreciated by the recipients, and often much worthwhile clinical work also results.

Chronic and rehabilitative care should not be overlooked, as the "tyranny of the acute" is all too real. In Canada these services are almost exclusively concentrated in urban areas, with government showing resistance to permanent or even transient extension to remote areas of such disciplines as physiotherapy, occupational therapy, speech therapy, prosthetics, or nursing homes. It is part of the travelling physician's responsibility to support the community councils and nurse practitioners in petitioning the relevant authorities to provide these services to remote areas.

The obvious must not go unnoticed, or allowed to be ignored. Interpreters are needed for those health workers who cannot speak the language of the clients. The cultural norms and expectations of the communities must be recognized and respected, even on those rare occasions when they are to be opposed by the practitioners. A willingness to learn from the local people is an essential attitude of any appropriate northern medical practitioner.

Health Education

There are many opportunities for the travelling physician to offer an educational service to health workers and the public. Provision of an "in-service" to the staff can be a routine part of the physician's visit, and this should include all support staff, such as interpreters, aides and community health representatives, as well as nurses. Relevant journal material can be sent to the stations on a regular basis. Visits to schools, community councils, day-care centers and alcohol control groups can all also offer a unique forum for influencing the public's view of illness and health.

Many universities send medical students, nursing students, interns, and residents to remote practice locations. Providing these practitioners-in-training are adequately stimulated, supervised, and supported by the local practitioners, the experience can be invaluable for them, fostering an awareness of the potential, resources, and problems of remote communities, and occasionally stimulating an interest in working in such a practice in the future. The trainees also inevitably stimulate and challenge the local practitioners, introducing new ideas and offering alternative approaches to recurrent problems.

Research

The need for research relevant to the needs and problems of remote communities is obvious, but the methods, priorities, and controls to be imposed on northern research are far from obvious (13,14). Studies relating to land use, wildlife management, waste disposal, energy options, water availability, violence, and alcohol abuse, as examples, are considered very relevant by most northern residents but are apparently often considered to be either too broad and nebulous, or too mundane and pragmatic, for many urban researchers who concentrate instead on topics which are more easily definable, but are often also more esoteric and less useful. In research, as in so many other aspects of northern health care, if the local people are to obtain maximum benefit from the service offered they must control the structure and function of the service, often to a degree and in a manner which might not be appropriate, or necessary, in other areas.

Administration

Service provision, and educational and research activities, all have administrative components. Administrators and practitioners both frequently attempt to negate or minimize the necessity for, and worth of, administrative input by local practitioners. In both cases, it is a shirking of responsibility, on one hand due to elitism and a fear of loss of "power," on the other due to an unfamiliarity with administrative procedure and the odd conceit that only clinical efforts can affect health. Administrative input by local practitioners, including travelling physicians, is essential.

Problems and Challenges

Problems do exist, and often appear to be insurmountable. The level of health in many remote areas of Canada is grim, especially in communities of indigenous peoples (15-19) and is only changing in type of problems present, not the frequency or severity of problems (20,21). Although "local control" has been advocated for years as a necessary prerequisite to improvement in health in remote areas (22-28), ethnocentric caution and vested-interest decisions (i.e. fear of local control in health care being a step toward control of land and resources) have kept any significant decision-making power out of the hands of local people.

Perhaps the greatest challenge for the travelling physician lies in attempting to encourage and support self-care and local control initiatives. It will be these initiatives, combined with the necessary

political and socioeconomic changes, and not the clinical efforts of health workers, which will be the main determinants of change in community health (29,30). Skilled medical care, however, can and should assist those changes which will promote people-centered health care.

As an influential health care advocate for the community it is crucial that the physician attempt to influence policy and budget priorities relating to health in the area, as these decisions are frequently made in distant "centers," often by administrators who have little understanding of the needs of remote communities. In spite of the fact that the physician is a salaried government employee, she or he should function as a health care advocate for the communities and not as someone whose primary responsibility is to government. This is occasionally a source of conflict between the physician and the bureaucracy.

Difficulties in funding "unorthodox" programs in remote areas which have little political strength, in maintaining public confidence in nurse practitioners and lay dispensers in the face of a powerful North American physician image, and in attracting staff to areas where urban "comforts" and options are not available, make the service fragile and often erratic. The greatest needs in the present provision of remote health care are for local control, for provision of professional service in a credible and locally acceptable way, and for practitioner and public flexibility during the inevitable awkward moments inherent in such a setting. Even if unlimited financial resources were available, and they obviously are not, the urban medical model simply would not provide adequate care and would not promote health. Innovation, administrative flexibility, and a willingness to encourage local control of the service all allow for appropriate approaches to diagnosis, therapy, and health worker utilization. The travelling physician service can be one of these approaches.

This paper is not intended to represent the policies or opinions of any government or government department.

ACKNOWLEDGMENTS

Both of us owe much to Jack Hildes, whose intelligence, caustic wit, scientific vision, and unyielding commitment to remote areas and indigenous peoples have provided guidance on many occasions.

REFERENCES

1. Wotton KA. Mental health of the native people of Labrador. Presented to the Canadian Mental Health Assoc., St. John's, Newfoundland, August, 1983.

2. Sarsfield P. Travelling physician in Labrador. Presented at the 5th International Symposium on Circumpolar Health, Copenhagen, Denmark, August, 1981.

3. Rumbolt I, Trees R. Primary health care in Port Hope Simpson, Labrador, Canada, 1970-1979. In: Harvald B, Hart Hansen JP, eds. Circumpolar Health 81. Nordic Council for Arct Med Res Rep 1982; 33:106-109.

4. Sarsfield P. Health care without health professionals: One option. In: Harvald B, Hart Hansen JP, eds. Circumpolar Health 81. Nordic Council for Arct Med Res Rep 1982; 33:103-105.

5. Hessler R, Griffard C. Community health paraprofessional: the occupation of not quite. Inquiry 1976; 13.

6. Columbus K. A study of the health issues of the Labrador Inuit. Privately published report for Labrador Inuit Association, Nain, Labrador, Newfoundland, 1982.

7. Black LM. Health care delivery in the Arctic. In: Harvald B, Hart Hansen JP, eds. Circumpolar Health 81. Nordic Council for Arct Med Res Rep 1982; 33:77-79.

8. Mahler H. The meaning of "Health for All by the Year 2000"... Geneva: WHO, 1979.

9. Van Der Minne D. Indian health: The profession can help. Brit Columbia Med J 1975; 17(5).

10. Black D. Training physicians to practice in remote Canadian communities. Can Fam Physician 1982; 20(10).

11. Lawrence D. Physician assistants and nurse practitioners: Their impact on health-care access, costs and quality. Health Med Care Serv Rev 1978; 1(2): 1,3-12.

12. Canadian Nurses Association Putting "health" into health care: Submission to health services review, 1979. Ottawa; 1980.

13. Association of Canadian Universities for Northern Studies. Ethical principles for the conduct of research in the north. Ottawa: October 1981.

14. Freeman N. Science and ethics in the North. Arctic 1977; 30:71-75.

15. Report on health conditions in the Northwest Territories. Health and Welfare Canada, Yellowknife, NWT: 1981/1982.

16. Rodgers D. Suicide in the Canadian Northwest Territories: 1970-1980. In: Harvald B, Hart Hansen JP, eds. Circumpolar Health 81. Nordic Council for Arct Med Res Rep 1982; 33:492-495.

17. Young TK. Mortality pattern of isolated Indians in northwestern Ontario: A 10 year review. Public Health Reports 1983; 98:467-474.

18. Spady DW, ed. Between two worlds. Boreal Institute, Occasional Publication 16, Edmonton, Alberta, 1982.

19. Evers SE, Rand CG. Morbidity in Canadian Indian and non-Indian children in the first year of life. Can Med Assoc J 1982; 126:249-252.

20. Seltzer A. Acculturation and mental disorder in the Inuit. Can J Psychiat 1980; 25:173-181.

21. Spady D, et al. The Northwest Territories perinatal and infant mortality and morbidity study: A report to the Government of Canada. Edmonton, Alberta, 1979.

22. Berger TR. Report of advisory commission on Indian and Inuit health consultation. Health and Welfare Canada, Ottawa, 1980.

23. Sarsfield P. Report to the Naskapi Montagnais Innu Association and the Labrador Inuit Association regarding the health care delivery system in northern Labrador. Privately published by NMIA and LIA, Labrador, 1977.

24. Registered nurses of Native ancestry. Towards local Indian health control. Symposium held at Brandon General Hosp, Brandon, Manitoba, November, 1977.

25. Sarsfield P, Andrew B, Rawlyk RP. Local control of health care amongst indigenous peoples. Presented at Annual Conference of Can Public Health Assoc, St John's, Newfoundland, June, 1983.

26. Coombs J. Community supportive health: Rebuilding the total health of Indian communities. Ottawa: National Indian Brotherhood, March, 1979.

27. Bain HW. Community development: An approach to health care for Indians. (Editorial). Can Med Assoc J 1982; 126:223-224.

28. Task Force of Canadian Psychiatric Assoc. Recommendations re Canadian Native peoples' mental health, Native perspective. 1978; 2(8).

29. Nuttall RN. The development of Indian boards of health in Alberta. Can J Public Health 1982; 73:300-303.

30. Globe and Mail. Modern medicine powerless to help natives... Toronto, Ontario, November, 1982.

Peter Sarsfield
Cambridge Bay
Northwest Territories X0E 0C0
Canada

Circumpolar Health 84:406-409

TWO REMOTE CANADIAN MEDICAL PRACTICES

PETER SARSFIELD

Portions of the last five years have been spent in two widely separated remote Canadian travelling physician medical practices: from 1979 to 1981 with a Euro-Canadian population in southern Labrador, and from 1982 to 1984 with a predominantly Inuit population in the Kitikmeot (Central Arctic) Region of the Northwest Territories.

In both practices daily and monthly records were kept. These included information on each patient seen, specifically the age, sex, primary body system leading to the consultation, who initiated the referral (patient, nurse of physician), whether the problem was acute or chronic, the primary diagnosis and therapy offered, and whether further referral occurred. The monthly and annual records also noted the frequency and mode of physician travel, medical long-distance telephone calls made or received, health education activities such as school visits and meetings with community councils, total number of patients seen, days spent in each community, and time spent on administrative duties.

Land

a) Labrador: The south Labrador practice area covers about 400 km of coastline from latitude 52°N to 54°N, with the polar waters of the Labrador Sea and northerly airmasses creating an arctic and sub-arctic climate at a relatively southerly latitude. All of Labrador is part of the granite mass called the Canadian Shield, the glacier-scraped rock surface which in south Labrador has mixed forest inland. Winter lasts from November to April, with midwinter temperatures averaging -15° to -20°C. Annual snowfall averages 450 cm. Break-up of the coastal ice and lakes occurs in late May or June, and the summer lasts from June to late August, with a usually stormy open-water autumn until November.

b) Kitikmeot: This practice covers 1,100 km on the mainland and islands of the Central Arctic, from longitude 67°N to 71°N. There is considerable variation in vegetation over this area, from the tundra of Victoria Island and the Boothia Peninsula, to the dwarf shrubs and grassland of the mainland at Bathurst Inlet. Freeze-up comes in October and lasts until June, with the coldest month average temperature being at about -35°C, and the summer monthly average not going above +10°C. Although snow covers the ground for nine months of the year, the annual snowfall is less than 75 cm.

People

a) Labrador: The people of southern Labrador are called "settlers," a term which symbolizes the history of their British immigrant ancestors having occupied lands previously used by Inuit and Innu (Naskapi/Montagnais) over 200 years ago. Inter-marriage in the 18th and 19th centuries of settlers with Inuit has led to an assimilation of many indigenous skills, but the Innu and Inuit cultures are now entirely displaced to north Labrador. The resulting identity of the south Labrador settlers is distinct from Newfoundlanders as well as from Innu and Inuit.

There are 11 permanent communities in south Labrador: Lodge Bay, Mary's Harbour, Fox Harbour (St. Lewis), Port Hope Simpson, William's Harbour, Pinsent's Arm, Charlottetown, Norman Bay, Black Tickle, Cartwright, and Paradise River, ranging in size from 50 to 800 people, for a total of about 2,500. About one-third of this population seasonally migrates to nearby summer fishing settlements, which are deserted in winter and range in size in summer from one family to over 100 people. The fishery is the economic mainstay of south Labrador, with wage employment, forestry, crafts, and tourism providing an additional minor contribution. This is the most isolated and least "developed" region in eastern Canada, a situation which has resulted in considerable community self-sufficiency and strength.

b) Kitikmeot: Inuit make up over 90% of the 3,500 people living in the central arctic communities of Holman Island, Coppermine, Bay Chimo, Bathurst Inlet, Cambridge Bay, Gjoa Haven, Spence Bay, and Pelly Bay, the people being the Copper and Netsilik Eskimos of European designation. Inukitut is the primary language in most of the communities, and hunting and fishing are the major Inuit occupations, with caribou, char, seal, and muskoxen being plentiful. Trapping, such as for fox and wolf, is a source of income, as are the few salaried occupations, craft and art production, and the minimal summer tourism. There is little "development" in the region. The population is young and rapidly growing, with the 1980 census showing Kitikmeot having 13% of its population between age 0 and 4, 27% between 5 and 14, 56% between 15 and 64, and only 4% over age 65.

Communication and Transportation

a) Labrador: Telephones are now present in all communities, although they are unreliable and occasionally lack privacy. A Radio-Telephone (RT) link-up is available at police and medical facilities, and radio and television are now available to most of the communities. There are no roads from this region to "outside" so all transportation to or from south Labrador in winter is by single and twin-engine bush planes to Goose Bay in central Labrador and to St. Anthony in northern Newfoundland. Travel by snowmobile is frequent within the region from December to May. In summer, coastal freighter and passenger ships provide occasional travel options both on the coast and to Goose Bay or Newfoundland.

b) Kitikmeot: This region of the Arctic is the least served by transportation and communication facilities. Telephones are frequently "out" for lengthy periods, as the equipment is not on the satellite link provided to most of the rest of the Canadian Arctic. RT is not utilized by government agencies, but Citizen Band (CB) radios are used extensively by the public. Radio and television are available to most communities.

Transportation is almost exclusively by aircraft, with occasional inter-community snowmobile trips. There is jet service from Edmonton to Cambridge Bay twice a week, with the rest of the communities being served from Yellowknife by DC-3 scheduled runs which provide an expensive, unreliable, and slow service. There is also one private twin-engine charter aircraft operating from Cambridge Bay.

Medical Services

a) Labrador: All service is provided by Newfoundland's Grenfell Regional Health Services Board (GRHS), which in 1981 took over from the International Grenfell Association, a private health service with a philanthropic missionary origin which had provided medical care to northern Newfoundland and all of Labrador since early in this century, at least 40 years before the Government of Canada provided the same service to the Arctic. The Grenfell Board has its administrative and medical headquarters in St. Anthony, Newfoundland. Seven of the 11 communities in south Labrador have nursing stations staffed by nurse practitioners who are the primary care providers, having full "physician" privileges of diagnosis, treatment, and referral. Four communities have lay dispensers. The physician in this nurse-physician team practice lives in the largest community and provides a visiting and telephone consultation service for the nurse practitioners.

The nursing stations provide ambulatory primary-care, including preventive and homecare, and the practitioners also visit the smaller communities and summer settlements on a regular basis. The coastal Labrador and northern Newfoundland region has two hospitals, one small general practice and obstetrics facility in central Labrador and a 200 bed consultant-care hospital in northern Newfoundland, with the

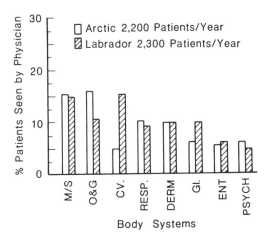

Figure 1. Morbidity patterns of patients seen by physician in southern Labrador, 1979-80 and Kitikmeot, 1983.

nearest tertiary-care facility being 1,000 km or 600 miles away, in St. John's, Newfoundland.

From the 1950s until 1979 all physician travel to the Labrador coastal communities originated from the hospitals, but in the 1980s physicians were again placed in residence in north and south Labrador. Subsequently, the villages with nursing stations were visited every 6 to 8 weeks, and the remaining communities every 8 to 10 weeks. The average length of stay was 48 hours, with occasional longer stays due to weather.

About 2,300 people were seen by the physician in patient contact each year from 1979 to 1981, of which 22% were children (age 16 and under), 31% adult males and 47% adult females. The main body systems involved were: cardiovascular (CV) 16%, indicating the high incidence of hypertension and coronary artery disease in the area, musculoskeletal (M/S) 15%, which reflects the strenuous nature of daily life, dermatology 10%, gastrointestinal (GI) 10%, respiratory 9%, gynecology 8%, ear nose and throat (ENT) 7%, psychiatry 5%, and obstetrics only 4%, as most babies are born in the referral hospitals (Figure 1). Of the patients seen by the physician, 9% were referred to a hospital. The acute/chronic status showed that 42% of the patients had acute illness, 32% chronic and stable illness, 17% an acute flare-up of a chronic problem, and 9% had no illness. It should be emphasized that this is a referral practice, with 78% of all patient contact by the physician being referred by nurse practitioners, 20% client-referred, and 2% physician-referred (Figure 2).

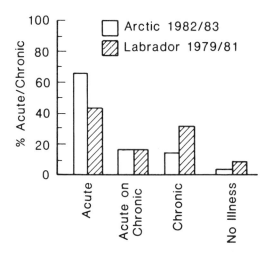

Figure 2. Acute/chronic status patients seen by physician in Labrador and Central Arctic.

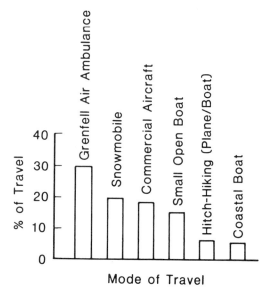

Figure 3. Travel options of physicians in southern Labrador, 1980.

The greatest demand of the south Labrador position lies in the frequency and difficulty of travel, accentuated by the absence of roads and scarcity of airstrips in the area. The health service utilizes single-engine air ambulances, on floats in summer and skis in winter, for patients and staff transport. There is also a small-plane commercial airline which flies three days a week "weather permitting," and coastal passenger ships from June to November. "Hitchhiking" opportunities exist via helicopters and freight boats, and snowmobile travel is utilized extensively in winter along the coast. Travel by the physician from one community to another occurred on an average of 144 days per year, by plane or helicopter 50% of the time, by boat 30% and by snowmobile 20% (Figure 3). Travel was cancelled due to weather about 30 days per year. While communities in both north and south Labrador are requesting more "local control" of health care, the province's responses are explicit in rejecting such options. The Grenfell Board persists in administering the entire area from northern Newfoundland to northern Labrador as one region, ignoring the vastly different cultural and medical needs of the people. The region of south Labrador does not face overt provincial or Grenfell opposition to its health care wishes in most instances, especially if the people accept the service offered without attempting to alter it.

b) Kitikmeot: All medical service is sponsored by the Canadian Government's Department of Health and Welfare, which directly operates the region's six nursing stations, and also provides funds to the Government of the Northwest Territories for

a resident physician and visiting consultants. Federal medical administrative headquarters for the Northwest Territories is in Yellowknife, which is also the main referral center for the Central Arctic, with several consultants and general practitioners working out of a small hospital. More complicated referrals go to Edmonton, a culturally and physically distant option. As in south Labrador, the physician lives in the largest community and is a consultant to the nurse practitioner.

This practice also involves considerable time spent in travel, which is complicated by the distances involved, the harsh climate, and the slow and unreliable air transportation service. The physician travelled on an average of 84 days a year, by scheduled flights 65% of the time and by charter 35%. An average of 119 days per year were spent away from the home community, not including holiday and study leave when locums were available. As in Labrador, this is primarily a referral practice, with nurses referring 76% of all patients seen, the remainder being self-referred. Although the population of the region is over 90% Inuit, only 77% of the people seen by the physician were Inuit. Nine percent of patients were referred to Yellowknife, and 2% were referred to Edmonton.

About 2,200 people were seen in patient contact each year, of which 24% were children, 29% adult males and 47% adult females. The main body systems involved were: obstetrics and gynecology 17%, reflecting the high birth rate in a young population, musculo-

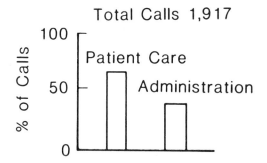

Figure 4. *Long distance health care tele-*
phone calls to and from physician
in the Kitikmeot Region, N.W.T.,
1983.

skeletal 16%, respiratory 11%, showing the
effects of endemic smoking and frequent
infections, dermatology 10%, gastrointestinal 7%, psychiatry 7%, ear nose and throat
6%, and cardiovascular 5%. Sixty-five
percent of the patients seen had an acute
illness, 15% chronic and stable illness, 17%
an acute-on-chronic problem, and 4% had no
illness. As in Labrador, about 25% of the
physician's time is spent in telephone
consultations with nurses and consultants.
An annual average of 1,900 long-distance
calls were made or received, 37% dealing
with administration, while 63% concerned
patient care (Figure 4).

An attempt is made by federal administrators to promote "consultation" with the
public, but much of this is merely rhetoric,
with little potential of actually changing
the service. At this time any local input
is provided by purely advisory and unfunded
health committees in some communities, as
well as by community councils and practitioners prodding government to increase the
level of commitment to the area. Although
more staff, increased numbers and different
types of health care programs, and improved
equipment are all needed, these are unlikely
to alter significantly the level of health
in the region. The main need now is for
local control of the service so as to make
it more relevant and responsive to local
needs.

CONCLUSION

While these practices are dissimilar in
their location, population profile, patterns
of ill-health, cultural pressures, and
medical service administrations, they do
share common concerns in their distance from
urban Canada, in their reliance on nurse
practitioners for primary care and on family
physicians for most consultations, and in
the need for aircraft evacuation for hospital and specialist care. They also share
the experience of the reluctance of government, in one case provincial and in the
other federal, to permit local supervision
of health care. The result in both cases is
a sustained and courageous effort at the
nursing station and community level, but
this effort is consistently hampered by
erratic transportation and communication
options, as well as by distant and culturally inappropriate referral facilities. It is
also often made irrelevant and occasionally
offensive by the striking absence of local
input to the service.

The overall result of a comparison of
these practices is that while there are
several obvious and important differences,
the similarities are more striking and also
more influential in determining the type and
efficacy of medical care offered to the
communities.

This paper does not intend to represent
the policies or opinions of any government
or government department.

ACKNOWLEDGMENTS

The nurses in both of these practices
have provided frequent support, stimulation
and guidance. The main debt of gratitude is
to the people of south Labrador and the
Kitikmeot for their kind and patient education of those providing medical care.

Peter Sarsfield
Cambridge Bay
Northwest Territories X0E 0C0
Canada

Circumpolar Health 84:410-413

PERFORMANCE OF DENTISTS WORKING WITH THE GRENFELL REGIONAL HEALTH SERVICES: PRODUCTIVITY AND SERVICES

JAMES G. MESSER

Since the early 1960s many isolated northern Canadian communities have depended on the services of travelling dentists. Since that time there have been many innovations within the primary delivery system and supporting facilities.

Grenfell Regional Health Services has remained with the travelling dentist concept for the small isolated communities within its area. Over the last 13 years, however, there have been many changes in equipment, facilities, and support staff, as well as a reduction in the number of communities covered by each dentist. The purpose of this study was to find out if treatment patterns have also changed.

There is little information in the literature concerning work output and work patterns of dentists. In 1982, however, a study of general dental services in the United Kingdom by Robertson and McKendrick (1) demonstrated that about 39% of income is derived from fillings and crown and root treatments whereas only 15% of income is from dentures and extractions. They also noted that only 10% of patients had radiographs taken and although orthodontic treatment was undertaken by 66% of the dentists, the median number of cases was one.

In a study of changes in dental treatment patterns in Norway in the 1970s Helöe (2) noted that fillings made up 55% of the treatment over the entire period from 1973 to 1977. Preventive services increased from 15% to 26% over the same period, while the percentage of dentures and extractions diminished from 34% in 1973 to 26% in 1977. It seemed that people increasingly sought dental treatment as facilities improved in rural areas.

METHODS

The monthly returns of 30 dentists over the period from 1977 to 1983 were analyzed to establish a division norm. Twenty-one of the dentists worked in permanently located dental clinics at health centers and hospitals while nine were located at bases with peripheral travelling clinics, four from the 1968 to 1977 period and five from the period 1978 to 1983.

The dentists in this study worked in small communities located on the northeastern and southern coasts of Labrador (Figure 1). These communities have no road connections with their base clinics and access is by bush aircraft and snowmobiles in winter and boats in summer.

The policy of the dental division is that travelling dentists should spend half of their working days at the travelling clinics. During this study only 37% of time was at the travelling clinics and 53% of time was spent at base. Adverse weather or transportation difficulties accounted for the remaining 10%.

In this study an item of treatment recorded on the dentist's monthly return was classified as a unit of work. The returns were tabulated in the major dental treatment groups.

The method of determining actual items of treatment such as a filling, extraction, denture insertion, root canal filling, or orthodontic appliance fitting were consistently applied throughout the period of the study. Intermediate procedures such as dressings, suture removal, or adjustments of appliances were regarded as miscellaneous procedures and were not included in this study.

RESULTS

Table 1 presents the work output in treatment groups for the Grenfell Regional Health Services Dental Division from 1977 to 1983 and for the travelling dentists both at their base clinics and travelling clinics for the periods 1968 to 1977 and 1978 to 1983. The following points arise from the data:

1) Travelling dentists in both the pre-1978 and post-1978 periods are slightly less productive than the norm, the average units of work per day being 14.5 and 15.0 compared to 16.1.

2) Both groups of travelling dentists are more productive at their travelling clinics than at their bases.

3) There are noticeable differences in the proportion of work in each discipline. The unassisted travelling dentists using portable equipment from 1968 to 1977 demonstrate a greater tendency towards extractions, dentures, and examinations compared to the 1978-83 group, who did fewer extractions and dentures and more fillings.

4) In both travelling groups there are fewer items of treatment in the preventive, endodontic, and orthodontic categories than the norm.

5) The number of dental examinations carried out is higher for travelling dentists, especially at the travelling clinics.

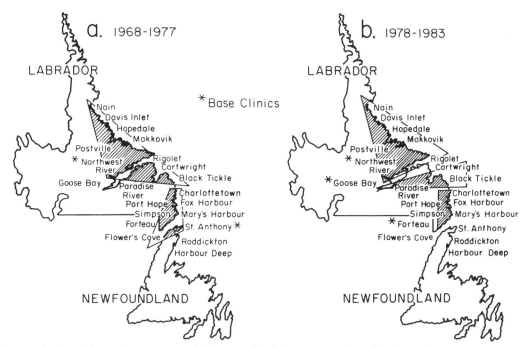

Figure 1. Location of the communities serviced by travelling dentists in 1968-1977 and 1978-1983, and the area covered by the Grenfell Regional Health Service Dental Division in 1977-1983.

Table 1. Average annual work output in major dental disciplines. Travelling dentists from 1968 to 1977 and from 1977 to 1983 compared with the Grenfell Regional Health Service Dental Division norm from 1977 to 1983.

	N=30 1977-1983 Dental Division norm	Travelling dentists					
		N=4 1968-1977			N=5 1978-1983		
		Base	Travel clinic	Total	Base	Travel clinic	Total
Patient visits	2660	776	1354	2130	1088	1193	2281
Units of work							
Examinations	759	302	667	969	424	1193	913
Radiographs	256	71	0	71	112	31	143
Extractions	1096	575	1024	1599	590	552	1141
Fillings	1167	220	277	497	574	477	1021
Prevention	259	57	63	120	62	93	155
Orthodontics	50	7	4	11	5	2	7
Prosthetics	80	24	59	83	30	45	75
Endodontics	57	12	5	17	22	7	29
Total units	3724	1268	2099	3367	1819	1695	3484
Av. units/day	16.2			14.6			15.1

Figure 2 illustrates treatment patterns for the Grenfell Regional Health Services Dental Division as a whole and the travelling dentist in the 1968-77 and 1977-83 groups. The patterns are expressed as a percent of total time. The items of work were time-weighted in order to present a more realistic comparison. The time-weighting is based on the Newfoundland Dental Association Fee Guide in which each item of treatment is awarded a time value. From this time analysis the following points emerge:

1) The pattern for the 1978-83 group of travelling dentists is more in line with the Grenfell Regional Health Services norm than the 1968-77 group.

2) There is a noticeably higher proportion of time spent doing examinations at the travelling clinics.

3) In the 1968-77 period, 31% of time at travelling clinics was used for extractions, while fillings only accounted for 15% of the time. In the 1978-83 period this ratio was reversed, with 29% of time being used for fillings and only 20% for extractions.

4) The treatment pattern at the base clinics in 1978 to 1983 is similar to the norm; however, orthodontic treatments and prevention are lower, a pattern also seen at the travelling clinics.

5) Other differences are less significant and may simply reflect a dentist's preferences or patient demand.

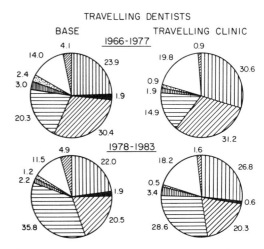

Figure 2. Treatment patterns expressed as a percentage of total time per work year. A comparison between the patterns of travelling dentists at their bases, travelling clinics and the Dental Division average.

DISCUSSION

From the results presented in Table 1 and Figure 2 it is obvious that the emphasis has changed from an emergency service (extractions and dentures) to a more restorative oriented service at the travelling clinics. Much of this could be attributed to improved equipment and the use of assistants, as recommended by McPhail (3). It may also be influenced by changes in patient demand and dentist's preferences. In general the trend agrees with some of the findings in the Norwegian study (2). Preventive services appear to be much lower in this study and may be due to the method of collecting the data.

The high proportion of examinations by travelling dentists is more difficult to interpret. It may be a result of a more frequent turnover in staff, who feel a need to examine patients prior to commencing a course of treatment. Treatment plans at travelling clinics are frequently not completed during the tenure of each dentist.

It is this author's experience that dentists working in the travelling areas can find it a frustrating experience. Professional and social isolation as well as cultural differences were discussed by Bedford (4), who advocated a need for careful assessment by all prospective dentists prior to working in northern clinics. He pointed out that not every dentist is suited to this type of work, although for some it can be a very rewarding experience.

It is also noteworthy that with the exception of denture services, patients are less likely to receive treatment requiring multiple visits. Orthodontic and endodontic treatment make up a very small proportion of treatment time at travelling clinics. This finding may reflect a reluctance to under take these forms of treatment when follow-up can be difficult. The reduction in the number of clinics covered by the travelling dentists does not appear to have significantly improved this situation so far, but, it is expected that more frequent visits in future will make it easier to provide such services. It could also be that fewer orthodontic and endodontic treatments at travelling clinics merely reflect a less educated demand. Another more likely explanation is simply the poor socioeconomic circumstances prevailing in the communities involved in this study, although this does not explain the low demand from children covered under the government program.

CONCLUSION AND SUMMARY

The conclusions to be drawn from this study are that improvements in facilities and backup assistance do influence treatment patterns. The earlier emphasis on extractions and dentures has been modified and restorative treatment has greatly increased. There are many other factors involved however, and it would be unwise to conclude that only these factors have influenced the change.

By using the treatment items as units of work it is noticeable that productivity has not significantly changed over the period. Nevertheless, the changes in treatment patterns show a significant move towards restorative treatment such as fillings, which normally require more time and skill than simple extractions. This shift could be interpreted as an increase in productivity.

This study does show that treatment patterns are changing and that the travelling clinics are showing a move towards the patterns observed for the whole Dental Division. It also indicates that the inhabitants of the small isolated communities covered by travelling dentists are gradually being given the opportunity to seek comprehensive dental care at a level similar to that of their more urbanized neighbors.

REFERENCES

1. Robertson BK, McKendrik AJW. Work output patterns of general service dentists. Brit Dent J 1982; 153: 227-232.
2. Helöe LA. Changes of dental treatment pattern in Norway in the 1970's. Community Dent Oral Epidemiol 1978; 6: 53-56.
3. McPhail CWB, Curry TM, Hazelton RD, Paynter KJ, Williamson RG. The geographic pathology of dental disease in the Canadian arctic population. J Canad Dent Assn 1972; 8: 288-296.
4. Bedford WR. In the news: Look before you leap. J Canad Dent Assn 1982; 2: 96-97.

James G. Messer
Dental Services
Grenfell Regional Health Services
St. Anthony, Newfoundland A0K 4S0
Canada

Circumpolar Health 84:414-415

HEALTH CARE EVALUATION IN A REMOTE SETTING

CHRIS GREENSMITH, JOSEPH DOOLEY, JUDE RODRIGUES and H. HODES

In recent years medical audit or peer review has become a fact of life in medical practice in North America. For example, in Canada the Canadian Council on Hospital Accreditation assesses the performance of individual institutions against preset standards (1). Similarly, within the Province of Manitoba the College of Physicians and Surgeons has a system of health care quality review for all physicians working in the province.

In Canada, responsibility for the provision of health care to Native peoples rests with the Federal Government. This responsibility is administered by the Medical Services Branch (MSB) of Health and Welfare Canada. In Manitoba, the Medical Services Branch contracts with the Northern Medical Unit (NMU) of the University of Manitoba for the recruitment and retention of physicians to several locations throughout the province. The NMU, in providing physician and consultant services, has always taken a strong academic interest in the health care of Native people.

Although there is a system of medical audit at each of the three hospital locations for which the NMU provides physicians, remote communities served only by nursing stations and travelling physicians have not received any attention.

During the summer of 1982 the NMU and the South Zone of the Manitoba Region agreed to develop and test a system of health care quality review for remote nursing stations.

Academic concerns aside, there are practical reasons for establishing an ongoing system of health care review. Although MSB has clear policies and protocols for dealing with almost every clinical eventuality in the north, our proposal would provide a more systematic method of establishing that these policies were adhered to.

Although some staff may stay at a remote location for one or two years, there is, in general, a fairly rapid turnover of staff. As rapid staff turnover equates with reduced continuity of care, it is in the best interest of each patient that the clinical record is as well documented as possible.

METHODS

Health care evaluation may be attempted by measuring the structure, process, or outcomes of a health care intervention (2). We used process evaluations, as they were easier to establish and are closer to outcomes than structure (3).

A committee was established of NMU and MSB personnel with the following objectives:

1. To develop abstracting forms which would provide a standard against which nursing station health care delivery could be evaluated;
2. To test the feasibility of using these forms in a field setting;
3. To identify problem areas in clinical care so that educational inservice programs could be appropriately directed.

As we began it became obvious that the nurses at the stations were apprehensive of the audit process and were afraid that they would be victimized when the results of the study became available.

This concern was addressed by including the three most senior zone nursing personnel on the audit committee and by the zone administration stating clearly that the outcomes of these studies would be used only to direct educational activities.

The committee decided that there were two clinical areas on which they would like to concentrate initially. These were: 1) antenatal care, and 2) the process of evacuating patients out of the community for treatment.

Abstracting forms for the evaluation of each area were developed based on the established MSB policies and the forms and documents completed by nursing station personnel in recording the management of each patient. For example, the form for the antenatal review was based on the universal antenatal assessment sheet used for all pregnancies in the Province of Manitoba. After several drafts our abstracting forms contained 75 questions which were asked of each antenatal record and 33 of each patient transfer.

In implementing this project two issues concerned with patient confidentiality had to be addressed:

1. The confidentiality of patient files had to be maintained at all times.
2. Patient files consisted of documents needed for the ongoing care of the patient and as such could not be removed from the nursing station.

A team of four reviewers (two NMU staff and two MSB staff) visited each nursing station to collect the data necessary for the project. Transportation and accommodation was provided by the MSB and printing, processing, and analyses were provided by the NMU. If any remedial action was found to be necessary this could only be taken by MSB.

Four nursing stations in eastern Manitoba were chosen for review initially. All stations are relatively remote from Winnipeg, being accessible by aircraft only. The stations are all modern and well-equipped structures with a complement of two or three nurses, depending on community size. A physician visits each community for approximately one week of each month.

RESULTS

Antenatal Audit

Seventy-two pregnancies were reviewed, representing all deliveries in each community during 1982. The age of the patients ranged from 15 to 38 years. Nineteen pregnancies were primiparous, 41 were for the second through fifth pregnancies and 12 were for later than the fifth pregnancy.

The medical history was completed on 75% of charts and we noted that 47% of our sample were smokers. In view of local concerns on the fetal alcohol syndrome, alcohol consumption was of particular interest, yet we found no specific place to record it on the charts.

Clinical assessment of patients was complete on most visits with only occasional slips from the recommended routine. Sixty percent of our sample received six or more antenatal checkups although only 15% received 12 or more visits. This sample was regarded as coming from a high risk population; however, almost 70% of pregnancies were not seen by a physician during the first trimester and although a well established system of antenatal risk assessment by numerical grading was available on every form, it was used only 75% of the time on the first visit and only 15% of the time at 36 weeks.

Two-thirds of all pregnant women received iron and vitamin supplementation, but very few received folic acid even though it was policy that it should be given.

In preparing our study we included several questions on the provision of antenatal classes and postnatal home visiting. On reviewing the charts, however, we discovered that there was no specifically designated part of the patient's chart to record that activity. As a result a directive was issued to staff on how to record such activities and new standardized forms were compiled by MSB.

The outcome of the 72 pregnancies followed was established. Although every attempt was made to have all deliveries take place in obstetric units we found, nevertheless, that six deliveries had occurred at the nursing stations. Of the other deliveries the outcome was found to be normal in 43, abnormal in 13 and not recorded in 10. There were no stillbirths but there were three congenital abnormalities.

Evacuation Audit

A representative sample of 100 charts were examined from the communities visited. All transfer documents were completed by the station nursing staff, although they themselves initiated only 54% of the transfers. There were several administrative concerns with the process of transferring patients. An adequate medical history was completed for 85% of cases and an appropriate record of the physical assessment was completed in 65%.

Of particular importance in the evacuation audit was that 80% of the time there was no indication of any exchange of information at the time of discharge. In only 15 cases did the discharge summary arrive within six weeks of discharge. In 42 cases it never arrived.

Once our field trips were completed the data we gathered were collated by computer using the Statistical Package for the Social Sciences (SPSS). Results were presented for each individual nursing station and for the group as a whole. All results were returned to MSB and a copy of results for individual nursing stations was returned to that station. MSB considered our results and then drafted and circulated a memo to all nursing stations specifically addressing any deviations from established policy. Proposals for new recording forms were drafted. Nursing supervisory staff provided inservices on any changes on their visits to the stations.

I believe that this project demonstrates that although health care evaluation is difficult and time-consuming, it is possible in a remote setting. Valuable information on policy implementation can be gathered and as a result remedial steps can be taken to ensure a standardized and effective approach to health care delivery in the north.

REFERENCES

1. Standards for the accreditation of Canadian health care facilities. Canadian Council on Hospital Accreditation, Ottawa, Canada, 1983.
2. Donabedian A. Quality of care: some issues in evaluating the quality of nursing care. Am J Public Health 1969; 59:1833-1936.
3. Sacket DL. Evaluation of health services. In: Last JM, ed. Public health and preventive medicine. New York: Appleton-Century-Crofts, 1980: 1815.

Chris Greensmith
Northern Medical Unit
University of Manitoba
61 Emily Street
Winnipeg, Manitoba R3E 1Y9
Canada

SECTION 8.   PROGRESS IN SELF DETERMINATION

Circumpolar Health 84:419-422

OBSERVATIONS ON THE "MEDICALIZATION" OF INUIT SOCIAL LIFE

JOHN D. O'NEIL

This paper should be considered more as a stimulus for discussion than as a fully researched and argued analysis of health service delivery in the Canadian North. This material is based on several years of resident ethnographic field work in a Canadian Inuit village where the general focus of that research was on health and health care services. It also incorporates observations based on a year's residence in an academic research unit where northern health is a major interest. It is not intended as a critical assessment of health care services nor is it intended to allocate responsibility for current problems. Rather, I hope to provoke a critical and reflective discussion of the role that northern medical discourse plays in determining health problems and policy in the Canadian North.

In my training as an anthropologist, I have learned to look for the meaning behind social and verbal behavior. Anthropologists are fond of telling the story behind the words. We often use the notion "thick description" to frame our attempts to understand how human actions and events are symbolically related to a deeper set of cultural premises and values. For example, we describe a particular ceremony or ritual and show how it is the public performance of an integrated set of understandings about role relationships, expectations, and obligations between genders and generations (1). Anthropologists also use a number of related concepts to facilitate this discussion of meaning.

At the level of everyday life, "praxis" is a term which describes the performance of customs, rituals, and other regularly patterned behavior which is infused with meanings drawn from deeper ideological levels of knowledge. "Ideology" refers to forms of knowledge that people depend on for understanding and controlling their life conditions. It is fundamentally embedded in institutional and historical structures and processes (2). And finally, "discourse" refers to organized and rationalized knowledge that is publicly available through a connected series of oral and written communications (3). Often the meaning that the analyst discovers at these various levels is difficult to perceive from the perspective of those involved in its production at either the everyday interactive or the institutional levels. The problem is akin to the ancient cliché of not being able to see the forest for the trees.

With this very brief theoretical framework in mind, I would like to ask the reader to consider a fundamental contradiction in the northern medical discourse. There is a growing perception amongst southern health care providers and other concerned professionals that northern people are over-utilizing health services and are increasingly demanding more technological, bureaucratic, and professional medicine. For many of us, these demands seem the antithesis of the public health, preventive medicine, health education, and community controlled primary care services that many health professionals feel is the direction that northern health services should take. This paper is intended to address this fundamental contradiction in the current northern medical discourse.

In discussions over the past several months with clinicians, consultants, administrators, and researchers, this particular topic has arisen on many occasions. There have been a number of reasons offered to explain this contradiction. One suggestion is that Canadian Inuit, in particular, have experienced a long history of forced evacuation to southern medical institutions for tuberculosis, obstetrical care, etc. Inuit now want northern medical institutions as a safeguard against future epidemics and mass evacuation to the south. A second suggestion is that northern communities involved in regional politics are expressing local self-interest in demanding to have their "own doctor" vis-à-vis other northern communities. A third suggestion has been that Inuit in northern communities have a "soap opera" understanding of southern medicine based on their observations of afternoon hospital-based soap operas which provide the dominant definition of what southern medicine is all about. A fourth suggestion has been that the colonial legacy and history of dealing with the erratic policy of southern institutions has created situations where northern community organizations will attempt any strategy that promises to increase local resources; whether that resource is a physician or a fire truck is immaterial. I think each of these suggestions has a certain degree of validity and when taken together with the argument to be presented here contribute to a better understanding of the contemporary health policy dialogue.

My argument is that when health services are transferred from the south prior to local political developments which would ensure local input into the design and operation of health services, a process is established where Inuit social life comes to be defined in medical terms by health care providers. The "medicalization" of social life and institutionalization of communities is then reflected in the "medicalized expectations" that increasingly characterize Inuit demands in the Canadian North. This argument hinges on a critical observation. When one is working "from the nursing station" in a northern Inuit community or when one looks at the community from the perspective of local nurses, one of the strongest impressions is that every house should have a "chart" hanging beside the front door. The community is analogous to a hospital ward where the nursing station is at one end of the village and the "patients" radiate out from the nursing station. Reflect for a moment on your first impressions when arriving at a nursing station in a northern Canadian community. Often conversations revolve around the health status of different families and good nursing care is defined as the ability to monitor the changing health status of the community.

With this analogy in mind, I would like to address what I feel are some of the reasons behind this impression and more importantly what are its implications for both health care productivity and the decentralization of control over health care services.

Northern medical discourse is consti- tuted in a fundamental way within the internal colonial heritage that characteriz- es the relationship of northern Canada to the nation state. This colonial relation- ship has been described in detail by Robert Paine and Hugh Brody in their excellent work from the mid-1970s (4,5). Paine uses the analogy of the nursery with Native people in the role of children and southern bureau- crats, educators, and other professionals in the role of nannies. He makes a strong argument that northern communities are "wards" of the larger society and that the southern institutional activity is to socialize northern people into the broader societal framework. While Paine's work addresses primarily other administrative and educational structures, I think his analogy is particularly strong in the area of health care. The nursery analogy is also rein- forced by the fact that many early northern nurses in Canada were British trained and in fact did not have public health backgrounds but were instead "ward sisters" with hospi- tal training.

The most fundamental aspect of contem- porary northern medical ideology is that northern Native societies are defined as sick societies. Indeed, the 1984 Circum- polar Health Conference is an excellent example of the way in which this element of the ideology is manifested in the public domain. Most of the papers emerging from the conference state in their first para- graph that morbidity and mortality rates for this or that particular disease are four or

five times the national average. And I would guess that the media reacts by issuing statements that sickness is rampant in northern communities. An important dimen- sion of this sick society discourse is the role that social science has played. The prevailing paradigm borrowed from social science is that sociocultural change produc- es social disintegration which produces a sick society. Finally, the bureaucratic and economic interests of health services and the various research industries are to a certain extent dependent on a perception that Native societies are sick societies. If more sickness can be discovered, more resources are necessary and the future growth of these institutions is assured.

At the community level, there are many processes that occur that contribute to a medicalized understanding of community life. Perhaps unique to the Canadian North is the combination of clinical and community health functions that local health personnel practice in the everyday performance of their health care responsibilities. This combination of functions means that nurses have detailed and intimate knowledge of people's social situations both inside and outside illness episodes. However, because of the clinical nexus of most health care interactions with Inuit, the nurses continue to perceive these people largely in the role of patients. Thus, when called upon to intervene at psychological or social levels, clinical perceptions continue to influence attitudes. At the same time, nurses often have community-based information available to them clinically that patients may not have provided. Particularly with the use of interpreters, nurses may have access to personal and privileged information about individuals or families through conversa- tions and interactions with their interpret- ers where the individual or family concerned has not consented to the provision of this information. Interpreters in this sense are used as informants and contribute to the general approach that nurses take to moni- toring the social and physical welfare of the community.

A second important dimension of meaning in action at the community level is related to the outpatient structure of health services organization. Nursing stations are not set up to monitor patients on an inpa- tient basis; consequently much clinical care occurs in the homes of individuals. This structural situation again reinforces the need for nurses to monitor the day-to-day health status of individuals and families in the community.

A third dimension is related to the nurses' perception of the way in which Inuit are able or not able to monitor their own health status. In conversations with many nurses, there seems to be a consensus that many Inuit have difficulty in determining when a particular condition requires medical attention. This perception is derived largely from a tendency for some people to make use of health services outside working hours. A common complaint voiced by many northern nurses is that a person will bring a child to the nursing station at 3:00 in the morning with a running ear that could have easily been treated during the after-noon. This situation reinforces nurses' feelings that they must monitor individuals and families in order to prevent minor complaints from becoming major problems.

What are some of the implications of this northern medical ideology? The tenden-cy on the part of health care professionals working in the north to see social life in medical terms has implications on political and economic levels. Health care profes-sionals are generally regarded as credible and influential commentators on social life generally. Their perception of Native societies as sick societies therefore may have powerful implications in undermining the self-determination dialogue. For exam-ple, the relationship between alcohol abuse and political self-determination can be argued in two directions. From the Native perspective, political self-determination is an essential first objective which will do much to reduce the political and economic stresses that are responsible for alcohol abuse. On the other hand, if alcohol abuse is considered as a characteristic of a sick society, it can be used as a rationale for delaying self-determination negotiations. That is, if people can't control their alcohol use, how can they be trusted with the responsibility to handle their own political and economic affairs. As an example, consider the controversy that surrounded the release of the Foulks and Klausner Report on alcohol use in Barrow, that emerged at the 1981 Circumpolar Health Symposium (6).

A second implication is that northern communities come to be understood as total institutions (7). Under the influence of this perspective, community residents become non-persons; they are seen instead as inmates of a medically managed institution and as such, forfeit normal rights of privacy, independence, informed consent and more basically, self-respect and personal dignity. They may be visited in their homes without prior consultation and their medical records, which include much non-medical information, may be scrutinized by anonymous visiting health professionals without their consent. This institutional attitude also inhibits movement towards community control over health services. Do you turn over control of the hospital to patients, or of the asylum to inmates? A similar under-standing constrains efforts to restructure

community health services according to local priorities.

A related implication is that a certain portion of any northern community will resist this institutionalization process by avoiding any contact with health services, with the result that they may place them-selves at increased risk by adopting such an extreme attitude. In the Inuit village where I conducted research, I recorded several cases where potentially serious morbidity was not reported to the nurses and those involved indicated that this decision was related to their desire to avoid becom-ing dependent on professional health servic-es. In other northern communities, there are situations where certain households in the community do not appear in nursing station records and maintain invisibility vis-à-vis medical services.

To return to the contradiction in the northern health dialogue stated at the beginning of this paper, what implications does this northern medical ideology have on Inuit expectations about health care servic-es? Ideologies of powerful, dominant groups in societies have a way of converting others to their cause, irrespective of either the validity of the ideological premises to local realities, or of their relevance to the interests of the converts. In this case, northern people are beginning to believe their social problems are medical problems, and that more medical resources, narrowly defined in technical and profes-sional terms, are necessary to alleviate these problems.

This demand for sophisticated technolo-gy and highly trained professionals, we all realize, is not likely to have any signifi-cant impact on the ecological and economic sources of most of the "real" health prob-lems in the modern North, and it will also delay meaningful Inuit involvement in health care services. The "total institution" surveillance orientation of health services is perceived by young people as intimidating and impossible to participate in. Mastering the technical skills to become a nurse or doctor is difficult enough for young people from isolated northern areas, but then to become involved in monitoring the lives of their co-residents in a northern village is seen as impossible. In local terms, only respected elders can assume this sort of relationship with a community. Similarly, meaningful involvement in administrative aspects of northern health services is hindered by a similar local perception that, unlike other institutional activities such as education or municipal services, health care is less a service to be tailored to meet local needs, than it is a system of surveillance and control that stands apart from community life. The demand for more doctors and hospitals seems to indicate that northern communities have accepted the argument that their societies are sick societies, a situation which can only be improved through bigger and better monitoring and control systems.

There is really no conclusion for this paper. I have tried in a somewhat polemical way to raise a series of issues which I believe are relevant to northern health and hope this presentation will encourage those involved in providing health services to northern communities to reflect on the labelling power that their activities have on people's ideas and actions. I am certainly as guilty as anyone else of contributing to a northern medical ideology that emphasizes sickness as a dominant characteristic of northern society, and I would like to suggest that we begin to document health as intensively and systematically as we now study disease as one way of modifying the potentially damaging aspects of our ideology.

ACKNOWLEDGMENT

I would like to acknowledge the financial support of the National Health Research and Development Program, Health and Welfare Canada, and the Arctic Institute of North America, Firestone Foundation.

REFERENCES

1. Geertz C. The interpretation of cultures. New York: Basic Books, 1973.
2. Foucault M. The birth of clinic: An archaeology of medical perception. New York: Vintage Books, 1975.
3. Young A. Rethinking ideology. Int J Hlth Serv 1983; 13:203-219.
4. Brody H. The people's land: Eskimos and whites in an eastern Arctic. New York: Penguin Books, 1975.
5. Paine R, ed. The white Arctic: Anthropological essays on tutelage and ethnicity. Newfoundland Social and Economic Papers No. 7. Toronto: Univ of Toronto Press, 1977.
6. Foulks EF, Klausner SZ. Alcohol, cultural continuity and economic change in north Alaska. In: Harvald B, Hart Hansen JP, eds. Circumpolar Health 81. Nordic Council for Arct Med Res Rep 1982; 33:506-510.
7. Goffman E. Asylums: Essays on the social situation of mental patients and other inmates. New York: Anchor Books, 1961.

John D. O'Neil
University of Manitoba
750 Bannatyne Avenue
Winnipeg, Manitoba R3E 0W3
Canada

Circumpolar Health 84:423-425

OVERSTUDY OF THE INUIT? AN ETHICAL EVALUATION

ROY J. SHEPHARD

INTRODUCTION

Scientists often undertake major studies of small circumpolar populations without giving great thought to the costs that their observations may impose upon the subjects examined. This paper makes a brief but critical retrospective examination of the impact of the International Biological Program (IBP) upon the community of Igloolik (69° 40'N), a settlement of some 500 Inuit that was visited by up to 30 White investigators in 1969 and 1979.

Knowledge Gained

The visitors were occasionally able to offer the benefits of medical and dental treatment, but their main contribution to the community was of knowledge about itself, particularly its current fitness status and the likely impact of modern technology and related changes of lifestyle upon this status.

Probably because of sampling problems and limitations of field methodology, it was previously believed that both fitness and lung function were poor in the Inuit (1,2). IBP funding allowed us to fly modern laboratory equipment to the Arctic for the first time, and it thus became possible to make accurate measurements of cardiorespiratory performance, muscular strength and body composition on an entire Inuit community, many of whose members were still following a traditional lifestyle.

New findings demonstrated by the IBP research (3) included (i) a high level of aerobic fitness in both men and women, but especially in hunters, (ii) a limited relationship between aerobic fitness and success in hunting, (iii) above average pulmonary function, with a relatively low prevalence of respiratory disease, (iv) a late growth spurt compared to White children, (v) good general nutrition (with high average hemoglobin readings), (vi) very thin skinfolds, apparently with an altered ratio of deep to subcutaneous body fat, (vii) an unusual distribution of sweat glands, (viii) slow aging in young adults, but rapid functional loss after the age of 50 years, and (ix) an ability to satisfy no more than 30 to 40% of community energy needs from hunting, trapping, and fishing resources.

Costs to the Community

Direct Costs: Safety procedures during physiological testing matched the best available in metropolitan laboratories, and no injuries or other complications arose despite repeated examination of almost the entire population.

Subjects were paid an hourly rate as compensation for loss of hunting time. Agreement on compensation was an important early step in negotiations with the village council. In the absence of a clear policy, some investigators could pay excessive sums for simple tests. This not only jeopardizes future studies, but also puts an undesirable pressure upon subjects to participate.

Indirect Costs: Indirect costs are hard to measure. The cultural impact of the White visitors was slight, since they lived in a separate building and cooked their own meals. Moreover, although a large group came to Igloolik for a short period, for most of the two years the White component of the village was only boosted by some 10% relative to the normal influx of teachers, health care workers and government administrators.

The Western concept of times was strongly reinforced by reminders of laboratory appointments and a gift of alarm clocks for participants in a study of circadian rhythms (4). Field tests of performance--particularly the all-out 12 minute run--stressed Western concepts of competitive play (2), while the laboratory tests focussed on Western concepts of maximal performance and "high-tech" medicine rather than more fundamental concerns of public health. However, individual contacts with the physiologists were brief, and they probably had only a minor impact upon attitudes already shaped by regular exposure to Hollywood movies. Moreover, the elemental needs of shelter, nutrition, education, and health were well met in Igloolik, so that no great harm resulted from stressing a technically advanced type of health care.

A previous generation of Whites brought a disastrous epidemic of measles to the Arctic. Perhaps because of the segregation of living quarters, the IBP team did not initiate any major epidemic of infectious disease. One investigator proved to be an alcoholic, however, and on occasion this person unfortunately involved members of the Inuit community in drinking sprees.

Direct Benefits to the Community

How did our new knowledge translate into benefits for the Inuit community? Several specific examples might be cited.

Accurate Growth Curves: Health promotion depends on knowledge of health potential. Growth standards for southern Ontario (5) or Canada (6) were not appropriate to the Inuit community. Development of accurate curves for the Inuit allowed better assessment of items such as child development, with a potential not only to gauge the health of the individual child, but also to make more appropriate choice of furniture for the school classrooms (7). In 1970, a steep curve of adult height versus age seemed to suggest that the younger Inuit were making good the height deficit relative to their White counterparts (2). A ten-year longitudinal follow-up, however, indicated that much of the steep age gradient seen in 1970 was environmental, possibly caused by a combination of calcium deficiencies and snowmobile induced injuries; adults aged 20 to 29 years in 1970-1971 were 2 cm shorter when measured again in 1980-1981 (8).

Urban Lifestyle: We were able to demonstrate to the Inuit the adverse biological effects of acculturation to an urban lifestyle (Table 1). An arbitrary index of acculturation showed a positive correlation with body fat, and (in the men) a negative correlation with aerobic power and leg extension strength. A ten year follow-up study demonstrated a similar deterioration in the fitness status of the entire community as the community members became progressively acculturated to a "western" lifestyle (8).

Respiratory Disease: Fears had been expressed that exposure of the Inuit to severe cold might cause the "Eskimo lung" syndrome of chronic respiratory disease, pulmonary hypertension, and right bundle branch block. Our survey covered active hunters with a high frequency of cold exposure, and we were able to show that EKG abnormalities were rare, both at rest and during vigorous exercise, while lung function scores compared quite favorably with White subjects of the same age (9,10).

Thermoregulation: Studies of thermoregulation demonstrated local cold acclimatization (3), with an unusual distribution

Table 1. The adverse biological effects of acculturation to an urban lifestyle. Coefficients of correlation between an arbitrary index of acculturation from Dr. Ross McArthur (2) and selected indices of physical fitness (2).

	Men	Women
Age	n.s.	n.s.
Skinfold sum	p<0.001	p<0.001
VO_2(max)	p<0.009	n.s.
Leg strength	p<0.068	n.s

of sweat gland activity in the traditional Inuit. Localization of the active glands to the face (1,11) is an important adaptation to cold, minimizing the risk that clothing will become saturated with sweat and thus lose its insulation when it becomes necessary for the hunter to take a rest.

Fitness of the Hunter: While the hunters met the rigors of the arctic environment and the physical demands of hunting with a high aerobic power, we rejected the IBP hypothesis that this represented a genetic adaptation to the arctic habitat (1). The observed changes were explicable more simply as a conditioning response, and were lost after a few months of acculturation to a sedentary Western lifestyle (1,8).

Fat and Cold Protection: Extremely low skinfold readings were found to be compatible with a good cold tolerance, providing sufficient energy reserves for prolonged work (1). We concluded that adjustable layers of clothing provided better cold protection than a thick layer of subcutaneous fat (which might cause overheating and thus sweat saturation of clothing during vigorous physical effort).

Community Energy Reserves: Perhaps the most important of our findings concerned the prospects of overall energy balance for the settlement (12). We looked at the energy cost of each type of hunting and the corresponding food yield, concluding that 30 to 40% of community needs were being met by hunting. Future prospects for those Inuit wishing to conserve a traditional lifestyle were discouraging, in that hunting trips were covering about 40,000 square kilometers of territory to satisfy less than half the requirements of a young and rapidly expanding population (1).

Health Baseline: At the time of the IBP survey, Igloolik was affected relatively little by the "southern" lifestyle problems of overeating, underactivity, and cigarette, alcohol, and drug addiction. Our data thus provided a yardstick of health standards that could be reached by other arctic communities, and (by comparison with such settlements) a warning of the potential consequences of a worsening of lifestyle.

Indirect Benefits to the Community

Employment Opportunities: Young Inuit were able to apply their high school skills as interpreters and laboratory technicians during the study. Some of these individuals found continuing employment, as a permanent scientific laboratory was established in the settlement.

Athletic Opportunities: Demonstrations of a high aerobic power among the Inuit also attracted the attention of Sport Canada, and a number a young Inuit were subsequently trained to high levels of competition, particularly in cross-country skiing. Governmental support was forthcoming for both Western style athletic competition (the Northern Games) and traditional Inuit gatherings such as the Arctic Games.

CONCLUSIONS

Most human endeavors have some unfortunate side effects, but it seems fair to conclude that the good has outweighed the bad in the physiological testing of the Inuit. A practical consumer proof of this view is seen in the willingness of the Village Council to accept a repetition of the physiological test procedures when this was proposed for the winter of 1980-1981. Nevertheless, the concerns raised in this paper have potential application to many studies of the circumpolar habitat, and if the cooperation of the indigenous peoples is to be assured in the future, the costs of research should be weighed very carefully against potential benefits to both the investigator and the community.

REFERENCES

1. Shephard RJ. Human physiological working capacity. London: Cambridge University Press, 1978.
2. Shephard RJ, Rode A. Fitness for arctic life: The cardiorespiratory status of the Canadian Eskimo. In: Edholm OG, Gunderson EK, eds. Polar human biology. London: William Heineman Medical Books, 1973.
3. Milan F, ed. The human biology of circumpolar populations. London: Cambridge University Press, 1980.
4. Lobban MC. Seasonal variations in daily patterns of urinary excretion in Eskimo subjects. In: Shephard R, Itoh S, eds. Proceedings of the Third International Symposium on Circumpolar Health. Toronto: University of Toronto Press, 1976:17-22.
5. Stennett RG, Cram DM. Cross-sectional height and weight norms for a representative example of urban school-age Ontario children. Can J Publ Health 1969; 60:465-470.
6. Pett LB, Ogilvie GF. The Canadian weight-height survey. Hum Biol 1956; 28:177-188.
7. Shephard RJ. Men at work. Springfield, IL: CC Thomas, 1974.
8. Rode A, Shephard RJ. "Future Shock" and the fitness of the Inuit. In: Fortuine R, ed. Circumpolar Health 84. Seattle: University of Washington Press, 1985. (This volume.)
9. Rode A, Shephard RJ. Pulmonary function of Canadian Eskimos. Scand J Resp Dis 1973; 54:191-205.
10. Rode A, Shephard RJ. Lung function in a cold environment--a current perspective. In: Fortuine R, ed. Circumpolar Health 84. Seattle: University of Washington Press, 1985. (This volume.)
11. Schaefer O et al. Regional sweating in Eskimos. In: Shephard R, Itoh S, eds. Proceedings of the Third International Symposium on Circumpolar Health. Toronto: University of Toronto Press, 1976:46-48.
12. Godin G, Shephard RJ. Activity patterns of the Canadian Eskimo. In: Edholm OG, Gunderson EK, eds. Polar human biology. London: William Heinemann Medical Books, 1973:193-215.

Roy J. Shephard
School of Physical and Mental
  Health Education
University of Toronto
320 Huron Street
Toronto, Ontario M5S 1A1
Canada

Circumpolar Health 84:426-427

USE OF A FUNCTIONAL MATRIX FOR RESEARCH IN NATIVE COMMUNITIES

NORMA LING and B.D. POSTL

Health status of Canadian Indian and Inuit peoples remains below that of other Canadians by almost all health indices. On their part, Indian/Inuit peoples are advocating their increased involvement in the planning and provision of health services (1). A means of responding to both health status and Indian/Inuit concerns is by community-based needs assessments. This goal may best be reached by the conduct of community-based research, with Indian/Inuit people functioning as full partners to the research team. This concept has been described or implied in the scientific literature (2,3).

The involvement of Indian/Inuit people improved the likelihood of community acceptance of cohort or longitudinal studies, the desired method of community-based research. In the case of survey (interview) research, the involvement of Indian/Inuit people in the design and administration of questionnaires has likewise improved compliance with their use.

In the conduct of research involving Indian and Inuit people, the researchers must be aware of the many levels of acceptance that must be assured prior to institution of the study.

(i) Individual informed consent by the Indian and Inuit people remains the cornerstone of the ethical conduct of community-based research. To accomplish this, all explanatory letters and standard materials must be presented orally in the local dialect and in syllabics understandable at that level. The need for Indian/Inuit liaison personnel is crucial in this regard.

(ii) Community leaders and council members must also be approached to ensure their understanding and informed consent. These leaders must be involved in the priority-setting of research projects involving their communities.

(iii) At a slightly broader level, regional Indian/Inuit political and cultural agencies must be approached to ensure their cooperation and positive involvement. This level of organization has assumed an increasing role in health advocacy, program planning, and program evaluation for Indian/Inuit communities, and is an important resource to the effective conduct of research. In the conduct of projects with broad health perspectives or implications, the involvement of national Indian/Inuit forums may be likewise necessary and beneficial.

(iv) Health services to Indian/Inuit are provided by the Medical Services Branch of Health and Welfare Canada. These services include treatment programs, preventive programs and health education services. The federal government supplies and staffs all nursing station facilities and a number of hospitals in Indian/Inuit communities of Canada.

The involvement of federal agencies in the planning and conduct of health-related research is therefore vital to its success. As the main resource provider, federal agencies must be aware of the likely and projected impact on resource allocation of proposed research, both in the short and long terms. Moreover, applied research may potentially have an impact on health programs, and therefore requires full involvement of these agencies, if successful programs are to follow.

(v) University-based researchers must also submit research to peer review and acceptance procedures. Most university-based ethical standards committees are not well provided with members aware of the cultural and political sensitivities of Indian and Inuit people. The University of Manitoba Committee on the Use of Human Subjects in Research has, therefore, invited First Nations Confederacy/Manitoba Keewatinowi Okimakanak to provide a committee representative to be involved in the consideration of all proposed research involving Indian people. It is hoped that this member will increase the cultural awareness of ethical committees in the consideration of grants.

(vi) In addition to these five levels of clearance appropriate to the conduct of research involving Indian and Inuit people, ancillary clearance is sometimes necessary by other agencies. Examples include funding and data resource agencies such as the Manitoba Health Services Commission of N.W.T. Health Care Plan. Research in the N.W.T. also requires the approval and licensing of the Science Advisor of the N.W.T.

To satisfy the clearance maneuvers as described, we have developed a personnel matrix that increases the involvement of Indian/Inuit people.

Field Worker Position

Following the above clearance procedures, local community councils are approached to assist with the hiring of a suitable candidate to function as a field worker. The communities consider such qualities as interpersonal relationships, communication skills, fluency in the local dialect, length and quality of residence in the community, initiative and judgement, plus the relation of past work and living experiences.

The field worker performs "technical" duties specific to each project. More importantly he or she becomes an identified agent within the community to whom all questions and concerns may be directed. The constant presence of such a person enhances the acceptability of a project by facilitating a type of immediate "service" element to the research. Concerns that relate to daily "health" experiences may be immediately directed to the field worker for resolution. In this regard, the field worker evolves as an advocate for individuals, ensuring that promised action occurs and that pertinent information is fed back to the community.

Prior to the initiation of duties the field workers participate in a training and awareness program varying from two to six weeks, located in a major center. Throughout the duration of a project, their abilities become enhanced through on-going information and demonstration by project investigators. Dependent on individual ability and motivation, a field worker will develop into an adept worker possessing specific skills and information in the particular health-related area.

Regional Coordinator Position

The regional coordinator functions as a supervisor for the field workers, as well as coordinator of educational activities. This position requires more developed skills than that of the field worker. The regional coordinator must have previously demonstrated relevant skill, usually having acquired the experience in a health or education-related field. The individual requires fluent knowledge of local dialect, traditions, and lifestyle, preferably being of Indian/Inuit origin. This person serves as a major resource to the field worker. In essence, the regional coordinator provides liaison between the research study group and the communities, including political leaders and service agencies.

Project Coordinator Position

The project coordinator provides the central coordination and direction of the project. So far, we have utilized individuals with experience as a nurse practitioner. The position requires an ability to establish and maintain thorough communication lines among all parties, compile data and interpret results, provide direction to regional and field workers, evaluate regional coordinators' performance, and compile interim and final reports.

The coordinator must be accessible on a daily basis to address questions and concerns from all levels of personnel. A major responsibility is the maintainance of information flow so that the study has the required incoming information and all involved parties remain informed of study progress.

The project coordinator reports to the principal investigator or co-investigators who maintain responsibility for ethical clearance and maintenance, study design, data evaluation, and project reporting at meetings or in the scientific literature. The principal investigator also assumes ultimate responsibility for liaison and community interaction through the personnel matrix. They are accountable for all ethical, financial, and scientific aspects of the project.

The use of this matrix has allowed the scientific investigators to increase their role in study design, data analysis, and project evaluation. It has also provided an optimal environment for the involvement of Indian/Inuit people in research and in priority-setting for their communities.

REFERENCES

1. Young TK. Indian health services in Canada: A sociohistorical perspective. Soc Sci Med 1984; 18:257-264.
2. Bain HW. Community development: An approach to health care for Indians. Can Med Assoc J 1982; 126:223-224.
3. Nuttall RN. The development of Indian boards of health in Alberta. Can J Public Health 1982; 73:300-303.

Norma Ling
Northern Medical Unit
University of Manitoba
61 Emily Street
Winnipeg, Manitoba R3E 1Y9
Canada

Circumpolar Health 84:428-430

INNU HEALTH: THE ROLE OF SELF-DETERMINATION

BEN ANDREW and PETER SARSFIELD

Up until the 1950s the Innu, called Naskapi and Montagnais by Europeans, lived a life of relative self-sufficiency, healthfulness and political independence in the territory known to Innu as Ntesinan. Various colonial powers made claims to Ntesinan in the 18th and 19th centuries, a country they had in most cases never set foot in and of which they knew next to nothing. However, these claims did not intrude until the prospect of hydroelectric, lumbering, and mining exploitation motivated the newcomers to intervene directly and attempt to assert control over Innu people and Innu land.

In the 1920s a quarrel developed between Canada, specifically Quebec, and what was then the separate British colony of Newfoundland over the ownership of Labrador, a term which at that time described an area roughly equal to Ntesinan. This region stretched from the Saguenay River east along the north shore of the St. Lawrence River, and included all the land between the north shore and Ungava Bay eastward to the Atlantic coast of Labrador. In 1926 this colonial dispute was brought to the Privy Council in London and in 1927 the British partitioned Ntesinan, granting that which was not theirs to give to Quebec and Newfoundland. The term Labrador then came to refer to that part of Ntesinan "awarded" to Newfoundland, while the rest of Innu country went to Quebec. In 1949 the settlers of Newfoundland voted to join with Canada, and the Labrador portion of Ntesinan was brought with them into Canada.

In 1951 Canada instituted the Indian Act and shortly afterwards began a program, in their words, to civilize the Innu. In the Labrador part of Ntesinan, where the Government of Newfoundland refused to recognize the existence of the Innu people even from a genetic or cultural standpoint, Canada began in 1953 to sponsor the same settlement and "civilization" programs already underway in the more southerly areas of Canada. The approach adopted is well illustrated by the following typical extract from a report written in 1957 by the chief Newfoundland Government official charged with implementing these policies in the field, Walter Rockwood, Director of the Division for Northern Labrador Affairs:

"Although the Indians of Labrador are still more primitive than the Eskimos, this is probably not because of any inherent quality of the race but rather, unwittingly or otherwise, because of less intimate contact with our civilization.... One fact seems clear, civilization is on the northward march and for the Eskimo and the Indian there is no escape. The only course now open, for there can be no turning back, is to fit him, as soon as may be, to take his full place as a citizen in our country.... Towns will spring up and ultimately the entire population of coastal Labrador will flow into a growing industrial area.... The days of the primitive hunting economy are numbered and these minorities must be prepared to pass over into the industrial society now ready to burst upon them." (1)

This ethnocentric and primitive view of the Innu and Inuit culture and options persists into the 1980s. This man's government, and others since, have busily set to work on their crude attempts at social engineering. The colonial governments instituted repressive hunting restrictions and enforced them with harsh penalties; they leased the major Innu salmon rivers to tourist fishing clubs and repeatedly drove off Innu fishermen at gunpoint; they encouraged the opening of iron ore mines, the construction of hydroelectric dams, and the initiation of lumbering operations. The Mishikamau Lake complex in central Ntesinan was flooded in 1971 and became an inland sea to feed the turbines of the Churchill Falls hydroelectric project. In a single grant the American-based corporation ITT received the logging rights to 25,000 square miles of Ntesinan. Laws were enforced requiring the attendance of Innu children at newly erected schools run by the English and French staff imported for the purpose.

So it has been that over a period of 30 years the Innu have been transformed from a society which expected a high degree of individual initiative, self-reliance and responsibility, and which offered in return a life of extraordinary liberty, to that of a powerless and dependent population in a northern colony. In one generation the Innu have been brought from political and economic independence and dignity to a state of destitution and humiliating dependency.

In these circumstances the health of the Innu people has deteriorated rapidly (2,3). The strain on Innu social systems imposed in the government villages has led to widespread alcohol abuse, and violent delinquent and antisocial behavior previously unknown.

Innu people are sick and dying, however, not because of inadequate supplies of drugs, not because of a shortage of public health nurses, not because the nursing stations are old or poorly equipped, and not because of ineffective and insensitive health programs. The Innu are sick and dying because of a well documented syndrome of collective ill-health brought on by the enforced dependency and attempted accultur- ation of an entire people. This ill health will improve or worsen not according to fate or the level of health care funding but only as a result of a political choice by those now engaged in the extension of control over Innu land and Innu lives.

The reaction of those who imposed this catastrophe on Innu society has not been to admit any error or to question their premis- es and priorities, because to do so would be a challenge to the basis on which Canadian northern policy has been built, which is the assumption that the pioneering European has an inherent right to claim the countries of the non-European peoples to the north. The response has instead been simply to try to adjust the reserve and community environment in an attempt to produce the results antici- pated in the original plans.

In this attempt health care programs have been playing a role. We are equally dependent in the area of medical care as we are in others, but we cannot be enthusiastic over the offer of control of a few health programs when control over the areas that matter so much to Innu people, such as land, resources, education, and immigration, re- main out of Innu control. For those who have sought to take Innu land to attempt to separate the business of medical care from those factors which largely provoke its employment is useless and dishonest. Beyond this recognition is the reality that even the highly conditional sharing of responsi- bility in a few isolated programs has been met with opposition by other levels of government. It is quite apparent that even if the Innu were to achieve total control and direction of the medical system, we would not be much further ahead in being able to influence those factors that deter- mine the health of the Innu people.

The fact is that for the Innu health and ill-health are profoundly political issues, inseparable from social and economic considerations. The arrival of an elaborate health-care system among the Innu has coincided with a rapid overall worsening of Innu health. This is not to imply that one has led to the other but rather to emphasize that the health or ill-health of the Innu has been decided by factors that have very little to do with the health-care system. We feel that those who are sincere in wanting to promote Innu health, rather than merely developing a larger self-serving medical system, must be prepared to address problems to which the traditional medical disciplines do not have the answers.

The World Health Organization has recognized that individual good health can best be assured through maintainance of healthy socioeconomic and cultural systems, and that conversely, the exploitation and humiliation of societies will inevitably lead to both collective and individual ill-health.

For the Innu the real health system will be one which will allow Innu society to function properly again, one which will remove foreign domination, and one which will offer the Innu respect as a distinct people. Above all it would permit the Innu the freedom to live unmolested in the Innu country of Ntesinan.

In recent years more Innu than at any time since the beginning of the settlement policies in the 1950s and 1960s are abandon- ing the government villages and reserves to live in mobile family camps in the interior of Ntesinan for a period of about seven months in each year. Once such village, Sheshashit, and the government school are now almost empty. The change in the health of Innu families when living away from the environment of the government villages is remarkable. Alcohol abuse suddenly stops. A combination of improved diet, a rigorous lifestyle, and the stable emotional and social environment offered by a functioning Innu society, make for a startling contrast to life in the villages. It is initiatives such as this which represent the health-care system on which Innu energies and attentions are focused today.

The Innu are not willing to play the part cast for them, nor do the Innu accept the ranking of hunting people as on the bottom rung of human development. The Innu ask that the health professions challenge with us the myths and assumptions that attempt to make Ntesinan someone else's frontier. We ask that you work with us to develop concepts of health and health-care which are appropriate to the Innu People.

This paper is not intended to represent the opinions or policies of any government or government department.

ACKNOWLEDGMENTS

This paper and its presentation would not have been possible without the involve- ment of Peter Penashue and Antony Jenkinson. The advice of Lorna Medd and Kay Wotton was very useful.

REFERENCES

1. Rockwood W. Memorandum on general policy in respect to the Indians and Eskimos of Northern Labrador. Govern- ment of Newfoundland, Division of Northern Labrador Affairs, St. John's, Newfoundland, 1957.

2. Wotton KA. Mental helath of the Native people of Labrador. Presented to the Canadian Mental Health Association, St. John's, Newfoundland, 1983.
3. Wotton KA. Mortality of Labrador Innu and Inuit, 1971-1982. In: Fortuine R, ed. Circumpolar Health 84. Seattle: University of Washington Press, 1985. (This volume.)
4. Sarsfield P. Report to the Naskapi Montagnais Innu Association and the Labrador Inuit Association regarding the health care delivery system in northern Labrador. Privately published by NMTA and LIA, Labrador, 1977.
5. Sarsfield P et al. Local control of health care amongst indigenous peoples. Presented to Canadian Public Health Association, St. John's, Newfoundland, 1983.

Ben Andrew
Naskapi Montagnais Innu Association
Sheshashit
Labrador, Newfoundland AOP 1MO
Canada

Circumpolar Health 84:431-435

THE ORAL HEALTH OF THE FIRST RESIDENTS: WHO'S IN CHARGE?

JOHN T. MAYHALL

Carl E. Mindell, a U.S. Public Health Service psychiatrist, has been quoted as admitting:

> We really don't believe it is important to involve the people we are serving in the provision of the service. We fail to talk with them enough as equals which, of course, means our seeing that they have something to contribute to the relationship, and allowing them to make mistakes. (1)

Although this quotation is 16 years old, I believe it is still worth examining the sentiment behind it today. The three countries I propose to discuss have involved their First Residents to differing degrees when oral disease, its prevention, and its treatment have been under consideration. By any measure of oral health, Alaska's, Canada's, and Greenland's arctic and subarctic residents have an unenviable record. Most health workers will, upon reflection, agree that dental caries and periodontal disease are probably the most prevalent diseases of arctic residents.

It is not my intention to offer specific recommendations for the alleviation of oral disease or its prevention. As the Citizen's Advocate Center noted in their report entitled, "Our brother's keeper: The Indian in White America":

> [We do] not offer recommendations. We offer this observation: that the Indians do not need one more white man's plan for their betterment. Thousands of recommendations are on the shelves and in files, probing every corner of Indian life, every facet of Government policy. Recommendations have come to have a special non-meaning for Indians. They are part of a tradition in which policy and programs are dictated by non-Indians, even when dialogue and consultation have been promised. (1)

First, let us take a very brief look at the problem of oral disease. Reports by dental epidemiologists noted the oral health conditions in Greenland beginning 70 years ago when the Danish dentist, Budtz-Joergensen (2) reported that 58% of the population at a main trading station had caries, while at an outpost only 10% were affected. Then, in the mid-1930s, P.O. Pedersen visited Greenland and laid the foundation for subsequent studies. Pedersen not only examined the living inhabitants, but compared their oral health with that of the skeletal material in the National Museum of Copenhagen. The pre-colonization skulls revealed a caries rate of 38%. Without detailing Pedersen's results, a dramatic increase in caries was seen from the isolated east coast outposts with about 4.4% of the population affected to approximately 88% of those living in the main trading stations on the west coast (3).

By 1945, Baarregaard (2) had found up to 95% of the population affected by caries in the large communities. In the outposts the rate had climbed dramatically to over 40%. Baarregaard also stated that the condition of the periodontium deteriorated in the main trading post residents when compared with the outpost residents. Since these early studies, Jakobsen has continued to observe the oral health of Greenland. In 1978, at the Fourth International Symposium on Circumpolar Health in Novosibirsk, he reported the results of a 1974 study (4) noting:

> Dental caries has been clearly spreading in Greenland over the past decades, parallel to the social changes which have taken place within the same period. The picture of dental disease we see in Greenland today is the result of an extremely high carbohydrate consumption ... forced almost suddenly upon a population which had developed no tradition for oral hygiene in the previous way of life.

In the mid-1970s, Jakobsen and Hansen (5) reported the prevalence of caries in first grade children and seventh grade adolescents to be one and one-half to two times higher than in Denmark. Untreated caries was 4 to 5 times higher than in Denmark.

Moving westward to Canada, we see the same progress of oral disease from a historical perspective. As late as 1937, a physician travelling through the eastern Arctic of Canada noted a caries rate in which only about 1 tooth per individual was affected by dental caries (6). Earlier studies of pre-contact skeletal material had revealed no caries present (7). As in Greenland, the oral disease rates have climbed since with 82% of the children in Rankin Inlet having apparent caries in 1981 (8). Of these, one-fifth had rampant caries (more than six carious teeth).

Gershman (9) has estimated that in the last ten years the prevalence of dental caries in the eastern Arctic has doubled almost universally. While this figure may sound extreme, I have no doubt that it is conservative, as I found a 66% increase of the rate in only four years in the Foxe Basin residents about ten years ago (10). At the same time, periodontal disease has increased as well, but the Canadian figures are not hard and fast as yet. I am hopeful that the next few years will reveal the "true" facts about the oral health of Canadian Inuit and Indians, since a large study is now being suggested. These results will for the first time provide a basis for decisions about the delivery of care to the Natives of Canada.

There have been numerous well-founded studies of the oral health status of the Alaska Native population over the last 60 years. In 1925, R.W. Leigh (11) examined over 300 Eskimo skulls in the U.S. National Museum. While Leigh's sample included skeletal material from Greenland and Canada, it appears that most were from Alaska. Less than 1% of the skulls showed evidence of caries. Leigh suggests that the Eskimos he studied were "afflicted with a high incidence of destructive degeneration of the investing dental tissues," although it is difficult to ascribe all of this to periodontal disease as presently defined. In 1939, Rosebury and co-workers (12,13) found unusually low caries rates for the Yukon-Kuskokwim area of Alaska. Then, in 1961, Russell and his colleagues (14) stated that, "Dental caries prevalence was found to be high in the principal villages [of Alaska] ...; intermediate in men from relatively remote villages and very low in men from coastal villages in the Yukon-Kuskokwim delta area. In the last two groups, prevalence seemed to be rising." Russell et al. (15) also studied periodontal disease in the Eskimo Scout Battalion of the Alaska National Guard and stated that "Men from about half the villages represented showed very little indication of bone resorption, despite a high prevalence of active gingival disease."

In 1955, the U.S. Public Health Service assumed responsibility for the dental health of the Alaska Native population. In the first ten years, the number of decayed, missing, or filled teeth for 6 to 17 year olds increased slightly from 8.69 permanent teeth per individual to about 8.82 teeth (16). By 1970, (17) this figure has been reduced to 7.50 teeth, probably because of an extensive preventive program consisting of large numbers of topical fluoride treatments. But, as Zitzow (18) noted in 1978, the once admirable low caries rate has "...deteriorated to a level comparable to that of their fellow Americans."

Probably one of the most extensive surveys yet undertaken in Alaska was published for the Yukon-Kuskokwim Health Corporation in 1980 by John White (19). Remember that this was the area that over two decades earlier had one of the lowest oral disease rates in Alaska. The 1978 decayed, missing or filled teeth (DMFT) rates for those under six years of age were comparable to those of the general U.S. population, while those between six and seventeen had significantly higher rates. For subjects 45 years and older, the rates were lower than the national average. Significantly higher periodontal disease rates were seen in all age groups when they were compared with national norms.

With this brief overview of the oral "health" of arctic residents we can see that, while there have been efforts--in some cases, massive ones--to alleviate and prevent dental pathology, these have had, at best, a stabilizing effect. The situation is as it is partly because of the trust that First Residents, historically, placed in the modern health care system. But, as Germaine Greer states in her recent book:

> All technological change causes social problems; the impact of Western medicine in traditional societies is one of the most problematic areas of Modernization. The prestige of the white-coats is enormous, the respect for their miraculous hypodermics total. (20)

If the system of the past has not been effective in preventing oral disease, should it be changed? If the answer to this question is in the affirmative, then how should it be altered, and who should make these decisions? In Alaska, Greenland, and Canada, there have been major changes to the dental delivery systems in the past ten years, with more still to come. In general, at least in Canada and Greenland, the changes have been orchestrated by the government. This is probably also true for Alaska, although the advent of health corporations has altered the decision-making process somewhat.

By asking who should make the decisions about the prevention and treatment of oral disease, the initial response of most would be that those whose health is affected should make the decisions. If we accept this premise, let us look at the pitfalls of such "consultation." I noted at the beginning of this paper that some doubt that governments are able to do this in a meaningful way (1). Driben and Trudeau, in a case study of a northern Ontario Indian band (21), pointed out that, as government involvement in the affairs of the Indian increased, so did dependency on the government to the point that today about 90% of the Indians' income is government-derived. Now, if that dependency is to be curtailed, the Indian band is in an extremely vulnerable position. Hugh Brody (22) also observed that, while people from southern Canada went north to assist the Inuit of Canada--most with the highest of intentions--they increased the dependency of those they were "helping" to a point where the Inuit find it difficult to maintain their own lifestyle.

Thus, until recently, we non-Natives have felt that we had the answers to the alleviation of disease, pain, and suffering. In many cases, medical science has had the answers--tuberculosis control being a good example. But we have usurped the authority of the First Residents in providing these measures generally without consultation.

What about more consultation? If there is to be planning for the control or eradication of oral disease, then we should consult with the residents in a meaningful way. Jago (23) cites the work of Arnstein, who set out a typology of participation as if it were a ladder of eight rungs. The bottom rungs are manipulation and therapy. In these cases, the real objective is to enable the holders of power to educate or cure the participants. As one progresses up the ladder, one approaches levels of tokenism. At the fifth rung, placation, the have-nots are allowed to advise, but the power holders still make the decisions. The next level, partnership, allows for negotiation and some trade-offs. Only at the top do citizens obtain a majority position in decision-making or full managerial power.

But as Jago points out, the participation of consumers in the decision-making process of providing health care will not necessarily guarantee more adequate care. He feels, "It is clear, therefore, that the consumer may influence the quality of care, but not determine it." (23) But there is some hope if true consultation is achieved. Dr. Carruth Wagner, the former Chief of the Division of Indian Health in the U.S., is quoted as saying:

> ... I think we can state without equivocation the fact that every significant health advancement the Indian has achieved has been where the Indian himself is taking the primary responsibility for planning and assuming a job in that health endeavour. The sanitation and water supply construction program, everywhere the Indian has taken a very active role in planning these, it has been successful: where the Indian didn't take it and where we went into the reservation and put it on there without any consultation with the Indian, it has been completely valueless. (1)

Dr. John White, in the Yukon-Kuskokwim Health Corporation dental feasibility study (19), entitled one chapter, "Just a shifting in the winds." He cautions that laws governing all of us, and especially those First Residents who are ostensibly accorded special status by their governments, have a history of change depending on the government in power. He notes that the concerns of the American public, and its representative Federal government, vacillate from one generation to the next. He cautions that "... today's well-funded programs may lose American public and Congressional support."

Certainly, White's caution applies to Canada. Using the example of the Fort Hope band of Indians (21), we see that at the signing of their treaty in 1905, the band was promised a reserve and a cash settlement which is paltry by today's standards. The treaty commissioners also promised not to interfere with the band's economy--a promise that lasted for 50 years. In the 1960s, schools were built which were the nidus of village life, a lifestyle inconsistent with successful trapping, thus the advent of an economy based on welfare and social assistance.

Then, in 1969, the Canadian government released a White Paper on Indian policy. This policy resulted in massive make-work projects, job training and other dependency-producing programs. Its goal, however, was to replace a dependence of the Indian on the government with a role of equal status, opportunity and responsibility. Driben (21) points out that the White Paper initiatives could be withdrawn without notice. By 1971, the government had stated that they did not intend to continue with the initiatives outlined in the White Paper, although Driben notes that parts of the policy had already been implemented.

Now, the Canadian government is suggesting that the Indians and Inuit become responsible for their health care. Will this mean a loss of funding? Who will actually make the decisions about health care? And who will be responsible for any failures that will inevitably occur? If the First Residents are able to control completely their dental delivery systems, two very difficult problems must be addressed. Who will be responsible for the service, and who will deliver the services? White addresses these problems succinctly by stating, "It is a difficult task to be a provider of health services and a simultaneous advocate for the consumer of these services." (19)

I would like to spend more time, however, on the second problem--the personnel needed to deliver oral health care. I feel it is important that given cultural, environmental, and linguistic barriers between the present providers and the consumers, we must at least examine the possibility that the First Residents should provide their own care. It is naive to believe that there will be enough First Resident dentists available in the next generation to staff all of the needed positions for dentists. But there are alternatives to the use of dentists in large numbers that have proven successful in some parts of the world. I refer here to the dental nurses of New Zealand and those of Saskatchewan, Canada. Jakobsen (4) noted that the reorganization of the dental care delivery system in Greenland would concentrate on preventive measures and the utilization of indigenous auxiliary personnel. Any additional personnel would consist of increased numbers of chairside assistants and Greenlandic hygienists, while the numbers of dentists would remain constant. These local auxiliary personnel may be able to influence local residents in preventive measures such as better dietary selection and oral hygiene. In Canada, the emphasis for preventing oral pathology and treating routine problems has increasingly fallen to the dental therapists in the Arctic (9). These individuals live in a small community after they finish a two year training program and undertake restorations, extractions, etc., working from a treatment plan devised by a supervising dentist who consults with the therapist on a regular basis. Up to 20% of their time is to be spent on education and preventive services (24). Of the 117 graduates and current students in the program, 36% are Natives and another 25% are non-Native northern residents (9). Thus, about two-thirds are familiar with the environment, culture, and languages of the First Residents in the North.

While I do not have exact figures for Alaska, Dr. David Jones has informed me that almost all dental assistants with the Alaska Area Native Health Service are First Residents. At most, two dentists are in this category. Alaska appears to be ahead of Canada and Greenland in the management of dental services by the consumers themselves. To quote David Jones, "The major change which is occurring is the exercise of self-determination by the Alaska health corporations in assuming management of dental delivery programs. In four years, eight programs have been assumed or initiated statewide, with three more programs slated for turnover in the next 24 months. This change of management, while it is relatively recent, appears to be improving the dental health of Alaska Native people. More services are being provided, additional providers hired, preventive dental programs strengthened and expanded, and facilities expanded."

If we look at the examples that each of the three nations considered here offer, there appears to be hope for better dental health in the First Residents. In Alaska the people are taking charge. In Canada the people are providing a large amount of the services. And in Greenland prevention has become the highest priority. Each country can benefit from the initiatives of the others in preventing, controlling, and rehabilitating oral pathology.

The North American countries tend to be ethnocentric and ignore some of the recommendations of the World Health Organization, but their goals for the year 2000 may be worth invoking here. The Fédération Dentaire Internationale (25) and the WHO (26) have, jointly, proposed a set of dental health goals to be aimed for by the end of this century. While there are six of these, I want to bring only three to your attention. First, 50% of the 5 to 6 year olds should be caries-free by the year 2000. Second, the average number of decayed, missing, or filled teeth should be no higher than three per individual 12 year old. Finally, 85% of the population should retain all of their permanent teeth at the age of 18 years. To attain these goals, the First Residents must be involved as never before; preventive measures must increase immensely; all consumers and providers must be aware of the pain and suffering, loss of productivity and of personal worth that accrue from dental caries and periodontal disease. But we must also remember, as George Bernard Shaw stated (27), "Do not do unto others as you would have them do unto you--their tastes may be different."

REFERENCES

1. Cahn ES, Hearn DW, eds. Our brother's keeper: The Indian in White America. New York: New American Library, 1969.
2. Baarregaard A. Dental conditions and nutrition among natives of Greenland. Oral Surg 1949; 2:995-1007.
3. Pedersen PO. Investigations into dental conditions of ancient and modern Greenlanders. Dent Rec 1938; 4:191-198.
4. Jakobsen J. Recent reorganization of the public dental health service in Greenland in favor of caries prevention. J Comm Dent Oral Epidem 1979; 7:74-81.
5. Jakobsen J, Hansen ER. Cariessituationen: Grønland. Tandlaebladet 1974; 78:839-853.
6. McEuen CS. An examination of the mouths of Eskimos in the Canadian eastern Arctic. Can Med Assn J 1938; 38:374-377.
7. Ritchie SG. The dentition of the Western and central Eskimos. In: Cameron J. Osteology of the Western and Central Eskimos. Report of the Canadian Arctic Expedition 1913-18: Vol 12, part C. Ottawa: King's Printer. 1923:C59-67.

8. Gelskey SC, Hando-Lowes PG. Assessing the oral health status of Rankin Inlet's schoolchildren. Canad Dent Hygienist 1981; 15:54-57.

9. Gershman DM. Inuit dental health and dental services in the Northwest Territories. D.D.P.H. essay, University of Toronto, 1984.

10. Mayhall JT. Canadian Inuit caries experience 1969-1973. J Dent Res 1975; 54:1245.

11. Leigh RW. Dental pathology of the Eskimo. Dent Cosmos 1925; 67:884-898.

12. Rosebury T, Waugh LM. Dental caries among Eskimos of the Kuskokwim area of Alaska. I. Clinical and bacteriological findings. Am J Diseases Child 1939; 57:871-893.

13. Rosebury T, Maxwell K. Dental caries among Eskimos of the Kuskokwim area of Alaska III. A dietary study of three Eskimo settlements. Am J Diseases Child 1939; 57:1343-1362.

14. Russell AL, Consolazio CF, White CL. Dental caries and nutrition in Eskimo Scouts of the Alaska National Guard. J Dent Res 1961; 40:594-603.

15. Russell AL, Consolazio CF, White CL. Periodontal diseases and nutrition in Eskimo Scouts of the Alaska National Guard. J Dent Res 1961; 40:604-613.

16. Abramowitz J. Dental services for American Indians and Alaska Natives, fiscal year 1965. Washington DC: U.S. Dept Health, Education and Welfare, Public Health Service, Bureau of Medical Services, Division of Indian Health, 1964.

17. Dental Services Branch, Division of Indian Health. Dental services for Alaska Natives, fiscal year 1970. Anchorage: U.S. Dept Health, Education and Welfare, Public Health Service. Division of Indian Health, Alaska Native Health Area Office. 1970.

18. Zitzow RE. The relationship of diet and dental caries in the Alaska Eskimo population. Alaska Medicine 1979; 21:10-14.

19. White JR. Yukon-Kuskokwim Health Corporation dental feasibility study. Bethel: Yukon-Kuskokwim Health Corporation, 1980.

20. Greer G. Sex and destiny. Toronto: Stoddard. 1984.

21. Driben P, Trudeau RS. When freedom is lost: the dark side of the relationship between government and the Fort Hope band. Toronto: Univ of Toronto Press, 1983.

22. Brody H. The people's land. Harmondsworth: Penguin, 1975.

23. Jago JD. Issues in assurance of quality dental care. J Am Dent Assn 1974; 89:854-865.

24. Davey KW. The federal dental therapist. Canad Dent Hyg 1980; 14:87-88.

25. Fédération Dentaire Internationale. Global goals for oral health in the year 2000. Int Dent J 1982; 32:74-77.

26. World Health Organization. Planning oral health services. Geneva: WHO, Offset Pub 53, 1980.

27. Valentine AD. A community approach to the prevention of dental disease in the children of developing countries. Int Dent J 1981; 31:23-28.

John T. Mayhall
Faculty of Dentistry
University of Toronto
124 Edward Street
Toronto, Ontario M5G 1G6
Canada

Circumpolar Health 84:436-442

SELF-DETERMINATION AND INUIT YOUTH: COPING WITH STRESS IN THE CANADIAN NORTH

JOHN D. O'NEIL

The stress of social change in northern regions and particularly its impact on Native youth has received a great deal of scientific and popular attention in recent years (1-8). Although significant regional and local variation is acknowledged, this work generally concludes that where acculturative stress is high, young people are committing suicide, abusing drugs, experiencing emotional distress, and injuring themselves and each other at intolerably high rates. Suicide rates among young people have risen astronomically in the past decade. For example, in 1971 the suicide rate in the Northwest Territories was below or near the Canadian average of 10 per 100,000. By 1978 it has risen to 35 per 100,000 or three times the Canadian national average. The recent suicide epidemics in the Mackenzie Delta and the Keewatin District indicate rates as high as 170 per 100,000. Psychiatric observers have identified the individual at risk as a young man in his late teens recently returned from high school, often the first-born son and usually a family favorite, the suicide occurring in the context of romantic problems and drinking (4). Others have noted that when communities are under stress, it is usually young people who express the health consequences of that stress in the loudest terms (9).

The acculturative stress model, developed by Berry and his colleagues for work in northern Quebec, has been adopted generally to explain these circumstances (10). This model originally argued that when modern community pressures were at greatest variance from traditional cultures, identity confusion would be greatest and mental ill-health would be highest. It has since been modified to incorporate a political dimension as a result of findings in northern Quebec which indicate that the James Bay negotiations and land claims settlement have had a positive impact on young adult role modelling and identity integrity (2,3). Our current understanding of the relationship between social change and mental health accords considerable explanatory power to the extent to which communities and individuals have control over their daily lives and destinies. To put it another way, improvements in self-government and self-determination are fundamentally linked to reductions in social and mental health problems in northern communities.

This paper describes the situation of young adult men in one Canadian Inuit village where recent political changes related to the prohibition of alcohol and the resulting increase in the community's sense of political self-control, have created conditions where young adult men are coping constructively with the social, economic, and political stresses which continue to affect northern society (11).

The study was ethnographic in design and involved two years of resident fieldwork (1977-1978; 1980-1981) where participant-observation and life history interviews were combined with a questionnaire survey of the young adult population and a review of their medical records. The data from the study are available in dissertation form and are only briefly summarized here to support the argument advanced (15).

This study examined the situation of young adult men as members of three narrowly defined historical cohorts: 1) The Junior Team (15 to 19); 2) Polar Bear Hunters (20 to 24); and 3) Managers (25 to 29). The cohort concept as defined by anthropologists interested in aging and age boundaries is useful for disentangling historical, maturational, and contextual factors which affect people's experience of stress and their coping responses (12-14). That is, we need to separate the normal experience of social transition from the more historically situated experience of stresses arising from social change, modernization, and economic development. In the absence of a long-term prospective study, the cohort approach is also a useful way to examine the relationship between social change and individual adaptation.

The purpose of the study was to identify significant transitions in the life course during these important years and to identify differences in adjustments and adaptations made by young people to changing historical circumstances. As people mature through different life stages, they experience history differently. These experiences require different adaptations and adjustments and adaptational requirements or demands may differ significantly. Coping styles appropriate for one cohort at one point in time may be inappropriate for successive cohorts during later historical periods. Coping styles developed by one cohort may also persist into later life stages. Therefore, the adaptations made by one cohort as teenagers may appear inappropriate to successive cohorts and vice versa. The adaptation made by people in their early twenties when they were teenagers was quite different from that made by people presently in their late twenties and is likely to be different again from the present teenage cohort.

This important conceptual point was made dramatically clear to me when I began my second year of field work. In 1982 young people in their early twenties appeared to have strong family, land, and traditional orientations and appeared to be profoundly anti-White in their behavior and attitudes. (Anti-White is used here as a cultural reference and not in an interpersonal conflict sense. It indicates a resistance to adopting behavioral styles and attitudes that reflect southern Canadian cultural orientations.) These young people had few health problems and little evidence of social maladjustment. In 1978, however, those of this same cohort were profoundly alienated from their families. They were seriously experimenting with different drugs and appeared to be aggressively adopting the White lifestyle. My research, therefore, was directed towards an analysis of how changing historical circumstances led to this fundamental shift in identification and coping style. Major differences among the three cohorts are summarized in Table 1.

The cohort age boundaries are somewhat arbitrary but also reflect important transitional phases. The 24 year old boundary is perhaps less clearly defined and involves a whole series of changes indicating independence and self-sufficiency. The transition at 19 however, is a fundamental and clearly recognized transition in a young man's life. The demarcation was confirmed for me during a Hamlet Council meeting where councillors were discussing the formation of a youth club. While Council agreed that participation in youth club activities might benefit teenagers, they were adamant in insisting that its membership be limited to young people 19 years of age and under. They argued that young people over the age of 19 had structural access to other organizations and political bodies available in the community and should in fact be too busy supporting their families to engage in youth club activities. They also argued that if the youth club was to foster self-expression among the town's young people, older youth's participation would inhibit teenage involvement.

It was further evident that the Hamlet Council and some of the town's elders clearly considered the behavior of teenagers as evidence of a serious social problem. They argued that the years of 16 to 19 should be a very productive transitional period. It should be a time when young men concentrate on learning to hunt and begin to help their family economically. It should be a period where young people cease to act like children and begin to act like adults, or in Inuktitut terms, begin to use their reason. It is a time when the inuusuuqtuq label implies transition and active assumption of adult roles and responsibilities.

(Inuusuuqtuq translates literally as "the one who resembles a person" or "the one who is becoming a person." The word has a long history of use with reference to Inuit teenagers.)

From the older people's perspective it appeared that young men were not in the least engaged in the productive process. In behavioral terms most teenagers slept during the day, played games at night and showed little interest in either learning to hunt or finding work. They spoke Inuktitut poorly and infrequently and seemed to avoid normal social intercourse with their extended family. Their behavior was regarded as the continuation of childhood rather than the transition to adulthood.

The teenage reaction to this attitude was resentment. Teenagers felt they were being asked to behave according to impossible standards. While they did not fully understand the social forces responsible for creating the situations with which they had to cope, they were able to articulate a sense of frustration at being unable to express values and identifications that they held internally, in a public manner which would impress and satisfy the larger community. In the words of one young man:

It seems like old people are always saying we can't do anything. It's like they blame us because there aren't enough jobs in town. Without a job, how can I buy a ski-doo to go out hunting? Only kids ride on their father's komatik (sledge).

The result is that although the majority of teenage youth identify strongly with the Inuit way of life, they also perceive the older generations and local Inuit organizations (who are responsible for allocating employment opportunities), as the causes for the stresses they are experiencing. My argument here is that in fact Inuit teenagers are coping with the social conditions of life in northern Canada in a positive fashion. Their situation could be worse. The rates for suicides, drug abuse, and emotional disturbances could be higher. Young people could be more angry and more alienated. Contrary to outward appearances, most teenage Inuit in this particular village express a commitment to imummarik or "genuine Eskimo" principles. Their apparently alienated behavior instead reflects northern economic and political conditions and the consequent lack of opportunities for accumulating capital which is today necessary for pursuing land-oriented activities.

If we compare Inuit teenagers with their counterparts in southern Canada where the social and psychological consequences of high youth unemployment is a national concern, but where statistics indicate that even in so-called "disaster" areas, unemployment is still less than half of most northern communities, the situation of Inuit youth becomes clearer. Our own society substitutes education for young people as a strategy for keeping unemployment figures down. The education option however, is not available for Inuit youth in isolated communities. In strictly technical terms, of course, secondary and post-secondary education are as available for Inuit youth as for any young person in the country. In practical terms, however, the pursuit of higher education in the Canadian north requires personal adjustments that are themselves highly stressful. The only viable option is to leave one's family and community at the age of 15 to attend high school in Yellowknife, the territorial capital. This entails living with strangers in a totally foreign cultural context. If you were to suggest to a 16 year old boy and his parents in a small town in northern Alberta that the boy had to leave the community at age 16 for four or five years of boarding school in Montreal, I suspect the reaction would be extremely negative. A comparable situation exists in the Northwest Territories. As the numbers in Table 1 indicate, there has indeed been a drop in the percentage of each cohort completing secondary education over the past ten years. This decrease in part reflects greater self-determination on the part of communities and young people. The older cohort had little choice but to accept a policy that required them to spend considerable portions of their childhood and adolescence in residential schools away from home. Young people today reject this option.

This decision by Inuit youth not to pursue education outside the village context is related as well to a more fundamental historical issue. The Junior Teamers are the first cohort to be raised entirely in the village context. Previous cohorts spent the early part of their lives either in camp on the land, or away at residential schools. In either case they often had early exposure to southern society or to other northern

Table 1. Variation among young adult cohorts.

	Junior Team (20)	Polar Bear Hunters (17)	Managers (14)	
Historical/biographic factors				
1. Born in or near Sanctuary Bay.	60	41	36	*
2. Lived in Sanctuary Bay entire life.	50	35	14	**
3. Lived part of life outside Kitikmeot region.	20	24	64	**
4. Related to Whites by descent or marriage.	30	41	36	N.S.
5. Had experience with boarding school as a child.	0	18	36	**
6. Parents encouraged education.	75	41	21	**
7. Have no secondary education.	10	6	57	**
8. Completed secondary education.	5	6	14	**
9. Able to work as a translator.	10	18	21	N.S.
10. Prefer English to Inuktitut in everyday conversation.	80	59	36	**
Domestic context				
1. Majority of kindred lives in Sanctuary Bay.	55	71	36	**
2. Currently residing with older relatives.	90	76	14	**
3. Father still alive.	80	88	43	**
4. Father is very active hunter/trapper.	45	53	21	**
5. Father has full-time employment.	30	24	29	N.S.
6. Had first sexual experience younger than 15.	20	41	21	**
7. Marriage was arranged by parents.	N/A	29	43	N.S.
8. Wife is from another village.	N/A	41	36	N.S.
9. Child(ren) adopted by older relative.	N/A	41	50	N.S.

All numbers expressed as percentage of total population of each cohort (indicated in brackets).
*   indicates chi square statistic significant at alpha = 0.05.
**   indicates chi square statistic significant at alpha = 0.01.
N.S. not statistically significant.

towns. As Table 1 indicates, the Junior Teamers had had limited exposure to other towns or the south and identify strongly as villagers. Much of their everyday conversation is related to being from a particular village. Their identification with the sports teams is village-oriented. In the same manner as an older person might view himself as Netsilingmiut (people of the area where there are seals), teenagers see themselves as the people of a particular village. This village identification supercedes other social criteria, such as religion and tribe, which characterize the social identifications of older Inuit.

The consequence of this identification is that Inuit villager role models are perceived by most teenagers as the lifestyle to be emulated. White identities are considered dangerous. Many have older brothers in so-called managerial positions who seem to be very unhappy. Teenagers are aware of the stress this older cohort experiences in their functions of mediating between White bosses, Inuit clients, and

Inuit boards of directors. This emulation of village role models also suggests that teenage Inuit aspire to be like their fathers. Although a normal situation in most communities, in the context of the contemporary Canadian north, they are perhaps the first cohort whose fathers are truly villagers. In the other young adult cohorts now in their twenties, most of the fathers are still Nunamiut or people who continue to be oriented primarily to a land-based subsistence. While the distance between fathers and sons in these older cohorts may appear to be greater, in some ways there is less tension because these cohorts were freer to experiment with White identities and new social roles. Indeed, parents of these cohorts often encourage their sons to learn White skills and behavior for economic reasons. For teenagers today, the greatest value is seen to be the ability to combine various land and village economic strategies in the same manner as their parental cohort. They want to be carpenters, heavy equipment operators and

Table 1.   (Continued)

	Junior Team (20)	Polar Bear Hunters (17)	Managers (14)	
Contemporary coping behavior				
1. Only travel is to nearby villages by snowmobile.	20	41	21	**
2. Have travelled out of Kitikmeot in past two years.	80	59	79	N.S.
3. Have visited at least four different villages in past two years.	75	41	36	**
4. Go onto the land at least twice per month.	55	71	57	N.S.
5. Never attend church.	55	59	43	N.S.
6. Earned more than $10,000 in 1981.	0	47	57	**
7. Had a full-time job in 1981.	15	41	57	**
8. Enjoy indoor jobs the most.	30	12	36	**
9. Worked only in indoor jobs in 1981.	45	12	36	**
10. Earned more than $250 carving in 1981.	10	24	43	**
11. Have been elected to political office.	N/A	47	29	*
12. Watch television news almost every night.	45	24	36	*
13. Go to the gym almost every night.	75	24	21	**
14. Go to almost every dance.	75	47	64	*
Health behavior				
1. Started smoking cigarettes younger than 14.	70	35	7	**
2. Smoke at least half package of cigarettes/day.	85	71	86	N.S.
3. Do not drink any alcohol.	70	41	36	**
4. Occasionally use alcohol illegally.	5	12	22	**
5. HOS score higher than 30 (at risk for psychiatric problems).	55	12	21	**
6. Frequent visits to nursing station as teenager.	25	47	43	*
7. More than 1/3 of visits to nursing station in past two years are stress-related.	5	12	29	**
8. More than 1/2 of visits to nursing station in past two years are minor injuries.	40	12	0	**

tradesmen. They see more value in manual outdoor labor than in "bookkeeping" functions. Their ambitions are to be able to integrate full-time village employment into a land-oriented lifestyle. These land aspirations are for both subsistence and cultural renewal.

Young men are only content to ride their fathers' sledge until they are 14 or 15, after which most feel their own snowmachine is essential for developing a sense of independence and manhood. The minimal capital investment for hunting equipment today in the Canadian north would be approximately $2,000.00. Accumulating such a large amount of money is nearly impossible, given the kind of jobs generally available to teenage Inuit. Make-work projects and part-time jobs provide little more than a weekly wage large enough to contribute to the purchase of family groceries with a little left over for movies and cigarettes. Opportunities for substantial capital accumulation exist only in major summer construction projects or through rotational shifting in regional mines. Access to either of these opportunities is largely controlled by Whites and there is little support for the one-time arrangements that are generally the preference of teenage Inuit. Whites want "career-oriented" young people to pursue better paying occupations. The tendency for teenage Inuit to work one long shift and then return to the village with their savings is considered inappropriate by White employers.

Consequently, the change from riding a father's sledge to becoming an independent, self-sufficient hunter can rarely be achieved before the transition at 19 to married status. Married status with dependents is perceived by older Inuit who control community employment as the primary consideration when allocating employment resources. The result is a four year hiatus where the only option to teenage Inuit is to become committed basketball and volleyball players. To the Junior Teamers, the team is everything. Daily matches in the school gym are the focus throughout the fall, winter, and spring months. Teammates provide primary socialization experiences and support, and the ultimate perception that work or hunting requirements intrude into sports activities in inevitable.

While the evening round of basketball and volleyball games are generally perceived by the rest of the community as a complete waste of time and evidence that youth are moving away from Inuit values and ideals, there is evidence that below the surface these games in fact are distinctly Inuit and may reinforce commitment to Inuktitut values. On several occasions I observed cases where young people who appeared too White in their competitive demeanor were ostracized by the remainder of the group. Also, the Inuit principle of never expressing anger was systematically enforced in young Inuit sporting activities. Young men who lost their temper were scorned by their teammates.

The teen dance, which is also perceived by the larger community as an indication of movement away from Inuit values, also provides evidence for young people's commitment to Inuit identifications. Tacit understandings concerning eye contact, body contact, seating arrangements, the extent of body movements during dance and many other features of the courtship ritual were clearly defined for Inuit youth in distinctly conservative terms and varied dramatically with the often flamboyant dancing styles of Whites who attended the dances. The stereotype of the promiscuous teenager (which has replaced the older and equally invalid stereotype of wife-swapping) is clearly either outdated or superficial. Relations between genders at rock dances are severely constrained and sexual relations occur usually after a prolonged courtship and when some indication of future commitment has been made. One young man, who returned to the village after several years in the south, commented frequently on the restraint expressed in teenage sexual relations and waited nearly five months before assuming a regular sexual relationship with a young woman.

The significance of these changes will perhaps be clearer if we shift our attention for a moment to the youth cohort now in their early twenties: The Polar Bear Hunters. As I indicated earlier, this cohort has shown a remarkable improvement in social and health status over a four year period. Are these changes simply due to maturational effects or has there been a significant change in the overall socioeconomic context?

In another paper, I have argued that the prohibition of alcohol in Inuit communities is symbolically representative of a growing sense of self-determination and political confidence in many Inuit communities. This new sociopolitical climate has occurred largely in the past four or five years, at a time when the Polar Bear Hunters were beginning to establish families. The previous cohort, the Managers, had gone through this transition during a period when Inuit self-confidence and esteem was generally low, and alcohol was exacerbating general community tensions and conflicts. They responded by attempting to delay marriage and family commitments, much to their parent's chagrin, and by pursuing White social identifications and concomitant economic strategies. The Polar Bear Hunters, on the other hand, made the transition in an alcohol-free context and into a community where traditional hunter imagery was again providing the primary social and political symbols for male self-definition. A simple example of the significance of this shift in cultural focus can be drawn from visiting patterns. In 1978, young men in their early twenties who are now the Managerial cohort, were frequent visitors in the homes of White teachers, administrators, etc. in the town. Their younger brothers in 1982 however, rarely visit Whites. When such visits do occur, they are more often with transient laborers and tradesmen, people who are usually co-workers, than with the local White elite.

These observations pose an obvious question. How have these wider sociopolitical changes affected the coping styles of Inuit teenagers and can we expect a similar transition from them as they pass into their early twenties? If we compare the present situation of Inuit teenagers to that of the Polar Bear Hunters when they were teenagers, the differences are dramatic. The Junior Team may indeed be alienated from assuming productive roles in community life, but their "recreational" solutions provide a context where important symbolic and moral dimensions of social expectations and obligations can be developed. While their older brothers in the Polar Bear Hunting cohort have focused their innovative energies on revitalizing a commitment to land activities and "family"; the Junior Teamers are focusing on general social interactional styles and cultural performance. Basketball games and dancing to rock music may not appear to have any serious connection to the wider social life of the community, but on close observation, these activities are "thick" with rules and restrictions regarding appropriate ways to express aggression, affection, competitiveness, leadership, cooperativeness, etc. On closer analysis, these cues are also strikingly Inuktitut or "in the manner of an Inuk."

This analysis has very positive implications for the future. The growing sense of confidence that the trend towards political self-determination has fostered in the larger community has had a differential impact on three successive teenage cohorts over the past decade. Those who are now in their late twenties participated aggressively in wresting control over local affairs away from Whites, but at the expense of losing their connectedness to the land, their families, and the wider community. Those who are now in their early twenties are actively engaged in a wide range of land-based activities and are focused socially on their families, but have little interest in community affairs and to some extent, have lost the ability to behave "in the manner of an Inuk." Contemporary Inuit teenagers, to paraphrase Gerald Berreman

paraphrasing Bob Dylan, appear to be in the process of "bringing it all back home" (16). They are assuming fully articulated villager identities and generating social interaction patterns that synthesize dimensions of tradition and modernity in a way which bodes well for the future integrity of the community.

ACKNOWLEDGMENTS

I would like to acknowledge the financial support of the National Health Research and Development Program, Health and Welfare Canada, and the Arctic Institute of North America, Firestone Foundation.

REFERENCES

1. Brody H. Land occupancy: Inuit perceptions. In: Milton Freeman Research Ltd., ed. Inuit land use and occupancy project. Ottawa: Supply and Services 1976; 1:185-238.

2. Wintrob RM, Sindell PS, Berry JW, Mawhinney T. The psychosocial impact of culture change on Cree Indian women: 1966-1980. In: Harvald B, Hart Hansen JP, eds. Circumpolar Health 81. Nordic Council for Arct Med Res Rep 1982; 33:467-480.

3. Berry JW, Wintrob RM, Sindell PS, Mawhinney T. Culture change and psychological adaptations among the James Bay Cree. In: Harvald B, Hart Hansen JP, eds. Circumpolar Health 81. Nordic Council for Arct Med Res Rep 1982; 33:481-489.

4. Rodgers DD. Suicide in the Canadian Northwest Territories 1970-1980. In: Harvald B, Hart Hansen JP, eds. Circumpolar Health 81. Nordic Council for Arct Med Res Rep 1982; 33:492-495.

5. Seltzer A. Acculturation and mental disorder in the Inuit. Can J Psychiat 1980; 25:173-181.

6. Atcheson JD, Malcolmson SA. Psychiatric consultation to the eastern Canadian arctic communities. In: Shephard R, Itoh S, eds. Proceedings of the Third International Symposium on Circumpolar Health. Toronto: University of Toronto Press, 1976:539-452.

7. Kraus R, Buffler PA. Sociocultural stress and the American native in Alaska: An analysis of changing patterns of psychiatric illness and alcohol abuse among Alaska Natives. Cul Med Psychiat 1979; 7:111-151.

8. Forsius H. Behavior. In: Milan FA, ed. Human biology of circumpolar populations. Cambridge Univ Press, 1980.

9. Eyer J, Sterling P. Stress-related mortality and social organization. Rev Radical Polit Econ 1977; 9:1-44.

10. Berry JW. Acculturative stress in northern Canada: Ecological, cultural and psychological factors. In: Shephard R, Itoh S, eds. Proceedings of the Third International Symposium on Circumpolar Health. Toronto: University of Toronto Press, 1976:490-496.

11. Dacks G. A choice of futures: Politics in the Canadian north. Methuen Publishing Co, 1981.

12. Nydegger C. On being caught up in time. Human Dev 1981; 24:1-13.

13. Eckert JK. Experiential cohorts among American men. Presented at the Annual Meeting of the Gerontological Society, Dallas, 1978.

14. Lazarus R. The stress and coping paradigm. In: Eisdorfer C et al., eds. Models for clinical psychopathology. Spectrum Books, 1981.

15. O'Neil D. Is it cool to be an Eskimo?: A study of stress, identity, coping and health among Canadian Inuit young adult men. Unpublished Ph.D. dissertation, University of California (San Francisco-Berkeley), 1983.

16. Berreman GD. Bringing it all back home: Malaise in anthropology. In: Hymes D, ed. Reinventing anthropology. Vintage Books, 1974.

John D. O'Neil
Department of Social and Preventive Medicine
University of Manitoba
750 Bannatyne Avenue
Winnipeg, Manitoba   R3E OW3
Canada

Circumpolar Health 84:443-446

THE ROLE OF HOSPITAL-BASED MEDICAL INTERPRETERS IN ADVOCACY FOR NORTHERN NATIVE PATIENTS AND COMMUNITIES

JOSEPH M. KAUFERT, WILLIAM W. KOOLAGE, MARGARET SMITH, ANDREW KOSTER, JOHN D. O'NEIL, ISABEL WHITFORD, JOSEPH CONNOR, LORNA GUSE, ESTHER MOORE and WINNIE GIESBRECHT

INTRODUCTION

This paper examines advocacy functions performed by Cree and Saulteau language-speaking interpreters working in two urban hospitals providing tertiary medical care to Native Canadians from remote northern communities. It will focus upon the roles played by medical interpreters in representing individual patients in tertiary care settings and their emerging involvement in representing the interests of remote northern communities in the urban health care system.

In their role as paraprofessional case workers in urban hospitals, medical interpreters represent the interests of individual Native clients. In our pilot study, hospital-based medical interpreters were also observed to assume the role of advocates for northern communities through: 1) working as contact persons and informants for patients from remote communities and urban migrants; 2) providing feedback on one situation, that is, consumer perception of primary care services on the reserve; and, 3) serving as unofficial spokespersons for political and economic concerns of northern communities.

Advocacy roles for hospital-based interpreters working with individual patients involve explaining biomedical concepts and hospital organization both to people evacuated for short-term care and to urban migrants (1). At both the individual and the community level, advocacy involves a process of interpreting and brokering understandings of biomedical concepts and organizational objectives between clinicians or administrators on the one hand, and Native patients or community groups on the other. In terms of concept of cultural brokerage described by Paine, this involvement of interpreters in advocacy may entail loyalty conflicts (2). In one situation, the interpreter may be called upon to represent the interests of the individual or community. In another situation the interpreter may be called upon to maintain biomedical definitions of a situation or represent the organizational or professional perspective of the hospital.

METHODS

Over an 18-month period, participant-observation and analysis of videotaped clinical consultations were utilized to develop an inventory of roles and situational contexts characterizing the work of Native interpreters in urban hospitals. Description of the role of urban medical interpreters in individual patient-centered and community-oriented advocacy utilized case examples derived from a series of audio-taped interviews with eight interpreters and participant-observation data from a pilot study in an urban hospital setting. Case material comes from an exploratory study which documented not only the interpreters' perspective, but included interviews with Native patients, physicians, and hospital administrators (3). This research is the preliminary stage of a multiphase project which will examine the roles played by interpreters within urban and rural medical settings, their contribution to medical care and the occupational stresses associated with their work. Briefly summarized, the overall program of research will include: (a) a task analysis of interpreter/patient encounters in two urban hospitals over a one year period; (b) a stratified sample of 100 sets of interviews with clinicians, patients, and interpreters before and after medical encounters; (c) content-analysis of a series of videotaped consultations in which an interpreter took part; and (d) the collection of data on the training and career patterns among 20 interpreters working in two urban hospitals through participant-observation and life history interviews.

Interpreting and Advocacy for Patients

During our preliminary investigation of the problems experienced by northern Native patients evacuated to southern urban hospitals, we were impressed by the pivotal roles played by Native Canadian interpreters as advocates for individual patients. In working with individual patients, it became clear that medical interpreters functioned as: (1) direct linguistic translators; (2) cultural informants providing explanations of Native culture and language to administrators and professionals in urban hospitals; (3) biomedical interpreters explaining biomedical concepts and hospital organizational structure to Native patients; and (4) as patient advocates representing the interests of the individual Native patient.

The interpreter's role as language translator frequently corresponds with the health care system's definition of the function of the interpreter as providing a channel through which biomedical concepts are translated into linguistically appropriate terms. Misunderstandings arose between health care practitioners and interpreters when the former view the latter's role as simply that of a "pragmatic translator." Many health care workers became frustrated when they felt the interpreters were censoring or inadequately translating a patient's reply. Since the clinicians did not speak Dene, Inuktitut, Algonkian (Cree, Saulteau), or Siouan, they had no way of knowing that the interpreters were establishing rapport, putting the patient at ease, or finding culturally appropriate analogies for complex western scientific terminology and concepts. Clinicians and administrators did not always recognize that the involvement of interpreters added a significant role to clinical encounters that directly influenced the overall social and cultural context of diagnosis and treatment. Examples of attempts to define the interpreter's role in terms of narrower language translation functions were observed in situations in which they were asked to find an equivalent concept in Cree or Saulteau for an anatomical term or physiological process. Although in some cases appropriate terms did exist in Native languages, the interpreters often found it necessary to move beyond the direct translation of the concept to explain the function of an organ or describe a procedure in lay language. The most effective collaboration between language interpreters and health care workers in translation involved a model of shared control over clinical communication in which both participants share in building a therapeutic relationship and establishing communication with the client (4).

The second major role performed by interpreters involves explaining the linguistic and cultural perspective of the Native patient and the environmental perspective of remote northern communities to clinicians and administrators in urban hospitals. For example, an interpreter may explain why interpretations of biomedical concepts may be unacceptable from a cultural standpoint, or why a treatment regimen may be unrealistic because of administrative barriers or resource limitations. As an intermediary, the interpreter is supposed to provide the clinician or administrator with objective information about the Native patient's culture and community background. Information about the patient and his or her environment are assumed to be directly translated, rather than altered to reflect the agenda of the patient or interpreter. As cultural informants, interpreters explained to clinicians the significance of the patient's home environment in achieving compliance. For example, in the case of a child with a skin infection, the interpreters were able to communicate to the attending physician in an urban hospital the

problems of obtaining water supplies for daily bathing and laundering.

Interpreters also act as intermediaries in facilitating information flows between clinicians, patients and their families by explaining biomedical concepts and providing information about the organizational structure of urban hospitals. This role involves sensitizing patients to the hospital milieu, explaining procedures, patient education, and obtaining meaningful informed consent. Although this type of function primarily involves translation of biomedical knowledge, interpreters must link their knowledge of health care procedures and human physiology with parallel knowledge of indigenous language and culture. An example of this function was observed in a situation in which an interpreter attempted to provide health education for a diabetic patient by referring to more familiar animal anatomy and making analogies between metabolic processes influencing a diabetic's diet and familiar mechanical processes such as maintaining a gas and oil balance for outboard motors.

Although the other three roles played by Native language interpreters in urban hospitals all involve elements of advocacy, their involvement in direct representation of the interests of the individual Native patient is a more direct and visible form of advocacy. As patient advocates, the interpreters were often faced with conflicts between their role of health system employee/practitioner and their involvement in maintaining their patients' rights. Direct involvement of interpreters in advocacy was observed in two cases in which meaningful consent for a procedure had not been obtained and the patient could not understand or accept the procedure within the context of their cultural values. Two cases were documented in which interpreters had been involved in attempting to explain a cardiologist's decision to implant a pacemaker while a patient was undergoing diagnostic catheterization. In these cases, the patient was unable to understand the function of the pacemaker and had a cultural aversion to having a foreign body implanted. In one case, interpreters were asked in after the pacemaker had actually been implanted. In another, the interpreter was involved in prospectively explaining the procedure prior to obtaining informed consent from the patient. In the second case, the failure of the clinician to communicate the nature of the male patient's cardiological problem and the function of the pacemaker before performing the implantation placed the interpreter in a direct loyalty conflict in which it was necessary to represent the interests of the less powerful Native patient, rather than the therapeutic objectives of the clinician.

In the process of retrospectively trying to explain the risks and benefits of the pacemaker to the patient, the interpreter moved from a role of language and cultural translation to one of direct advocacy for the patient.

Community Advocacy Functions
Among Urban Medical Interpreters

In addition to advocacy on behalf of individual northern clients within urban hospitals, Native language interpreters were also observed to perform the additional function of representing the interests of entire northern communities. This added function was significant because in some situations there was no single provincial or national Native organization which could represent the health concerns of reserve communities or communities in unorganized territories. In these situations medical interpreters were able to augment the work of regional and provincial Native organizations by using their informal networks to gain information about health policies and articulate the concerns of their home communities. Specifically, interpreters performed roles as: (a) urban contact persons for communities whose members were evacuated to urban hospitals or who lived as more permanent migrants in urban areas; (b) informal representatives of perspectives of band leaders and community perspectives on primary care services on reserves and the northern patient transportation system; and (c) as unofficial spokespersons for northern communities in urban policy-making.

Interpreters frequently became involved in advocacy functions for community groups through their involvement with individual clients. An example of the role of hospital-based interpreters as urban contact persons was observed in a case in which they worked with both band council and representatives of the urban welfare system to find housing and income support for the family of a teenage patient with renal failure. The patient and her family migrated to the urban center from a reserve community on the Ontario border initially in order to receive dialysis, and following a transplant operation, to facilitate continuous medical monitoring during the period of highest likelihood of tissue rejection. Urban contact and community liaison functions performed by urban health interpreters are of increasing importance because larger numbers of Native patients with chronic disease problems are required to remain in urban centers for extended periods in order to receive technically sophisticated treatment. In working with the family of the renal patient, the interpreters functioned as intermediaries between the community leaders and the urban welfare system. At an individual level, the interpreters explained basic features of urban living to the family and became involved in helping the family to search for appropriate housing. Interpreters were directly involved in attempting to clarify the eligibility of the client family who did not have treaty status by dealing directly with members of the band council and with representatives of four different urban agencies. The interpreters were able to explain ambiguous and conflicting messages about the family's eligibility to the band leaders, city income maintenance workers, and representatives of urban based Native family service organizations. As the interpreters encountered administrative barriers associated with the ambiguous eligibility criteria and overlapping jurisdictions, they moved into more direct political advocacy by raising the possibility of publicizing the case in the media and lobbying with leaders in the urban Native community. In helping the family to search for alternate housing, interpreters became involved in liaison with landlords and were able to confront and counter discriminatory rental practices. Ultimately, community liaison work clarified the eligibility of the family and assisted in finding urban welfare benefits. Finally, working as individual advocates, the interpreters used their own informal networks within the city to locate appropriate housing and settle the family.

The second type of community advocacy function involved the medical interpreters' role of representing the concerns of remote Native communities about local primary care services and the system of referral and evacuation to urban tertiary care centers. An example of this function was observed in a situation in which interpreters informally discussed the concerns of band leaders and clients from a remote reserve in terms of a community's concerns about the potential mismanagement of emergency cases in their nursing station. Interpreters became involved with the case of a pediatric patient who was evacuated from the community with an acute infection where members of the community felt there had been inadequate treatment and referral at the primary care level. Working through their informal networks and work-related contacts with clinicians and administrators serving the reserve, interpreters were able to communicate the community's concern about current practice in the nursing station. Using their informal networks to contact representatives of the community, the interpreters were able to convey more accurate information on the patient's medical condition and remedial measures which were being taken. In serving as a clearinghouse for information about health-related situations in remote Native communities through their informal networks, interpreters provide a significant but informal source of advocacy.

The third advocacy function performed by interpreters on behalf of remote communities involves communicating rural northern perspectives on policy-related issues such as economic development and administrative autonomy. Although regional and provincial Native organizations officially represent the perspective of reserve and unorganized communities in policy-making in the areas of economic development and local administration, these issues also become primary focuses of discussion in the informal networks of urban Native people in administrative and helping professions. Interpreter involvement in health-related issues associated with community development and local autonomy was observed in their participation as members of advisory boards for health and social service agencies. Pressure from some reserve and Métis communities for increased financial and administrative control over primary medical care services has primary implications for both community development and local autonomy. Urban-based interpreters were asked to serve as consultants by both the bands and medical administrators in developing two demonstration projects through which reserve communities have received special grants to develop locally administered primary care centers. A related issue involving community control of services was observed in the involvement of hospital-based interpreters in initiatives directed at improving the system of child welfare and foster home placement. Native medical interpreters have served as intermediaries between Native families and the child welfare system. In public policy forums considering ways for restructuring the system to make it more responsive to the cultural perspective of the Native family, medical interpreters have become directly involved in speaking for the policy perspective of urban and rural Native communities.

A final example of Native interpreters' involvement in political advocacy for rural communities was documented in their response to complaints from band leaders and individual clients about the lack of cultural awareness among the staff of a rural community hospital serving several reserve communities. Interpreters became involved in communicating the communities' concern to the provincial health bureaucracy and acting as consultants in helping the community hospitals to establish interpreting and advocacy services.

CONCLUSION

The involvement of urban-based medical interpreters in advocacy functions on behalf of individual patients and remote communities has direct implications for the emergence of the interpreter/advocate as a new health profession. However, the extension of their roles in cultural brokerage and advocacy also involves the potential for role conflict. Specifically, several interpreters indicated that they experienced cross-pressures and dissonance in attempting to combine their roles as health system employees with their roles as advocates for individual patients and communities.

ACKNOWLEDGMENTS

Ongoing research on the role of Native Canadian interpreters is being sponsored by a formulation grant from the National Health Promotions Directorate of Health and Welfare Canada (Grant No. 6607-1305-49). We gratefully acknowledge the contribution of the University of Manitoba Northern Medical Unit and Welfare Canada in supporting travel and community liaison. The ten authors of this paper comprise the Native Health Media Collective.

REFERENCES

1. Kaufert J, Koolage W. Role conflict among culture brokers: The experience of Native Canadian medical interpreters. Soc Sci Med 1984; 18:283-286.
2. Paine R. Patrons and brokers in the east Arctic. St. Johns: Univ Toronto Press, 1971.
3. Kaufert J, Koolage W, Kaufert PA, O'Neil J. The use of "trouble case" examples in teaching the impact of sociocultural and political factors in clinical communication. Med Anthro 1984; 7.
4. Bloom M, Hanson H, Fries G, South V. The use of interpreters in interviewing. Ment Hyg 1966; 50:214-221.

Joseph M. Kaufert
Department of Social and Preventive Medicine
University of Manitoba
Room S110-750 Bannatyne Avenue
Winnipeg, Manitoba R3E 0W3
Canada

Circumpolar Health 84:447-450

STAGES IN DEVELOPMENT OF A NATIVE HEALTH BOARD

JAMES A. HAHN and WILLIAM M. DANN

The current trend of federal and state policy regarding Native Americans promotes local control of health service delivery through regional corporations governed by consumer governing boards. (U.S. Public Law 93-638 Indian Self Determination Act.) Both crosscultural disparities with this corporate form, as well as lack of attention to developing board competency have compromised this potentially powerful tool for achieving self-determination. The concepts of representation, deciding on behalf of unknown others, argument in search of optimal solutions, majority rule, planning, and modeling have no precedent in Alaska Native culture. Government funding sources that set standards and the governing boards themselves have paid little attention to developing competence in governance.

The purpose of this paper is to examine the developmental process and lessons for the future of one Native board, that of the Norton Sound Health Corporation of Nome, Alaska, which was founded in 1970.

Stage I. *Advocacy*

The Norton Sound Health Corporation (NSHC) originated as an alternative health care delivery system to the Federal Indian Health Service. This unique federally-funded experiment sought to capitalize on current hostilities expressed by minority groups in order to generate program designs more responsive to local needs, or to coerce existing service agencies to alter their programs.

Board members were elected by each of 16 communities stretched over 25,000 square miles and encompassing 6,200 residents. Members were largely men, some with limited advisory board experience but few with management or governance background. Initially, staff of the Corporation advised village councils that interest in improved health, knowledge of village needs, and ability to speak out on issues were key characteristics for board member selection.

Staff members were liberal-minded young health professionals attracted to an opportunity to effect change in Federal health delivery to Alaskan Natives as well as effect self determination in health. Few staff members had experience in Alaskan Native culture or community development. Rather, they forged ahead on a somewhat "romantic" conception of the Eskimo and of "power to the people."

The purpose of the advocacy stage was to improve the quality and acceptance of existing services to the consumer. These services were external to the consumer, and therefore board structure operated as a single whole, lending "power in numbers," maximizing representation credibility to the advocacy effort. The role of the board member was to allow its members to confront, intimidate, and be of support to staff personnel who advocated positions similar to those held by the board. The board's leadership characteristics during this period were typically "grass roots," with the polished ability to be angry at appropriate times through verbal spokesmen.

This stage paralleled the Alaskan Native push for a settlement of land claims against the Federal government. Hence, spokesmen emerged in the culture to meet the need and the government, crippled by a national sense of liberal guilt over historic treatment of Native Americans, was quite receptive or threatened by Native political power.

The catalyst for transition out of the advocacy period was receipt of funding for programs the board had advocated.

To this day, elements of the advocacy stage or approach remain in board deliberations of whether to approve research on human subjects or of agency efforts they have not already contracted for. This legacy of unity based in the struggle of the have-nots and in clarity of purpose, retarded moving on to responsibility for service delivery and attendant realities of conflicting priorities, falling short of goals long advocated, and dealing with being beholden to those holding the dollars, etc.

Stage II. *Staff Dominance*

Staff dominance arose out of technological responses to program operations. There was a concentration on effectively operating the programs advocated in Stage I and ensuring that program designs were culturally relevant.

The staff preempted the board. Technological, financial, and legal complexities of contracting for health care delivery demanded a high level of expertise exercised in a timely manner. A few "bleeding heart" supporters of advocacy were overshadowed by a full range of professionals seeking to elevate their professional status. Increasingly, Western medical technology rather than village expectations determined program design. Life was taken out of the Stage I commitment to development of Native staff members. In essence, the tail wagged the dog in Stage II as program compliance of direct delivery overshadowed and ran the board.

The staff openly competed for program money. Leadership was dispersed throughout the programs rather than centralized in the executive director. Individual program directors gained access to the governing board of advocate for funding or favorable treatment.

Stage III. *Board Dominance*

Stage III emerged from board paranoia that the non-Native staff, which became dominant by default in Stage II, was building an ongoing power base and taking undue advantage of the Native contingency. In the case of NSHC, dominance was realized through emergence of a single antagonist on a mission of dethroning the "carpetbagger" staff. Comfortable in that role by virtue of a strong sense of self and bicultural life experience, he also sought to whip the Native board members for giving up control and not personally behaving responsibly.

The battle for control took the form of engaging upon day-to-day mechanics through demand for detailed documentation, reworking of material brought before the board, the launching of personal attacks upon staff members and an intrusion daily into the running of the office in search of violations of policies or board directives. The antagonist rapidly worked his way into a board delegate position for various meetings on local, state, and national levels. Becoming extremely well informed on issues and programs, he fostered board dependence upon him to regain the control he chided them for giving up. He became a trusted link to ongoing information apart from non-Native staff now suspected of having ulterior motives.

Management's response was removal of program staff from interaction with the board in an effort to preserve some vestige of their sinking morale. Controlling input to the board eliminated the advocacy for programs by their managers that characterized Stage II. During this period, management control became centralized in the executive director or point man in the battle. Retention of staff and morale during this period was difficult and the history or scars would serve to make it difficult in the future.

Stage IV. *Transition*

In Stage IV, an exponential increase in the business at hand forced the board to delineate and allocate responsibility in more precise terms. For NSHC, that quantum jump came in the form of new hospital construction and ominous future responsibility for operation of the hospital.

Stipulations of the federal construction grant required an expedient method of making on-the-spot decisions and mandated that those decisions be the responsibility of a single individual, the executive director. This forced empowering the director with fiscal power tens of times that previously granted.

The size of the Corporation and its complexity would double with assuming management of the hospital. The upcoming change from management of known grant or contract funds to reliance upon uncertain levels of patient revenue from insurance and private pay sources raised board anxiety about their competence for the task, as did fear of legal exposure. The corporate habit of seeking more and more funds for increasing expense budgets was now halted by the need to contain costs such that rates to the public were viewed as reasonable. Adding to the board's uneasiness was the need to comply with complex and varied state and federal regulations that restricted their decision-making prerogatives.

The board was forced to restructure itself into committees that would develop expertise in various program areas and expeditiously process business of the Corporation as they prepared to assume management of the hospital. The need to develop trust of fellow members through committees and responsible boardsmanship of each member both served to dilute the power of the antagonist.

The board as a whole for the first time urged that the staff find appropriate training on their new responsibilities. The redirection of previous interpersonal and organizational energies of the board toward reorganization was facilitated by a trainer with the insight and capabilities to promote managerial techniques and instill a sense of corporate performance. Critical to success was the focus of the training upon appropriate board/staff roles and board processing of staff material rather than technical skills or knowledge. The board was virtually on trial to the trainer who maintained an ongoing relationship with them.

The staff returned to an initiating role based on information flow. The staff, in turn, were now also on trial with the board and its trainer regarding its production and presentation of material to the board.

The catalyst for transition from Stage IV was the actual assumption of management responsibility for the hospital and concurrent development of a management-by-objectives planning and evaluation system.

Stage V. *Professional Management*

The combined pressures of the demands of operating the hospital coupled with increased public pressure forced the NSHC board to apply the theories learned in Stage

IV. Until now, a board member had simply been a functionary of the Corporation and ceased to be a board member when not in session. The takeover of hospital services made board members the target of consumer concerns regarding the quality and cost of care. From this point on, the responsibility of board participation went beyond the board itself, becoming a part of the consumer constituency.

The pressures upon the board brought more conservative behavior. Cost containment was a high priority, performance and efficiency its facilitator, and management-by-objectives the lever.

The board worked effectively through committees divided along major functional divisions of the Corporation, thereby dispersing power and leadership on the board. Staff were assigned to prepare material for committee deliberation, which served to establish positive board/staff working relationships on that level. Tasks were clear and shared. Board members were now called upon to carry out consumer surveys as part of the planning process and to follow through on village concerns. In addition, the board imposed strict rules of conduct upon members.

By giving planning and monitoring responsibility clearly to the board through its committees, Stage V in one sense saw the staff become more responsible to the board. However, the board also recognized its dependence upon management for execution, which swung the pendulum back to staff initiative.

Stage VI. *Enlightened Advocacy*

Stage VI of the NSHC board development is still under way. It is a continuing application of board management and coalescence of board and staff toward service-related goals.

As the board became proficient in carrying out its responsibilities and overcame its anxieties, it found itself returning to the concerns of Stage I, with an enlightened orientation. Rather than advocacy through confrontation, there is concern for an increased sense of ownership by constituencies. Programs return to a community or self-help design and villages seek greater control of programs. A regional consumer relations committee is established to insure responsiveness to patient concerns.

Enlightened advocacy brings with it an increased emphasis on Native hiring issues. This comes about through a board-generated revision of hiring policies favoring Native hire and training. Increasingly, a greater sense of ownership is defined in terms of Native control at the staff level.

This affirmative action is congruent with the underlying theme of reducing external dependence and fostering full local control.

DISCUSSION

The pattern of stages in development of the NSHC governing board parallels stages in the maturation of an organization as defined by management theorists (i.e. natural leader stage, corridor of crisis, professional management stage [Lewis Allen]). This process, largely inevitable, is dictated by the cadence and extent of crisis or internal and external pressures for change. The impact of the process upon organizational performance stems from the extent of resistance to change of both board and staff, the quality of training covering the gamut of board/staff relations, and the ability of the staff to remain focused on a long range, developmental perspective versus meeting their immediate ego needs.

Throughout its development, staff and board perspectives are often in conflict. Failure to resolve conflict precipitates stages in board development that retard growth toward competent governance, as exemplified in the NSHC experience. Conflict can be reduced or even avoided through increased emphasis on board/staff dynamics and training. Among developing Native corporations, much of existing education is vested in the staff rather than in the governing board. Yet, it is the governing board that has the responsibility to direct corporate affairs. The board's success will predetermine much of the success of staff responsible to it.

From the Norton Sound experience, the following are offered as elements of a successful training effort:

1. Reaching a clear operational understanding of board vs. staff roles.

2. Training on board operations, e.g. needs assessment, planning, program evaluation, use of committees, financial oversight, and staff evaluation.

3. Use of a facilitator/trainer to aid in definition of board and staff expectations as well as means to clarify and simplify written and oral communication.

4. Ongoing facilitation/evaluation of board performance on operations as well as member-to-member and member-to-staff interaction, utilizing preferably a continuous external facilitator/trainer.

5. An ongoing dialogue regarding the nature and extent to pressures for change in the board/staff dynamic.

The other critical lesson from the Norton Sound experience is that government is derelict in its duty to its citizens when it contracts with or regulates the affairs of organizations providing services but fails to address performance of the governing boards. Licensure, Joint Commission on Accreditation of Hospitals, contracting audits, etc. fail to prescribe that governing boards should have training while dictating the same for members of the professional staff. Yet, the performance of that governing board is critical to organizational performance. Further, while staff performance is monitored and evaluated there is no evaluation of governance. Like the staff, governing boards are susceptible to bad habits and loss of focus and would similarly benefit from external evaluation. Successful public policy seeking local, consumer, or Native control of service delivery must address itself to this developmental need.

James A. Hahn
Dann and Associates, Inc.
2440 E. Tudor Road
Suite 156
Anchorage, Alaska 99507
U.S.A.

APPENDIX: ABBREVIATED PROGRAM, SIXTH INTERNATIONAL SYMPOSIUM ON CIRCUMPOLAR HEALTH

OPENING PLENARY SESSION

OPENING SPEAKERS:
Frederick Milan, President, Circumpolar
    Health Conference
Bernard Kelly, Director, Region X, U.S.
    Department of Health and Human Services
Faye Abdellah, Deputy Surgeon General,
    United States Public Health Service
John Pugh, Acting Commissioner, Alaska
    Department of Health and Social
    Services
Jay Barton, President, University of Alaska
Dalee Sambo, Alaska Director, Inuit
    Circumpolar Conference
Baruch Blumberg, Nobel Prize Winner 1976,
    Medicine and Physiology
Lydia Novak, President, Central Committee,
    Soviet Medical Workers' Union, USSR

SCIENTIFIC SESSIONS

DENTAL HEALTH
Douglas H. Smole, Chair

Principal Speaker
John T. Mayhall

A Nationwide Survey of the Oral Health of
the Natives of Canada
    John T. Mayhall, John Stamm

The Microbiology of Nursing Caries in
Canadian Indian Children
    A.R. Milnes, G.H. Bowden, I. Lebtag,
    D. Gates

Enamel Thickness in 46, XY-Females'
Permanent Teeth
    Lassi Alvesalo, Erkki Tammisalo

A University Based Dental Care Delivery
Model for the Keewatin Region, Northwest
Territories
    Olva Odlum

Utilization Patterns of Available Dental
Services in Rural Alaska: A Model for
Behavioral Change
    Mim Kelly, Theodore A. Mala

Dental Caries Prevalence in School Children
from Two Ethnic Groups Living in Three
Labrador Communities: A Comparison of
Surveys Carried out in 1969 and 1983
    James G. Messer

Administration and Maintenance of a Long
Term 0.2% Sodium Fluoride Mouthrinse
Program: A Six Year Study Involving
Fifty-Five Schools in Northern Newfoundland
and Labrador
    James G. Messer

The Performance of Dentists Working with
Grenfell Regional Health Services: A
Comparison of Productivity and Range of
Services Depending on Supporting Facilities
    James G. Messer

Dental Health
POSTER SESSION

Nursing Bottle Dental Caries: Its Impact on
Infant Care in the North
    Howard Cross, Bonnie Trodden

Nursing Bottle Caries
    Howard Cross, Bonnie Trodden

Epidemiological Observation of Jaw Fractures
in Greenland
    P.K. Hansen, J.J. Thorn

COLD INJURY, PHYSIOLOGY AND ADAPTATIONS
William Mills, Chair

Principal Speaker
Jacques LeBlanc

Increased Tendency to Cold Induced Vasospasm
in the Fingers (Raynaud's Phenomenon) in
Copper Smelter Workers Exposed to Arsenic
(As)
    H. Linderholm, B. Lagerkvist

"Future Shock" and the Fitness of the Inuit
    Andris Rode, Roy J. Shephard

Seasonal Variation of Blood Pressure, Basal
Metabolism Rate and Skin Temperature in
Outdoor Workers in Northern Finland
    Juhani Leppäluoto, Juhani Hassi,
    Rauno Pääkkönen

Effects of Nasal Breathing at Different
Temperatures on Carbon Dioxide Sensitivity
Dyspnea and Alae Nasi EMG Activity
    K.R. Burgess, W.A. Whitelaw

Possible Mechanisms for the After-Drop of
Core Temperature upon Rewarming from Mild
Hypothermia
    Gabrielle K. Savard, K.E. Coopu,
    W.L. Veale

Environmental Cold May Be a Major Factor in
Some Respiratory Disorders
    E.LL. Lloyd

Immunologic Changes in Frostbite
    John Ninneman, George Stewart,
    Nuri Ozkan, William Mills

Lung Function in a Cold Environment-- A
Current Perspective
    Andris Rode, Roy Shephard

Thermal Biofeedback Training with Frostbite
Patients
    Bruno M. Kappes, William Mills

Effect of Cold Exposure on Exercise
Tolerance and Exercise ECG in Patients with
Effort Angina
    C. Backman, H. Linderholm

Effects of Diamide on Pulmonary Hypertension
Due to Cold and Hypoxia
    H. Kasprzak, J. Bligh, L. Peyton

Measurements of Human Vasomotor Function by
Color Thermography: Alcohol and Cold
Exposure
    Edgar Folk, Jr., P.R. Jochimsen,
    M. Edmund, T.L. Smith

Hypokalemia Following Moderate Hypothermic
Hemodilution
    Raymond A. Dieter, Jr.

Cold Injury, Physiology and Adaptations
POSTER SESSION

Fitness, Growth and Lung Function--A Ten
Year Follow-up of Canadian Inuit
    Andris Rode, Roy J. Shephard

Over-Study of the Inuit? An Ethical
Evaluation
    Roy J. Shephard

Acculturation and the Biology of Aging
    Roy J. Shephard, Andris Rode

Physical Loading in Downhill Skiing
    E. Rauhala, J. Karvonen, J. Venalainen

Physical Fitness and Training Programs on an
Antarctic Base
    Graham L. Hurst

Interbase Study of Some Physiological
Parameters at British Antarctic Survey Bases
    S. Bridgman, M. Green, G. Hurst, R.
    Parker

A Cooling Power Index Based on Human Heat
Exchanges
    Jean Rivolier

Acclimatization to Cold in Antarctic
S.C.U.B.A. Divers
    S.A. Bridgman

INFECTIOUS DISEASES
Brian McMahon, Chair

Principal Speaker
Peter Skinhøj

Hepatitis B in the Baffin Region of Northern
Canada
    B. Larke, G. Froese, R. Devine, V. Lee

Hepatitis B Viral Markers in Two
Epidemiologically Distinct Canadian Inuit
(Eskimo) Settlements
    G.Y. Minuk, N. Ling, B. Postl,
    J.G. Waggoner, C. Pokrant, L. Nicolle,
    J.H. Hoofnagle

Use of Hepatitis B Vaccine in a General
Population at High Risk of Infection
    W.L. Heyward, T.R. Bender,
    B.J. McMahon, D.P. Francis, D.B. Hall,
    W.L.M. Alward, J.E. Maynard

A Comprehensive Program to Control the
Spread of Hepatitis B Virus Infection in
Alaskan Natives
    B.J. McMahon, W.L. Heyward,
    G.R. Brenneman, E. Tower,
    W.B. Hurlburt, T.R. Bender,
    M.L. Cartter, G.H. Ivey, E.R. Rhoades

Immunoregulation in Inuit Infants with
Recurrent Pneumonia
    Elena R. Reece

Lower Respiratory Tract Infections among
Canadian Inuit Children
    J. Carson, B. Postl, O. Schaefer,
    D. Spady

Reactivation of Tuberculosis in Manitoba
1976-1981
    I. Johnson, M. Thomson, J. Manfreda,
    E. Hershfield

The Epidemiology of Nasopharyngeal Carriage
of *N. meningitidis* in an Isolated Northern
Community
    L.E. Nicolle, B. Postl, G.K.M. Harding,
    W. Albritton, A.R. Ronald

Bunyaviruses Throughout the Western Canadian
Arctic
    Donald M. McLean

A Statewide Surveillance of Invasive
Haemophilus influenzae Type b Disease in
Alaska
    Milton Lum, H. Peter, D. Hall,
    M. Fitzgerald, J.I. Ward

The Current Status of Alveolar Hydatid
Disease in Northern Regions
    R.L. Rausch, J.F. Wilson

Microbiologic Investigations of the Barrow
Eskimo Specimens
    D.R. Silimperi, W.L. Alward,
    J.C. Feeley, W.W. Myers, W.L. Heyward

Communicable Disease Control in the Early
History of Alaska II. Syphilis
    Robert Fortuine

Regional Variation in Mortality from
Infectious Disease in Greenland
    Peter Bjerregaard

Infectious Diseases
POSTER SESSION

Acute Hepatitis B Virus Infection:
Relationship of Age to the Clinical
Expression of Disease and the Subsequent
Development of the Carrier State
    Brian J. McMahon, Wallace L.M. Alward,
    David B. Hall, William L. Heyward,
    Thomas R. Bender, Donald P. Francis,
    James G. Maynard

The Serologic Course of Hepatitis B Surface
Antigen and e Antigen and the Development of
Primary Hepatocellular Carcinoma in
Asymptomatic Carriers of Hepatitis B Virus
    Wallace L.M. Alward, Brian J. McMahon,
    David B. Hall, William L. Heyward,
    Donald P. Francis, Thomas R. Bender

Hepatitis B and Lower Respiratory
Infections: Evidence of an Association
    William Heyward, David Hall

The Spatial and Temporal Context of an
"Isolated" Outbreak of Hepatitis A
    Tom Kosatsky, John P. Middaugh

Observations on the Pattern of Spread of
Hepatitis B Infection in Yupik Eskimo
Villages of Southwestern Alaska
    Elizabeth A. Tower

Increasing Prevalence of Hepatitis B
Antigenamia during Pregnancy in Alaskan
Eskimos
    David Estroff, Jacqueline Greenman,
    William L. Heyward,
    H. Huntley Hardison, Brian McMahon,
    Tomas Bender

The Evolution of Chronic Otitis Media in the
Inuit of the Eastern Canadian Arctic and Its
Managerial Implication
    J.D. Baxter

Chronic Otitis in Greenland
    C. Brahe Pedersen, R. Vejlsgaard,
    B. Zachau-Christiansen

Bronchiectasis: An Epidemiological Study of
Pre-Disposing Factors
    David Hall, Joseph Wilson,
    Wallace Alward, Belinda Ireland

Pertussis: An Epidemiological Study of
Incidence and Mortality in the
Yukon-Kuskokwim Delta
    David Hall, Belinda Ireland,
    Wallace L.M. Alward, Ludlow Paap,
    Mathew Cartter

Tuberculosis in Inuit
    S. Grzybowski, E. Dorken

Long Term Evaluation of a Trial of
Chemoprophylaxis against Tuberculosis in
Frobisher Bay, Canada
    E. Dorken, S. Grzybowski, D. Enarson

An Investigation of the Immunogenetic
Susceptibility of *Haemophilus influenzae*
Type b (HIb) Disease in Alaskan Eskimos
    D.R. Silimperi, G.M. Peterson,
    D.B. Hall, E.M. Scott, J.I. Rotter,
    J.I. Ward

Communicable Disease Control in the Early
History of Alaska I. Smallpox
    Robert Fortuine

Evaluation of the Blood Marker Iophenoxic
Acid, and the Orally-Ingested SAD-BHK$_{21}$
Rabies Vaccine in the Arctic Fox
    Erich H. Follman, Donald G. Ritter,
    George M. Baer

GENETICS, ANTHROPOLOGY AND DEMOGRAPHY
Edward M. Scott, Chair

Principal Speaker
Gudrun Pétursdóttir

Paleopathological Investigations of
500-Year-Old Eskimo Mummies
    J.P. Hart Hansen

A Portrait of Alaska Native Health--1800
    Robert Fortuine

Demography in Historical Greenland
    Kristen E. Caning

Causes of Death, Age at Death, and Changes
in Mortality in the Twentieth Century in
Ammassalik (East Greenland)
    Joëlle Robert-Lamblin

Mortality among the James Bay Cree, Quebec
    Elizabeth Robinson

Mortality of Labrador Innu and Inuit,
1971-1982
    K.A. Wotton

Rural-Urban Differences in Lung Size and
Function in Iceland
J. Axelsson, J.G. Óskarsson,
S. Jonsson, G. Pétursdóttir, A.B. Way,
N. Sigfússon

Study of Contribution of Genetic and
Environmental Factors of Predisposition to
Coronary Heart Disease in Native and
Newcoming Population of Chukotka
Yu. P. Nikitin, T.I. Astakhova,
V.A. Koshechkin, M.I. Voevoda,
A.V. Tikhonov

Genetics, Anthropology and Demography
POSTER SESSION

Hereditary Polymorphic Light Eruption in
Canadian Inuit
P.H. Orr, A.R. Birt

Demographic Descriptors as Surrogates for
Structural Factors
Coralie Farlee

CANCER AND OTHER CHRONIC DISEASES
Anne Lanier, Chair

Principal Speaker
C.S. Muir

Prevalence of Diabetes Mellitus and Sequelae
in Indians of Eastern Manitoba
J. Dooley, J. Rodrigues

Prevalence of Diabetes among the Cree Ojibwa
of Northwestern Ontario
T.K. Young, L.L. McIntyre

Rheumatic Diseases in the Inuit Population
of the Keewatin 1974-1982
K. Oen, B. Postl, N. Ling,
I.M. Chalmers, M. Schroeder

Prevalence of Rheumatoid Arthritis and
Related Disorders in Yupik Eskimos
David Templin, Anne Lanier,
Ken Takegami, David Clement,
Betsy Weiss, David Hall, David Foster

Respiratory Health of an Inuit Population
R. Belleau, P. Durand, N. Tremblay,
B. Duval, P. Foggin

The Seasonal Occurrence of Peptic Ulcer
Disease among the Inuit of Northern Labrador
G. William N. Fitzgerald,
Joel R.L. Ehrenkranz

Angle Closure Glaucoma in Keewatin Zone
J. Speakman

Chronic Disease/Illness Survey of a Labrador
Community
Alison C. Edwards, John R. Martin,
G.J. Johnson, J. Green

Cancer Incidence in Northern Finland:
Environmental Effect and Diagnostic Patterns
Frej Stenbäck

Surveillance for Primary Hepatocellular
Carcinoma in Alaska Natives through a
Hepatitis B Registry and Serologic Screening
for Alpha-Fetoprotein
Anne Lanier, William Heyward,
Mathew Cartter, Brian McMahon,
Thomas Bender

Malignant Lymphoepithelial Lesions of the
Salivary Glands in Alaska Natives: Case
Report and Review of Cases from 1966-1980
Sarala Krishnamurthy, Anne P. Lanier,
Susan Clift, Kathy T. Kline,
Werner Henle, G. Bornkamm, A. Gown,
D. Thorning

Ultrastructural Investigations of Malignant
Salivary Gland Tumors in Eskimos
M. Sehested, B. Hainau, H. Albeck,
N. Højgaard Nielson, J.P. Hart Hansen

Space/Time Interaction Between Greenland NPC
Patients
H. Albeck, M.P. Coleman, N. Højgaard
Nielson, H. Sand Hansen,
J.P. Hart Hansen

Food Habits and Naso-Pharyngeal Carcinoma
Annie Hubert, Joëlle Robert-Lamblin,
Margarida Hermann

Cancer and Other Chronic Diseases
POSTER SESSION

Deaths Coded to Cirrhosis among Alaska
Natives 1974-1978
Anne Lanier, W.W. Richards, P.H. Dohan

Survelliance and Analysis of Trends in
Cancer Among Alaska Natives 1960-1983
Anne Lanier, David Hall,
Sarala Krishnamurthy, William Blot

Tobacco and Alcohol Use among Teenagers in a
Cohort of Southwest Alaskan Eskimos
Anne Lanier, David Hall, Lisebo Malatai

The Eye in High Altitude: Comparison between
Arctic Populations and 392 Adults in
Titicaca Region in Peru
H. Forsius, W. Losno

Current Trends in Cancer Incidence in
Greenland
N. Højgaard Nielsen, J.P. Hart Hansen

Antibodies to Epstein-Barr Virus-Associated
Antigens in Relatives of Alaska Native
Nasopharyngeal Cancer Patients
David Foster, Anne Lanier, David Hall,
Werner Henle, Gertrude Henle

The Refractive Errors of Young Adult Yupik
Eskimos
    Wallace L.M. Alward, David B. Hall,
    Thomas R. Bender, John A. Demske

Severe Familial Cholestatic Syndrome in
Greenlandic Children--Clinical, Histological
and Therapeutical Findings
    Inge-Merete Nielsen,
    Bendt Brock Jacobsen, Kim Ornvold,
    Bengt Zachau-Christiansen

TB in the James Bay Cree Population
    Lise Renaud, Charles Dumont

SOCIAL ENVIRONMENT, MENTAL HEALTH, AND
ALCOHOL AND DRUG ABUSE
William Richards, Chair

Principal Speaker
John Berry

Alcoholism and Mental Health Treatment in
Circumpolar Areas: Traditional and
Non-Traditional Approaches
    Theodore A. Mala

A Comparison of Substance Use and Abuse in
Alaska with United States National Data
    Janice Dani Bowman, Theodore A. Mala

Reducing the Incidence of Fetal Alcohol
Effects in Alaskan Villages
    Francia Schultz

"Here's Looking at You, II." Strategies for
Implementing Drug/Alcohol Education in
Elementary and Secondary Schools
    Carolyn F. Peter

Project North Star--An Organized
Comprehensive Approach for Reducing the
Risks Associated with Alcohol and Other Drug
Use among Adolescents in a Rural Community
in the State of Alaska
    Carolyn F. Peter

Village Alcohol Control: Traditional Methods
and the Local Option Law
    Thomas D. Lonner, J. Kenneth Duff

The Impact of Prohibition on an Inuit
Community
    John D. O'Neil

Drugs in Alaska: Patterns of Use by Adults
and School Age Youth
    Bernard Segal

The Medicalization of an Inuit Village
    John D. O'Neil

Acculturation and Mental Health Among the
James Bay Cree: Evidence for a Multivariate
Model
    J.W. Berry, R.M. Wintrob,
    T.A. Mawhinney

The Possibilities and Abilities of
Preventive Work for the Mental Health Care
Centers in Northern Finland
    Pekka Larivaara

Mental Health Service Delivery in Alaskan
Correctional Facilities
    Richard R. Parlour, David J. Sperbeck

Psychological and Cultural Aspects on Arctic
Hysteria among the Skolt Lapps
    Leila Seitamo

Teenagers in Greenland
    Grete Ulrich

Social Environment, Mental
Health, and Alcohol and Drug Abuse
POSTER SESSION

Health Behavior Change: An Experimental
Study at the Alaska Health Fair 1982
    Barbara Bathony

Assessing Health Behavior through the Key
Informant Approach
    Edward Deaux, John W. Callaghan

Perceptions of Stress and Patterns of Coping
among Inuit Youth
    John D. O'Neil

Alternate Methods of Measuring Life Change
(Psychosocial Stressors)
    Jan W. McLaurin

The Psychometric Component of the Infant
Mortality and Mortality Cohort Study
    Barbara Doak, Barabara Nachmann

Social Environment, Mental Health,
Alcoholism and Drug Abuse among a Colony of
Russian Old Believer Settlements Near Homer,
Alaska
    George T. Jermain

A Model for the Delivery of Alcohol and Drug
Abuse Treatment in Alaska
    Verner Stillner

Alcohol-Related Health Problems in
Alaska--Preventive Strategies
    Bill Richards

The Role of Ethnicity in the Predisposition
to Alcoholism
    Barbara Hoffmann

Mental Health and Self Determination in Areas of Forced Acculturation
Robert Alberts

Social Environment, Personality Structure and School Avoidance: A Study in a North-Finnish Rural District
Harriet Forsius

Determinants of Youth Suicide in the Canadian Urban North
Debrah Bray

Psychiatric Consultation and Diagnosis in Arctic Canada
Eric Hood, S.A. Malcolmson, J.D. Atcheson, R. Gleenie, G. White

Alcohol: Availability and Abuse
C. Earl Albrecht

Seasonal Variation in Suicide and Mental Health Depression of Finland
Simo Näyhä

A Psychological Survey of a Wintering Group, Using the MIPG Model
B. Bouvel, A. Abraham

ENVIRONMENTAL AND OCCUPATIONAL HEALTH PLANNING AND ENGINEERING
William Ryan, Chair

Principal Speaker
Daniel Smith

Health Hazards in Snowmobile Usage
J. Hassi, H. Virokannas, H. Anttonen, I. Järvenpää

Haddon's Strategy for Prevention: Application to Native House Fires
B. Friesen

Viruses in Sewage in the North of Finland
K. Lapinleimu, L. Soininen, M. Stenvik

The Effects of a Smoking Prevention Program for Alaskan Youth
John F. Lee

Industrial Hygiene
Stacie Pascal

Allergenic Airborne Pollen and Spore Research in Alaska
J.H. Anderson

HEALTH CARE DELIVERY AND INFORMATION SYSTEMS
Cynthia Schraer and Peggy McMahon, Co-Chairs

Principal Speaker
Sixten Haraldson

What Expectations Do We Have on Front-Line Health Services for Adversely Situated Populations?
Sixten S.R. Haraldson

The Community Health Aide Program in Alaska
P.J. McMahon, C.D. Schraer, R.D. Burgess, J. Sozoff, G. Brenneman

Health without Health Professionals-- Exploration and Implementation of One Option on the Labrador Coast
Janet S. Tuffy

Village Health Care: A Summary of Patient Encounters from Alaskan Village Clinics
Penelope M. Cordes

A System of Health Care Quality Review for Remote Northern Nursing Stations
C. Greensmith, J. Dooley, J. Rodrigues, H. Hodes

1/2 a Loaf is Better than None or Mini Bacteriology for Mini Facilities
Anne Gillan

An Economic Perspective on Teleradiology for Remote Communities
J.M. Horne

Innu Health: The Role of Self-Determination
Ben Andrew, Peter Sarsfield

Preparing Students of Native Ancestry for Entrance into the Medical Professions
M.C. Stephens, J. Silver

Alaska's Approach to Planning an Emergency Medical Services System: How Is It Working Three Years Later?
Gloria H. Way, Mark S. Johnson

Physician Recruitment to Remote Areas: A Canadian Model with International Application
Catherine J. Borrie

Medical Recruitment for the Australian National Antarctic Research Expeditions (ANARE)
D.J. Lugg

Support Systems for Remote-Site Health Care Providers
Philip O. Nice

Health Care Delivery and Information Systems
POSTER SESSION

Alaska's First Hospital
Robert Fortuine

Two Remote Canadian Practices
Peter Sarsfield

Stages in the Development of Native
Governing Boards: A Case Study
William M. Dann, James Hahn

Community Health in the Northern Regions:
From Conception to Application
Lise Gravel

Health Care Delivery and Cultural Diversity:
A Normative Model
Robert F. Eshleman

The Use of Functional Matrix in Research in
Native Communities
N. Ling, B. Postl

Variation and Convergence between Self-
Perceived and Clinically Measured Health
Status Variables of the Inuit in Northern
Quebec
Peter M. Foggin, Reger Belleau,
Bernard Duval, Jean-Pierre Thouez

Northwest River Health Committee--Response
to a Crisis in the Health Care Delivery
System of Northern Labrador
M. Baikie, K. Baikie-Pottle, B. Watts

Travelling Physicians in Northern Canada
Peter Sarsfield, Kathryn Wotton

Evaluation of Primary Health Care Delivery
in the Grenfell Region of Northern
Newfoundland and Labrador Canada
H. Onyett

A Unique Canadian Provincial Approach to
Special Services in the North: A Five Year
Experience of a Pediatrician Permanently
Based in the Grenfell Region of Northern
Newfoundland and Labrador, Canada
H. Onyett

The Role of Hospital-Based Medical
Interpreters in Advocacy for Northern Native
Patients and Communities
J.M. Kaufert, W.W. Koolage, M. Smith,
A. Koster, J. O'Neil, I. Whitford

Portable Diagnostic System for Acute
Abdominal Pain
A.C. Harvey, P.F. Moodie,
J.R. Kirkpatrick

Referral Pattern Study in Northern
Newfoundland and Labrador
J.H. Williams, Alison C. Edwards

A Report on a Conference on Hearing
Impairment in the Baffin Zone: Motivating
Factors and Conclusions
Henry J. Ilecki, J.D. Baxter,
Fiona O'Donoghue

Eye Care in Canadian Northwest Territories
J.G. Gillan

MATERNAL AND CHILD HEALTH
George Brenneman, Chair

Principal Speaker
Holger L. Hultin

Northern Infant Syndrome: A Deficiency
State?
John C. Godel

Low-Valid Paracerivical Block (Lo-va-PCB)
Anesthesia in Obstetrics with 10 mg of
Bupivacaine Hydrochloride
Louenivo Reijo

Changing Pattern of Parturition in Northern
Finland From 1950 to 1982
J. Puolakkta, P.A. Jarvinen,
A. Kauppila

Darkness-Related Secondary Amenorrhea
Martha Stewart, Effie Graham

Developmental Milestones in James Bay Cree
Children Ages 12-30 Months
M.E.K. Moffatt, C. Kato

Follow-up Perinatal/Infant Morbidity and
Mortality Study I. Demography, Utlilization,
Morbidity, Mortality
B. Postl, J. Carson, D. Spady,
O. Schaefer

A Cohort Study of the Yukon-Kuskokwim Delta
Eskimos: An Overview of Accomplishments and
Plans for the Future
Thomas R. Bender, Christopher Williams,
David Hall

Maternal and Child Health
POSTER SESSION

Follow-up of Tympanoplasties in Three N.W.T.
Communities 1975-1980
P.H. Orr, D.W. McCullough

Length, Weight, and Head Circumference in
Quebec Cree Children
M.E.K. Moffatt, C. Kato, G.V. Watters

Follow-up of the Perinatal Infant Morbidity
and Mortality Study (PIMM) II. Physical
Assessment
D. Spady, B. Postl, J. Carson,
O. Schaefer

Prenatal Program Evaluation--Alaska Native
Medical Center, (ANMC) Anchorage Service
Unit Deliveries 1979, 1982, 1983
Jackie Pflaum, Nancy Sanders,
Teresa Wolber, Jacqueline Greenman

Evaluation of Alaska's Improved Pregnancy
Outcome Project
Marti Dilley

Fertility Rates in Greenlandic Inuit
Teenagers
P.K. Hansen, S.F. Smith

NUTRITION
Elizabeth Nobmann, Chair

Principal Speaker
Leif Hallberg

Survey of Dietary Factors Which May
Contribute to Iron Deficiency among Bristol
Bay Area Alaska Eskimo Children
Elizabeth Nobmann

Risk Factor Levels of Coronary Heart Disease
and Their Determinants in Finnish Children
and Adolescents
Hans K. Åkerblom

Lipoprotein and Fatty Acid Profiles in
Alaskan and Greenlandic Eskimos: Possible
Implications for Cardiovascular Disease. A
Review of the Literature
Knut Kielland

Low Incidence of Urinary Calculi in
Greenland Eskimos as Explained by a Low
Calcium/Magnesium Ratio
Bjarne Bo Jeppesen, Bent Harvald

Endogenous and Exogenous Sources of
Nitrate/Nitrite and Nitrosamines in Canadian
Inuit with a Traditional or Western
Lifestyle
H.F. Stich, P. Hornby

Infant Feeding Practices on Manitoba Indian
Reserves
G. Marchessault

Nutrition
POSTER SESSION

Seasonal Variation in Serum 25-Hydroxy
Vitamin D in a Fairbanks Community: Relation
to Variations in Diet and Sunlight Exposure
Meredith Tallas

A Nutrient Analysis of Twenty Southeastern
Alaska Native Foods
Helen M. Hooper

An Evaluation of Household Country Food Use
in Makkovik, Labrador, during One Food
Supply Cycle
M.G. Alton Mackey, R.D. Orr

Mercury Surveillance in Several Cree
Villages of the James Bay Region, Quebec
Charles Dumont, Russell Wilkins

Epidemiologic Aspects of Some
Gastrointestinal Diseases with Special
Reference to Hypolactasia in Skolt Lapps
Timo Sahi, Mikko Kirjarinta

Comparison of Total Serum Cholesterol in
Genetically Comparable Town-Dwelling and
Farm-Dwelling Icelandic Youngsters
A.B. Way, J. Axelsson, G. Pétursdóttir
N. Sigfússon

Prevalence of Iron Deficiency Anemia Among
Alaskan WIC Participants
Joan Pelto

Birthweight and Maternal Age Specific Infant
Mortality Rates in Alaska
Joan Pelto

MEDICAL AND HEALTH ASPECTS OF INDUSTRIAL
DEVELOPMENT IN ARCTIC AND COLD REGIONS
Robert Rigg, Organizer

Louis Rey, Comité Arctique International,
Monaco, Chair and Guest Speaker

Alfred S. McLaren, USN (Retired) Guest
Speaker, Applications of Undersea
Transportation in Arctic Development

Work Stress of Norwegian Coal Miners in
Spitsbergen
N.O. Alm, K. Rodahl

Industrial Development and Morbidity: Native
People in Alaska and the Canadian Arctic
Charles W. Hobart

The Prevalence of Peripheral Articular
Symptoms and Signs in Two Adjacent Iron Ore
Mines in Labrador
John R. Martin, Alison C. Edwards

Some Comparisons about Perception in Extreme
Environments: Antarctica, a Submarine and a
Tropical Island
Jane S.P. Mocellin

Beyond Hypothermia and Frostbite:
Occupational Health Issues of the Arctic
Worker
Lawrence D. Weiss

REPORT OF THE INTERNATIONAL BIOMEDICAL
EXPEDITION TO THE ANTARCTIC
J. Rivolier, Organizer

PANELS AND POLICY SESSIONS

SPECIAL SESSION
ARCTIC HEALTH SCIENCE POLICY

United States Arctic Science Policy
Moderator: John Middaugh

Susan Addiss, President, American Public
Health Association
The Need for a Health Component of an Arctic
Science Policy

Juan Roederer, Director, Geophysical
Institute, University of Alaska-Fairbanks,
Polar Research Board, National Academy of
Sciences
U.S. Arctic Science Policy: A National
Perspective

Dael Wolfle, Chairman, University of Alaska
Foundation, Scientific Advisory Commisssion
Science Policy Development--The Process and
the Future

SEARCHING FOR A BETTER LIFE
Carl Hild and Theodore Mala, Co-Chairs

A discussion of the interactions between
Native-oriented cultures and Western
European culture, and how these affect
successful delivery of health services.

ALASKA HEALTH EDUCATION CONSORTUIM SEMINAR

Five panelists' descriptions of their
successes in promoting health education at
local, regional and governmental levels.

Moderator: Nancy Bill, President, Alaska
Health Education Consortium

Panel Members:
Paul Gregory, Community Relations
    Specialist, Bethel Regional Hospital
Patrick B. Hefley, Coordinator, Health
    Education/Risk Reduction Project, State
    of Alaska
Robert Imire, Coordinator, School Health
    Program, Yellowknife, Northwest
    Territories
Curt Mekemson, Coordinator, Coalition for
    HB84 (Alaska Indoor Air Act)
Jan Schoellhorn, Coordinator, Accident and
    Injury Control Program, Yukon-Kuskokwim
    Health Corporation

NATIONAL ARCTIC HEALTH SCIENCE POLICY--
AMERICAN PUBLIC HEALTH ASSOCIATION TASK
FORCE
Moderator: Mim Dixon

John Middaugh, Chairman, APHA Task Force;
State Epidemiologist, Division of Public
Health, State of Alaska
National Arctic Health Science
Policy--APHA's Role

Fredrick McGinnis, Department of Human
Resources, State of Georgia
National Arctic Health Science
Policy--Findings

Robert Fordham, Associate Deputy Director,
National Center for Health Services
Research, National Arctic Health Science
Policy--Recommendations

INTERNATIONAL ARCTIC HEALTH SCIENCE
POLICY--FUTURE DEVELOPMENT
Moderator: Wayne Myers

David Martin, Director, Indian and Inuit
Health Services, Medical Services Branch,
Health and Welfare, Canada

Hannu Vuori, Regional Office for Europe,
World Health Organization

Per-Ola Granberg, Chairman, Nordic Council
for Arctic Medical Research

Chester Pierce, Chairman, Committee on Polar
Biomedical Research, Polar Research Board,
National Academy of Sciences

Eugene Brower, Mayor, North Slope Borough

Dalee Sambo, Alaska Director, Inuit
Circumpolar Conference

Dael Wolfle, Alaska Director, Chairman,
University of Alaska Foundation, Scientific
Advisory Commission

CLOSING PLENARY SESSION

Otto Schaefer, Director, Northern Medical
    Research Unit, Medical Department,
    National Health and Welfare, Canada
Yu. P. Nikitin, Deputy Chairman, Siberian
    Branch of the Academcy of Medical
    Sciences of the USSR
Hannu Vuori, Regional Office for Europe,
    World Health Organization
Per-Ola Granberg, Nordic Council for Arctic
    Medical Research
C. Earl Albrecht, American Society for
    Circumpolar Health

MISCELLANEOUS SYMPOSIUM EVENTS AND MEETINGS

Breakfast Meeting
Canadian Society for Circumpolar Health

Alaska Public Health Association Breakfast

Alaska Public Health Association Business
Meeting Including Resolutions
Speaker: Susan Addiss, President,
American Public Health Association

Breakfast Meeting
American Society for Circumpolar Health

Symposium Luncheon
Speaker: S. Chandrasekhar,
Visiting Professor of Demography,
University of Alaska-Fairbanks

Symposium and Alaska Public Health
Association Luncheon
Speaker: Victor Sidel, President Elect,
American Public Health Association

Dinner Meeting
International Committee on
Circumpolar Health

Alaska Public Health Association
Awards Banquet
Guest Speaker:
William H. McBeath, Executive Director,
American Public Health Association

Cultural Program
Inuit Spirit Night